An Introduction to
MEDICAL
SCIENCE

An Introduction to
MEDICAL
SCIENCE

A Comprehensive Guide to Anatomy, Biochemistry and Physiology

by Ned Durkin

MTP PRESS LIMITED
International Medical Publishers

Dedication

To my late father, my mother and all my other good teachers.

Knowledge is like a garden: if it is not cultivated, it cannot be harvested.
—Guinean proverb

Published by
MTP Press Limited
Falcon House, Cable Street
Lancaster, England

British Library Cataloguing in Publication Data
Durkin, Ned
   An introduction to medical science.
   1. Human physiology
   I. Title
   612   QP34.5
   ISBN 0-85200-072-3
   ISBN 0-85200-154-1 Pbk

Printed in Great Britain by Spottiswoode Ballantyne Ltd.,
Colchester and London

Contents

Preface

This is a book for beginners. I have tried to write a text that would be helpful to students of diverse backgrounds who are starting basic science studies in preparation for work in one of the many health fields.

In some ways this is a conventional text. It clearly states, for instance, that most people have but one heart, two kidneys and 12 pairs of cranial nerves. In some ways it is different from other texts. First, it begins with the basic physics, chemistry and biology necessary for understanding anatomy, biochemistry and physiology. Secondly, it tries to stress the relevance of these sciences to health, disease and patient care.

Medicine is the science and art concerned with the preservation and restoration of health and with the care or cure of the person with disease. Today, for every one physician, there are more than nine other medical professionals, although the ratio varies from country to country. These "helping people" include nurses, therapists, technicians, pharmacists, medical assistants and even the caring family and friends of those who are ill.

Unlike music and mathematics, medicine has never had any child prodigies. Professional excellence in a medical field has always been achieved slowly, by hours of study and work, and has been built on a rock-solid foundation of basic science. Students today begin their professional studies with varying amounts and quality of preparation. Too often the students' foundation of basic science is shaky, and for them the process of knowledge building is nearly impossible. Even bright, well-motivated students can have difficulty and almost drown in what seems to be a sea of unrelated and incomprehensible facts.

You simply cannot understand how people breathe unless you know about some of the physics of gases. To learn how the kidneys function you must first know osmosis, as well as hypotonic and hypertonic solutions. Metabolic pathways can be memorized, but it is not easy to make much sense of them unless you have a grasp of elementary chemistry. To deal with this problem of student preparation I have added, where appropriate, mini-reviews of basic science principles, and have attempted to define or explain unfamiliar or complex scientific terms as their use arises. The first Chapters, for example, contain material on the atom and elements, chemical classes, osmosis, the cell, scientific units and anatomical terms.

Most people who study the basic health sciences do not intend to become professional scientists. Generally they want to learn how to provide a service for a patient or the community. In turn, most people who seek medical help do not voice their complaints in precise anatomical, biochemical or physiological terms. It would be an unusual patient who complains that something is wrong with his or her DNA synthesis, that his or her systolic blood pressure is too low, or that his or her blood sugar concentration is too high. Still, for students, the basic sciences are essential not only for knowing how the body functions in health, but also for understanding the signs and symptoms of disease, the how and why of laboratory tests and clinical procedures, and the logic of correct diagnosis and treatment of disease. Knowledge precedes care.

As more and more people become involved in providing health care, the necessity increases for learning and sharing this vital knowledge. To conclude on a real note of hope and encouragement, I believe that students can — with perseverance — learn the material, see its beauty and worth, and enjoy doing it.

Many persons have helped me with this book. I am grateful to Virginia Carlson, Stina Miller, Peres Owuor and Elaine Parthanais for their expert typing and other kindnesses. David Horrobin, DPhil, MRCP, Doris Arnold, RN, and Margaret Nishakawara, PhD, have read various chapters and made excellent suggestions. Gregory Nicolosi, PhD, and Joseph Foley, MD, also have helped generously. Dr Horrobin initiated the project and provided invaluable advice. I am most indebted to him.

Mr D. G. T. Bloomer and his staff at MTP Press Limited are to be commended for their expertise and their patience. I would like also to thank all my students in the United States, the West Indies and East Africa for their encouragement and insights. And finally, thanks to my friends and my family, too, for their generous and loving assistance. All errors are exclusively my own.

Teaching is a communal experience. A teacher can always tell from the puzzled looks and shaking heads that it is time to erase, to begin again. Writing is a solitary act. It lacks the interaction of the classroom, and the finished textbook does not come with an eraser. Because I cannot see my readers' reactions I would like to hear from them, to be told what is or isn't clear and useful, and what might be added to make this a better book. I shall endeavour to reply to all correspondence sent to me at the following address:

Ned Durkin, PhD, MD
PO Box 18182
Cleveland Heights, Ohio 44118
USA

1. An Introduction to Anatomy, Biochemistry and Physiology

INTRODUCTION

Anatomy is the geography of the body, the study of all its parts, their names, structure, location, description and relationship to one another. What is the direct route from London, England, to Timbuktu in Mali, Africa? What arteries take blood from the left ventricle of the heart to the cortex of the brain? To answer such questions correctly, you must give full and accurate names, locations and descriptions, and you must have an understanding of relationships between various places and parts. Geographers can study giant land masses and oceans was well as isolated valleys and street maps of small towns. Anatomists can also shift perspective in their studies. Gross anatomy refers to the study of the body by dissection or by cutting it apart. The first anatomists were gross anatomists; in fact, the word anatomy is derived from the Greek word *anatome* which means, literally, cutting apart. Beginning in the seventeenth century and continuing to the present, the study of optics and the development of different types of microscopes have made it possible to study smaller and smaller parts of the body, so what had previously been invisible to the naked eye can be enlarged many times, observed and studied. The branch of anatomy study that uses microscopes is called micro-anatomy, though the word histology is used interchangeably with micro-anatomy.

Biochemistry is concerned with the atoms, molecules and compounds which make up the body or provide it with energy. In a sense, it begins with the study of the composition of the foods and fluids we eat and drink and ends with the composition of the wastes we excrete. Those chemical processes, between eating and excretion, in which the foods are broken down and then used for growth, maintenance or energy, are what the biochemist tries to understand and explain.

Physiology is the study of how the cells, organs and systems of the body work and function together so that the body can stay alive. This is a very dynamic subject, for life can maintain itself only by continuously changing. These changes are called responses; anything that causes a response is called a stimulus. A stimulus may come from the external environment which surrounds the body, or may arise from within the body in its own internal environment. A physiologist tries to explain the relationship between stimulus and response in terms of the controlling mechanisms and their causes and effects.

Anatomy, biochemistry and physiology all overlap. You cannot know one without knowing the other two. Neat separations are made only by those who write specialized textbooks and by the librarians who must file them. They are all sciences, and in reality there is only one science. Dictionaries define science as "an orderly knowledge of material things or events based on observation and experiment". Science is this and more. It can be a force for both good and bad. It has made possible penicillin to kill disease-causing agents; has been the source of some pollutants killing life in our streams and waters; has put together powerful bombs to kill and wound; and has taught how blood transfusions can save the wounded. Scientists have helped more people to live longer, healthier lives and thus have been responsible for the increase in population, and yet, at the same time, have been responsible for the wasting of the limited resources of a sometimes too crowded world.

As a student of science, you should understand both the method of science and the limitations of science. A good scientist begins his or her work with a question or a problem — an admission that the scientist does not know how to explain a particular observation that he or she has made, or does not understand the mechanism by which some particular thing works or fails to work but he or she wants to find out.

Next, the scientist constructs an hypothesis — a possible solution or explanation for the problem. Occasionally, this hypothesis is arrived at after hours of reasoned study, but more often than not it results from imagination or simply guesswork. No matter how brilliant the hypothesis is, it must be tested so that it can be accepted or rejected. (An experiment is a test of a hypothesis.) The experiment has to be designed so that the matter or event in question can be observed under different conditions and measurements of some sort made. These measurements (the results of the experiment) are called the data. Finally, the scientist must make a judgment and decide whether the data support or contradict the hypothesis. A crucial point to remember is that the results of an experiment can never actually confirm the way things are; they can only confirm or contradict the way a scientist thinks they are.

Once there was a scientist who had a hypothesis that grasshoppers hear with their legs. To prove his hypothesis he designed an experiment in which he trained 200 grasshoppers to jump every time he said the word "jump". He would stick his head into the grasshoppers' cage, say "jump", and all 200 grasshoppers would simultaneously jump 5 cm into the air. The scientist carefully repeated this procedure 100 times, and every time he said "jump" the grasshoppers jumped 5 cm into the air. The scientist then chopped off all the legs from all the grasshoppers. Next he put his head into the cage and said "jump". Nothing happened. He whispered, then shouted the word "jump" 1000 times and still not a single grasshopper jumped. The scientist concluded that the data supported his hypothesis: grasshoppers hear with their legs. He believed that without their legs the grasshoppers were deaf and could not hear his instructions to jump.

Though the story is fanciful it does illustrate how the experimental method and data can be used to support an erroneous conclusion. Did the scientist's experiment prove that grasshoppers are not able to hear with their legs? Is it possible that grasshoppers could hear without their legs? Is there any evidence to support this? In fact, there is some evidence which shows that grasshoppers really do have receptors for sound on their front legs. If you really want to know though, you will have to find out for yourself. Such is the way of science.

Scientists are human, and often change their minds and make mistakes in both their thinking and the interpretation of their experiments; this is why science textbooks do not only get thicker and thicker as time passes, but also change as old ideas are *disproved* and new ideas are *proved*.

Many of the changes in scientific thinking lead to changes in the way patients are treated. In the not-too-distant past, it was common practice to bleed patients as this was thought to be good treatment for a variety of disorders. Similarly, giving fluids intravenously was looked upon as being harmful. Today the situation is reversed. Alfred North Whitehead summed up the rapid rate at which scientific thinking changes. He said, succinctly, "Knowledge keeps no better than fish".

The method of science has implications for you as a student. If you were to memorize this textbook word-for-word, picture-for-picture, but failed to understand what you were learning, your efforts would be wasted. Facts change, memories fade, and in time you would be left with nothing. But if you study the material carefully, really think about it and try to understand the principles involved, you will find they will remain with you long after your studies have finished.

WHY STUDY ANATOMY, BIOCHEMISTRY AND PHYSIOLOGY?

Your body has been with you a long time. You should know the names of its parts and what they look like, just as you know the names of your friends and can easily recognize them. A knowledge of anatomy will give you a basic vocabulary so that you can precisely define and locate the parts of the body. Anatomy is a practical necessity for nearly all your work. When giving injections it is necessary to know where the nerves are as well as where they are not. Sticking a needle into a nerve may cause severe damage to the nerve and may even cause paralysis.

Because biochemistry deals with life from a molecular viewpoint, it often frightens students and at times seems irrelevant to their work. It shouldn't. After all, you are what you eat; all that separates the food on your dinner plate from the proteins in your blood, the fat beneath your skin and the sugar nourishing your brain, is your appetite, and your digestive system which includes your liver. Biochemistry is also very necessary in your work for at least two other reasons: some diseases can be understood only at the

molecular level; some diseases are really chemical mistakes that the body makes. The treatment and prevention of many diseases is also chemical; that is, drugs are used and their action can only be understood if you understand the normal biochemistry of the body.

You have been breathing all your life, yet you probably do not know all the reasons why, or the mechanisms involved in breathing. Physiology will help you understand your body and how it works and also help you understand your patients, and why their bodies are not working properly. You should use your knowledge of physiology every time you take a temperature or blood pressure, test urine for sugar, or help a patient exercise his or her muscles.

There was a poet who said that a poem, like love, should begin in delight and end in wisdom. The same can be said hopefully of your study of anatomy, physiology and biochemistry. You should end by growing in wisdom, by gaining some understanding of the body so that you can serve well and effectively those who need your skills.

WHAT IS LIFE?

A good question; everyone asks it at least once in their life. Unfortunately, the question is too big, the answer too complex and too mysterious for scientists to answer fully. We really do not know, other than to repeat that life is the sum of all the forces that resist death.

There are, however, some characteristics always associated with living things. These characteristics do not really define life, they are simply found wherever we find living things. You know these characteristics. An easy way to bring them to mind might be to imagine that you came across a motionless animal and wanted to find out if it were dead or alive. If you pinched the animal and it was irritable or responsive to the stimulus of pinching, and moved, you would know the animal was alive. You would have to look closely at the animal to see if it were carrying out respiration, taking in oxygen and giving out carbon dioxide. If you felt the animal and it was alive, it would probably be warmer than the environment around it because it was carrying on metabolism, breaking down foods and storing their energy, using some of it and releasing it as heat. Finally, if you watched it a long time and it never changed except to decay or break down into something unrecognizable as an animal, you would be certain that it was dead; for one of the characteristics of life is its ability to regulate its life processes in different conditions, to change in changing conditions and survive. The characteristics of life are so important it might be good to look at them in detail.

a. Growth. If you are on the beach and keep shovelling sand into a pile it will get bigger; it will grow. Human growth is quite different.

You began your life as a single small cell, but this did not grow or develop into one giant 70-kilogram cell. That one cell divided and kept on dividing into many different types of cells by the processes of cell division and differentiation.

There are certain words commonly used to describe growth. If tissues get bigger without an increase in the number of cells, but only an increase in the size of existing

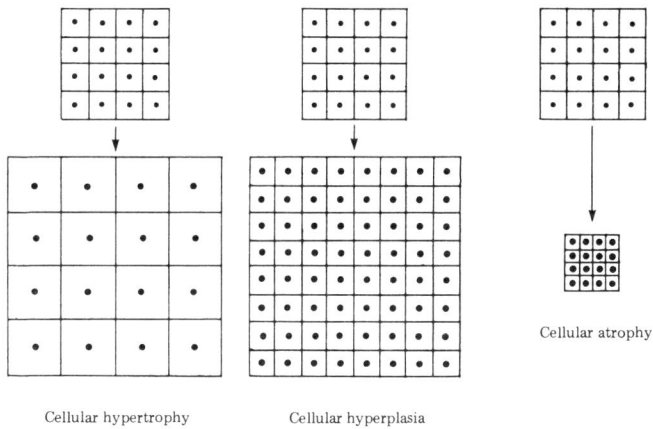

Figure 1.1 Cell growth: hypertrophy, hyperplasia and atrophy.

cells, this is called hypertrophy. If tissues or organs get bigger because of the formation of new cells through cell division, this is called hyperplasia. Atrophy is the reduction in the size of cells or organs after they have reached full development (see Figure 1.1).

There are many things we do not understand about growth. Some cells become liver cells, others become kidney cells; both are very different types of cells yet they have a common parent cell.

Another problem is the cessation of growth in an organ; the liver, the kidneys and other organs retain the potential to grow throughout life, yet they do not increase in size. The growth of an organ, the growth of cells, is very carefully controlled. When this control breaks down and cells grow uncontrollably, the disease is known as cancer — a hyperplasia. Although human growth is carefully controlled, it does not occur at a constant rate. Normally, the rate of growth in length is greatest during the first 2 years of life; it then slows down, but increases again during the early teen-years or the years immediately preceding them. Growth in height is almost always completed in the late teens or early twenties.

b. Reproduction. You are here because your parents reproduced. The pages of this book have been reproduced also, for there are many identical copies of it produced from a single printing plate. Human sexual reproduction differs from this, for what is reproduced is not a duplicate of what produced it, just as you are different from your father and your mother. Sexual reproduction ensures not only that the species will be continued, but that no two members of it will be exactly alike. The great Bengali writer, Rabindranath Tagore, once said that "with the birth of every child comes again the hope that God will not be too disappointed". In a scientific sense he was right, for every individual is unique, a new biological beginning.

c. Irritability. This property of life has nothing to do with personality but refers to that characteristic of life by which an organism can respond to a stimulus, can change because of a change in the environment. If you push a rock it will move, but if you push a man (stimulus) he might not only move but he may also push back at you (response), thus illustrating the property of irritability.

d. Contractility. Contractility is the scientific name for the ability to contract — to become shorter. This property is most highly developed in muscle tissue. If cells could not contract, there would be no movement, no life.

e. Absorption. The epithelial cells, which form the inner-most lining of the digestive tract, are specially developed for absorption — for taking molecules or particles into themselves across their membranes. All cells of the body share this property to some extent. Absorption is a selective property as the cell is a most discriminating host. Not all the molecules that call are "invited in", and some of those which do manage to enter for example, sodium ions, are quickly pumped out.

f. Metabolism. This is the name given to all the chemical reactions occurring in the body. There are millions of them. To simplify matters a little, these reactions are classified as being either anabolic or catabolic. Anabolism refers to those reactions in which molecules are put together or bigger molecules are made from smaller ones, and can be thought of as chemical addition. Catabolism covers those reactions in which molecules are broken down, and can be thought of as chemical subtraction. Anabolic reactions *require* energy; whereas catabolic reactions *release* energy. In a healthy adult, the anabolic reactions are approximately equal to the catabolic ones; while in a growing child there is more anabolism. Metabolism has been called "the fire of life" because the energy released from the burning of foodstuffs (catabolic breakdown) is necessary for those anabolic reactions by which the body maintains itself.

g. Respiration. Wherever there is human life, oxygen must be present. For energy to be supplied to the body, food must combine with oxygen and burn. You can perform a simple experiment showing the importance of oxygen-to-fat catabolism by taking a burning candle and placing a glass over it. (Candle wax is a type of fat.) As soon as the oxygen is consumed, the fire is extinguished. Respiration is really the combination of oxygen with a food substance so that carbon dioxide and water are produced and energy is released. All your cells are undergoing respiration all the time that they are alive.

h. Excretion. Living organisms must not only take in food, they must also eliminate the leftovers and get rid of any substances which might be harmful or toxic to them. They must excrete them. In a human, waste disposal is fairly complex, for the waste materials simply cannot diffuse out through the skin. The kidneys contain cells which are specialized for the excretion of acids and other waste materials.

i. Homeostasis. This word refers to the ability of the body to maintain a certain stability despite changing environmental conditions. This stability is maintained because of the body's ability to react and compensate for internal and external environmental changes, not because everything in the body is fixed or locked in place. An example of this ability can be offered. The temperature around you can vary drastically, going from freezing cold in the Arctic Circle to boiling hot in an Equatorial desert. In both locations your body compensates for these changes so that your blood neither freezes nor boils, and your body temperature remains relatively constant. This stability is maintained only at the expense of much energy.

When death occurs, homeostasis is no longer possible. The

body cannot maintain its stability and order and therefore decays. Claude Bernard, the famed French physiologist, summed it all up when he said that "a free and independent life in a changing external environment is dependent on the maintenance of a constant internal environment", that is, the body must keep its temperature relatively constant and have adequate oxygen, nutrients, etc. He compared the body to a flame, continually changing only to remain the same.

j. Death. Fire begets ashes. Death is the final certainty shared by all living organisms.

WHAT ARE LIVING THINGS MADE OF?

The answer is easy. Living things, just like the sea, soil and stars, are made of matter. But what is matter? Matter is anything that has a mass and occupies space.

The basic unit of matter is the atom. Today we know of about 300 different kinds of atoms which occur in nature. These different atoms are called nuclides. Nuclides are grouped into elements. An element is a chemical which cannot be broken down to give another chemical substance. You know the names of many elements: hydrogen, oxygen, iron, tin. There are at least 105 and possibly 107 different elements that are known today. Many of these elements are only rarely found in the crust of the earth or have only a brief existence in a physics research laboratory. Fortunately there are only 13 or so elements that are biologically prominent (see Table 1.1). Scientists abbreviate the names of the elements and these abbreviations are taken from the first letter or letters of the Latin name for the element. Usually the Latin name and the English name are the same — the abbreviation for carbon is C and for calcium it is Ca. There are three important exceptions however; the abbreviation for sodium is Na, for potassium it is K and for iron it is Fe.

Table 1.1   Some of the elements that are biologically prominent.

Element	Symbol	Atomic number	Atomic weight
Carbon	C	6	12.011
Hydrogen	H	1	1.008
Oxygen	O	8	15.999
Phosphorus	P	15	30.974
Potassium	K	19	39.102
Iodine	I	53	126.904
Nitrogen	N	7	14.007
Sulphur	S	16	32.064
Calcium	Ca	20	40.08
Iron	Fe	26	55.847
Magnesium	Mg	12	24.305
Sodium	Na	11	22.990
Chlorine	Cl	17	35.453

There is a mnemonic which can help you remember the thirteen most important elements. (A mnemonic is a memory help in code form.) The mnemonic is *CHOPKINS CaFe Mg NaCl.* C is for carbon, H for hydrogen, etc. You can recall the elements by thinking of CHOPKINS Cafe, a small restaurant which serves mighty good (Mg) steaks; most people like salt (NaCl) on their steaks.

There are other elements in the body in smaller con-

centrations and these are sometimes referred to as trace elements. Less is known about these trace elements because of the difficulty of measuring their concentration in living tissue. Some of the most important trace elements include: copper (Cu), zinc (Zn), fluorine (F), manganese (Mn), molybdenum (Mo), cobalt (Co) and selenium (Se).

When two or more elements combine, they form a compound. The basic unit of the compound is a molecule. A molecule is the smallest unit of a compound which exists and has the chemical characteristics of the compound. Water is a molecule you should be familiar with. It contains two hydrogen atoms and one oxygen atom. Water can be abbreviated as HOH or H_2O. These atoms are held together by chemical forces called bonds which are extremely important, for they are a source of potential energy, an energy bank where the ability to do physical or chemical work is stored. When a molecule is broken down so that the atoms are no longer held together, some of the energy which has been stored in this bond is set free or harnessed into doing work.

A mixture is two or more substances which are not joined together by chemical bonds. Salt and pepper together on your plate make up a mixture.

Now that we have some definitions, it is necessary to go beyond the definition and get some understanding of what an atom is. It is going to be difficult to explain, for even physicists who have spent their entire lives studying the atom are not so sure. We know that atoms are small. It has been calculated that in an average man there are seven octillion atoms (one octillion is the number one followed by 27 zeros!). An atom is defined as the smallest quantity of an element that can exist and still retain the chemical properties of the element. All the atoms of an element are alike, though not necessarily identical, i.e. there may be some variation in the number of certain particles within.

A single atom is made up of 200 or more small, sub-atomic particles, but it is necessary to know only the three basic particles. The first two particles — the proton and the neutron — are bound together very tightly in the nucleus (centre) of the atom, while the electron can be thought of as travelling around the nucleus. The proton and neutron are very big when compared to the electron and are about 1840 times as heavy. An electron can absorb energy and can change the pathway along which it orbits. It can leave one atom and go to another or it can travel around two different atoms, never belonging completely to one. Chemical bonds are formed by the exchange or sharing of electrons between two atoms. An electron is a negatively charged particle and will therefore be attracted to positive particles and be repelled by other negative particles. Electrons can flow through certain substances called conductors, carrying an electric current. Electricity is a flow of electrons. An atom or molecule which has more electrons than protons is called a negative ion while one that has fewer electrons than protons is called a positive ion. Bio-electricity is a flow of ions.

In the nucleus of the atom we have the tightly bound neutrons and protons. The nuclear force holding these particles together is greater than the repellent force which tends to repel the like-charged positive protons. The neutron is slightly bigger than the proton and has no charge, whereas the smaller proton has a positive charge which causes the

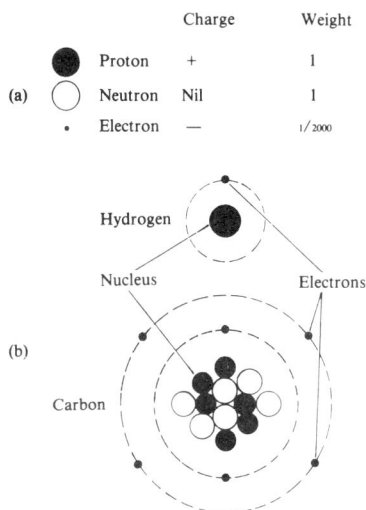

Figure 1.2 (a) The particles which make up the atom. (b) Diagrammatic sketch of the atom showing its parts. Negatively charged electrons circle the nucleus composed of protons and neutrons. The diagram represents a working model of the atom. It does not in any real sense represent a "picture" of the atom.

whole nucleus to have a positive charge. This positive charge acts as an attractive force and "holds" the negatively charged electrons in their orbits. Figure 1.2a shows the three basic particles which make up the atom. Figure 1.2b is a working model of the atom and is not an actual picture. Physicists who try to measure an electron can only tell one of two things about it at the same time. They can either measure how fast the electron is going, or where the electron is; they can never know both at the same time. This is one reason why a better representation or more realistic picture of an atom would show the electrons represented by a "cloud".

Since all atoms have only three basic parts, and since there are 105 different elements, the number and arrangement of these basic particles are what make the elements different. Silver is different from gold. The differences are caused by the different numbers and arrangement of the neutron, proton and electron and not because it has any new or different particles.

There are three ways to separate the atoms and identify them on the basis of their atomic arrangement: (a) the atomic number, (b) the mass number and (c) the atomic weight.

a. The atomic number gives the number of protons in the nucleus of the atom. Hydrogen has one proton in its nucleus and therefore has an atomic number of 1; carbon has six protons and will have an atomic number of 6. In an electrically neutral atom (one that is not an ion), the number of protons will be equal to the number of electrons in that atom. Hydrogen, with an atomic number of 1, will have one proton and one electron. Carbon, with an atomic number of 6, will have six protons and six electrons.

b. The mass number also identifies atoms. The mass number is always a whole number, for it is determined by adding the number of protons to the number of neutrons. The mass number gives the number of particles in the nucleus of the atom; electrons are ignored because they weigh so little.

The number of neutrons in the nucleus is not necessarily the same as the number of protons; hydrogen has an atomic

number of 1 and, as it has no neutrons, a mass number of 1. Carbon has six protons and six neutrons in its nucleus, so it will have a mass number of 12. An atom of sodium with an atomic number of 11 and a mass number of 23 will have 11 protons and 12 neutrons in a nucleus at the centre of the atom and 11 electrons in motion around the nucleus. If the number of protons does not equal the number of electrons, the positive and negative charges will not balance; the atom will have an electric charge and will be called an ion. An atom of uranium has 92 protons and 146 neutrons; it will have an atomic number of 92 and a mass number of 238.

Scientists have a special way of writing the atomic number and the mass number. The carbon atom, which has six protons and six neutrons, is written with the atomic number (the number of protons) below and to the left of the symbol for the element, and with mass number (the sum of neutrons and protons) above and to the left of the symbol — $^{12}_{6}C$. A uranium atom can be written $^{238}_{92}U$.

c. The atomic weight is the third identifying number. It is possible to give the weight of a single atom. A single atom of hydrogen (^{1}H) weighs:

$$0.000\ 000\ 000\ 000\ 000\ 000\ 000\ 001\ 673\ \text{grams,}$$

or, if written in scientific shorthand:

$$1.673 \times 10^{-24}\ \text{grams.}$$

The mass of one hydrogen atom (1.673×10^{-24} grams) is said to have a mass of 1 dalton. Keeping track of all those zeros can be a little too complicated at times, so a different system of expressing weights has evolved. In the new system an atom of carbon with six neutrons and six protons is assigned an atomic weight of 12.000. An atom of hydrogen with one proton and no neutrons is assigned an atomic weight of 1.000. The atom (nuclide) of carbon which has 12 neutrons and protons has 12 times the weight of hydrogen which has only one proton. The uranium atom $^{238}_{92}U$ has an atomic weight of 238.000 because it has nearly 20 times as many protons and neutrons as the carbon molecule.

But looking closely at Table 1.1 (see page 4) we notice that the atomic weights are not all whole numbers; they don't just have zeros after the decimal point. Why is this? Why aren't all the numbers whole numbers, for aren't we just adding the neutrons and protons together and don't they each have a value of one? The mass number is determined by adding neutrons and protons but the atomic weight is an indication of all the atoms which make up the element, not just a single atom. Carbon has an atomic weight of 12.011 but a mass number of 12.000 because not all the carbon atoms have six protons and six neutrons. A few carbon atoms have six protons and eight neutrons and so will be heavier than most carbon atoms, which have only six protons and six neutrons. Most atoms of carbon are $^{12}_{6}C$, while a few are $^{14}_{6}C$. The following example should make it clearer.

We have a sample of pure carbon. In this sample there are 10 000 different carbon atoms. On estimating the different kinds of carbon atoms in the sample we find that of the 10 000 carbon atoms 9945 have six protons and six neutrons and are therefore $^{12}_{6}C$. The remaining 55 atoms are of the $^{14}_{6}C$ and are heavier because they have six protons and eight neutrons. To get the atomic weight of this sample we have to consider all the atoms and so calculate an average:

$$9945 \times 12 = 119\,340$$
$$55 \times 14 = 770$$
$$\overline{120\,110}$$

$$120\,110 \div 10\,000 = 12.011$$

We can now say that the atomic weight of carbon is 12.011. All the atoms of an element will have to have the same number of protons but they can have a different number of neutrons.

Atoms of the same element which have differing weights because of differing numbers of neutrons in the nucleus are known as isotopes; $^{12}_{6}C$ and $^{14}_{6}C$ are isotopes of carbon. Isotopes of the same element behave identically in most chemical reactions and some isotopes have important medical uses.

If we know the atomic weight of an element we can calculate the atomic weight of a molecule. To calculate the atomic weight of water (HOH or H_2O) simply add the weight of each element in the molecule as many times as it is present:

Hydrogen	H	$1.008 \times 2 =$	2.016
Oxygen	O	$15.999 \times 1 =$	15.999
Water	H_2O		18.015

In many working situations the numbers after the decimal point are ignored, so the atomic weight of water is roughly 18. Another example is glucose (grape sugar). The formula for glucose is $C_6H_{12}O_6$:

Carbon	C	$12.011 \times 6 =$	72.066
Hydrogen	H	$1.008 \times 12 =$	12.096
Oxygen	O	$15.999 \times 6 =$	95.994
Glucose	$C_6H_{12}O_6$		180.156

In many calculations the atomic weight of glucose is taken as 180.

There are two more definitions you should learn now because they both relate to atomic weights. The first is gram molecular weight (the mole). That quantity of a substance, the weight of which in grams is numerically equal to its molecular weight, is called a gram molecular weight (a mole). One mole of calcium weighs 40.08 grams; if you have 16.000 grams of oxygen you will have 1 mole of oxygen, while if you have 32.000 grams you will have 2 moles of oxygen. One mole of salt (NaCl) is 58.443 grams (the atomic weights of sodium and chlorine added together). Although there are two atoms here, they form one molecule. One mole of any substance has 6.0222×10^{23} atoms, ions or molecules in it. The 16.000 grams of oxygen and the 40.08 grams of calcium both contain 6.022×10^{23} atoms. One mole of calcium weighs more than 1 mole of oxygen, for the same reason that 10 stones are heavier than 10 feathers — the

individual calcium atom has more neutrons and protons than the individual oxygen atom. The mole expression thus gives an indication of the number of atoms, ions or molecules present.

The other very important definition is that of *a molar solution*. This is a means of expressing the amount of solute which is dissolved in a solution. A solution is a fluid which contains a dissolved substance and the solute is that which is dissolved in the solution. If you dissolve a teaspoon of sugar in a cup of water, the sugar is the solute, the water is the solvent and together they make up a solution. To make a molar solution, you take 1 mole of a substance (the number of grams of solute is equal to the molecular weight) and place it in a measuring container. Add distilled water to the container until you reach the 1 litre mark (1 litre is 1000 cubic centimetres, about $1\frac{3}{4}$ pints and is abbreviated l). If you wanted to make up a 0.5 molar solution of the sugar, glucose, you would first find its atomic weight. Glucose is $C_6H_{12}O_6$ so it will have a molecular weight of 180. One mole of glucose would be 180 grams, but since we are interested in $\frac{1}{2}$ a mole, we want only 90 grams of glucose. We take the 90 grams of glucose, place it in a measuring container, add distilled water and start to stir. We stop adding the water when the level of water in the container reaches the 1000 cc or the 1 litre mark.

In clinical work one frequently sees the expressions millimole (mmol) or milliequivalent (mEq). There are 1000 millimoles in 1 mole, and 1000 milliequivalents in one equivalent. Many laboratory values are expressed in mmol or mEq because the concentration of many substances is so very small that it is easier to express them this way rather than as a fraction of a mole.

One mmol is 1/1000 of a mole, and there are 1000 mmol in 1 mole or 1 gram molecular weight of a substance. Suppose you had a sample of fluid and the glucose concentration was 1 gram/l. How many millimoles of glucose would there be in the 1 litre? We know that 1 mole of glucose has 180 grams of glucose. We know also that since there are 1000 mmol in 1 mole of glucose, 180 grams of glucose = 1000 mmol. In the solution we have 1/180 of 1 mole of glucose, so we also have 1/180 of 1000 mmol of glucose. If we set an equation and let X equal the unknown number of millimoles in 1 gram of glucose, we can answer the question:

$$\frac{1 \text{ gram}}{180 \text{ grams}} = \frac{X \text{ mmol}}{1000 \text{ mmol}}$$
$$180\,X = 1000 \text{ mmol}$$
$$X = 5.55 \text{ mmol/l or}$$
$$0.00555 \text{ mol/l}$$

After going through the calculation you might be interested to know that the concentration of glucose in your blood is probably around 5.55 mmol/l. In the Chapter on units, definitions, etc., there is more information about the conversion from one type of unit to another.

The concentration of potassium in a typical patient's plasma might be 0.004 moles per litre (mol/l). This can be expressed as 4 mmol. To make a 4 mmol solution you must consider that this solution contains 4/1000 of 1 mole. In 1 mole of potassium there are about 39.1 grams; therefore, in a

4 mmol potassium solution there are about 0.156 grams of potassium:

$$4/1000 \times 39.1 \text{ grams} = 0.156 \text{ grams.}$$

The concentration of ions is sometimes expressed as mEq/l. The equivalent weight of an ion equals the molecular weight divided by the absolute value of the charge of the ion. There are 1000 mEq in one equivalent weight. If the concentration of sodium ions in a typical patient's plasma is 145 mEq/l, you can calculate how many grams this is. In a solution with 145 mEq/l there are:

$$145/1000 \times 22.99 \text{ grams} = 3.33 \text{ grams.}$$

Because sodium, potassium, chloride and bicarbonate ions all have a charge with an absolute value of 1, the value of their concentration in mEq will equal their concentration in mmol. To convert mEq to mmol, divide the number of mEq by the absolute value of the ion's charge. For example, the absolute value of the charge of the calcium ion (Ca^{++}) is 2. Two mEq/l of calcium will have the same concentration as a solution having 1 mmol/l.

WHAT ARE THE CHEMICALS OF LIFE?

A. Water

Water is the most common and important molecule in your body. It is the chief constituent found inside your cells, and it also bathes them on the outside. Hair, bone and adipose (fat) tissue are the only tissues in which the water content is not greater than 50%.

A dramatic example might help to illustrate this point. The average adult human brain weighs approximately 1350 grams or about 3 pounds. The brain has been compared to a telephone switchboard or a computer. An equally invalid but instructive comparison would be to compare the brain to an aquarium. If you take the human brain and carefully remove all the water, leaving everything else, what remains would weigh less than 300 grams. Most of the human brain is water. The fact that water makes up so much of your body is an advantage. Water is a very good solvent. This means that many chemicals are soluble in it; they will dissolve in it. If the molecules are dissolved in solution, they can move about freely within the solution so that in time their concentration will be equal throughout the solution. More important, they will have the chance to "bump into" other molecules and, perhaps, react with them and form a new molecule. Another advantage of water is that it takes quite a bit of heat to raise its temperature. You learned this while waiting for the water to boil for your tea. Because it takes so much heat to change the temperature of water, the body with its high water content has an easier time regulating its temperature.

"Man is like a fountain", said Heraclitus, "always the same but never the same water". Water molecules are always coming in or going out of our bodies, about 1.5–3 litres every day. A healthy individual is said to be in water balance; this means that the intake of water is approximately equal to the output. A healthy individual can live only 3 or 4 days without any water. Disease also comes if he or she cannot eliminate water. This is why the fluid intake and output of many patients is so carefully monitored.

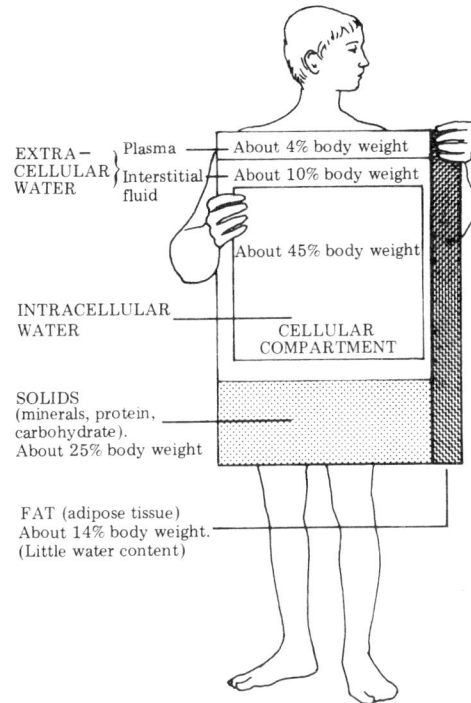

Figure 1.3 Typical composition of the adult body.

Figure 1.3 shows in schematic form some of the body relationships. If you were to consider the lean body mass of an individual, that is, his weight without his adipose tissue, you would find that water makes up 60%. This is because fat tissue contains little water. Body water is named after its location in the body. About twice as much water is located inside the cells of the body as is located outside the cells. Water within the cells is referred to as the *intra*cellular water; water which is outside the cells is the *extra*cellular water.

The extracellular water has two major divisions or compartments: the plasma, which is the fluid portion of the blood; and the interstitial fluid, which is the water which bathes and surrounds the cells of the body. The volume of the interstitial fluid is about three times greater than that of the plasma. These fluid compartments will be discussed again but it should be pointed out now that water can move from one compartment to another.

You might want to calculate how much of your body is water. If your total bodyweight is 70 kg (154 lbs), let us assume that 60% of your weight is water. Therefore:

$$70 \text{ kg} \times 60/100 = 42 \text{ kg of water.}$$

One kg of water is equal to 1 litre of water, so there are approximately 42 litres of water in your body. Of course, if you are in water balance, you will probably take in 2–3 l/day of water and eliminate 2–3 l/day of water. An understanding of water balance is necessary for many situations involving patient care. Health personnel are often faced with questions like these: how much water should be given to a dehydrated infant, and how much water should be given to a patient who has just had surgery and can't eat or drink?

Water's importance is not restricted to the body. Three quarters of the earth's surface is covered by water. Water is therefore a vital necessity for all life. Safe drinking water is indeed essential for individual survival and community health.

B. Carbohydrates

Carbohydrates (and water) are the chief constituents of bread, potatoes, sugar, cassava root and rice, and make up at least 45% of your diet. Chemically, carbohydrates are simple molecules made up of carbon, hydrogen and oxygen.

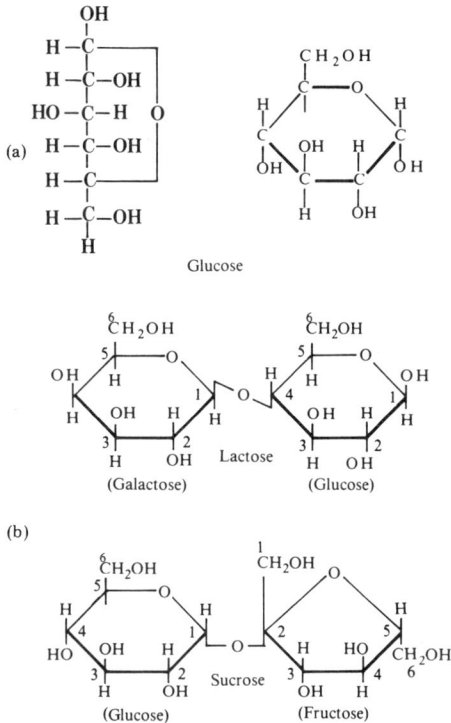

Figure 1.4 Carbohydrates. (a) Two ways of diagramming the structure of the carbohydrate, glucose — a monosaccharide. (b) Disaccharides — lactose, sucrose.

a. Monosaccharides. An extremely important carbohydrate in your body is the sugar, glucose (see Figure 1.4a). There is glucose in your bloodstream right now and even if you did not eat anything overnight there would still be 70–100 mg of glucose in every 100 ml of your blood tomorrow morning. Glucose is important in your metabolism, in fact your brain normally derives nearly 100% of its energy from the metabolism of glucose. Diabetes is a disease in which the amount of glucose in the blood is not properly regulated. The glucose molecule is called a monosaccharide because there is only one sugar unit present. In a monosaccharide there is one atom of oxygen for every carbon atom, and two atoms of hydrogen for every oxygen atom: $C_xH_{2x}O_x$.

b. Disaccharides. Two monosaccharides linked together form a disaccharide (see Figure 1.4b). A disaccharide with which you are familiar is sucrose. Sucrose is the sugar that is sold in the stores, that you put in your cakes and tea. It is made up of two (monosaccharide) sugar units: glucose and a molecule somewhat like glucose called fructose which is found in honey.

Another disaccharide is lactose which is the carbohydrate found in milk, and for this reason is particularly important for babies and children. It is made up of two monosaccharides: glucose and galactose.

Maltose is another disaccharide. It is made up of two glucose units joined together and it is formed when starch is broken down.

c. Polysaccharides. The final important carbohydrate in our diet is starch. Starches are polysaccharides because they are made up of many monosaccharides linked together. Starches are found in plants. A potato is little more than water and starch wrapped up in a skin. Cereals, grains and rice are mostly starch.

Man does not have any starch in his body, but he does have a compound like starch which is called glycogen. Glycogen is also a polysaccharide and is made of many glucose units hooked together. It is one giant molecule made up of many little glucose molecules. The difference between glycogen and the starch is in the way the glucose molecules are linked together. Glycogen is also a very important molecule. It can best be thought of as a glucose bank. If you have eaten a lot of carbohydrate, some of it will be saved and converted into glycogen. Then if you go for a time without eating, or your body has a special need for extra sugar, the glycogen is broken down, releasing glucose into your bloodstream. This is one of the ways of ensuring that there will always be glucose in your bloodstream.

Carbohydrates are really the prime source of energy for the body. After being digested, they can either be immediately used for energy, converted to glycogen for later use or converted to fat.

C. Fats

Fats, like carbohydrates, are made up of carbon, hydrogen and oxygen; however, the ratio between the carbon, hydrogen and oxygen molecules is not the same as for carbohydrates, and their structure is more varied. Fats, like carbohydrates, are burned in the body to release energy and produce carbon dioxide and water. In terms of energy storage, fats are more important than carbohydrates. If you go for more than 48 hours without eating, all your glycogen will be broken down. However, as every dieter knows, you can starve yourself for 48 hours and your fat will not disappear. Fat is a very concentrated energy source and it takes much longer for it to disappear.

Another name for fats is lipids. We find fats or lipids in our diet in the cream on top of milk, the oil or dripping we fry our meat in and the white part of meat. Generally, most lipids will not dissolve in water. Lipid is a very large classification and we must be more specific.

a. Glycerides. Glycerides are molecules made from two other types of molecules: glycerol and fatty acids (see Figures 1.5a and b). Usually three fatty acids are joined to one glycerol molecule; this is called a triglyceride. Glycerides are to fats as glycogen is to carbohydrates. They are energy storage forms of fats. Put your hand over your stomach and, if there is a big bulge, most of it will be caused by stored triglycerides.

b. Steroids. Cholesterol is the name of a steroid you might be familiar with. The birth control pills are likewise steroids (see Figure 1.5c). Steroids are also secreted by the adrenal glands and reproductive tissues of the body. The basic steroid

(a)

$$H-\overset{H}{\underset{|}{C}}-OH + HO-\overset{O}{\overset{||}{C}}-CH_2-(CH_2)_6-CH_3$$

$$H-\overset{|}{C}-OH + HO-\overset{O}{\overset{||}{C}}-CH_2-(CH_2)_6-CH_3 \longrightarrow$$

$$H-\overset{|}{C}-OH + HO-\overset{O}{\overset{||}{C}}-CH_2-(CH_2)_6-CH_3$$

$$\underset{H}{\overset{|}{|}}$$

Glycerol   3 Fatty acids

$$H-\overset{H}{\underset{|}{C}}-O-\overset{O}{\overset{||}{C}}-CH_2-(CH_2)_6-CH_3$$

$$H-\overset{|}{C}-O-\overset{O}{\overset{||}{C}}-CH_2-(CH_2)_6-CH_3 + 3\,H_2O$$

$$H-\overset{|}{C}-O-\overset{O}{\overset{||}{C}}-CH_2-(CH_2)_6-CH_3$$

$$\underset{H}{\overset{|}{|}}$$

Neutral fat
(triglyceride)

(b)

$$H-C-C-C-C-C-C-COOH$$

Saturated fatty acid

$$H-C-C=C-C=C-C-C-COOH$$

Unsaturated fatty acid

(c)

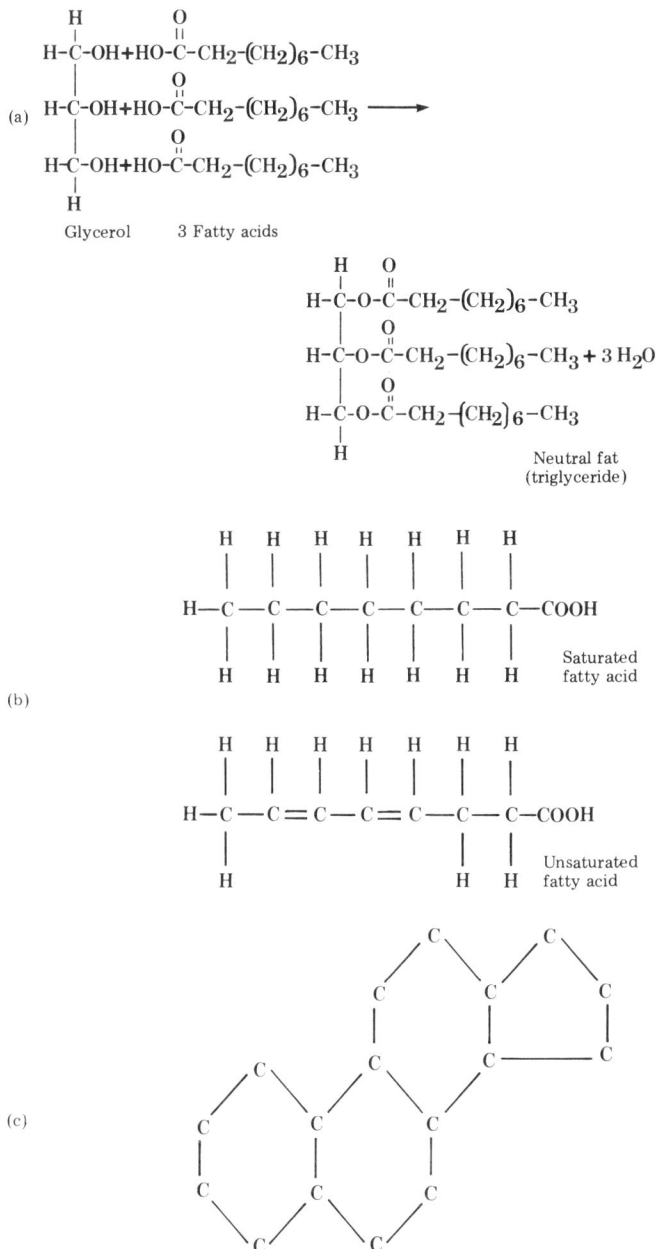

Figure 1.5 Fats. (a) Neutral fat (triglyceride) consists of three fatty acids attached to three hydroxyl groups of glycerol. (b) The hydrocarbon structure of saturated and unsaturated fatty acids. (c) Carbon-ring structure of various steroids, including the female and male sex hormones — estrogen and testosterone.

structure is four rings of carbon, arranged much like chicken wire.

c. Phospholipids. The third class of lipids is known as phospholipids because they contain the element, phosphorus, in addition to carbon, hydrogen and oxygen. They have very complicated structures, are important parts of all cell membranes and are of special importance in the nervous system.

d. Prostaglandins. These are the "newest" members of the lipid family. Prostaglandins are synthesized from fatty acids and have two hydrocarbon chains attached to a hydrocarbon ring. They have a powerful influence on the contraction of smooth muscle and activity of certain enzymes, though research into their actions is just beginning. Prostaglandins are found both inside cells and outside cells in the fluids which bathe and nourish them.

There are many diseases related to fats and their metabolism but perhaps the most important consideration is that people who eat too much and store too much fat are not as healthy and do not live as long as thin people do.

In addition to its metabolic role, the fat beneath the skin serves as an energy insulator, reducing the loss of heat to the outer environment. Animals which face the coldest environments have the most fat beneath their skin.

D. Proteins

Proteins are produced only in living organisms and are perhaps the most important class of chemicals in the human body. They are made up of carbon, hydrogen, oxygen, nitrogen and, occasionally, sulphur. One reason that proteins are so important is that many of the proteins in human beings are different from the proteins found in animals. The fats and carbohydrates in your body are not different from the fats and carbohydrates of animals. The glucose molecule nourishing the brain of the elephant is no different from the glucose molecule in your bloodstream, but the proteins in the cells of that brain are different. Proteins are so unique that you have proteins in your body that are not found in any other body — proteins can be more specific than your fingerprints.

So how can proteins be unique if they are made of only carbon, hydrogen, oxygen and nitrogen? These four elements are arranged in 21 different molecules known as amino acids. A protein is really just a lot of amino acids linked together by chemical bonds; amino acids are the building blocks of proteins (see Figure 1.6 for a typical amino acid, alanine).

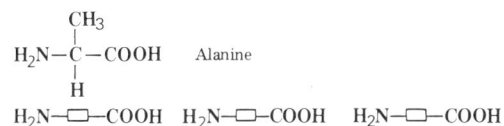

$$H_2N-\overset{CH_3}{\underset{|}{\overset{|}{C}}}-COOH \quad \text{Alanine}$$
$$\underset{H}{}$$

$$H_2N-\square-COOH \quad H_2N-\square-COOH \quad H_2N-\square-COOH$$

Figure 1.6 Alanine. Formation of proteins by linking amino acids together by peptide bonds formed between the carboxyl group of one amino acid and the amino group of another.

The order or sequence in which these amino acids are arranged is of extreme importance. If an error is made in the sequence in which the amino acids are linked together, the resulting protein may not be able to function properly. An average protein has 500 amino acids in it. Since there are 21 different amino acids which can make up this protein, the number of different proteins that can be made is fantastic. In fact, the number is so large it would have over 600 zeros in it. Table 1.2 lists the different amino acids.

The amino acids are classified as either essential or non-essential. The adjective non-essential is actually misleading, for all the amino acids listed are essential for life. They are all necessary for the synthesis of protein, cellular structures and certain hormones. The distinction between essential and the so-called non-essential amino acids is somewhat arbitrary.

Essential amino acids cannot be synthesized by the body or cannot be synthesized in adequate amounts. For example,

Table 1.2 Essential and non-essential amino acids.

Amino acids	
Essential	*Non-essential*
Phenylalanine	Alanine
Valine	Aspartic acid
Threonine	Cysteine
Tryptophan	Cystine
Isoleucine	Glutamic acid
Methionine	Glycine
Histidine	Hydroxylysine
Arginine	Hydroxyproline
Leucine	Proline
Lysine	Serine
	Tyrosine

the body lacks the enzymatic machinery to synthesize tryptophan and lysine. These amino acids are therefore called essential amino acids and must be included in the diet. Because tryptophan and lysine are not very plentiful in foods like maize, they can be added to certain foods to supplement the diet, particularly for those people for whom maize is the staple diet. The essential amino acids, histidine and arginine, can be synthesized by the body but only to a very small extent. During conditions of rapid growth the amount synthesized by the body is inadequate, so these amino acids must be included in the diet of growing individuals.

The body has enzymes to convert the essential amino acid, phenylalanine, to tyrosine. Tyrosine is often called a *non-essential* amino acid because it can be synthesized in the body. Tyrosine is an essential component of hormones and necessary proteins. In fact, if the levels of phenylalanine are not adequate, sufficient tyrosine can't be synthesized, and so tyrosine has to be added to the diet. Thus a *non-essential* amino acid can become an *essential* amino acid.

Again, all amino acids are important for protein synthesis and metabolism, although the body does require some amino acids more than others. The following mnemonic should help you to remember the essential amino acids:

PVT. TIM. HALL.

P stands for phenylalanine; V for valine . . .

Good sources of all amino acids are milk, meat, fish, fowl, cheese and eggs. Kwashiorkor is a disease resulting from a deficiency of proteins in the diet. The name comes from the Ga people in Nigeria who noticed that when a mother stopped breast-feeding one child so that she could breast-feed another baby, the older child became sickly. This was because he was no longer getting sufficient protein in his diet, which had been previously supplied by the mother's milk.

More of this material is covered in the Chapter on metabolism and nutrition.

Since proteins contain carbon, hydrogen, oxygen and nitrogen, they cannot be completely burned, unlike fats and carbohydrates, to give only CO_2 and H_2O. When proteins are broken down, some CO_2 and H_2O are produced, and the nitrogen is left in the form of ammonia (NH_3). Ammonia is very harmful to cells, so it is rapidly converted to urea

$$NH_2-\overset{\overset{\displaystyle O}{\|}}{C}-NH_2$$

Most of the ammonia and urea synthesis occurs in the liver. Within normal limits, urea is not harmful and is excreted in the urine.

Proteins are broken down for energy only when fat and carbohydrate stores are gone; they are important as energy sources only when there is an inadequate supply of fat and carbohydrate; their real job in the body is to provide specific structures. The part of a muscle responsible for the shortening of the cell is protein. Some of the chemical messengers in the blood (the hormones) are proteins, as are the antibodies, which are specific chemicals made by the body to defend it from attack by invading micro-organisms. Proteins also function as enzymes.

An enzyme is defined as a protein catalyst. A catalyst is a substance that speeds up a chemical reaction but is not permanently changed by the reaction. An analogy might help. Suppose you had a small picture-puzzle and wanted to put the pieces together. You might try to put it together standing up, holding each of the pieces in your hand, but it would be far easier if you had a table or a surface to work on. The table does not play any part in the choosing or moving of the different pieces, it just makes it easier for you to fit the right pieces together. In your body, molecules are always coming together forming bigger molecules, or bigger molecules are being broken down into smaller molecules. Glucose units are being linked together to make glycogen; fatty acids and glycerol are being joined together to form triglycerides; amino acids are being hooked together to form proteins; fats and carbohydrates are being broken down to give CO_2 and water; essential amino acids are being converted to non-essential amino acids. None of these reactions could occur in the body unless there was present a very special and unique surface to enable the right molecules to come together and change. By functioning as a specific surface for chemical reactions, the energy required for the reaction to take place is reduced. The diagram of an enzyme might help (see Figure 1.7).

Only those molecules which fit the enzyme will react. A fat molecule can never be added to glycogen because there is no enzyme for that reaction. Another point the diagram illustrates is that the chemical reaction can go either way, from one molecule to two, or from two molecules to one.

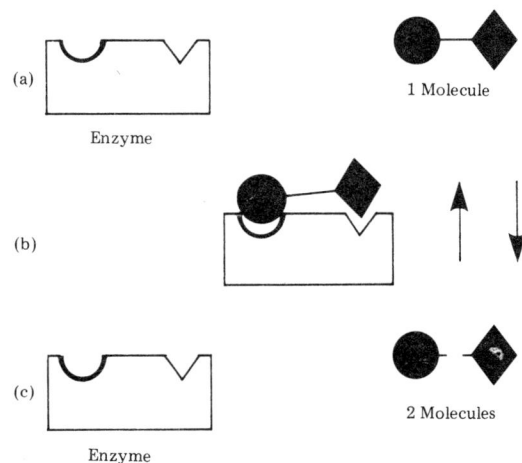

Figure 1.7 Model of an enzyme.

Which way the reaction will go depends upon the concentration of the various molecules and on the energy that is available for the reaction. If there are a lot of the large molecules, there will be many of these bumping into the enzyme and as a result the enzyme will tend to form many of the small molecules. An enzyme is a protein (many amino acids linked together) and occasionally an ion or another molecule contributes to the structure of the enzyme. When the enzyme is put together, the amino acids are hooked together one-by-one in a straight line, but they ultimately get twisted and coiled up upon themselves so a complex shape evolves. In recent years, the word "glycoproteins" has appeared in the medical literature with ever greater frequency. Glycoproteins are proteins that have short chains of carbohydrate attached to them. The carbohydrate portion is made up of from two to six different sugars, some of which have a nitrogen-containing amino group. Glycoproteins are found on the surface of membranes, in secretions, serum and other body fluids. In fact, many of the plasma proteins and hormones do have a small carbohydrate component and can be considered to be glycoproteins. Examples are fibrinogen, ceruloplasmin and follicle-stimulating hormone. Ordinarily, the carbohydrate is added after the protein has been synthesized.

E. Nucleic acids

Nucleic acids are the newest class in the chemicals of life. The more we find out about them, the more important they become. They are called nucleic acids because they were first found in the nucleus of the cell, but now we know that nucleic acids are found both in the nucleus and in the cytoplasm outside the nucleus. (More about these terms when we talk about the cell.) Nucleic acids contain carbon, hydrogen, oxygen, nitrogen and phosphorus.

Two common nucleic acids are deoxyribonucleic acid (DNA) and ribonucleic acid (RNA). Every cell in your body contains DNA and RNA. The DNA in your body is unique to your body. In fact, your body is the way it is because of your DNA and RNA. There is an exception to this. If you are one of a pair of identical twins, you and your twin will have identical DNA. Identical twins are two individuals formed from the same ovum. After fertilization, the fertilized ovum divides and separates into two sets of cells and the two individuals begin their separate development. Since they both develop from the same source, they will have the same DNA and the same appearance.

a. Chromosomes and genes

One of the questions that has troubled scientists for a long time is why is it that pregnant humans have little humans and pregnant rhinoceroses have little rhinoceroses? When a friend of yours is pregnant, you expect the baby to look something like his or her parents, and no doubt the proud rhinoceroses expect their offspring to look something like them.

But why is there this universal expectation? After all, both we and the rhinoceros began our lives as a single cell called a zygote. This zygote was formed from the union of a single male sperm cell and a single female egg (ovum). Even with a microscope it would not be possible to predict which zygotes were potential humans and which were potential animals.

You do already have hints as to the reasons for these developmental differences. Remember, many of your proteins, that is human proteins, are unique to humans and different from those of other animals. If two zygotes synthesize different enzymes and other proteins, they will develop different metabolic pathways, will synthesize different structures and will become different creatures.

The crucial question is: why are different proteins synthesized? Protein synthesis is under the control of the genes. Many human genes are unlike the genes of the rhinoceros or any other form of life, just as many of the genes of the rhinoceros are unique to rhinoceroses. Genes are the chemical carriers of heredity. Your resemblance to your parents has a chemical basis which began at conception when the paternal genes in the male sperm cell came together with the maternal genes in the female ovum. The genes themselves are located within the nucleus of the cell in rod-like bodies called chromosomes. Each chromosome consists chiefly of many long, tightly coiled DNA molecules. The DNA molecules making up the chromosomes are very large; in fact, they are the largest molecules in the cell. Each chromosome contains thousands of genes arranged in a line (linear sequence). With one exception, each cell has 46 chromosomes arranged in 23 separate pairs. The chromosomes of each pair are similar to one another but different from the other chromosomal pairs. Because of the constant number of chromosomes, the number of genes and the amount of DNA in each cell is also constant. The exception refers to the number of chromosomes found in sperm cells and ova. The nuclei of these cells contain half the DNA found in other cells of the body, as sperm and ova possess only 23 chromosomes or one half of each chromosomal pair. More about this will be said subsequently. Of your total of 46 chromosomes, you received 23 from your father and 23 from your mother.

So far it has been established that genes are: (1) Made of DNA. (2) The chemical basis for heredity. (3) Located on chromosomes within the cell. (4) Ultimately responsible for protein synthesis.

Still more needs to be said. It may be useful to think of DNA as a molecule containing information or a plan that enables the genes to function as the carriers of heredity and as the ultimate regulators of protein synthesis. Some evidence for this concept can be drawn from the following facts. Bacteria, plants, birds, crocodiles and man are all biological organisms and are listed in order of increasing complexity. Associated with this increasing complexity is an increased content of DNA in each cell. A single human cell is potentially capable of carrying out many more complicated metabolic syntheses and functions than a single bacterial cell, so it is not surprising that a human cell would require more information and have many times the DNA content of a bacterial cell.

More compelling evidence comes from the study of chromosomal disorders. In the condition known as Down's syndrome, grossly abnormal offspring are formed. Some die before birth, and many of the infants who do survive have a very shortened life expectancy. Abnormal development of the heart and digestive system are frequently seen in these infants, but the most common characteristic is an abnormal brain development causing impaired mental development.

There is no cure or treatment for this mental retardation. It must be emphasized that although these infants are retarded, they are no less than human. If they survive into childhood, they usually develop gentle and affectionate natures, and are seldom vicious or belligerent.

Study of the chromosomes of infants with Down's syndrome shows that they have a total of 47 chromosomes. It is not yet known how the extra chromosome causes this disorder. Down's syndrome is a relatively rare disorder, however the likelihood of giving birth to this type infant is greater in older mothers, specifically those over 40 years of age when the chances of this occurring is approximately 1 out of 50. Other diseases of differing severity may result from deletions of chromosomes or parts of chromosomes, or the inclusion of additional chromosomal material.

It should not be thought that a disease process requires deletion or addition of a whole chromosome or a large portion of one. In fact, many more disorders result from errors within a single gene. This error or chemical defect within the gene causes the gene to carry or express misinformation which leads to some fault in protein synthesis and/or development. This is best explained by an example — phenylketonuria. There is a gene on a chromosome which contains the information necessary for the cell to synthesize the enzyme, phenylalanine hydroxylase (see Figure 1.8a).

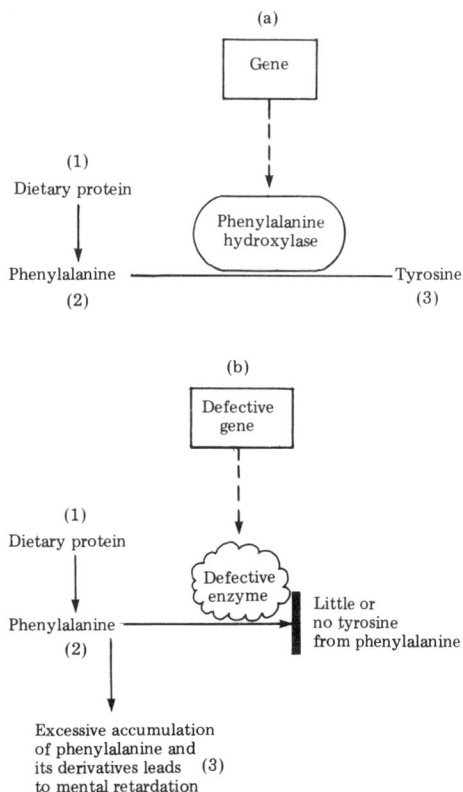

Figure 1.8 The development of phenylketonuria. (a) Normal conditions. (b) Conditions in phenylketonuria.

This enzyme, like all other enzymes, is a protein and converts the essential amino acid phenylalanine to the amino acid,

tyrosine. Since tyrosine can be synthesized from phenylalanine, it is classified as a *non-essential* amino acid.

In some cases, there is a defect within the gene controlling the synthesis of the enzyme, phenylalanine hydroxylase, so that the enzyme synthesized under the direction of the faulty gene is not functional and lacks the ability to convert phenylalanine to tyrosine (see Figure 1.8b). As a result of this deficiency, tyrosine will not be synthesized from phenylalanine, and phenylalanine and other metabolites derived from phenylalanine will accumulate in the blood. This condition is called phenylketonuria (PKU) and is characterized chiefly by a severe mental retardation which develops in the infant after the first 4–6 months of life. Newborn infants with PKU may also have inflamed skin, difficulties in eating and frequent vomiting spells. It is thought that the mental retardation is caused by the excessive amount of phenylalanine and its derivatives which interfere with the brain chemistry necessary for normal mental development.

You might think that the way to treat PKU would be to withhold all phenylalanine from the diet, but you will recall that phenylalanine is an essential amino acid which cannot be synthesized by the body. Taking away all this amino acid would also lead to very serious problems. In practice, PKU is treated by giving commercial protein diets containing less than normal amounts of phenylalanine and supplemented with tyrosine. The amounts of phenylalanine in the commercial diet are adequate for the synthesis of cellular proteins but small enough to prevent the excessive accumulation of the harmful metabolites.

Of course PKU must be diagnosed early in life if it is to be treated successfully. This is usually accomplished by pricking the infant's heel to draw blood and then measuring the amount of phenylalanine in the blood. Elevated levels of phenylalanine may indicate PKU. It is of more than passing interest to note that one of the major developments in PKU research did not come from the research lab but originated from an alert mother of a child with PKU. She claimed that the diapers of her sick infant had a different smell from those of her other children, who were well. This strange smell was traced to a metabolite of phenylalanine in the urine, and this discovery led to an investigation of phenylalanine metabolism that later proved fruitful.

b. Structure of DNA and RNA and the genetic code for protein synthesis

Previous sections have indicated that there is a relationship between DNA, genes, the synthesis of proteins and development. The purpose of this section is to show how the chemical structure of DNA and RNA confers upon these molecules the information or plans necessary to direct the synthesis of complicated proteins from 21 different amino acids. More precisely, the relationship between the molecular structure of DNA and RNA and specific amino acids will be discussed.

Both DNA and RNA are made up of a series of repeating units called nucleotides. Each nucleotide molecule has three components:

(1) One phosphorus and four oxygen molecules combined to make up a single phosphate molecule.

(2) A 5-carbon sugar — in DNA the sugar is deoxyribose and in RNA the sugar is ribose.

(3) One of five nitrogenous bases:

Base name	Symbol	Found in
Thymine	T	DNA only
Adenine	A	DNA and RNA
Guanine	G	DNA and RNA
Cytosine	C	DNA and RNA
Uracil	U	RNA only

The nitrogenous bases are small molecules containing carbon, hydrogen and nitrogen, and, with the exception of adenine, oxygen. The particular structure of these nitrogenous bases is not of critical importance. What is significant is the way in which individual base fits into the molecule as a whole. A diagram of a nucleotide is given in Figure 1.9.

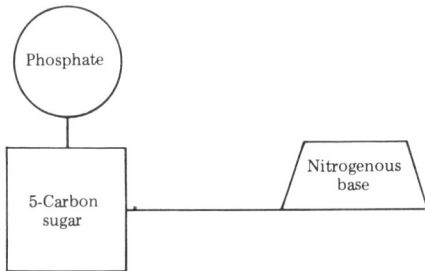

Figure 1.9   A nucleotide.

DNA and RNA are formed by linking many nucleotide units into a single molecule. DNA nucleotides will contain either adenine, guanine, cytosine, or thymine. RNA nucleotides will contain either adenine, guanine, cytosine or uracil. Figure 1.10 indicates the nucleotide sequence in a real DNA molecule.

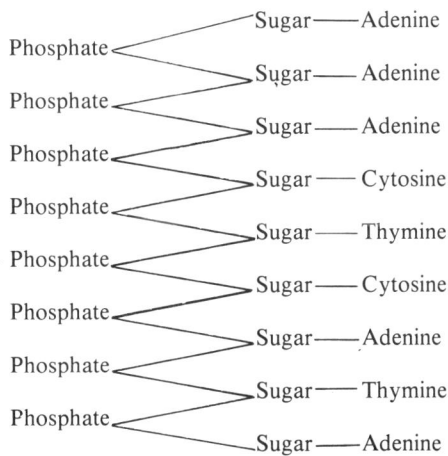

Figure 1.10   The nucleotide sequence in a DNA molecule

Actually, DNA does not exist as a single molecule in a straight line, but two DNA molecules exist together in a double helix. Figure 1.11 shows the double helix. One way to

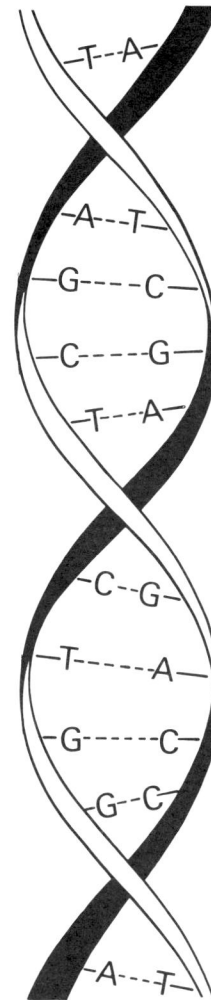

Figure 1.11   Base pairings between the two nucleotide chains forming the double helical structure of DNA.

think of a helix is to compare it with a spiral staircase that twists and turns upon itself so that one part of the staircase is always above another part. In a double helix, the two DNA molecules are twisted around one another and held together by weak chemical bonds. Figure 1.10 shows the base sequence of only one of the two DNA helixes, because only one DNA molecule is used during the synthesis of a protein. The relationship between the two DNA molecules is said to be complementary. This follows from the fact that adenine in one helix is always paired opposite thymine in the other helix and *vice versa*. Guanine is similarly paired with cytosine. Thus:

1st helix		2nd helix
A	opposite	T
T	opposite	A
G	opposite	C
C	opposite	G

This can be diagrammatically represented as follows:

1st helix		2nd helix
C	. . . . .	G
A	. . . . .	T
T	. . . . .	A
G	. . . . .	C
A	. . . . .	T
T	. . . . .	A

This relationship means that the sequence of one DNA molecule can be converted into that of its partner molecule by replacing each thymine with adenine, and *vice versa*, and each guanine with cytosine, and *vice versa*.

Before going further it might be helpful to show why information is often dependent upon the order of a sequence. Take, for instance, this list of words: kiss, would, Peter, only, Malaika. See for yourself what a variety of sentences can be made with these five words:

> Only Peter would kiss Malaika.
> Would Peter only kiss Malaika?
> Peter would kiss only Malaika.
> Malaika would only kiss Peter.
> Would Malaika kiss only Peter?
> Only Malaika would kiss Peter.
> Malaika would kiss only Peter.
> Would Peter kiss only Malaika?
> Would Malaika only kiss Peter?
> Would only Peter kiss Malaika?
> Peter would only kiss Malaika.

Each of these 11 sentences contain the same five words but, by rearrangement, each sentence can express a different idea or ask a different question. More different ideas can be expressed than there are words.

The above example could be useful to you if you think of a protein as a "sentence" formed by 21 different "words" (amino acids). The plan for each sentence is contained in the arrangement of four different "code letters", A, T, C and G, located in the chromosomal DNA.

Let us review the pertinent facts and restate the problem of how DNA contains the plan for the synthesis of specific proteins. For life to develop or maintain itself proteins must be continually synthesized. Proteins are built by linking amino acids together; most proteins contain hundreds of amino acids. There are 21 different amino acids usable in the synthesis of a single protein and many amino acids are used more than once. If the protein is to be functional, the proper amino acids must be linked together in the correct sequence. This synthesis requires information, which is contained in the chromosomes in DNA molecules.

DNA is formed by repeating units called nucleotides. Each nucleotide contains a phosphate group, a sugar and one of four nitrogenous bases; A, T, C or G. The essential problem is to determine how these four bases can plan or direct the synthesis of a protein containing 21 different amino acids. Nature's solution to this problem is remarkable and simple: a code which is carried by the nucleotide sequence of the DNA molecule and is ultimately expressed or translated in protein synthesis.

The simplest way for you to work out this code would be to get a pencil and paper and do some figuring on your own. Write the numbers from 1 to 21 and let each number stand for a different amino acid. The trick is to determine an arrangement whereby the four different bases in a nucleotide can stand for, or code for, each of the amino acids. If you take one base or "code letter" at a time you can identify four separate amino acids:

$$A = 1$$
$$C = 2$$
$$G = 3$$
$$T = 4$$

But stop, this cannot be the basis of the code, for there are no code words for most of the amino acids, numbers 5 to 21. Try again, this time taking two bases at a time. By taking two at a time you can rearrange the sequence to provide additional code words, just as we can spell either "on" or "no" if we have the two letters n and o. Here is the way to try the two bases at a time:

1 = AA	5 = GA	9 = CA	13 = TA
2 = AG	6 = GG	10 = CG	14 = TG
3 = AC	7 = GC	11 = CC	15 = TC
4 = AT	8 = GT	12 = CT	16 = TT

You must be getting closer, for there are now code words for 16 of the 21 different amino acids. The next step would be to take three bases at a time. Figure 1.12 lists 64 different code words, listing all the combinations of four bases, three at a time, from AAA to TTT. Since there are 64 code words and 21 amino acids, we shall have more code words than are necessary. The three bases which code for a particular amino acid are called a codon. There are more code words (codons) than there are amino acids.

These additional code words are not wasted though. One amino acid can have more than one code word standing for it, just as in the English language you often find more than one word with the same meaning, and so it is with these additional code words — others are used as "punctuation"

AAA	AAG	AAC	AAT
AGA	AGG	AGC	AGT
ACA	ACG	ACC	ACT
ATA	ATG	ATC	ATT
GAA	GAG	GAC	GAT
GGA	GGG	GGC	GGT
GCA	GCG	GCC	GCT
GTA	GTG	GTC	GTT
CAA	CAG	CAC	CAT
CGA	CGG	CGC	CGT
CCA	CCG	CCC	CCT
CTA	CTG	CTC	CTT
TAA	TAG	TAC	TAT
TGA	TGG	TGC	TGT
TCA	TCG	TCC	TCT
TTA	TTG	TTC	TTT

Figure 1.12 Triplet code (64 words).

and indicate in code where one complete protein molecule ends and another begins. In effect these "punctuation" codons say, "Begin the synthesis of a protein here" and "This is the end of the protein" and "Synthesize a different protein starting here".

If you refer back to Figure 1.10 you will see a total of nine bases from which three code words can be formed. In fact, the figure is really the code for the beginning of a protein: AAA for phenylalanine, ATA for tyrosine, and CTC for glutamic acid. These three DNA bases, which code for a particular amino acid, are called the DNA codons; thus, AAA is a DNA codon for phenylalanine.

So far, the DNA code for protein synthesis has been established, but the steps between the plan and the actual synthesis have been omitted. To consider these steps it is necessary to consider RNA in detail. Some of the terms used here to describe cellular anatomy will be given more fully in the section on the cell. There are three types of RNA:

(1) *Messenger RNA.* This molecule is like DNA in that it contains a series of nucleotides linked together and has information necessary for protein synthesis. RNA merely copies or transcribes the DNA message. Three RNA nucleotides with their bases act as a single code word for one of the 21 amino acids or serve as "punctuation" in protein synthesis. The three bases which code for an animo acid are sometimes referred to as an RNA codon. Structurally, messenger RNA is unlike DNA in three respects:

(a) Messenger RNA contains the sugar ribose rather than the deoxyribose in DNA.

(b) Uracil in RNA replaces thymine in DNA.

(c) Messenger RNA exists as a single helix.

Most DNA is found in the nucleus, while most RNA is found outside the nucleus in the cytoplasm. The cytoplasm is the watery part of the cell outside the nucleus. It is in the cytoplasm that the amino acids are joined together to form the protein. Messenger RNA functions to take the plan or information from the nucleus to the cytoplasm. The information contained in the genes, in the DNA code, is transcribed to RNA, and the molecule acts as a messenger, relaying the information from the nucleus to the cytoplasm.

The chromosomal DNA contains all the information necessary to synthesize all the proteins ever made by the body. Naturally, all these proteins are not made at the same time. DNA molecules in the nucleus are very stable, whereas messenger RNA is short-lived and synthesized only when a particular protein or proteins are being synthesized. When RNA is being synthesized it uses DNA as a model or template. This ensures that the DNA information corresponds to the RNA message. It appears that the initiation of messenger RNA synthesis is one of the key steps in the initiation of protein synthesis.

In conclusion, information contained in chromosomal DNA is stable and always present in all cells, but only a small portion of this information is transcribed to messenger RNA at any one time, so only a few of the proteins which can be synthesized by a cell are synthesized.

(2) *Ribosomal RNA.* Ribosomal RNA is found in the ribosomes, which are located in the cytoplasm of the cell. These are small, dense granules containing about 50% ribosomal RNA and 50% protein. The ribosomes are often associated with a part of the cell known as the endoplasmic reticulum. Although ribosomal RNA has the same composition as messenger RNA, it is very tightly coiled, is not an "information" molecule and contains no codons. Instead, the ribosomes function at the site of protein synthesis; they bind the messenger RNA and the specific enzymes necessary to join the individual amino acids together. The precise role of the RNA in the ribosomes is not known. It is known that messenger RNA leaves the nucleus and comes to the ribosomes and binds to them. The attachment of a single messenger RNA molecule to a series of ribosomes results in the formation of a long, bead-like string, often called a polysome.

(3) *Transfer RNA.* Each transfer RNA molecule can transfer one particular amino acid from the cytoplasm to the appropriate site on the messenger RNA molecule at the ribosome, where the amino acid is incorporated into the growing protein chain (see Figure 1.13). There is a particular transfer RNA molecule for each amino acid — an alanine transfer RNA for alanine, a tyrosine transfer RNA for tyrosine and so on. Each amino acid will bind only its particular transfer RNA molecule.

Transfer RNA molecules are small and are not information molecules like DNA and messenger RNA. One end of each transfer RNA contains three nucleotides, which are complementary to, and can therefore recognize, the three appropriate nucleotides or the codon on the messenger RNA molecule. Because of this specific recognition, the three transfer RNA nucleotides (bases) that relate only to a certain messenger RNA codon are called the anticodon (see Figure 1.14). This correspondence between the messenger RNA codon, the transfer RNA anticodon and the particular amino acid coded for by the messenger RNA, permits the message contained in the messenger RNA molecule to be read at the

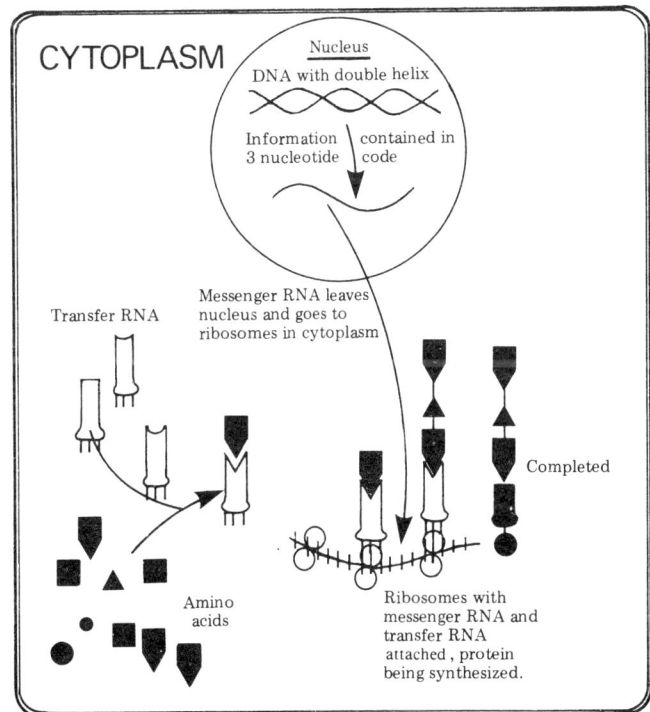

Figure 1.13 Outline of DNA–RNA–protein relationship.

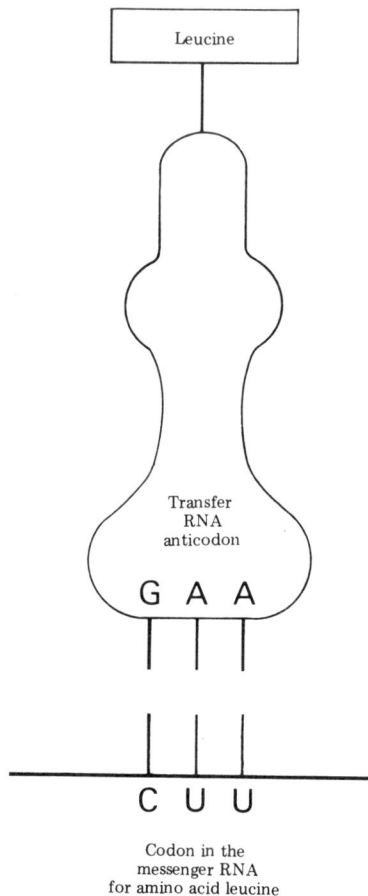

Figure 1.14 The relationship between the codon, the anticodon and amino acid.

it could form a thread that would reach from the earth to the sun and back to the earth again, many times.

There is an impressive amount of information contained by the sequential arrangement of nucleotides; each DNA nucleotide contains any one of the following four molecules:

adenine, cytosine, guanine or thymine.

The information contained in DNA is in coded form and contains the instructions for protein synthesis.

Proteins give structure to cells, form enzymes and have many other functions. The function of a protein depends upon the order in which the amino acids are linked together.

Three adjacent nucleotides in the DNA molecule form a codon (code word) for a particular amino acid. There are different codons for each amino acid. The order of codons in the DNA molecule corresponds to the order in which the specific amino acids are to be joined together to form a specific protein. All the codons which contain the information or instructions necessary to synthesize a particular protein constitute a structural gene.

In the nucleus of the cell the instructions for synthesis of a protein are chemically transcribed into a messenger RNA molecule. It is not known what initiates this transcription. The instructions contained in the DNA code are preserved by the sequential arrangement by the nucleotide triplets (anti-codons) of the messenger RNA. These messenger RNA molecules leave the nucleus, journey to the cytoplasm and attach to the ribosomes. The instructions contained in the DNA molecule are carried out jointly by the transfer RNA molecules and messenger RNA molecules which translate the instructions into a complete protein.

There are specific transfer RNA molecules for each amino acid; they can bind or carry only one of the different amino acids. Each of the transfer RNA molecules, which carry a particular amino acid, has a three-nucleotide base anticodon. This anticodon can recognize and bind only the messenger RNA codon, which is the code for the amino acid carried by the transfer RNA molecule. This correspondence between the particular amino acid called for by the messenger RNA codon, and the particular amino acid carried by the transfer RNA with its codon, functions to join the amino acids together in the correct sequence and thus form a functional protein. In essence:

DNA → RNA → protein.

Some recent research shows that certain viruses can synthesize DNA from RNA. The full significance of this finding is not known.

c. Importance of DNA, RNA, protein synthesis and pertinent examples

Students sometimes have difficulty in seeing the relevance of this material to their work. While it is true that medicine was practiced long before the discovery of the genetic code, its discovery has really revolutionized medicine and the understanding of disease processes and has greatly influenced the search for new ways to treat and prevent disease.

Antibiotics are chemical substances which suppress the growth of bacteria and other micro-organisms. There are certain antibiotics which work because they combine only with bacterial ribosomes and thus interfere with protein

ribosome and translated into a protein molecule. The amino acids called for by the messenger RNA codons are brought to the ribosomes by transfer RNA and are linked together in the order dictated by the sequence of codons in the messenger RNA molecule. The correct amino acid called for by the messenger RNA is brought to the ribosome because of the correlation between the codon and the anticodon of the transfer RNA which carries the required amino acid. Because protein synthesis is an anabolic reaction, energy will be required. This energy is usually supplied by ATP molecules, or molecules similar to ATP, about which more will be said later.

Perhaps the material in the preceding section can be summarized and put in a slightly different perspective.

DNA is an information molecule. If all the DNA in the human body could be isolated, it would just about half fill a teacup. DNA is the chief chemical constituent of the approximately 100 000 different genes that each cell has, and which functions as the chemical basis for heredity.

The DNA in the cell is tightly coiled in chromosomes. Most human cells have 46 chromosomes arranged in 23 chromosome pairs. One set of 23 chromosomes comes from each of the two parents. Scientists have "guesstimated" that if all the DNA in the body were unravelled and joined together, synthesis in the bacteria, but leave protein synthesis in the human relatively unaffected. If the micro-organisms cannot synthesize new protein, they will not be able to reproduce themselves, and the infection will be limited.

A virus is essentially strands of DNA or RNA wrapped up inside a specialized protein coat. A distinguished physician and virologist tells the story of a student who was asked; "What do viruses do?" The student thought, then replied; "Viruses cause the diseases that nobody knows the cause of". There is a certain logic to the answer. As we really don't know all that viruses do, we can often blame them for diseases we don't understand. There are, however, some things that are known about viruses. Viruses cannot reproduce outside cells. Viruses can infect bacteria, plant, animal and human cells. Outside of cells, viruses are inactive, but once inside a cell a virus can remain inactive or begin to function.

Using its own DNA or RNA and the chemicals and synthetic machinery of the infected cell, the virus can duplicate itself many times over. The virus can synthesize protein within the cell, as the nucleic acid of the virus codes for protein and nucleic acid just as the nucleic acid of the cell's nucleus does. The information in the viral nucleic acid contains information necessary to synthesize more viruses. With both the virus and the cell's DNA trying to direct protein synthesis in the cell, disastrous results can occur. The cell may be destroyed because so much of it is occupied by virus particles that have been reproduced from the first virus which has entered the cell.

The common cold is caused by a virus. The virus enters the upper respiratory tract and infects many of the cells lining the respiratory epithelium of the nose and possibly the cells lining the throat. There is inflammation, swelling of tissue, nasal secretion increases, the infected cells die and are soon replaced by new cells. Polio is known to be caused by a different virus which infects certain cells of the nervous system. Some other diseases known to be caused by specific viruses include measles, mumps, shingles, hepatitis and influenza. Certain types of cancer might be caused by viruses. You could prevent a virus from duplicating itself inside a cell if you could prevent all protein synthesis within the cell. Of course, this would kill the cell.

Researchers are trying to develop drugs which will prevent viruses entering cells. If the virus can't enter the cell, it can't infect the cell. Other aspects of the body's defences are discussed in the Sections dealing with immunity and the immune system.

A classic illustration of the relationship between DNA and protein synthesis comes from a study of the condition known as sickle cell anaemia which results from a mutation. (A mutation is a permanent, inheritable change in the chromosomal material.) The chief characteristic of this hereditary condition is the existence of abnormal haemoglobin molecules in the red cells. Haemoglobin is an iron-containing protein, which helps to carry oxygen to the tissues. Each haemoglobin molecule has two sets of different protein chains; the larger contains 146 amino acids and the smaller contains 141.

In the sickle cell mutation there is a change within one codon in the DNA molecule. This new codon codes for a different amino acid and this different amino acid is inserted into the protein. In the case of the abnormal haemoglobin in sickle cell anaemia, the change in a single codon causes the amino acid, valine, to be inserted into the larger of the protein chains in place of glutamic acid. The substitution of this one amino acid in the protein has effects on haemoglobin and the red cell, and these cells assume a sickle shape when the oxygen content of the blood is reduced. These distorted red cells are more rapidly removed from the circulation than cells with normal haemoglobin, so an anaemia or insufficiency of red cells results. The abnormally shaped cells can often become stuck and block the flow of blood through the capillaries, the smallest channels of the circulatory system. This blockage will interfere with the delivery of oxygen to the tissues supplied by the capillaries, and this lack of oxygen may cause injury or death to these tissues.

Before going on, you should consider that, although a cellular process due to a molecular substitution is being described, this sickling phenomenon occurs in a living human being. When the oxygen is reduced and a large number of red blood cells assume the abnormal elongated sickle-shape, a pain crisis results. This is due to the reduced blood flow, lack of oxygen and subsequent cell injury and death. The sickle cell pain crises are self-limiting, but, as the name suggests, very painful. They may be brought on by strenuous exercise, infection, cold and other unknown causes. There are effects throughout the body as a result of the sickling of the cells containing abnormal haemoglobin. Since the cause of this abnormal protein is genetic, the individual with sickle cell disease has a life-long disease. This disease is most common in Africans and peoples of African origin. It is found also, but to a lesser extent, in Greeks and in people of the Middle East and India. At present there is no way to cure the disease, and persons with sickle cell disease generally have a shortened lifespan.

The severity of sickle cell disease depends on the percentage of normal and abnormal haemoglobin molecules (see Figure 1.15). As the presence of the abnormal protein in the haemoglobin molecule depends on the presence of the mutant gene, the amount of abnormal or sickle haemoglobin depends on the number of mutant genes. Each person receives one gene from each parent with instructions for haemoglobin synthesis. If neither parent has the mutant gene, then the individual will have two normal genes and all haemoglobin will be normal. If one, or both, parents carry the mutant gene, the person may have the sickle cell trait. The chances of this happening are worked out in the box diagram in Figure 1.16. If a person has a gene N (normal haemoglobin) and a mutant gene S (sickle haemoglobin), he or she will synthesize both normal and sickle haemoglobin. These individuals with the genes NS, who synthesize both normal and abnormal, are said to have the sickle cell trait. This is a distinct entity and is not equivalent to sickle cell anaemia or sickle cell disease (SS) in which both genes are S and in which nearly all the haemoglobin is sickle haemoglobin. It is only under exceptional circumstances that persons with the sickle cell trait will have their red cells sickle, as most of their haemoglobin is normal haemoglobin. Individuals with sickle cell trait (NS) will not become anaemic because of their small amount of abnormal haemoglobin. One study has shown that about 10% of black Americans have the sickle cell trait and also that about 10%

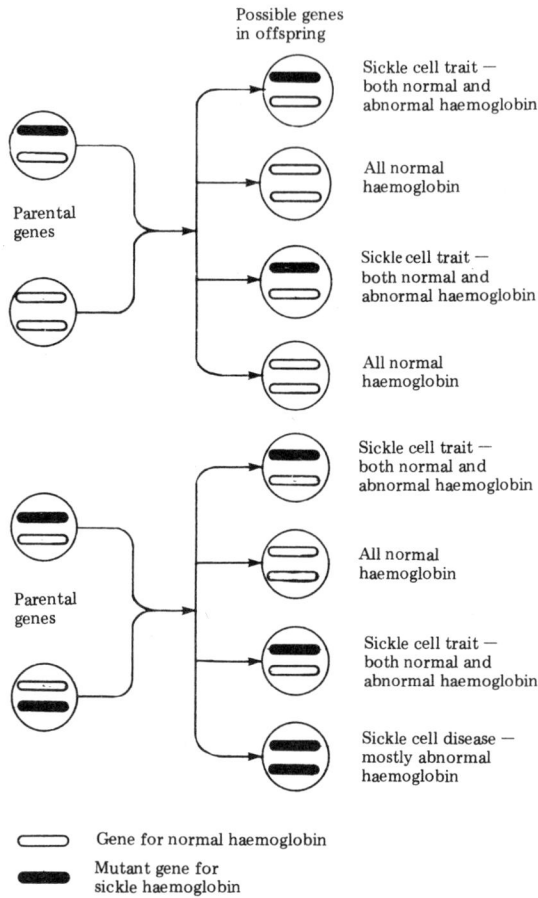

Figure 1.15 Genetic patterns in sickle cell disease.

Let N stand for the gene for normal haemoglobin
Let S stand for the mutant gene for sickle haemoglobin

Put the genes of each parent outside the box and the
product (possible genetic combinations of the offspring)
in the box

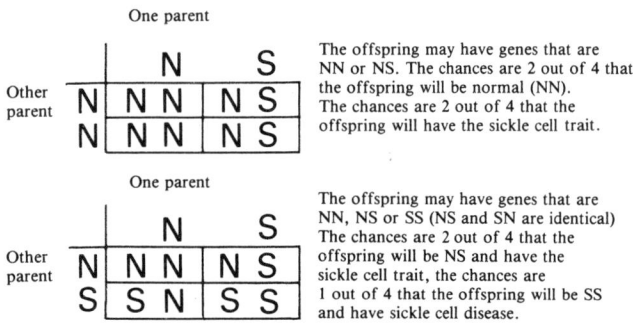

Figure 1.16 Genetic determinants for sickle cell disease.

of the black American football players in the professional
National Football League have the sickle cell trait. Having
the sickle cell trait did not hinder participation in this rugged
league. Inasmuch as sickle cell disease is a genetic disease, it
is possible to tell prospective parents the probability, if any,
of their offspring having sickle cell disease by examining a
sickle blood sample taken from each parent.

There is evidence that the sickle haemoglobin confers
protection against malaria. Thus, in endemic malaria areas of
the world, the so-called abnormal haemoglobin would

actually be beneficial. It should be noted that there are other
haemoglobin disorders besides sickle haemoglobin and that
there are many other genetic diseases.

F. ATP

We have used the word energy frequently. Energy is the
ability to do work. In the body energy is needed to do the
work of sending signals from the brain to the muscles, to
make the muscles move, to breathe, to put molecules together
and to excrete wastes. The cells of the body work 24 hours
a day and require a great deal of energy. The immediate
source of energy for all these different jobs is a high energy
compound called adenosine triphosphate (ATP). Chemically,
ATP is formed from the base adenine (A), the sugar ribose,
and three phosphate (TP) molecules all linked together in one
molecule.

We said earlier that fats and carbohydrates were the chief
energy sources, and now we say it is ATP. The energy
contained in food molecules is released and stored in ATP as
the food molecules are catabolized to CO_2 and water. An
analogy might help. Suppose you were fortunate enough to
have a £1000 note in your pocket and had to go to market for
food supplies. You might not really be so fortunate, for what
shopkeeper would have change for so large a note? It would
be more convenient if you had many small notes. ATP is the
"small change" of energy compounds, for it can easily be spent
in the body. When a large fat molecule is metabolized, the
energy within that molecule is transferred to over 100 ATP
molecules. The energy in each ATP molecule is just the right
amount for the body's needs and can be easily spent. ATP is
also an "internationally recognized currency" for it can be
spent in different cells. Brain cells, heart cells, liver cells, all
have different metabolic patterns, yet the final source of
energy for all them is ATP. An active cell can spend more
than a million ATP molecules in a second. The amazing ATP
molecule is used throughout the kingdom of Life, for it
supplies energy to the elephant's muscles, to bacteria enabling
them to synthesize protein and even to the firefly so that it
can give its brief flash of light. ATP has been compared to
electricity, a simple form of energy that makes light.

ATP is important, but how can a molecule store energy?
The energy is stored in the bonds or arrangement of electrons
which keep the two or more atoms together. It might help to
think of the atoms being linked by very tight springs. When
the springs are cut or the bond is broken, a great deal of
energy is released. In the body, the end phosphate group is
cut off from the other two phosphate groups on the side of
the ATP molecule by the enzyme, adenosine triphosphatase
(ATPase), leaving adenosine diphosphate (ADP) and releasing energy which is put to biological work. When fat and
carbohydrate molecules are broken down, the energy that is
stored in their bonds is transferred to a system which puts
that energy into making ATP from ADP and phosphate. If
energy is released when ATP is broken down, it will obviously
take energy to build up the ATP from ADP and phosphate.

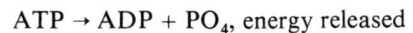

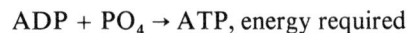

$$ATP \rightarrow ADP + PO_4, \text{ energy released}$$

$$ADP + PO_4 \rightarrow ATP, \text{ energy required}$$

Close your book now, get some rest and save your ATP;
you will need it for the rest of the book.

2. Units, Definitions and the General Organization and Systems of the Body

INTRODUCTION

The purpose of this Chapter is to list some of the units of measure, to consider in general the organization of the body and to introduce some definitions and anatomical terms. It contains facts and descriptive terms with which the uninitiated student may not be acquainted but which are necessary for further study. There may, however, be some students who are already acquainted with much of this material and for them this Chapter will serve as a review.

A. UNITS OF MEASURE

A number of professional groups and societies have recommended that the same units and terminology be used throughout the world. Many countries such as the United Kingdom, Australia, Canada and India are moving to adopt the units and principles of the Système International d'Unités (SI units). The basic SI units are the metre (m) for length, the kilogram (kg) for mass, the mole (mol) for the amount of substance and second (s) for time.

Before continuing, I would like to mention two historical footnotes. Many of us today know that ice just begins to melt at 0° Centigrade (°C) and water boils at 100°C. The temperature scale was, however, originally set up so that water was considered to boil at 0°C and freeze at 100°C! That system was changed to the present system after better methods of freezing water became known.

Immediately after the French Revolution it became a criminal act in France to ask for, or buy, a dozen oranges or a dozen of anything. The basis of this concept of criminality was the fact that units like the dozen, the yard or the pound (lb) were the units of kings and monarchs, whereas the gram, the metre, the litre and their multiples of 10 or $\frac{1}{10}$ were considered to be units of logic, revolution and the people.

The lessons that you might derive from these notes are: firstly, that scientific conventions change; and secondly, that you can get into trouble if you don't change with them. I plead guilty to not using the SI units exclusively in this text because, as a practical matter, I believe that some of the older conventional units should be retained until the newer SI units have gained wider use. I have included formulas for converting to the new units when necessary.

Some SI prefixes and symbols and their meanings are listed in the following table:

Prefix	Symbol	Meaning or multiplication factor	Example
mega-	M	1000 000 or 10^6	megametre (Mm)
kilo-	k	1000 or 10^3	kilogram (kg)
hecto-	h	100 or 10^2	hectogram (hg)
deca-	da	10 or 10^1	decagram (dag)
deci-	d	1/10 or 10^{-1}	decilitre (dl)
centi-	c	1/100 or 10^{-2}	centimetre (cm)
milli-	m	1/1000 or 10^{-3}	millimetre (mm) milligram (mg)
micro-	μ	1/1000 000 or 10^{-6}	microgram (μg)
nano-	n	1/1000 000 000 or 10^{-9}	nanometre (nm)

a. Length. The next table lists some SI units derived from the metre and an Anglo-Saxon unit — the inch:

Metric length	Inches
1 kilometre (km) = 1000 m	39370.0
1 metre (m) = 100 cm	39.37
1 centimetre (cm) = 1/100 m = 10 mm	0.3937
1 millimetre (mm) = 1/1000 m = 1000 μm	0.03937
1 micrometre (μm) = 1/1000 000 m = 1000 nm	0.00003937
1 nanometre (nm) = 1/1000 000 000 m = 10 Å	0.00000003937
1 Angstrom (Å) = 1/10 000 000 000 m = 1/10 nm	0.000000003937

Measurements of length and circumference are so frequently made by health workers that, occasionally, proper care is not taken. This is unfortunate, as accurate measurements do frequently provide essential information. For example, one useful indicator of an infant's normal development comes from measurements of the circumference of his or her head and chest. At birth, the average head circumference is 34–37 cm and the chest is about 2 cm less. After 2 years, the chest grows faster and surpasses the circumference of the head. For these measurements to be useful they must be made with precision and accuracy.

In clinical work there is often a subtle difference in the use of the words "length" and "height". Length refers to the measurement made when the individual is lying down. You cannot simply tell an infant or young child to stand up straight — you cannot be assured that they will be able to or will make the same effort every time you wish to measure them. For this reason, infants and young children are measured lying down.

19

Height refers to the measurement made when the individual is standing erect. It is interesting to note that there can be 1 cm difference in an individual's height over the course of a single day. This is because of the compression of weight-bearing structures, particularly those of the spine, which takes place when the person stands erect all or most of the day.

A statistician has made a rough calculation that if you measured all the people in the world — infants, young people and adults — and determined an average height, this would turn out to be about 1.5 metres. This also illustrates the usefulness and the limits of the term average. Are you and your friends average and are you and they about 1.5 metres tall? One and one half metres is 1500 cm — about 59 inches. The size of the human heart is about 9 cm by 13 cm or 90 mm by 130 mm. The diameter of a liver cell is about 15 μm. A virus is about 50 nm in diameter.

(Some textbooks use the terms micron (μ) and millimicron (mμ) to refer respectively to the micrometre (μm) and the nanometre (nm). In 1967, the General Conference of Weights and Measures recommended that the terms micron and millimicron should no longer be used.)

b. Weight or mass. In the SI units the basic unit of mass is the kilogram. Weight is expressed in kilograms or multiples or fractions of the kilogram. When you weigh something, you simply put it on the scale and read a number. In actuality there is a formula for weight:

$$\text{Weight} = \text{mass} \times \text{gravity.}$$

If you were to weigh yourself on the moon, your weight, but not your mass, would be considerably reduced because the force of gravity would be reduced on the moon.

In these unusual circumstances, when it is necessary to differentiate between weight and mass, and therefore to consider the influence of gravity, mass would be expressed in kilograms (kg) and weight would be expressed in newtons or dynes. (A newton is that unit of force which would produce an acceleration of 1 m/s^2 in a mass of 1 kg. One dyne is equal to 10^{-5} newton; there are 100 000 dynes in 1 newton. One kilogram, with an acceleration due to gravity of 9.8 m/s^2 exerts a force of 9.8 newtons.)

Don't be upset if you are not familiar with the above units. At the present time they have not achieved widespread use. If some new, proud parent asks you what the weight of their infant is, you could tell them that the weight is 32.34 newtons! Most likely they would not know whether to be pleased or worried, and they might not be interested in the mathematics of multiplying the infant's mass (3.3 kg) by the acceleration due to gravity (9.8 m/s^2) to get the answer in newtons. Parents, and nearly everyone else, would be pleased if you merely said that the infant's weight is 3.3 kg.

Measurements of weight are an important part of a person's health record. Life insurance companies have found that the most useful single statistic for a person of a given age, sex and height is the person's body weight.

Many texts make reference to the fact that a typical adult male weighs 70 kg (154 lbs). Older texts use 65 kg as a figure; this illustrates the effects of improved nutrition and also the greater tendency towards obesity. A typical human heart weighs 240–310 grams, while the pituitary gland weighs a little over 600 mg.

SI units	United States
1 kilogram (kg) = 1000 g	= 2.2 pounds (1 pound avoirdupois = 16 ounces)
1 gram (g) = 1/1000 kg = 1000 mg	= 0.0022 pound (lb)
1 milligram (mg) = 1/1000 g = 1000 μg	= 0.000 0022 lb
1 microgram (μg) = 1/1000 000 g = 1000 ng	= 0.000 000 0022 lb
1 nanogram (ng) = 1/1000 000 000 g	= 0.000 000 000 0022 lb

Note: 0.0684 grams = 1 grain = 1/7000 lb

A careful record of a patient's weight is often very useful. An unexplained loss of weight, in spite of a good appetite, can indicate disease, just as the regaining of weight following surgery may indicate recovery. In certain types of heart, kidney or respiratory failure the patient may not be able to eliminate water. This retained water adds to the patient's weight, so a careful weight record can be useful in monitoring the patient's condition.

c. Volume and amount of substance. In the SI units, the official unit of volume is the cubic metre (m^3). In the health professions, the unofficial but most used unit of volume is the litre (l). A litre is a cubic decimetre (1 dm^3), and is one decimetre (0.1 metre or 1 dm) in length, 1 dm in width and 1 dm in depth. There are 1000 millilitres (ml) in one litre (1 l). The cubic centimetre (cm^3) was originally defined as that volume occupied by one gram (1 g) of water at 4°C and one atmosphere pressure. Accurate measurements show that:

$$1 \text{ ml} = 1.000\ 03 \text{ cm}^3,$$

so there is an effort to use millilitres rather than cubic centimetres.

SI units	United States
1 litre (l) = 1000 ml	= 1.06 US liquid quarts = 34 fluid ounces
1 decilitre (dl) = 100 ml	= 3.4 fluid ounces
1 millilitre (ml) = 1/1000 l = 1000 μl	= 0.034 fluid ounces
1 microlitre (μl) = 1/1000 000 l	= 0.000 034 fluid ounces

Note: 1 US gallon = 0.83 English (Imperial) gallon.

A typical adult female might have a total blood volume of 4 litres and her heart might pump 65 ml with each beat.

One litre of water weighs approximately 1 kg.

If you have a sample of blood and someone asks you how much sodium, potassium, calcium, glucose and cholesterol are present in it, you have to know how much of the substance is present and the correct units to express the amount. Clinical laboratories make these determinations daily, and express their results in several ways. Usually lab results are expressed as concentrations — so much substance in a particular volume of fluid such as blood plasma or serum, urine or cerebrospinal fluid. (Plasma is the fluid portion of the blood; serum is plasma from which certain proteins have

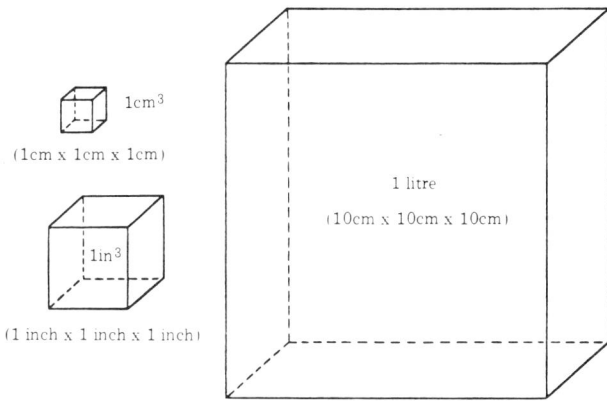

Figure 2.1 Comparison of United States and SI units of volume.

been removed. Again, these terms are described more fully in the Chapter on the blood.)

In the SI units, the preferred way to express concentration is moles per litre (mole/l). You remember that 1 mole is the molecular weight of the substance expressed in grams. The mass of the substance expressed in grams, divided by the molecular weight of the substance expressed in grams, gives the number of moles:

$$\text{Moles of a substance} = \frac{\text{mass of the substance in grams}}{\text{molecular weight of the substance in grams}}$$

Let's go through some examples to show how they might be expressed and how they might be converted to SI units.

(1). The glucose concentration in the blood plasma is 90 mg/100 ml (90 mg/dl). What is the concentration in moles/litre?

We are given the weight in 1/10 of a litre, which tells us that there will be 900 mg of glucose in 1 litre of plasma. Next we have to convert 900 mg into grams. Since there are 1000 mg in 1 gram:

$$900 \text{ mg}/1000 \text{ mg} = 0.9 \text{ gram}.$$

The formula states that the number of moles is found by dividing the mass expressed in grams by the molecular weight expressed in grams.

The formula for glucose is $C_6H_{12}O_6$; from the table in the first Chapter you can calculate that the molecular weight is 180 and in 1 mole of glucose there are 180 grams. To find the number of moles of glucose present we have to divide 0.9 g by 180 g:

$$0.9 \text{ g}/180 \text{ g} = 0.005 \text{ moles glucose}.$$

In 1 litre of our sample there would be 5/1000 of a mole of glucose. It would be better to express this result in millimoles/litre (mmol/l).

There are 1000 mmol in 1 mole, and each millimole is 1/1000 of a mole. We have 5/1000 of a mole in 1 litre, so we have 5 mmol in 1 litre. The final result is expressed as 5 mmol/l.

(2). In the same sample we have 90 mg of cholesterol in 100 ml of plasma. Again how many millimoles of cholesterol would be present in 1 litre?

The formula for cholesterol is $C_{27}H_{45}OH$: one molecule of cholesterol contains 27 carbon atoms, 46 hydrogen atoms and 1 oxygen atom. Using the table of atomic weights in the first Chapter, we can calculate the molecular weight of cholesterol is about 387 and that there are 387 grams of cholesterol in 1 mole of cholesterol. In our sample there would be 0.9 g cholesterol/litre. Therefore:

$$0.9 \text{ g}/387 \text{ g} = 0.00232 \text{ moles cholesterol}.$$

By using SI units, though, you realize that the molecular concentration of glucose (5 mmol/l) is greater than that of cholesterol (2.32 mmol/l), even though there are 90 mg of glucose and 90 mg of cholesterol in 100 ml. In essence, the sample contained more glucose molecules than cholesterol molecules, but the individual cholesterol molecule had a greater mass than the individual glucose molecule.

(3). The laboratory reports the concentration of the sodium ion (Na^+) in the plasma is 140 mmol/l, the concentration of potassium ion (K^+) is 4 mEq/l, and the concentration of the calcium ion (Ca^{++}) is 10 mg/100 ml.

Since the sodium concentration is already expressed in mmol/l it does not need any conversion. If you wanted to find out how many grams of sodium would be in 100 ml of plasma, you would not have much difficulty. You know that 1 mole of sodium has 22.990 g, and that you have 140/1000 of 1 mole of sodium in 1 litre. Therefore:

$$22.990 \times (140/1000) = 3.22 \text{ g in } 1000 \text{ ml } (0.322 \text{ g/dl}).$$

Since the charge of the sodium ion is plus one ($^+$), 140 mmol/l will equal 140 mEq of Na^+/l.

Since the potassium ion has a charge of plus one (K^+), a concentration of 4.0 mEq/l is equal to 4.0 mmol/l. (Milli-equivalents (mEq) are not part of the SI units.)

To convert 10 mg Ca^{++}/100 ml, we multiply by 10 to get the concentration of 1 litre. There are 40.08 g in 1 mole of calcium, therefore:

$$\frac{0.1 \text{ g}}{40.08 \text{ g}} = 0.00250 \text{ moles}.$$

Thus:

$$10 \text{ mg } Ca^{++}/100 \text{ ml} = 2.5 \text{ mmol}/1.$$

Since the charge of the calcium ion is plus two (Ca^{++}), 2.5 mmol/l will equal 5 milliequivalents per litre (5 mEq/l).

Perhaps these examples will help you see how to convert the units from one to another. There are some benefits derived from expressing concentrations in mmol/l.

d. Temperature. Temperature ranges over millions of degrees throughout the universe. Human life can survive only within a small segment of that spectrum. There are two temperature scales in clinical use throughout the world. The Fahrenheit scale (°F) is named after the eighteenth century scientist who introduced the mercury thermometer, and the Centigrade scale (°C), which was discovered by the Swedish astronomer Celsius.

The Centigrade scale uses two standard points determined under standard conditions: 0 °C is the temperature at sea level at which ice melts, and the temperature at which water boils is assigned 100 °C. There are 100 equal divisions between the two points. On the Fahrenheit scale the melting point is 32 °F while the boiling point is 212 °F.

Thermometers in chemical usage cover a much smaller scale. Oral temperature in healthy, resting adults varies from 36.3 to 37.1 °C (97.3–98.8 °F). Different parts of the body have different temperatures (rectal temperature is 0.5 °C higher than oral temperature). There is a normal fluctuation in temperature each day of 0.5–0.7 °C, being lowest in the morning and highest in the evening. Strenuous exercise causes temperature to rise. A fever is an elevation of temperature above the normal range.

To convert Centigrade into Fahrenheit multiply °C by $\frac{9}{5}$ and add 32. To convert Fahrenheit into Centigrade subtract 32 from °F and multiply the answer by $\frac{5}{9}$:

$$°F = (\tfrac{9}{5} \times °\dot{C}) + 32$$

$$°C = (°\dot{F} - 32)\tfrac{5}{9}.$$

In SI units, the temperature scale is expressed in degrees Kelvin (°K). The formula for temperature in degrees Kelvin is:

$$°K = °C + 273.15.$$

It is expected that temperature will continue to be expressed in degrees Centigrade for most medical uses. The Centigrade scale is sometimes called the Celsius scale.

e. Pressure, work and energy. These concepts are discussed again in the appropriate Chapters, but it might be well to jump the gun and discuss the units used for pressure, work and energy. By doing this now you will know where to look if you ever need to convert to SI units.

Pressure is defined as force per unit area. Medical apparatus, such as the sphygmomanometer used for measuring blood pressure, expresses pressure in millimetres of mercury (mmHg), i.e. the force that will support a column of mercury (Hg) so many millimetres high. Other instruments measure pressure in centimetres (cm) of water.

In SI units, the unit of force is the newton. One newton is the force that causes 1 kg to accelerate at a rate of 1 metre per second per second (1 m/s²). A force of 1 newton acting on 1 square metre equals 1 pascal (pa). Thus, in SI units, pressure is expressed in pascals. Under standard conditions the following relationships hold:

1 mmHg = 13.6 mm H_2O
1 mmHg = 1/760 atmosphere = 1 torr
1 mmHg = 133.32 newtons/m²
1 mmHg = 133.32 pascals (pa)
1 mmHg = 0.13332 kilopascals (kpa)
1 kpa   = 1000 pa = 7.50 mmHg

Energy is defined as the ability to do work; while work is defined as force multiplied by distance. In SI units, the force is the newton, and the distance is expressed in metres (m). Both work and energy can be expressed in the same unit — the joule:

1 joule = 1 newton × 1 metre.

It appears that the calorie is ingrained in the popular consciousness as the unit of work and energy. The conversion factors for joules and calories are listed below:

1 calorie = 4.18 joules (J)
1 joule = 0.239 calories
1 kilojoule (kJ) = 1000 joules (J) = 239 calories
1 000 000 joules = 1000 kJ = 1 megajoule (MJ)

B. Definitions

The anatomical position refers to the position of the body assumed in all anatomical descriptions. Its use is a convention, in that there is no rigid logic behind the choice of the particular position, but this use is a convenience and aids clarity and communication.

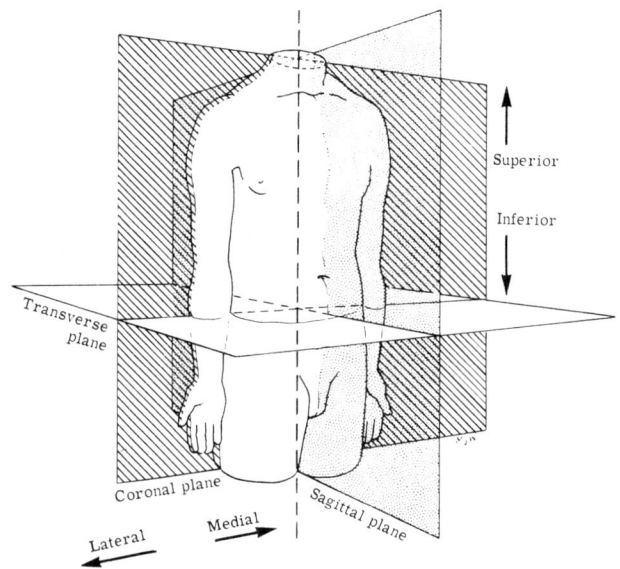

Figure 2.2 Terminology in human anatomy.

Figure 2.2 shows an individual in the anatomical position. The body is upright, with the palms facing forward. The visible surface in the figure is the anterior (ventral) surface. The back surface, not represented in the figure, is the posterior (dorsal) surface.

If a line is drawn longitudinally down the midline of the body dividing it into two equal parts, the body has been divided in a median plane. If structure A is described as being medial to structure B, A is closer to the midline than is B. If structure X is described as being lateral to structure Y, X is farther from the midline than Y.

The terms proximal and distal are usually used when describing the bones of the limbs. The proximal end of a limb is closer to the point of attachment, while the distal end is further away. Thus the elbow is at the proximal end of the forearm and the ankle is at the distal end of the leg. Superior (cranial) means closer to the head, while inferior (caudal) means further away from the head and closer to the tail end.

A section (plane) through the midline, which divides the body of a structure into a right and left half, is called a sagittal plane. A plane which divides the body or structure into an upper and lower part is called a transverse plane. A plane which divides the body or structure into an anterior and a posterior half is called a frontal (coronal) plane.

C. General organization

The body is built around the bony framework (skeleton) and consists of:
(1) The head and neck.
(2) A trunk divided into the chest (thorax), the abdomen and the pelvis.
(3) The upper and lower limbs.

The main organs of the body are contained in one of the four main body cavities. These are:
(1) The cranial cavity.
(2) The thoracic cavity.
(3) The abdominal cavity.
(4) The pelvic cavity.

The abdominal cavity is the largest cavity, and for descriptive purposes it is often divided into nine regions. This is done by drawing imaginary lines over the surface of the abdomen. Two lines are vertical, two horizontal, and the nine areas formed are named as in Figure 2.3.

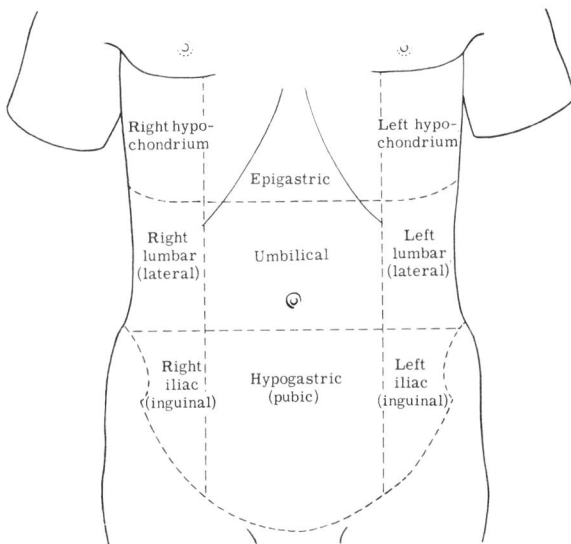

Figure 2.3   Regions of the abdomen.

It might be good now to shift perspective and to begin with the cell, working our way back up to the body as a whole.

The cell is the basic unit of life. Some of the parts of the cell have been mentioned in the previous Chapter: the nucleus and the cytoplasm. Included in the cytoplasm are organelles. An organelle is an organized particle or structure within the cell which carries out a specific function or functions. The ribosomes are an example of a cellular organelle. A group of cells performing a particular function or functions is called a tissue. There are four basic tissues: epithelial, connective, muscular and nervous. A group of tissues which are organized into a structural unit and perform a certain function or functions make up an organ. A group of organs which work together to perform some common function or functions make up a system.

One system is the cardiovascular (circulatory) system. The heart, arteries, capillaries and veins are the organs which make up the cardiovascular system. With the exception of the capillaries, all these organs contain all four tissues. These tissues contain different types of cells such as red and white blood cells, cardiac or smooth muscle, sensory neurones and endothelial cells. There are 10 major systems.

D. The systems

A brief outline of the major systems is given here and is, by necessity, an oversimplification. The purpose is merely to provide an overview of topics covered in greater detail in subsequent Chapters of this book. The student should not be discouraged because of any unfamiliarity with the terms and structures. Although each system is listed separately, no such isolation or independence is possible in the body. Each system interacts and co-operates with, and is dependent upon, the other systems.

a. The skeletal system. This consists of the bones, and the ligaments and cartilage which keep the bones together. The system provides support and protection to the body.

b. The muscular system. The skeletal muscles make up the muscular system. Most skeletal muscles are attached to the skeleton and function to enable the body to move and maintain an upright position.

c. The cardiovascular (circulatory) system. This system functions as a transportation system to deliver oxygen and nutrients to the tissues, and remove CO_2 and metabolic wastes from them. It consists of the heart, arteries, capillaries, veins and the blood.

d. The lymphatic system. This system consists of the lymph, lymphocytes, the lymph capillaries, the lymph nodes and the large lymph vessels. The spleen and the thymus also contribute to the lymphatic system. The lymphatic system returns fluid to the circulatory system and plays an important part in the defence of the body against bacteria and viruses.

e. The respiratory system. The lungs, the air passages leading to the lungs and the structures associated with them are the organs of the respiratory system. The chief function of the respiratory system is to bring O_2 into the lungs and remove CO_2 from them. Oxygen diffuses into the blood, and CO_2 diffuses out of the blood as the blood circulates in the lungs.

f. The urinary system. This system consists of the two kidneys (which form urine), the two ureters (which transport urine to the urinary bladder where urine is stored) and the urethra (through which the urine is discharged). The urinary system functions are to remove metabolic wastes such as urea and to help regulate the composition of the blood.

g. The digestive system. The alimentary tract (digestive tube) begins with the mouth and ends with the anus. The organs of the tract are the mouth, the pharynx, the oesophagus, the stomach, the small intestine and the large intestine, including the rectum and the anus. Other organs associated with the digestive system include the salivary glands, the liver and the pancreas. They all function to prepare ingested foods and fluids for absorption into the blood stream.

h. The endocrine system. An incomplete list of the organs in the endocrine system includes the pituitary gland, the thyroid gland and the adrenal glands. Other organs such as the pancreas, the testes and the ovaries have endocrine functions.

All these structures are glands because they produce and secrete hormones. Hormones function as metabolic regulators. Analogy might help. A traffic policeman working at an intersection regulates the flow of traffic. He can direct the cars to go in one direction and stop them from going in another. The policeman doesn't move any cars but accomplishes his end by signalling. Hormones can direct the flow of chemical reactions, starting some reactions and inhibiting others. The hormones usually interact with the membrane, enzymes, or the nucleus, of the target cell, and this acts as a signal which leads to the metabolic change. Hormones are made in the endocrine glands and are usually released into the bloodstream, which transports them to the target organ or organs, where they exert their effects. Because the hormones are made in one place and work in another they can be thought of as chemical communicators which help to co-ordinate and integrate the functions of various organs and systems. Finally it should be pointed out that the synthesis of hormones is a continuing process as most hormones have a short metabolic life. Insulin is a protein hormone with a half-life of about 30 minutes. This means that 50% of the insulin molecules are metabolized or destroyed within 30 minutes of their entering the bloodstream.

i. The reproductive system. The male reproductive system consists of: the testes (which produce both sperm and hormones), the accessory glands and the tubes transporting the sperm from the testes. The female reproductive organs are: the ovaries (which produce hormones and ova), the uterine tubes, the uterus and the vagina. The reproductive system produces hormones essential for normal development and permits the species to perpetuate itself with unique individuals.

j. The nervous system. The organs in the nervous system include the brain, the spinal cord, the nerve ganglia and receptors. The brain is located in, and protected by, the cranial cavity. Receptors translate stimuli from either the external environment, the internal organs or the internal environment into signals which are sent via sensory nerves to the brain or spinal cord. These signals are called impulses. The brain or spinal cord receives these impulses, processes them and may respond by sending impulses to other nerve cells, glands or muscle tissue. These impulses can signal the glands to secrete, the muscles to contract or relax, or can have some effect on nervous tissue. The nervous system is like the endocrine system, in that it integrates and communicates; however, the nervous system can integrate and process more complex information and can communicate it more rapidly than the endocrine system can. Finally, human consciousness, awareness of the future and capacity for choice are somehow contained within the nervous system.

Sometimes reference is made to the reticulo-endothelial system. This refers to isolated cells within the liver, the spleen and lymph nodes which remove certain substances from the blood.

3. The Cells and Tissues

INTRODUCTION

The word cell originally came from a Latin word *cella* meaning little room. In biology, the cell is the basic unit of all organisms and can be considered the home of life, for life cannot exist outside cells. The human organism begins as a single cell, the zygote, which divides into two cells, then the two cells divide into four cells, eight cells ... possibly into more than 1 000 000 000 000 000 cells.

These cells are not all alike. Mature red blood cells contain no nucleus, whereas sperm cells contain little more than a nucleus, surrounded by a membrane which has a tail. Many skin cells live for only a month, while most heart cells live for the life of the individual. Epithelial cells are thin and flat, ova are large and round and some nerve cells can be more than a metre long. The endocrine cells of the pancreas secrete protein hormones; nearby, the cells lining the intestine absorb amino acids. Osteoblasts build strong bone tissue, while rod-shaped cells in the retina of the eye can respond to light many miles distant.

Despite the large number of cells and their great diversity, the body exists as a community of cells rather than as a chaotic collection of them. This community arises from the organization of cells into tissues, organs and systems. This Chapter will consider the cell, its parts and their function, and the organization of cells into tissues.

WHAT ARE THE PARTS OF A CELL AND WHAT DO THEY DO?

The first published drawing of a cell was drawn by Robert Hooke in the year 1665. Today we have photographs taken through an electron microscope capable of enlarging the cell thousands of times. Some of the newer microscopic and photographic techniques give added dimension and texture to the pictures and have taught scientists a great deal. It is unfortunate though that you cannot see a film showing what happens in a cell, the movement and changes that take place within the cell. Since there are so many different types of cells it is not possible to describe any one that is typical. The structures common to most cells will be described here and their functions explained (see Figure 3.1).

Cells have three major divisions: the membrane, the cytoplasm and the nucleus. Some scientists prefer to term these divisions "phases" in order to emphasize that the cell is an integrated unity with connections and interactions among its parts.

A. The membrane

The membrane surrounds the cytoplasm of the cell. The chemical structure of the membrane has been compared to a

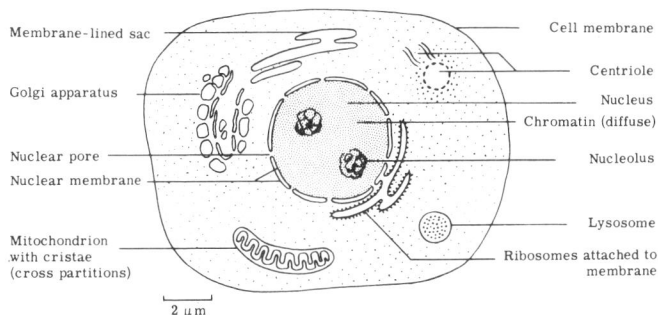

Figure 3.1   Some common organelles and structures of cells.

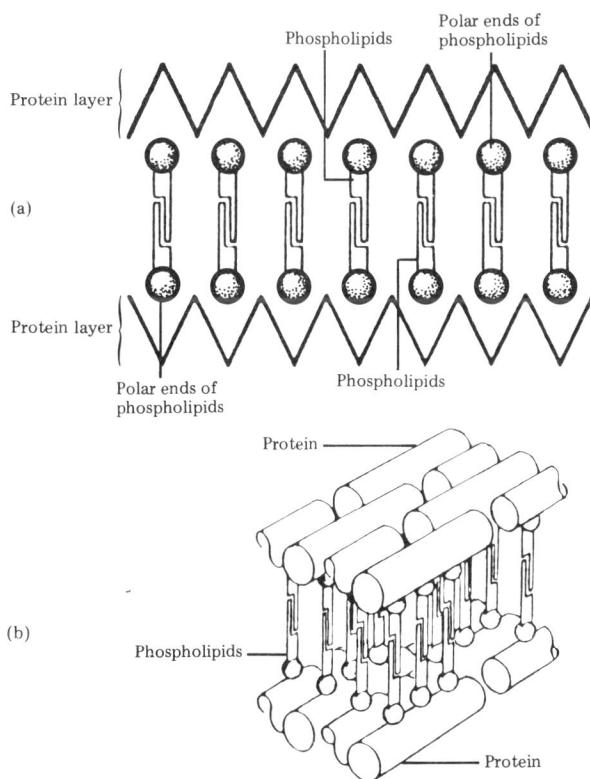

Figure 3.2   Model of membrane structure. (a) Cross-section and (b) Three-dimensional structure of membrane.

butter sandwich. This is because the membrane is a double-layered structure and each layer contains a protein component and a lipid component (see Figure 3.2). The lipid component is mostly phospholipid, and the two lipid layers are "sandwiched" between the two protein components. The membrane is not a simple homogeneous structure. It contains

25

enzymes and glycoprotein and is continually being broken down and renewed.

The outermost layer of protein and glycoprotein forms structures that are specific and give an identity to each cell. These specific protein–glycoprotein structures can be thought of as functioning as an address or box number inasmuch as they identify cells so that they are able to recognize one another during development and can ensure that chemical messages in the form of hormones are delivered to and received by the proper cells. Many viruses have been shown to combine with specific chemical groups on the surface of the cell before they enter and infect the cell. These receptors are known to be glycoprotein.

More will be said about receptors and hormones in the Chapter on the endocrine system, but the importance of receptors on the membrane should be emphasized now. Most hormones, with the exception of the thyroid gland hormones and the steroid hormones, begin their work at the cell membrane by interacting with the appropriate hormone receptor. Some scientists use the analogy of the automobile ignition lock and key. To start the engine the ignition key has to fit the ignition lock. The hormone (key) cannot do anything until it fits its receptor (ignition lock). If there is no receptor for the hormone, or hormone does not fit the receptor, the hormone cannot have any effect.

Perhaps the most important functional characteristic of the cell is its selective permeability. Molecules like oxygen and carbon dioxide can diffuse in and out with the greatest of ease. Other molecules, like glucose, cannot enter some cells unassisted and need insulin to facilitate their entry into the cell. Some small molecules like sodium ions can penetrate the membrane but are rapidly pumped out of the cell back to the extracellular fluid. Some molecules cannot cross the membrane at all and some large molecules, particles and even other cells can enter still other cells only by a process known as phagocytosis. In this process the molecule, particle or cell is wrapped in the cell's membrane and surrounded by the cell. This membrane-bound particle is then taken within the cell. More will be said later about phagocytosis.

The cell membrane is also involved in active transport. This process refers to the movement of substances from areas of low concentration to areas of high concentration. Since the direction of movement is the opposite of the diffusion gradient, the work of active transport requires the expenditure of considerable amounts of energy. The relative stability of the concentration of many intracellular and extracellular substances is dependent upon active transport.

Certain cells have many fine hair-like projections protruding from the membrane. These are called cilia and they function like brooms, sweeping particles across the surface of the cells. Cilia originate within the cytoplasm of the cells.

Certain other membrane adaptations are called micro-villi. These are small finger-like extensions of the cell and stick out from the membrane. The micro-villi help the membrane to make contact with other molecules by increasing the surface area of the membrane — think how much easier it is to catch or hold something with an open hand than with a fist. Many of the cells which line the gastrointestinal tract have numerous micro-villi, thus increasing the cell surface area by more than 20 times and therefore increasing the likelihood that a food particle will come into the cell and be absorbed.

B. The cytoplasm

Within the cell membrane is a fluid substance called the cytoplasm which contains the organelles (small intracellular structures). The cytoplasm can be as much as 85% water by weight, and it contains enzymes, nutrients and the following organelles:

a. Mitochondria. From the outside, mitochondria are shaped something like a peanut, averaging 0.5 μm in width and 1.2 μm in length, and are comparable in size to a bacterium. In a liver cell, there can be from 500 to 1000 mitochondria. Mitochondria, like some cells, are constantly being destroyed and constantly being renewed. If there were 1000 mitochondria in a liver cell, about 500 old mitochondria would be destroyed every two weeks and 500 new mitochondria would be formed. There would always be 1000 mitochondria, but not the same thousand. Again, this illustrates how dynamic, how changing life is.

The inside of the mitochondrion has an inner membrane arranged like shelves. These shelves contain enzymes arranged in a very specific order. This makes it possible for molecules to be broken down slowly, in a series of chemical reactions. A glucose or fat molecule is not broken down or oxidized in a single reaction to CO_2 and H_2O molecules, but in a series of enzymatic steps, many of which are located in the mitochondria. Since these are catabolic reactions, energy will be released. Some of this energy will be given off as heat, but a significant portion will be channelled into an anabolic reaction:

$$ADP + P \rightarrow ATP.$$

Because ATP is synthesized in the mitochondria, these structures are often referred to as the "powerhouse of the cell".

Cyanide is a very powerful and usually fatal poison. Its lethal effects are exerted on mitochondrial enzymes so oxidation cannot take place. The effects of cyanide poisoning are similar to those brought about by suddenly removing oxygen; both cyanide and the absence of oxygen would prohibit respiration in the mitochondria, stop the synthesis of ATP and kill the cells.

Mitochondria also play a role in controlling the concentration of some ions in the cytoplasm, but this function is not completely understood.

b. Lysosomes. Lysosomes are circular, about 0.5 μm in diameter and are wrapped in a single membrane. Inside this membrane are many powerful digestive enzymes which are so powerful that if the lysosome membrane were to be ruptured or torn and these enzymes released into the cytoplasm, they would start to digest the cell.

One author has referred to the lysosome as the cell's suicide bag. Normally, lysosomes are important in breaking down large particles which have undergone phagocytosis and cannot be handled by the cytoplasmic enzyme systems. These particles are digested only after the lysosome membrane has completely surrounded the particle, ensuring that the enzymes will not escape into the cytoplasm.

There are some rare genetic diseases in which the lysosomes, and some of the enzymes contained therein, are deficient. As a result, large particles or certain metabolic products can accumulate, since the cell's usual digestion and disposal system is not working. When the accumulation of particles or metabolic products becomes too great, the other functions of the cell are interfered with and the life of the cell is extinguished.

c. The endoplasmic reticulum. The endoplasmic reticulum is a series of hollow tubules that zig-zag and twist and turn throughout the cytoplasm of the cell. Some of these are continuous with the cell membrane, while others begin in the area around the nucleus and go outwards from there, suggesting to anatomists that the tubules might serve as a transportation system for molecules within the cell.

In some places the outer surface of the endoplasmic reticulum tubules is covered with granules of protein and ribonucleic acid. These granules are called ribosomes and that part of the endoplasmic reticulum which is covered with ribosomes is called the rough endoplasmic reticulum.

Messenger RNA attaches itself to the ribosomes and transfer RNA brings the amino acids to the appropriate position on the messenger RNA–ribosome complex. Thus, the rough endoplasmic reticulum is the site of protein synthesis. Cells that synthesize much protein will have more ribosomes than those cells which synthesize little protein. As an example, a liver cell has more rough endoplasmic reticulum than a nerve cell because a liver cell makes many more proteins.

That portion of the endoplasmic reticulum which does not contain any ribosomes is referred to as the smooth endoplasmic reticulum. Certain enzymes are located on the smooth endoplasmic reticulum; these enzymes detoxify — break down drugs and certain other harmful molecules.

d. The Golgi apparatus. This organelle gets its name from Camillo Golgi, who first discovered it in 1898. The Golgi apparatus is continuous with the endoplasmic reticulum and is formed from a series of membranes folded back upon one another. Newly synthesized proteins are channelled into the Golgi apparatus, where they are "packaged" so they will be protected against destruction by other enzymes in the cytoplasm. This protection is provided by part of the Golgi membrane surrounding the stored product.

The pancreas has cells that make many digestive enzymes which work within the gastrointestinal tract. The cells which make these enzymes have a well-developed rough endoplasmic reticulum and Golgi body. The enzymes are synthesized almost continuously and stored within membranes from the Golgi body until they are released from the pancreatic cell when food enters the intestine.

e. The centrioles. Each cell contains two centrioles which are at right angles to each other and are found just outside the nucleus. They are hollow cylinders, approximately 400 Å long and 1500 Å wide, the walls of which appear to be composed of nine hollow tubules or nine groups of tubes in a circle. The centrioles play an important part in cell division. The cilia of cells are anchored to the centrioles.

f. Inclusions. Strictly speaking, inclusions are not organelles; they are large collections (aggregates) of similar molecules which are insoluble in the cytoplasm and do not have fine structures like the other organelles. Glycogen is an inclusion in some cells, as are fat globules which are little balls of triglycerides.

Another important inclusion is a giant molecule called melanin. Melanin gets its name from the Greek word *melas*

which means black. The exact structure of the molecule is not known, but the molecule is found in parts of the eye and throughout the cells of the skin. The colour of your skin depends on the amount of melanin found in the cells of the outer layers of your skin. Black skins have more melanin than white skins. All people have some melanin in their skin except those individuals known as albinos who are completely white. This is a genetic disease in which the genes responsible for making the enzymes, which make melanin, are defective. This example should reinforce the importance of genes, enzymes and protein synthesis.

C. The nucleus

Heretofore, the continuously-changing nature of life and living material has been emphasized. Examples have shown how an organism responds to stimuli, constantly synthesizes new protein to replace the old and continuously renews some structures and organelles; however, it is true that, to quote the French saying: "Plus ça change, plus c'est la même chose" — the more things change, the more they are the same. And so it is with the cell. There is stability as well as change, particularly in the basic unit of life which is the cell.

One of the reasons why there is such constancy is found in the stability of the information contained in the DNA of the genes. The genes are located on the chromosomes and the chromosomes are located within the nucleus of the cell. Two important points must be stressed regarding the genetic information contained in the nucleus.

(1) The information contained in the chromosomal DNA is involved, directly or indirectly, in the production of all new materials used for the growth and maintenance of both the cell as a unit and the organism as a whole. The amount of information contained within a single nucleus is truly fantastic. The efficiency of information storage within the nucleus far exceeds that of the most recent computer.

(2) There is a great deal of duplication of information. The zygote, the brain cells, the liver cells and the intestinal epithelial cells all contain the same amount of DNA and the same information, even though they perform different functions. Not all the information is expressed or translated into protein synthesis at any one time, and different cells use different parts of the genetic information available to them. Scientists have "guesstimated" that a typical liver cell might use 5% of the information contained in its DNA. A brain cell would likewise use a small percentage of the DNA information, but parts of the information which it uses would be different from that used by the liver cell.

a. Components of the nucleus

Structurally, the shape of the nucleus is variable though usually it is round and about 2 μm in diameter. The nucleus has a double membrane called the nuclear membrane which separates the nucleus from the cytoplasm. Within the nuclear membrane is a clear fluid area called the nuclear sap; within the nuclear sap is chromatin. The 23 pairs of chromosomes in each cell are not visible unless the cell is dividing or is about to divide. The chromosomes usually exist in tightly-coiled threads of DNA and are called chromatin. It is thought that when specific information for protein synthesis is required in a cell that is not dividing, that portion of the chromatin containing the information uncoils or straightens out so that messenger RNA can be transcribed from DNA. Just as you cannot read your newspaper when it is crumpled up in a ball, so it is that the DNA message cannot be read and transcribed to messenger RNA when the DNA is in the tightly coiled chromatin form. The forces causing the chromatin to uncoil and to enable messenger RNA to be transcribed are not yet known.

Another component of the nucleus is the nucleolus. This is a small, discrete structure in the nucleus and contains clumps of RNA. It is thought that ribosomal RNA is synthesized in the nucleolus and then migrates to the cytoplasm. A nucleus may contain more than one nucleolus.

b. Mitosis

Much has been previously made of the fact that the entire complement of genetic material is contained in the nucleus of every cell. This duplication of information is not as inefficient as you might think. It is far better to have a surplus of information than to have a deficiency. Consider how much easier it is to buy a dictionary containing all the words of a certain language than it is to buy a book containing only the words you need to know at that time.

Mitosis is the process by which two cells containing identical genetic information are formed from one parent cell; it is cell division accompanied by information duplication. Mitosis is important not only in the development from zygote to adult, but also in the continuous cycle of cell death and cell renewal which goes on in certain tissues throughout the life of the individual.

A pathologist looks for mitotic figures in a tumour to find out if there is a malignant hyperplasia, and uncontrolled growth indicating cancer.

(1) The time between the end of one cell division and the beginning of another cell division is known as interphase. Even rapidly-growing cells can divide only once every 24 hours and the actual process of mitosis takes about an hour. This means that most of the time (23 hours), the cells are in interphase. Interphase precedes mitosis but is extremely important because it is during interphase that the DNA is duplicated. The DNA double helix splits apart and each strand serves as the model for its complementary strand. This synthesis requires enzymes, phosphate, deoxyribose and the four bases — A, T, C and G. The rules of base pairing are followed:

$$A + T, T + A, C + G, G + C$$

In principle, DNA synthesis is similar to the transcription of messenger RNA from DNA. After the completion of DNA duplication, the DNA threads remain together as uncoiled chromatin but are still not recognizable as chromosomes. Mitosis can now begin (see Figure 3.3).

(2) The first phase in mitosis is called prophase. During prophase, the centrioles duplicate themselves and move to opposite sides of the nucleus. The centrioles on opposite sides of the nucleus are connected by very fine thread-like structures called spindles. The nuclear chromatin rearranges itself and begins to take shape as chromosomes. These chromosomes are really double chromosomes because they

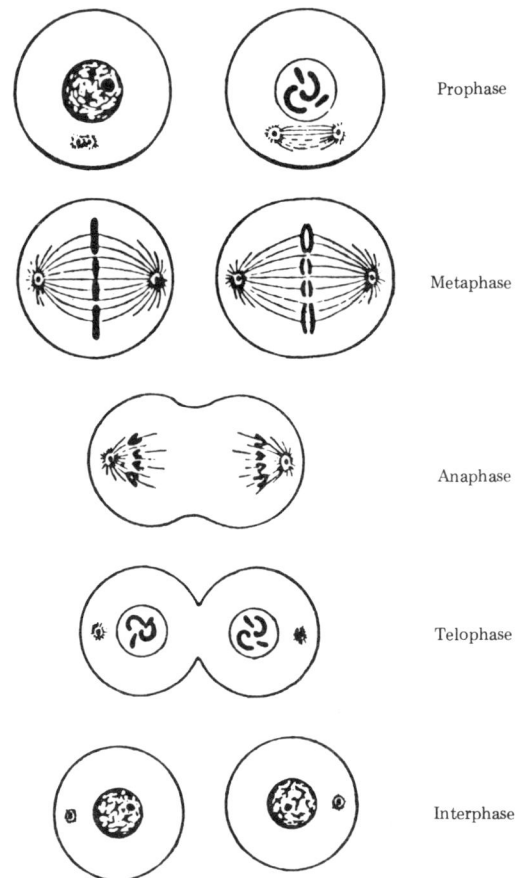

Prophase

Metaphase

Anaphase

Telophase

Interphase

Figure 3.3 Mitosis.

contain twice as much DNA as usual. The DNA was duplicated during interphase.

(3) In metaphase, the nuclear membrane begins to disappear while all 46 chromosomes begin to arrange themselves on the spindles between the centrioles, on the spindles which have become well developed.

(4) The chromosomes divide length-wise into identical parts, pull apart and move on the spindles to the centrioles; half of them migrating towards the left, and half towards the right, so that each half of the cell will have 46 chromosomes or 23 chromosomal pairs. This phase is called anaphase.

(5) The final phase is called telophase. During telophase the chromosomes lose their distinct shape and become chromatin, the spindle disappears and the beginnings of a membrane which will ultimately separate the cytoplasm of the two cells can be observed.

All textbooks have pictures of mitosis and explanations of it, but in fact it is still a mysterious phenomenon. Because scientists can photograph it and draw pictures of it does not mean they can fully understand it. There are still a great many problems concerning mitosis and questions arising as a result of mitosis. For example, why is it that if all the genetic instructions are the same in all cells, all cells do not look alike and do just the same things? What controls the different expression of DNA in different cells? This process by which cells become different, become either liver or pancreas or muscle cells, is called differentiation, and it is one of the great problems in biology.

Not all cells are capable of undergoing mitosis. The heart muscle cells and many cells in the brain cannot divide once these organs have formed. This helps to explain why injury to these organs is often so serious: because the cells cannot undergo mitosis, the organs cannot regenerate.

c. Meiosis

This will be mentioned now because it is often confused with mitosis, a very different phenomenon. Most cells contain 46 chromosomes, 23 maternal and 23 paternal chromosomes. If the sperm and ovum each had 23 chromosomal pairs, their union would result in a zygote with 92 chromosomes. Meiosis is the process by which the sperm and ovum reduce their chromosomal number to 23, leaving only one chromosome from each of the original chromosomal pair.

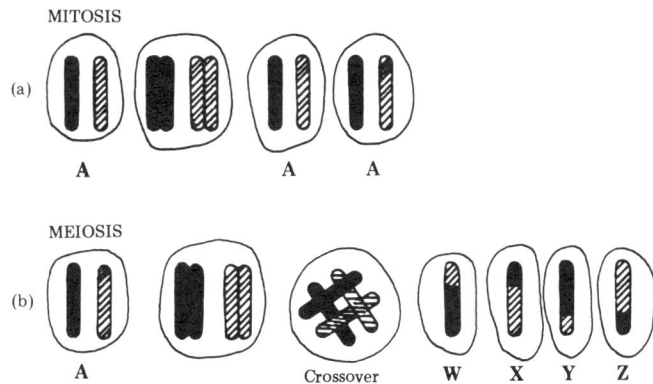

Figure 3.4 Comparison of mitosis and meiosis. In meiosis the cells formed have half the chromosomal number of the parent cell and different chromosomes. In mitosis the cells formed have chromosomes identical to the parent cell.

Meiosis is more complicated than mitosis. An essential feature of meiosis is the mixing or crossing-over of genes on matching chromosomes of the maternal and paternal pair. Figure 3.4 shows how a pair of similar maternal and paternal chromosomes interact during meiosis and exchange genetic material with one another to form two new chromosomes. This crossover occurs before the cellular divisions, which reduce the chromosomal number by half, and ensures that the genes in the sperm and ovum are different from the chromosomes of the other cells.

Because of this crossover of genes between paired chromosomes and the resulting formation of new chromosomes, every individual has a unique genetic constitution, different from that of his or her mother and father.

A cell having 46 chromosomes (23 chromosomal pairs) is said to be diploid; whereas a cell which has undergone meiosis and has 23 chromosomes is said to be haploid.

HOW ARE CELLS CLASSIFIED?

Cells are classified into four tissues; the study of tissues is called histology. The word tissue comes from the French word *tissu* which means "weave". The fabric of the body is woven from four different tissues. This separation or classification is based on the appearance of the cells, where they come from and where they are located, and to a certain extent on their function. The four tissues are: (A) epithelial tissue, (B) connective tissue, (C) muscle tissue and (D) nervous tissue. Every cell in the body will belong to one of these four tissues.

A. Epithelial tissue

Epithelial cells cover the surface of the body and line the tubular structures within it. They also cover most of the organs within the body, line the body cavities and form glands. The fundamental tendency of epithelial tissue is to maintain itself in tight-fitting sheets of cells; epithelial tissue is distinguished from connective tissue by the fact that epithelial cells are packed close together. (Connective tissue cells are separated from one another and supported by intercellular cement and other substances.) Epithelial cells have little intercellular cement between them but have special adaptations on adjacent cell membranes called desmosomes, which enable the cells to stay together and withstand mechanical stress. If you burn your skin and a little bubble of skin forms, called a blister, you are seeing a sheet of epithelial cells rise up and separate themselves from the connective tissue beneath.

Older texts refer to the supporting layer between epithelium and connective tissue as the basal membrane. Evidence from electron microscope pictures has shown that the basal membrane is very different from the typical cell membrane and so the term basal membrane is being replaced by a newer term, the basal lamina. It is thought that the epithelial cells contribute to the basal lamina and give off many thread-like filaments which may add to the attachment of the two tissues.

Epithelial tissues serve a variety of functions. The epithelial tissue which covers the surface of the body serves a protective function. It reduces the loss of moisture from body tissues and prevents micro-organisms from entering them. This protective function is enhanced because sheets of epithelium are arranged or stacked one on top of the other. If there is one layer of epithelial cells it is classified as a simple epithelium. If there are two or more layers it is classified as a stratified epithelium.

Epithelial cells also function in secretion and absorption. All substances that enter or leave the body must cross through epithelial tissue. Secretions are also produced by epithelial cells. The lungs, the gastrointestinal tract, the urinary and reproductive tracts are all lined with epithelial cells. The heart, the blood and lymph vessels are lined with cells that are epithelial in nature but customarily called endothelial cells. Similarly, the epithelial cells covering certain organs and lining some body cavities are called mesothelium.

A classification of epithelia is given below (see also Figure 3.5):

Simple epithelia	Stratified (compound) epithelia
squamous	squamous
cuboidal	transitional
columnar	

a. Simple epithelia. Squamous epithelial cells are thin, flat and shaped somewhat like the scales of a fish (see Figure 3.5a). They are found in parts of the kidney and in the small ducts of some glands. Mesothelia and endothelia are formed from simple squamous epithelia.

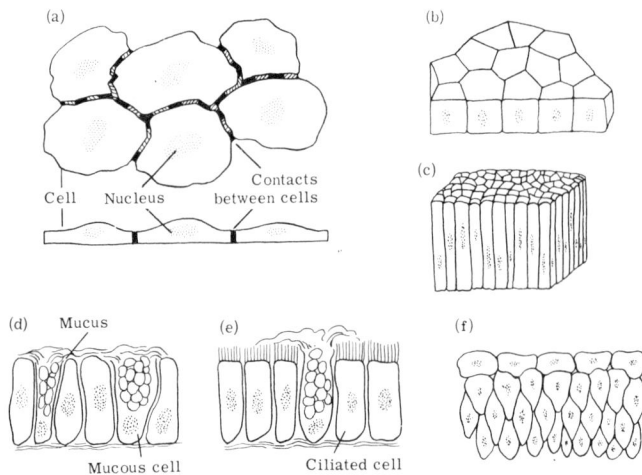

Figure 3.5 Epithelial tissue. (a) Squamous epithelium. (b) Cuboidal epithelium. (c) Columnar epithelium. (d) Mucous columnar epithelium. (e) Ciliated columnar epithelium. (f) Stratified (compound) epithelium.

Cuboidal epithelial cells are, as their name suggests, cube-shaped (see Figure 3.5b). The cuboidal epithelial cells of the thyroid glands help to produce thyroid hormone in the thyroid gland. The cells are also found in other glands and their ducts.

Columnar epithelial cells are taller than they are wide (see Figure 3.5c). Most of the gastrointestinal tract, from the stomach to the anus, is lined with this type of epithelium which functions in both secretion and absorption. Many columnar epithelial cells are specially adapted for the production of mucus (see Figure 3.5d). Some simple columnar epithelial cells have cilia (see Figure 3.5e). These ciliated columnar epithelial cells are found lining part of the respiratory tract and lining part of the uterus and uterine tubes. Some columnar epithelium is referred to as pseudo-stratified columnar epithelium. This is really a simple (one-layer) columnar epithelium, but under the microscope it may give the appearance of having more than one layer of cells because the nucleus is at different levels in the cells. The epithelium that lines the trachea leading to the lungs is columnar, ciliated and pseudo-stratified. Mucus-producing cells are also located in this ciliated pseudo-stratified columnar epithelium.

b. Stratified (compound) epithelia. The appearance of transitional epithelium is variable (see Figure 3.5f). This is because it is found in hollow structures which can change their shape. Think how the appearance of a balloon changes when it is blown up and then when the air is let out. The urinary bladder, which is lined with transitional epithelium, changes size and shape as it fills with urine. Figure 3.6f shows the stratified epithelium of the skin. Although it is called stratified squamous epithelium, only the outermost layers are squamous in shape. Compound epithelia are named by the shape or appearance of the cells closest to the surface of the external environment.

The epithelial cells at the base of the stratified epithelium have both a high metabolic and a high mitotic rate. The greater the distance between the inner and outer layers, the greater the distance which oxygen and nutrients must travel. The outermost cells cannot be adequately supplied, so these cells die. The inner layer with its high mitotic rate replaces the dead cells as they are sloughed off. This cell death and regeneration continues throughout life.

The stratified squamous epithelium in the skin of the palms of the hands and on the soles of the feet is exceptionally thick. Stratified squamous epithelium has a protective function and is found in those structures subject to frictional wear and tear. These include the skin, mouth, oesophagus, vagina and parts of the eye.

B. Connective tissue

This tissue includes groups of widely-differing cells which serve a variety of functions. The distinguishing feature of connective tissue is that the connective tissue cells are separated from one another by a substance, an intercellular matrix. This intercellular matrix is variable and may be jelly-soft, bone-hard or even a liquid. A classification of connective tissue is given below:

- (a) connective tissue proper
  - (1) loose connective tissue
  - (2) dense connective tissue
  - (3) adipose tissue
  - (4) lymphoid tissue
- (b) cartilage
  - (1) hyaline cartilage
  - (2) white fibrocartilage
  - (3) yellow fibrocartilage
- (c) bone
- (d) blood and lymph

Connective tissue includes bone tissue itself as well as the structures which connect bones to one another and attach muscles to bones. In addition to connecting the structures, connective tissue functions in supporting and separating the structures, also in the transporting of materials and nutrients and defending the body against infection. Bone, blood and lymph will be covered in separate Chapters.

a. Connective tissue proper

(1) Loose connective tissue. This is sometimes referred to as areolar tissue and is made up of different types of cells, fibres and a formless intercellular matrix containing extracellular fluid, often referred to as ground substance (see Figure 3.6a).

Loose connective tissue is similar to a dried-up sponge, in that it contains many potential spaces. These potential spaces are normally occupied by ground substance but may fill up and expand with fluid. Many times when a tissue is infected and swells, the increase in size is due to expansion of the loose connective tissue. All nutrients and wastes must pass through the ground substance which comes between the loose connective tissue cells and the blood.

The fibres in the ground substance give the tissue its strength. These fibres are either collagen or elastin. Collagen is the most abundant protein in animal tissues, white in appearance and of great strength. (Meat that has a high collagen content is very tough.) Collagen fibres get their strength from the unique and regular arrangement of amino acids within a molecular chain and the intertwining of these chains into strong fibrils. In principle, this is similar to the

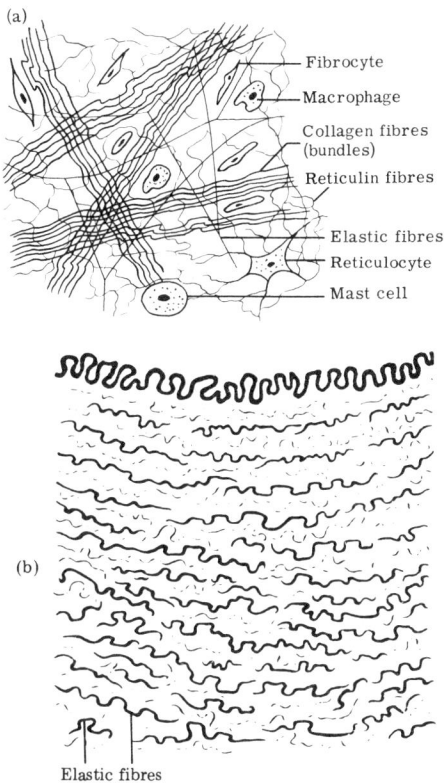

Figure 3.6 (a) Diagrammatic representation of the cells that may be seen in loose connective tissue. The cells lie in intercellular substance which is bathed in fluid that originates from capillaries. (b) Elastic fibres.

formation of a strong rope from many slender threads. Collagen is formed by cells in loose connective tissues called fibroblasts. After a deep cut or surgery, the scar which forms is made of collagen produced by fibroblasts.

The origin of elastic fibres is not understood. Fresh elastic fibres are yellow and differ from collagen because of the elasticity — they will stretch if pulled and then return to their normal length when the force is removed. Elastic fibres are important in tissues which must change size, stretch and contract (see Figure 3.6b).

Many other cells besides fibroblasts are found in loose connective tissue. Some of these cells are said to be "fixed" because they remain in place; while others are "wandering" and can migrate between the loose connective tissue and the blood and lymph.

Adipose cells are fixed cells and often scattered throughout loose connective tissue. These cells store fat; eventually they accumulate so much fat that the nucleus is pushed against the cell membrane.

Mast cells are wandering cells found in loose connective tissue and produce heparin and histamine, two compounds whose significance will be discussed later.

Some macrophages found in loose connective tissue are fixed, others are wandering. The word macrophage comes from two Greek words; *macro* meaning big, and *phago* meaning eat. Macrophages are able to "eat" bacteria and other large particles.

Plasma cells produce antibody which can react with viruses, bacteria and their products and can prevent them from exerting their harmful effects. Plasma cells develop from lymphocytes. Macrophages, plasma cells and antibody will be discussed in much greater detail in subsequent Chapters.

All these cells and antibodies share in defending the body against invasion by micro-organisms. This is significant when you consider that loose connective tissue is found beneath the stratified epithelium of the skin and beneath the epithelial lining of the digestive and respiratory tracts and parts of the urinary and reproductive tracts. Thus the macrophages and antibody-producing plasma cells form a second line of defence, should the bacteria or other micro-organisms penetrate the epithelium.

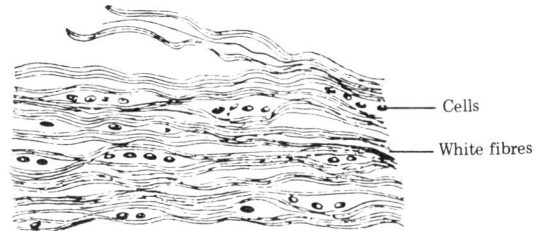

Figure 3.7 Dense connective tissue.

(*2*) *Dense connective tissue.* This tissue is much tougher than loose connective tissue because it contains very few fibroblasts and is usually formed from collagen fibres. Unlike loose connective tissue, collagen fibres are tightly packed and they run parallel to one another (see Figure 3.7). (Leather is dense, irregular connective tissue that has been processed from the hides of cattle.)

Because of its great strength, dense connective tissue forms the ligaments, which bind bones together and support many organs, and the tendons, which attach muscles to bones. When dense connective tissue forms a protective layer surrounding bone, it is called the periosteum; when it surrounds muscle, it is called fascia. It also forms protective coverings for the brain and spinal cord, the heart and the kidneys.

There is some dense connective tissue formed from elastic fibres. This tissue is found in the ligaments between bones in which there is a great deal of movement.

(*3*) *Adipose tissue.* Adipose (fat) cells are found scattered in loose connective tissue, but when they are gathered together in large groups or lobules, the result is termed adipose tissue (see Figure 3.8). A fat cell has a thin wall made of cytoplasm and a nucleus surrounding an island of fat stored in the form of triglyceride.

Besides being an energy storehouse, fat cells help insulate

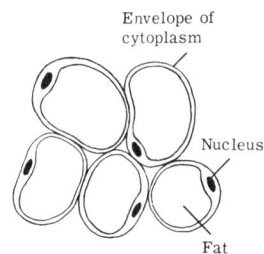

Figure 3.8 Adipose or fatty tissue.

the body by keeping the body's heat within the body. People who live in cold climates have much subcutaneous adipose tissue or fat stored beneath the skin. Women also have more subcutaneous fat tissue than men.

Adipose tissue is also found around some organs, for example on top of the kidneys and behind the eyes, and it serves to protect all of these vulnerable areas against mechanical injury. Adipose tissue has a high level of metabolic activity with fat being synthesized, stored and released into blood when needed.

(4) *Lymphoid tissue.* This is a type of loose connective tissue found in lymph nodes of the lymphatic system, the spleen, the tonsils and within the gastrointestinal tract. Lymphoid tissue should not be confused with lymph which is the fluid found within the vessels of the lymphatic system. This delicate-appearing lymph tissue contains a net-like arrangement of fibres called reticular fibres (see Figure 3.9). These are similar in composition to collagen fibres but they are much finer and not as strong.

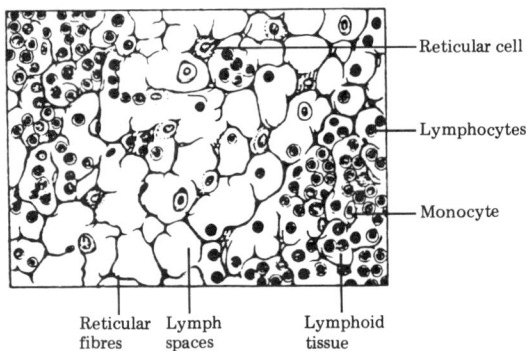

Figure 3.9 Lymphoid tissue.

The essential difference between loose connective tissue and lymphoid tissue is that lymphoid tissue contains dense aggregates of lymphocytes, and more plasma cells and macrophages. All these cells are important in defending the body against invasion by micro-organisms. This topic is covered more extensively in the Chapters on the blood and the lymphatic system.

Frequent reference has been made to the coverings and linings of the organs and body cavities. The word membranes is frequently used to describe these linings and coverings. They are formed from a combination of epithelial and connective tissues. Generally, there are three types of membranes:

(i) *Mucous membranes.* These line the digestive and respiratory tracts and parts of the urogenital tract. Mucus is a thick, sticky fluid containing water, salts, protein and carbohydrate and which is secreted by modified columnar cells (sometimes called goblet cells) and functions to moisten and protect the tissues beneath it.

(ii) *Serous membranes.* These membranes line the thoracic and abdominal cavities and cover the structures within them. Serous fluid, secreted by mesothelial cells, is clear and watery. Its chief functions are to moisten, reduce friction and permit easy movement of structures contained within cavities.

(iii) *Synovial membranes.* These are made of fibrous connective tissue and squamous epithelial cells, and they line

the joint cavities and the surrounding tendon sheaths and ligaments. Synovial fluid is thicker than serous fluid and mucus and it lubricates the joint to ease the movement of bones on one another.

b. Cartilage

Cartilage is the first of the connective tissues mentioned so far that can give support to the body; however, cartilage does not have the strength of bone. Cartilage is a strong tissue because it contains, in addition to the fibres, a mucopolysaccharide (protein plus carbohydrate) which makes the intercellular matrix strong and gives cartilage characteristics similar to plastic — easy to bend but more difficult to break. There are three types of cartilage: hyaline cartilage and white and yellow fibrocartilage (see Figure 3.10).

(1) *Hyaline cartilage.* Under the microscope, hyaline cartilage appears to be made-up of little islands of cells surrounded by a homogeneous matrix (see Figure 3.10a). There are collagen fibres in this matrix which are not visible because they are surrounded by mucopolysaccharide. The cells which produce the hard matrix are called chondrocytes. Hyaline cartilage makes up the temporary cartilage which later becomes bone, and also the articular cartilage which covers the bones at joint surfaces. It is also found in the trachea (windpipe) and in the attachment of the ribs to the sternum.

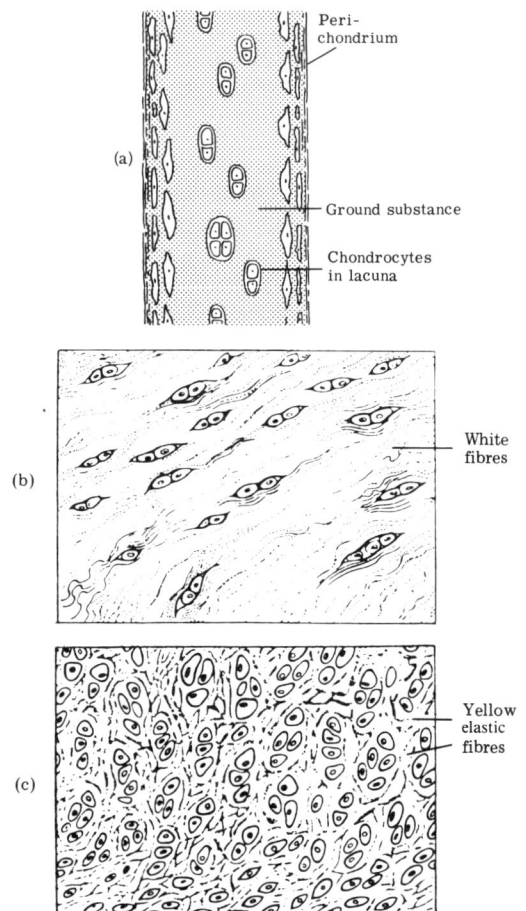

Figure 3.10 Cartilage. (a) Hyaline cartilage. (b) White fibro-cartilage. (c) Yellow fibrocartilage.

(2) *White fibrocartilage* is similar to hyaline cartilage except that the white collagen fibres are clearly visible (see Figure 3.10b). This is the cartilage which joins bones together in moveable joints. The vertebrae of the spine (backbone) are separated by pads of white fibrocartilage.

(3) *Yellow fibrocartilage* is like white fibrocartilage except that it has bands of elastin, rather than collagen, running through it (see Figure 3.10c). Place your finger behind your ear, push it forward, then let it go. It snaps back because of the elastin in the yellow fibrocartilage.

C. Muscle tissue

Muscle tissue makes up more than 40% of the body's weight. Muscle cells develop tension and can pull when they contract (shorten); they make movement possible. They also make it possible for a person to stand still. The contraction of muscle tissue also causes air to enter the lungs, blood to leave the heart, food to be propelled through the gastrointestinal tract and the muscular uterus to contract "squeezing" a baby out of the womb into the world at birth. There are three types of muscle tissue: (1) skeletal muscle, (2) cardiac muscle and (3) smooth muscle (see Figure 3.11).

(1) *Skeletal muscle* is usually found attached to bones, though there are a few exceptions like the lips, the facial muscles and the diaphragm. Skeletal muscle is often called voluntary muscle because it responds to the direction of the will; you can snap your fingers or blink your eyelids any time you choose to do so, because the acts of the will are transmitted to skeletal muscles via the nervous system.

Skeletal muscle is dependent on stimuli from the nervous system. Each place where the nervous system and the skeletal muscles come into contact is referred to as a myoneural junction. For a skeletal muscle to contract, a signal must be transmitted from the nervous system across the myoneural junction to the skeletal muscle. If there is some block or serious defect in the nervous system at the myoneural junction or within the muscle itself, the muscle will not be able to contract and will be paralyzed.

Under the microscope skeletal muscle appears to be striped or striated (see Figure 3.11a). These striations are the result of the orderly arrangement of two structural proteins, a thick myosin molecule and a thinner actin molecule, within the long multi-nucleated cell. More details on muscle structure and function are presented in the Chapter on the muscular system.

(2) *Cardiac muscle* is found only within the heart. It is striated like skeletal muscle, for there is an orderly arrangement of actin and myosin molecules within cardiac cells. The cells themselves, though, do have a different arrangement for they are not rigidly stacked but bend, branch and interlace with one another.

The ends of cardiac muscle cells have specialized thickenings called intercalated discs (see Figure 3.11b). These discs help communications between different cardiac cells. In fact, communications between separate cells are so good that, although the heart is made up of many cells, it behaves as though it were just a single giant cell. The heart beat results from the co-ordinated contractions of the cardiac muscle cells. The heart, unlike skeletal muscle, can beat without neural stimulation; it is involuntary. If you removed the

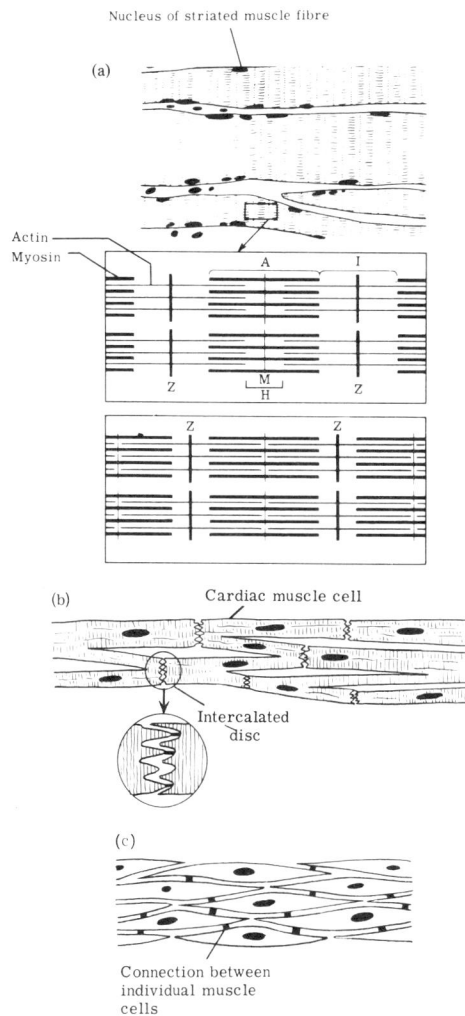

Figure 3.11 Muscle tissue. (a) Skeletal muscle. (b) Cardiac muscle. (c) Smooth muscle.

nerves going to the heart, the muscle would not be paralyzed; it would still beat and pump blood; the foetal heart pumps blood even before it is supplied with nerves. However, the nerves which do go to the heart are important, for they control its rate of beating or cause it to work more efficiently. The heart muscle has an inherent, spontaneous contractility, a rhythm of its own; but nerves and/or hormones are necessary to change the rate in response to the needs of the body.

(3) *Smooth muscle* gets its name because it does not show the striations that skeletal and cardiac muscle do. The cells contain myosin and actin, but their arrangement is not that ordered. The cells are wide at the centre, tapering at the ends, and are packed together so that the thick, middle part of one cell is next to the thin, tapered end of another (see Figure 3.11c). Smooth muscle, like cardiac muscle, is involuntary and can contract without the nervous system, but it needs nerves to work efficiently. Smooth muscle is unusual in that it can maintain itself in a contracted state for a long period of time without fatigue. This state of maintained tension is called tonus and is influenced by many hormones. Smooth muscle cells also have membrane specializations like desmosomes

and the intercalated discs of cardiac muscle which permit impulses to pass from cell to cell.

Smooth muscle is found within the tubes of the body; the walls of the arteries and veins, the respiratory, urinary and genital passages and in the gland ducts. It is also found in the eye and in the wall of hollow organs like the urinary bladder.

This muscle has the unique property of plasticity — as the bladder fills and the muscle is stretched, the muscle tonus is reduced and the muscle relaxes instead of increasing its tension.

D. Nervous tissue

It was stated earlier that the nervous system functions in communications, receiving signals from the internal and external environment, processing and storing information and sending instructions to glands, muscles and other nerve cells.

The basic unit of the nervous system is the neurone, which is the basic unit in the nervous system's communication processes because the properties of irritability and conductivity are uniquely developed in this cell. Neurones are irritable and can respond to a variety of stimuli, e.g. to sound and light, to changes in the concentration of salt and sugar in the blood and even to chemicals released by other neurones.

A response to a stimulus that is conducted from one end of the neurone to the other is called an impulse. Impulses are bio-electric conducted signals that neurones use to communicate with other neurones, glands and muscles. More will be said about impulses in the Chapter on the nervous system.

Structure of the neurone

Neurones in the brain and the spinal cord are multipolar. This means that the cytoplasm is drawn out into many small segments like branches from the trunk of a tree. A neurone receives signals from other neurones by means of its dendrites (see Figure 3.12). The greater the number of dendrites a neurone has, the greater the number of other neurones that will be in contact with it. The cell body of the neurone contains a nucleus, the other typical organelles and some fine protein threads called neurofibrils. The Nissl's granules which are seen in the cell body are masses of densely-folded rough endoplasmic reticulum.

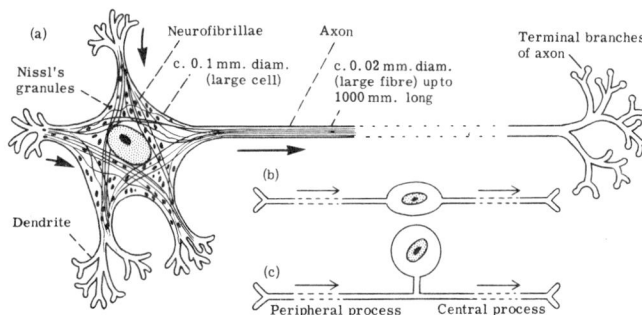

Figure 3.12   (a) Multipolar neurone. (b) Bipolar neurone.

In contrast to dendrites, a multipolar neurone has only one axon, which conducts impulses away from the cell body of the neurone. The axon begins from a part of the cell known as the axon hillock and the membrane of the axon is called the axolemma; the axon may then extend anywhere from a millimetre to more than a metre. Impulses which are conducted to the muscles of the foot are generated in a neurone whose dendrites and cell body are in the spinal cord; the long, thin axon leaves the spinal cord and travels the length of the leg before reaching the muscle tissue it stimulates. The axon branches before it ends and forms many small end feet (end bulbs). The end feet contain granules which are released when the impulse reaches the end feet. These granules contain the chemical transmitter which diffuses from the end feet across a very small space to reach another nerve, gland or muscle cell. The small space separating the two cells is called the synaptic space, and the area of functional contact between the end feet and the adjacent cell is called a synapse (see Figure 3.13). An impulse is conducted down to the end feet of the axon but does not cross the synaptic space; the signal is transmitted at the synapse from one cell to another by means of the chemical transmitter released by the axon's end feet. The processes of impulse conduction and synaptic transmission will be discussed in detail in the Chapter on the nervous system.

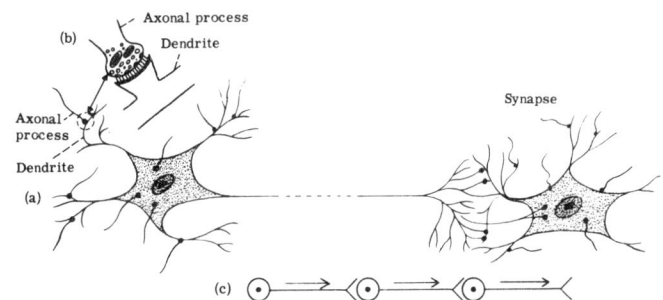

Figure 3.13   (a) Synapses between neurones. (b) Diagram of the electron microscopic appearance of one type of synapse. (c) Conventional diagrammatic representation of a chain of neurones.

Neurones which have only one long dendrite (and one axon) are called bipolar neurones. The dendrite of a bipolar neurone receives sensory stimuli, which are converted to impulses and conducted down the dendrite and axon of the cell. Sensory information is conducted to the brain and spinal cord by means of afferent, bipolar neurones. Efferent neurones conduct impulses away from the brain and spinal cord. These neurones are multipolar and send information to other neurones, instruct glands to secrete or muscles to contract. An efferent neurone whose impulses cause skeletal muscle to contract is called a motor neurone.

A neurone is not a nerve; the word *nerve* refers to a collection of nerve fibres. Nerve fibres may be the long dendrites of bipolar neurones or the axons of multipolar neurones.

Axons are surrounded by Schwann cells. Most Schwann cells produce layers of a fatty substance called myelin, which forms a large sheath around the axon. Myelin is essential for rapid impulse conduction. There is a large group of neural disorders which have degeneration of the myelin sheath as a common pathological feature. Disseminated sclerosis (multiple sclerosis) is perhaps the most common of these. The myelin in the brain and spinal cord degenerates so that sense perception and the ability to communicate instructions to muscles are interfered with. The space between adjacent Schwann cells is often called the node of Ranvier. Impulse conduction in long myelinated axons is accelerated because the impulse jumps from one node of Ranvier to the next.

The area surrounding the axon is called the endoneurium and contains collagen, fibroblasts and macrophages. The outermost layer of connective tissue surrounding many groups of nerve fibres is called the perineurium.

In the morning, sensory information is conducted over afferent sensory nerve fibres to the brain, which is informed that it is time to get up. The brain receives this information and processes it, then sends impulses to motor neurones in the spinal cord. These neurones send impulses via efferent nerve fibres, causing the appropriate muscles to contract, so the bed-covers are thrown back, the person stands up and the blood is redistributed — less blood to the legs and more to the brain. This is, of course, an oversimplification. The neurophysiological processes by which you remember who you are in the morning or why and how you decide to get up or stay in bed are not yet fully known.

4. The Blood

INTRODUCTION

We are all familar with the word blood. It is frequently used in speech because of its dramatic effect. Churchill said he had nothing to offer the British people in World War II but "blood, toil, tears and sweat". The word may, perhaps, derive some of its power from the knowledge that blood is the most important fluid of life. Blood is a complex fluid because it has cells and fragments of cytoplasm suspended in it. The fluid portion of blood is called plasma. Blood is classified as a connective tissue because it contains cells separated by a fluid matrix, and, in a sense, it connects all the cells of the body bringing them oxygen and nutrients, taking away carbon dioxide and wastes and helping cells to maintain proper ion concentrations.

The blood makes up approximately 5.5–8% of your body weight. If you weigh 70 kg, then roughly 4.9 kg of that weight is blood. In infants and children, blood makes up a higher percentage, while in obese people it makes up less.

WHAT ARE RED BLOOD CELLS AND WHAT DO THEY DO?

Another name for red blood cells is erythrocytes. The erythrocytes are the most common cells in the blood. The number of red cells and their volume in relation to plasma are extremely important in clinical medicine. If you were to take a sample of blood, place it in a test tube and spin it in a centrifuge, the heavier red cells would be quickly forced to the bottom and there would be a distinct separation between the cells and the clear plasma. For example, a tube 10 cm long is filled with blood and spun in a centrifuge. If the red cells are packed into the bottom 4.5 cm of the test tube and the clear plasma makes up the rest, the haematocrit is 4.5/10 or 45%. (The haematocrit is a measure of the volume of red cells per unit of blood.) The average haematocrit for an adult man is 47% with a normal range of from 42 to 50%; the average haematocrit for an adult woman is 42% with a normal range of from 39 to 48%. Having too many red cells (a haematocrit greater than 55%) is called polycythaemia, while having too few red cells is called anaemia. Anaemia should be suspected in a man if his haematocrit is 41% or below, and in a woman if it is 38% or below. People suffering from severe anaemia usually get tired very quickly, get short of breath and often appear pale.

The number of red blood cells is important. Obviously, it would be foolish to count all the red cells in the body, so the number in a small volume, a cubic millimetre (mm^3), is counted. In a healthy adult man the average number of red cells is 5.4 million/mm^3, and in a healthy adult woman the average is 4.8 million/mm^3. You can suspect anaemia if the man's red cell count is below 4.4 million/mm^3, and if the woman's is below 3.9 million/mm^3.

A red cell is generally described as a biconcave disc, meaning that the cell is circular in shape, thinner in the centre and thicker at the edges. A red cell averages about 7 micrometres (μm) in diameter (one μm is 0.001 mm), though this measurement is not critical as the red cell membrane can change size and shape. The inside of the red blood cell is unusual, for it contains no nucleus; the nucleus left the cell before maturation. Because of this it has more room for haemoglobin molecules. In addition to haemoglobin, the red cell contains water, some cytoplasm and enzymes.

To understand the function of haemoglobin, you have to understand the oxygen-carrying capacity of the blood. The plasma is 93% water while the red cell is more than 70% water. Gases such as air, which contains about 79% nitrogen and 20% oxygen, can dissolve in water. Although water can contain dissolved oxygen, the amount of oxygen which is usually dissolved in the water part of the blood is inadequate and would not support life. The haemoglobin molecule overcomes this difficulty because it has a special affinity for oxygen and readily combines with oxygen molecules, increasing the oxygen-carrying capacity of the blood by over 200 times. This fact is important and requires an example to illustrate its significance.

If a man is doing heavy work he can consume more than 4 litres of oxygen in 1 minute. If there were no haemoglobin in the blood, the heart would be required to pump more than 1200 litres of blood in 1 minute to deliver the necessary 4 litres of O_2 to the tissues. The bond between O_2 and haemoglobin is not strong, for the O_2 must be quickly released in the tissues. The relationship between O_2 and haemoglobin (Hb) is one of "friendship", a handshake of coming together in the lungs, followed by release in the tissue capillaries. As soon as O_2 has been released, CO_2 takes its place on the Hb molecule to begin its journey to the lungs. This will be discussed in more detail in the Chapter on the respiratory system.

Each red cell contains millions of Hb molecules. The normal adult Hb molecule is formed from two identical half molecules; each molecule contains two polypeptide chains made up of various amino acids linked together in different sequences. These chains are called the alpha (α) and beta (β) chains and constitute the globin portion of the molecule. There are four haeme molecules in each Hb molecule, and each haeme molecule contains an atom of iron. The iron is in the form of ferrous ions (Fe^{++}).

There are more than 120 genetic variants that code for

abnormal globin molecules. Sickle cell disease, discussed earlier, is an example of a haemoglobin disorder; the amino acid, valine, is substituted for glutamic acid at the sixth position of the β chain. There are also disorders of haeme synthesis. Since iron is required for haeme synthesis, an anaemia may result if the person becomes iron deficient. It is estimated that 10–30% of the world's population is deficient in iron. In developing nations, iron deficiency is a public health problem, while in industrialized societies it affects mainly women, children and the poor. Although women have fewer red cells than men, they have a greater need for iron because of the menstrual cycle. Pregnancy greatly increases the woman's need for iron. Some people have an adequate dietary intake of iron but are not able to absorb it. There is also a possibility of overdosage. Young children have been poisoned through eating their parents' iron supplements.

The amount of haemoglobin in the blood is an important clinical indicator. In adult men, the average is 15 grams of Hb/100 ml of blood, with a normal range of 14–18 grams. In adult women, the average is 14 grams of Hb/100 ml of blood, with a normal range of 12–16 grams. In men, values below 14 grams/100 ml, and in women, values below 12 grams/100 ml indicate anaemia.

Another clinical test is the sedimentation rate. In many disease conditions, the red cells will tend to stick together, one on top of another like a stack of plates. This is called a rouleaux formation and is caused by abnormal proteins or very high concentrations of certain proteins in the blood. If a sample of blood is drawn, treated with chemicals to prevent clotting and placed in a test tube, the rate of fall of the red cells can be measured. If there is rouleaux formation, the big protein particles will sink quicker than the isolated red cells. In men the area of clear plasma at the top of the test tube is 1–3 mm at the end of 1 hour, and in women it is 4–7 mm. The sedimentation rate is a general indicator of disease. In diseases like cancer, rheumatoid arthritis, tuberculosis and other infectious diseases it increases. It is also useful as a screening test for it is impossible to falsify a high sedimentation rate.

Another important point about red cells is their life span, usually 120 days. A red cell is formed in the centre core of marrow in the long bones and is destroyed in the reticuloendothelial system which includes the liver, spleen and lymphoid tissue. These tissues are very active; every second approximately 2.5 million red cells are destroyed and 2.5 million are being formed.

If, for some reason, there is a need for more blood cells, for example after haemorrhage or on moving to a higher altitude where there is less oxygen, the rate of red cell formation can be increased. This increase is brought about by a hormone called erythropoietin. It is believed to be produced in the kidney, travels to the bone marrow via the blood and speeds up the rate of red cell formation. Another hormone, testosterone, is also involved. The stimulus for erythropoietin synthesis appears to be low levels of oxygen in the blood flowing to the kidney. Much more will be said about hormones in the Chapter on the endocrine system.

WHAT CAUSES ANAEMIA?
Anaemia is a common clinical finding and illustrates mechanisms of red cell production and destruction. It is indicated by a low haematocrit, red cell count or haemoglobin concentration. Anaemia is not a disease but a sign of a disease, like fever it indicates that something is wrong. The presence of anaemia must initiate a search for the underlying cause of the anaemia. Anaemia can occur if the red cell production is inadequate, if destruction exceeds production or if blood is being lost through haemorrhage.

a. Impaired red cell production. Iron is necessary for red cell production, so a deficiency can cause anaemia. Inadequate supply of vitamin B_{12}, vitamin C and/or folic acid can also cause anaemia. Vitamin B_{12} presents special problems because, although the diet often contains adequate B_{12}, the gastrointestinal tract may not be able to absorb it. Red cells are produced in the bone marrow, so infections or tumours within the bone marrow can hinder production. Certain drugs, such as the antibiotic, chloramphenicol, and chemicals like lead and benzene, as well as certain drugs used in the treatment of cancer, can depress the marrow. There must be a proper metabolic environment for red cell production and this is not possible with certain endocrine and metabolic disorders. The above list of causes is by no means complete.

b. Excessive red cell destruction (haemolytic anaemia). The escape of haemoglobin from the red cell is called haemolysis, though in common clinical usage the term is used to refer to the premature destruction of red cells. The anaemia which occurs in sickle cell disease, and occasionally with the sickle cell trait, arises because cells containing abnormal haemoglobin have a shortened survival rate, particularly under conditions of reduced oxygen, acidosis or infection. There are certain diseases in which red cells with abnormal membranes are synthesized; these cells are rapidly destroyed by the spleen. A hyperactive spleen can also cause anaemia.

Other haemolytic anaemias can be caused by drugs, diseases of red cell metabolism and by immunological disorders; this last group is discussed later in this Chapter.

c. Excessive blood loss. Some people may be anaemic even though their red cell production and destruction rates are not abnormal. Some women lose unusually large amounts of blood when they menstruate. Hookworms (parasites that may inhabit the intestinal tract) derive their nourishment by sucking blood out of the intestinal tract. Tumours and ulcers (erosions of the lining of the intestinal tract) can bleed into the intestinal tract. These haemorrhages may be occult (hidden) because the blood mixes with the faecal contents. The stool guaiac test detects blood in the faeces and is often used if injury to the intestinal tract, or bleeding ulcers or tumours in the intestinal tract, are suspected.

The bone marrow of the adult produces red cells at about 20% of its total capacity so it can compensate for many increases in red cell destruction or red cell loss. If the marrow is stimulated to produce additional red cells it may release not only red cells into the circulation but also reticulocytes. The reticulocyte is a precursor (immature form) of the red cell, has lost its nucleus, contains RNA but does not have its full complement of Hb. Reticulocytes are usually about 1% of the red blood cells but this increases when the marrow is being stimulated. If the marrow is damaged and cannot respond to the need for increased red cell production, both the red blood cell count and the reticulocyte count will be depressed.

Other information pertinent to determining the cause of anaemia is derived from calculating the average size of the red cells and their average concentration of Hb. The concentration of red blood cell breakdown products in the blood and urine is also important.

WHAT IS OSMOSIS?

Osmosis is usually taught in introductory science courses and is often poorly understood. This is unfortunate, for this phenomenon has tremendous biological and medical importance. The red cell can be used to illustrate osmosis, but osmotic phenomena apply to more than red cells.

Osmosis is defined as the attempt by free-moving particles to equalize their concentrations on both sides of a semi-permeable membrane by diffusion. Let us go beyond the definition and really understand the process. A situation in which osmosis can occur must have three things:

The first is a semi-permeable membrane. This means that the membrane allows certain molecules to cross through the membrane, while other molecules are prohibited from doing so.

Next, there must be molecules which can cross through the membrane; these molecules are called free-moving molecules. Water and urea are examples of molecules which can cross most biological membranes, are therefore "free moving". Free-moving molecules have the characteristic of equalizing their concentrations on both sides of the membrane. All molecules have an inherent tendency to diffuse until their concentrations are equal but not all molecules can achieve it. Think of perfume molecules. If you take a bottle of perfume and place it in the centre of the room, open the top and wait a few minutes, it will not be long before the perfume molecules diffuse out of the bottle, moving from a high concentration to a low concentration. In time, the concentration in all parts of the room would become equal.

The third requirement is molecules which cannot cross through the membrane. These molecules are called osmotically active molecules because they exert an osmotic pressure. Like free-moving molecules they have a tendency to diffuse from areas of high concentration to areas of low concentration; however, they cannot follow their diffusion gradient because of their size or electric charge which prevents them from crossing the semi-permeable membrane. The osmotic pressure exerted by osmotically active molecules refers specifically to the force by which free-moving molecules diffuse from areas of high concentration to areas of low concentration. These terms may be clarified by the following example.

Let us take two sucrose solutions of equal volume but different concentrations and separate them by a membrane which is permeable to water but impermeable to sucrose. Solution A is 20% sucrose and solution B is 10% sucrose. Solution A has a greater osmotic pressure than solution B because solution A has more osmotically active (sucrose) molecules and fewer free-moving (water) molecules. (Figure 4.1a). This means that the concentration of the free-moving water molecules in solution A is less than in solution B; the water "concentration" in A is 80% and in B is 90%. The

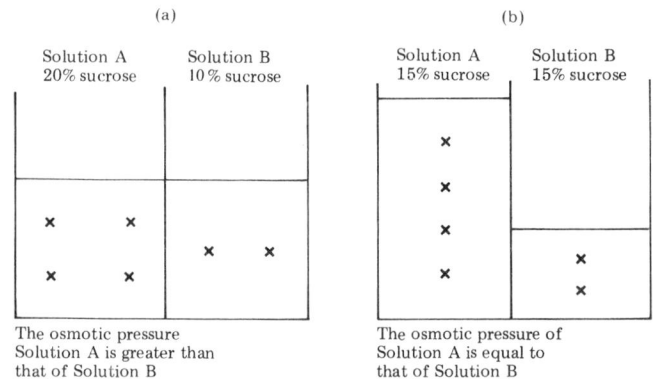

Figure 4.1 Osmosis.

concentrations of the free-moving (water) molecules are not the same and they must equalize. As B has more free-moving molecules that can cross the membrane than does A, there will be a net movement of free-moving molecules from B to A. The free-moving molecules will diffuse from B to A till their concentration on both sides of the membrane is equal, 85% and 85%, and equilibrium is reached (Figure 4.1b). If the concentration of water is the same on both sides, the concentration of sucrose molecules must be the same, as must be the osmotic pressure. At equilibrium the difference in height between solutions A and B will be indicative of the original differences in osmotic pressure between the two. If, after equilibrium has been reached, more sucrose molecules are added to A, the osmotic pressure of A will be increased and more water will move from B to A. The amount of water which moves will be directly proportional to the number of osmotically active molecules added.

If we were to take red blood cells and place them in a volume of distilled water, we would have an unstable osmotic situation. (The red cell membrane is semi-permeable.) The protein, enzymes and haemoglobin within the cell are osmotically active, because they cannot leave the inside of the red cell. The water molecules on both sides of the membrane are free moving and can easily pass through the membrane. The inside of the red cell can be said to have an osmotic pressure as it contains osmotically active particles, while the bathing medium has no osmotically active particles and therefore no osmotic pressure. 100% of the molecules outside the cell are water while, because of the osmotically active molecules inside the cell, the water content is much less than 100%. There are more free-moving water molecules outside the cell so they will tend to diffuse inside the cell, trying to achieve equal concentrations within the cell and outside it; this is impossible since there will always be some osmotically active molecules inside the cell. As the water moves into the cell, the cell starts to get bigger, to swell and change shape just as a balloon changes shape when air is put into it. As the cells get bigger and bigger, the membrane will be stretched, "pores" will develop and, as a result, enzymes and haemoglobin inside the cell will leak out, giving the whole solution a pinkish colour. A solution in which the osmotic pressure of the solution inside the cells is greater than that outside the cells is called a hypotonic solution (see Figure 4.2a).

But why don't the cells in your bloodstream haemolyze? They do not haemolyze because the plasma which bathes

x = Osmotically active molecules

Before

After

(a)

Water diffuses into the cell because the water concentration outside the cell is greater.

Cell swells

(b)

The concentration of the water and osmotically active molecules is the same inside and outside the cell.

No movement of water. No change in cell size.

(c)

Water diffuses out of the cell because the concentration of water inside the cell is greater than that outside the cell.

Cell shrinks

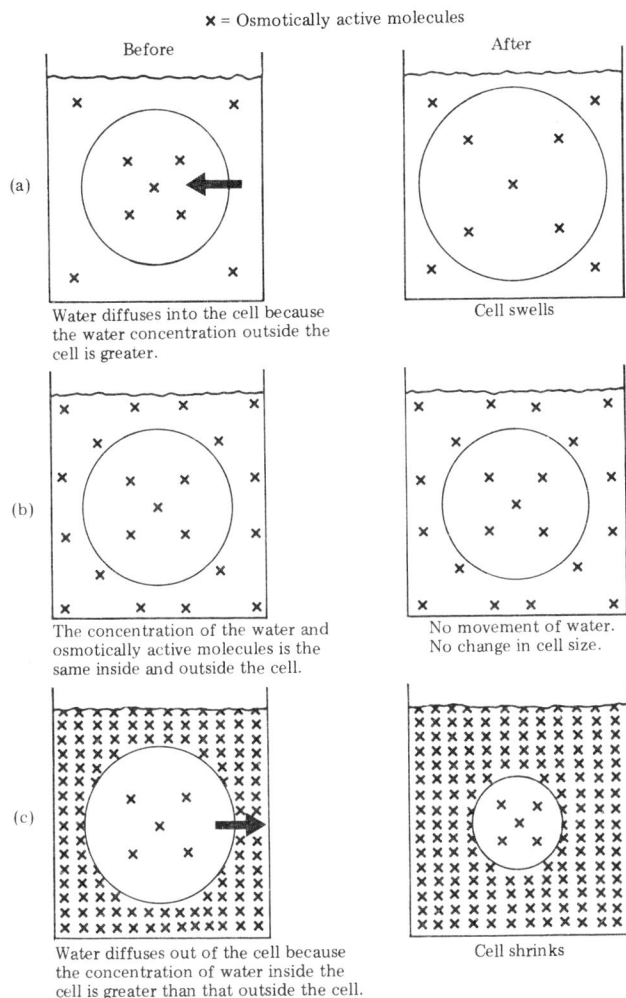

Figure 4.2 Osmotic pressures in solutions. (a) A hypotonic solution. (b) An isotonic solution. (c) A hypertonic solution.

them is isotonic; this means that the osmotic pressure inside the cell and outside the cell is equal (see Figure 4.2b). Thus, there will be no net movement of water or other free-moving particles across the cell because their concentrations are equal. Although the red cell contains by weight less water than the plasma, the solutions are still isotonic because the concentration of osmotically active particles is the same on both sides of the membrane. Many of the osmotically active molecules inside the cell are big and heavy, e.g. haemoglobin, while many of those outside the cell are small and light. It is the number of osmotically active particles that count and not their size.

If you add 9 grams of sodium chloride to 1 litre of water you have a 0.9% salt solution. This solution is called saline and it is isotonic to red blood cells. The concentration of osmotically active salt molecules is equal to the concentration of osmostically active molecules inside the cell. Inasmuch as there is no difference in osmotic pressure, the red cells will neither shrink nor swell. (This is a good place to point out that a 0.9% NaCl solution, a 0.15 molar NaCl solution and a 0.3 molar sucrose solution are all isotonic to red blood cells because all three solutions have the same number of osmotically active molecules.) In a 1.0 molar solution of

NaCl there is about 58 grams NaCl. In a 0.15 molar solution there is: $58 \times 0.15 = 9$ grams NaCl, just as in the saline solution. But why should a 0.15 molar NaCl and a 0.3 molar sucrose solution exert the same osmotic pressure? This is because osmotic pressure is a function of the number of osmotically active molecules and because one molecule of NaCl will give two osmotically active particles, Na^+ and Cl^-, in solution. Sucrose does not form two particles in solution, so the molarity of a sucrose solution or any other sugar solution must be twice the molarity of the NaCl solution if it is to have the same number of molecules in solution.

Because of this disparity between the number of moles and the number of osmotically active particles, the term osmole is used. The osmole represents the product of the number of moles and the number of particles contributed by 1 mole. To illustrate:

1 molar glucose × 1 particle/mole = 1 osmolar glucose
1 molar KCl × 2 particles/mole = 2 osmolar KCl

Inasmuch as the concentration of most substances in biological fluids is low, the term milliosmole (mOsm) is commonly used. There are 1000 mOsm in 1 osmole. The osmolarity of blood is about 0.3 osmoles (300 mOsm). A 300 mOsm solution of NaCl and a 300 mOsm solution of glucose will be isotonic to one another because they will both have the same concentration of osmotically active molecules.

If you take 1 litre of water with 15 grams of NaCl dissolved in it and place red cells in it, changes take place. The osmotic pressure of the bathing solution will be greater than the osmotic pressure inside the cells and thus the concentration of free-moving molecules inside the cells will be greater than outside the cell. The water molecule will diffuse from an area of high concentration to one of low concentration, trying to equalize the concentrations on both sides of the cell membrane and, therefore, water will leave the cell, causing the cell to shrink and change its shape.

The process by which water leaves red cells and distorts their shape is known as crenation. You can think of a raisin or sultana as a crenated grape because some of the water has left the grape, leaving the wrinkled raisin. A solution in which the osmotic pressure of the bathing solution is greater than that inside the membrane is known as a hypertonic solution (see Figure 4.2c).

WHAT ARE WHITE BLOOD CELLS AND WHAT DO THEY DO?

White blood cells are also called leucocytes. They are bigger but fewer in number than red cells, have nuclei and are not concerned with gas transport. If white blood cells were removed from the body and placed directly under a microscope, they would all look pretty much alike and many of the organelles within the cell would not be visible. To differentiate between the various kinds of white cells and their organelles, it is necessary to stain them with different dyes. Cells are smeared upon a glass slide, allowed to dry as they stick to the glass and then passed through a series of solutions of different dyes. Different kinds of cells and parts within them respond differently to different dyes, depending upon whether the dye is acidic or basic.

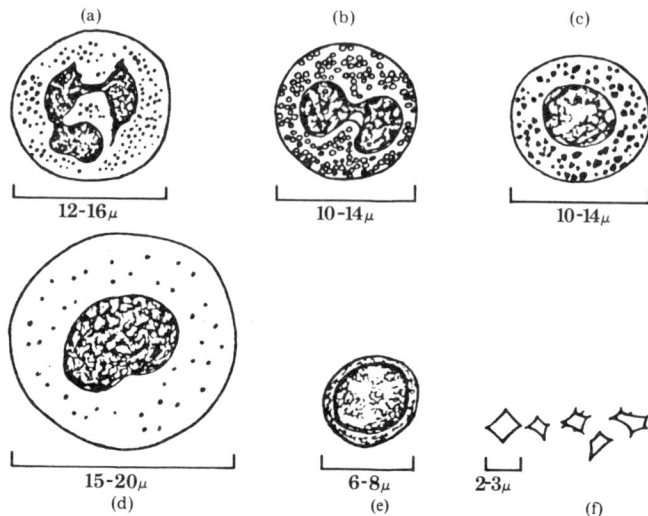

Figure 4.3 White blood cells. (a) Polymorphonuclear neutrophil.
(b) Eosinophil. (c) Basophil. (d) Monocyte. (e) Lymphocyte.
(f) Platelets (thrombocytes).

With these staining techniques and the use of a microscope, we can differentiate the types of white cells on the basis of their size, nuclear shape, colour and whether or not they have large granules in the cytoplasm.

The first way to differentiate among the leucocytes is to look for large granules in the cytoplasm of the cells (see Figure 4.3). Neutrophils, eosinophils and basophils all have large granules, a nucleus with a complex shape and belong to the subclass of leucocytes known as polymorphonuclear granulocytes. Polymorphonuclear granulocytes (polys) are differentiated from one another by their different colours after staining, for each of the types of granulocyte takes up the various dyes in different amounts, and therefore each has a different colour.

Monocytes and lymphocytes do not have large cytoplasmic granules and therefore belong to the subclass known as agranular leucocytes. The nuclei in monocytes and lymphocytes are usually round and differ from those found in the mature granulocytes. Structurally, lymphocytes are differentiated from monocytes on the basis of their size; lymphocytes are smaller than monocytes.

A white blood cell count includes the total number of neutrophils, eosinophils, basophils, monocytes and lymphocytes in 1 cubic millimetre (mm^3) of blood. The normal adult range is 5000–10 000 leucocytes/mm^3. It is possible to count separately the number of neutrophils, eosinophils, basophils, monocytes and lymphocytes in 1 mm^3 of blood. This is not routinely done, however. Often a blood smear is made and stained, 100 leucocytes are counted and the types of leucocyte are noted and expressed as a percentage. Thus a lab report might state that the leucocyte count is 8000, and the differential count is monocytes 6%, neutrophils 55%, eosinophils 3%, lymphocytes 35% and basophils 1%.

Platelets are not true cells but fragments of cells.

A. Polymorphonuclear granulocytes

These are sometimes called polymorphs or granulocytes because after staining they show small clumps of granules in the cytoplasm. The name, polymorphonuclear, refers not to the cytoplasm but to the shape of the nucleus of these cells, which is not small and round like that of the typical cell, but has an irregular shape, sometimes looking like a "C" or an "S" or sausage-shaped with bulging lobules connected with little strands. The nuclei stain dark blue. All granulocytes are formed in the marrow of the bones. There are three types of granulocytes: neutrophils, eosinophils and basophils.

a. Neutrophils. The majority of leucocytes in the blood of the normal adult are neutrophils. The normal range of neutrophils is about 3000–6000/mm^3. Neutrophils are so called because of their staining properties. The granules stain with either acidic dyes and/or basic dyes. Many of these granules are lysosomes, which contain powerful digestive enzymes and antibacterial chemicals. The nucleus of the mature neutrophil is large, has from two to three lobes and stains dark blue.

The production, circulation and destruction of neutrophils is much more dynamic than that of erythrocytes. Neutrophils circulate for several hours rather than for a few months as erythrocytes do. Because granulocytes can be produced and released into the circulation so quickly, the number of granulocytes in circulation can dramatically increase in a short period of time. Some neutrophils adhere to the lining of the capillaries and small veins. They can be released into the circulation in seconds.

When the neutrophil count exceeds 10 000/mm^3, this condition is called a neutrophil leucocytosis. This is seen in acute infections and in disorders associated with inflammation or cell death, such as after a "heart attack" with the death of heart cells. Other causes of a neutrophil leucocytosis include metabolic conditions, certain drugs and sometimes even after strenuous exercise.

Neutrophils are uniquely important in the body's defence against bacteria. If you have ever cut yourself and the site of injury became "infected", you have some insight into the process of inflammation and the role of neutrophils. What probably happened was that you cut your skin, broke down one of the body's barriers, bacteria entered, came in contact with connective tissue and caused a response to it. The redness, swelling and pain were caused by the increased volume of blood flowing to the injured area, the leaking of some plasma out of the capillaries into the cut causing a swelling and the resulting pressure that this puts on the nerves, causing pain. Into this infected area come the neutrophils which have passed out of the circulatory system drawn to the site of injury by chemical attraction known as chemotaxis. Chemotaxis is the movement of cells in a particular direction in response to certain chemicals. Many bacteria contain chemicals that induce chemotaxis, and similar-acting chemicals are released during antigen–antibody reactions involving complement.

Since neutrophils are mobile cells they can pass through capillaries and surround and engulf the bacteria. The process by which the bacteria are eaten by the neutrophils is called phagocytosis. Inside the cell, the lysosomes may digest the bacteria, or the bacteria may continue to grow inside the neutrophil, ultimately causing it to burst, releasing the lysosomes and so allowing them to begin their digestive work outside the cell. The pus that is often found at the site of an infection is really the remnants of exploded neutrophils and their contents.

There are diseases in which the number of white cells is reduced or their ability to kill bacteria is depressed. These patients are troubled by recurrent infections and even mild infections may be serious, possibly fatal to them. Ethanol (alcohol) is known to inhibit the release of neutrophils from bone marrow and this factor is thought to contribute to an alcoholic patient's increased susceptibility to infectious diseases.

Finally, neutrophils can be stimulated to release a fever-causing agent — a pyrogen. If the leucocytes come into contact with certain bacteria or bacterial products, some metabolic activity in the cells is stimulated, which leads to the release of pyrogen. Pyrogen is thought to be a special protein or groups of proteins in the neutrophils which exert their effect on the temperature-regulating centre in the brain. When pyrogen is released from the neutrophils, it enters the blood stream and reaches the brain. Pyrogen is one of the links between infection and fever.

The leukaemias are a group of diseases having as a common feature the unregulated production of white cells or their precursors. The cells that give rise to both red and white cells are called stem cells. Red cells and white cells go through a complex, controlled series of differentiations before reaching maturity. In leukaemia, immature white cells may be released from the marrow and will be ineffective in fighting infection. Sometimes the bone marrow is so diseased that neutrophil cells cannot leave the marrow, and the cell count is very low—this is called neutropenia. These facts explain why "simple" infections can threaten the life of a patient with leukaemia. As both red cells and white cells share a common site for development, and at some point a common parent cell, anaemia is a common finding in leukaemia.

b. Eosinophils. These cells get their name because their granules stain with a reddish-orange acidic dye named eosin (see Figure 4.3b). Less is known about eosinophils than neutrophils. They are able to act as phagocytes though it is thought they "eat" antigen–antibody complexes rather than bacteria. Their numbers increase in response to infestation with parasites and in such allergic conditions as hay fever and asthma. The normal range of eosinophils is 50–250/mm³.

c. Basophils are easily identified because their granules stain with a dark purple basic dye (see Figure 4.3c). Unfortunately, although they are easy to recognize, their function is not really known. Their numbers go from 0–100/mm³.

B. Monocytes

The second class of leucocytes is the monocytes. These are the largest of the leucocytes; they have a horseshoe-shaped nucleus and are phagocytic (see Figure 4.3d). Their cytoplasm is agranular.

Blood monocytes are the precursors of the macrophages found in loose connective tissue. The word macrophage comes from the Greek word *macro* meaning big, and the Greek word *phago* meaning eat; they are able to consume bacteria and swollen and dead neutrophils.

The movement of monocytes from the blood to an infected area is slower than that of neutrophils. The factors responsible for the conversion of a monocyte to a macrophage are not fully understood, but it is believed that the monocyte must first ingest a foreign protein. Recent evidence suggests that monocytes are drawn to an infected site by certain sensitized lymphocytes and the release of chemotaxic chemicals. In the presence of these lymphocytes and the foreign protein there is an increase in the metabolic activity of the macrophage, which is then referred to as an angry macrophage because of its increased ability to phagocytose and destroy cells. More will be said about this in the following section.

The normal range of monocytes in the blood is 300–600/mm³. Increased numbers of monocytes are often found in certain other conditions, e.g. in tuberculosis and in some of the leukaemias.

C. Lymphocytes

These cells have a large oval nucleus which fills most of the cell and leaves little room for the small amount of agranular cytoplasm (see Figure 4.3e). Numerically, lymphocytes are, after neutrophils, the second most common of the leucocytes. In a normal adult there are about 1500–4000/mm³, and this number makes up about one-quarter to one-third of the leucocytes. Lymphocytes are classified as being either T-lymphocytes or B-lymphocytes. This is, however, a functional distinction, for T-cells cannot be distinguished from B-cells with the light microscope.

Lymphocytes not only circulate in the blood but also circulate in the lymph and are attracted to sites of infection. Lymphocytes are important in providing immunity to the body by defending the body against infection. If you have immunity against a certain disease you are usually safe from that disease.

The foremost characteristic of both types of lymphocytes is their ability to distinguish between what is of the body (the self) and what is foreign to the body (the non-self). Lymphocytes must protect the body against certain viruses and bacteria and harmful bacterial products, and at the same time must not interfere with the body, its tissues and their functions. For example, certain bacteria synthesize and release harmful products known as toxins. These toxins are protein. Many hormones are also proteins. The lymphocytes must be able to prevent the toxins (the non-self) from causing injury and at the same time not interfere with the hormones (the self). They must be able to distinguish between toxins and hormones though both are proteins.

There is a whole group of diseases known as the auto-immune diseases in which the lymphocyte attacks are directed against the body rather than against any foreign invader. More will be said about lymphocytes in the Chapter on the lymphatic system and lymph.

a. B-lymphocytes. The precursors of these cells are formed in the bone marrow, but early in development they may be processed by the lymphoid tissue associated with the intestinal tract, for instance, the appendix and Peyer's patches. (The cells are called B-lymphocytes because the discovery of the lymphoid cell processing was first made in chickens where the intestinal lymphoid tissue is aggregated into a structure known as the bursa of Fabricius.)

B-lymphocytes are capable of becoming antibody-producing plasma cells when stimulated by antigen. These terms need to be defined: antigens are substances capable of

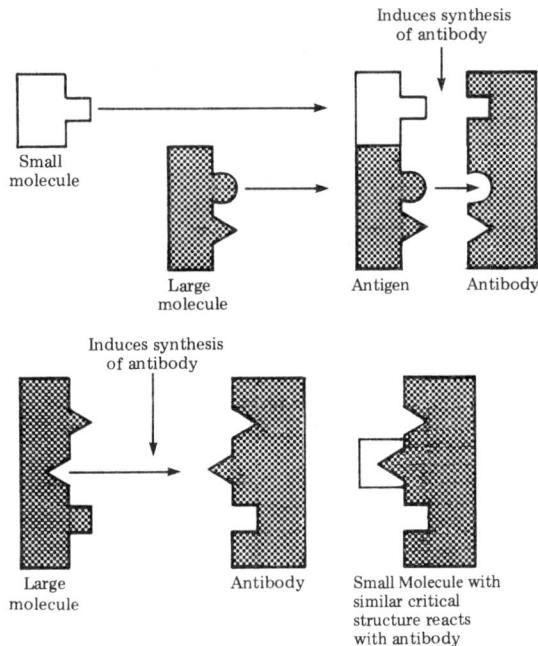

Figure 4.4   Antigen binding.

producing an immune response; they are usually complex macromolecules foreign to the body (however, almost anything, be it protein, carbohydrate or drug can be an antigen if it is properly introduced into the body). The immune response that the antigens generate in the case of B-lymphocyte and plasma cells is the production of antibody. An antibody is a protein, production of which is stimulated by a particular antigen. The antibody will react only with its particular antigen because the shape of the antibody is such that it can only bind ("fit") the antigen which initiated its synthesis (see Figure 4.4). Each molecule of antibody is capable of binding with at least two molecules of antigen. The antibody produced by the plasma cells does not destroy the antigen but may, by its binding, prevent the antigen from exerting its harmful effects.

There are many thousands of potential antigens and so the question arises; How can lymphocytes make specific antibodies to an antigen when there are so many different antigens? An analogy has been suggested which should be helpful. Once there was a man who wanted to purchase a dozen suits. These were to be special suits and were to fit only himself. He could go to a tailor who would take all his measurements and then make a suit which would be specifically for his shape. If this tailoring were not suitable, he could go instead to a store having thousands of different suits "ready-made", one of which would be certain to fit him. Once he came upon the suit that fitted him, he could order a dozen suits.

The production of antibody by B-lymphocytes is patterned like the selection of a "ready-made" suit. B-lymphocytes have receptors for antigen, though each cell will have receptors for only one particular kind of antigen and will produce only antibody to that one antigen. Before antigen can be produced, the B-cell must come into contact with the particular antigen that it is responsive to. There is some evidence that macrophages and/or T-cells may be required to present the

specific antigen to the specific B-cell. After the antigen has made proper contact with a specific B-cell, the B-cell undergoes a series of multiplications into daughter cells, some of which differentiate into antibody-producing cells. Other daughter cells become "memory" cells which will differentiate into plasma cells, will reproduce and rapidly produce antibody when the specific antigen is reintroduced at a later time. Plasma cells have more rough endoplasmic reticulum than do lymphocytes and are adapted for protein synthesis. With subsequent introduction of the specific antigen, the memory lymphocytes will rapidly differentiate, and reproduce themselves and release much larger amounts of antibody. This is referred to as the secondary response (see Figure 4.5).

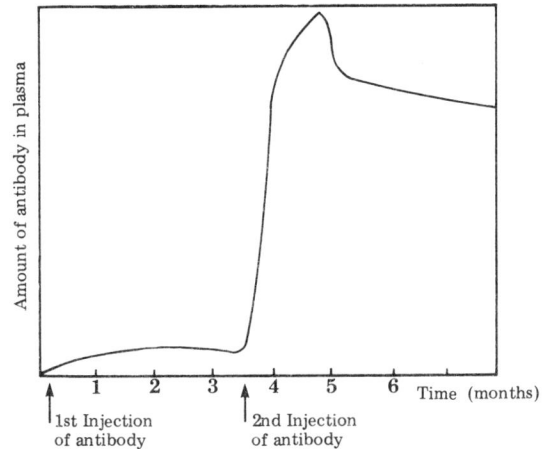

Figure 4.5   Antibody production. Rate following initial contact with an antigen and a subsequent contact with the same antigen.

These cellular activities can be illustrated by a specific example. Diphtheria is a disease caused by the toxin of the bacteria *Corynebacteria diphtheriae*. There was a diphtheria epidemic in Europe in 1944, when more than a million cases were reported, many of them fatalities. Today, diphtheria is not a threat in Europe or the United States because most infants are immunized against the disease. *C. diphtheriae* is cultivated, then its toxin is extracted and treated with formaldehyde and other chemicals. This treatment slightly alters the toxin molecule and reduces its virulence (its ability to cause harm). The altered toxin is called a toxoid. Infants usually receive injections of diphtheria toxoid simultaneously with tetanus toxoid and sometimes a suspension of killed whooping cough organisms. This is usually done in a total of three injections, each containing all three antigens. All this gives the infants immunity to these diseases for a number of years, after which a "booster" shot may be required. Should an immunized individual come in contact with diphtheria toxin, his "memory" cells are stimulated and his antibody production is great and rapid; the toxin is rendered harmless and disease does not occur.

Antibodies not only protect against viruses and bacterial toxins but may also lead to the destruction of bacteria. The walls of bacteria contain proteins and protein complexes which are capable of stimulating an antibody response. The combination of an antibody and bacterial cell wall antigen does not damage the bacteria unless there is present a series

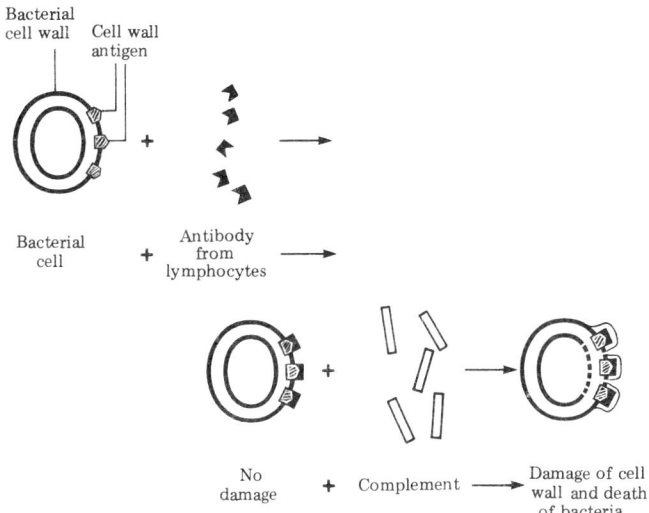

Figure 4.6 The bacterial-killing effects of antibody and complement.

of 11 plasma proteins which make up the complement system, more often called complement (see Figure 4.6). The combination of bacterial cell wall, antigen and antibody activate the complement system and lead to the lysis of the cell wall and death of the bacteria. The activated complement system also releases chemotactic factors which attract polymorphonuclear granulocytes. The complement system is also related to the blood clotting process. Activated Hageman factor will activate complement. Finally, complement, as well as antigens and specific antibodies, on the surface of a red cell membrane can lead to lysis of the red cell.

There are five different classes of antibodies made by the plasma cells. They all belong to the class of proteins known as immunoglobulins and are designated as IgG, IgA, IgM, IgD and IgE. All five classes of antibody may be made in response to a particular antigen.

(i) IgG. This is the most abundant of the immunoglobulins, having high concentrations in the blood and extravascular spaces. They provide most of the immunity to blood-borne infection, can activate complement and cross the placenta to provide a passively acquired immunity to the foetus. This immunity is, however, not lasting, for they cannot be supplied by the mother after birth and those immunoglobulins in the plasma will be destroyed in a matter of weeks.

(ii) IgA. This is the second most abundant of the immunoglobulins and is seen in many external secretions found in the respiratory, gastrointestinal and urogenital tracts.

(iii) IgM. Molecules of IgM are the largest of the immunoglobulins and can each bind ten antigenic sites. They are the first type to be synthesized in the immune response, can bind or agglutinate large particulate antigens such as bacteria and blood cells and can activate complement.

(iv) IgD. Little is known about this class.

(v) IgE. Like IgA this is found in the external secretions of the respiratory and gastrointestinal tracts. It has the ability to bind to mast cells. The combination of antigen and IgE antibody fixed to mast cells can lead to the release of histamine and other chemicals from the mast cells, leading to the allergic response.

b. T-lymphocytes. The precursors of these cells leave the bone marrow and are processed by the thymus gland early in development before being released into the circulation. They do not synthesize antibody but may co-operate with macrophages and help the B-cells to do so. T-lymphocytes have specific receptors for antigen, and when they make contact with it they release a variety of chemicals. The latter attract monocytes from the blood, stimulate their conversion to angry macrophages and inhibit the macrophages from leaving. Interferon may also be released, inhibiting the ability of viruses to reproduce.

Although the reaction between antigen and T-lymphocyte is specific, the net effects are destructive and not specific for that antigen. T-lymphocytes are important in immunity to tuberculosis and their activity is increased by the BCG tuberculosis vaccine.

T-lymphocytes have been implicated in graft or transplantation rejection. When a foreign tissue is grafted onto or into the body, the T-lymphocytes recognize the foreign antigens and may initiate a sequence of events leading to the destruction and possible rejection of the transplanted tissue. This may be prevented by treatment with immunosuppressive drugs or certain steroid hormones from the adrenal gland. Such treatment itself may cause problems, for, if the immune system is inhibited or suppressed, the patient is much more susceptible to infection.

Many tumour cells have specific antigens on their cell membrane. The role of T-lymphocytes in searching for these cells and possibly destroying them is currently being investigated. Research in immunology has made dramatic advances in the last few years. There are still major unanswered questions however. Why is it that immune response can be directed against one's own body or a transplanted organ, and yet it does not usually attack the foetus or a malignant tumour?

D. Platelets

The final category of cell is the platelets. The platelets are the smallest of all the blood cells, oval in shape, without a nucleus (see Figure 4.3f). They are really cytoplasmic fragments which have budded off the giant megakaryocytes which are found in the bone marrow. Their function is to stick to a blood vessel if it has been injured. Just as a patch on a tyre keeps the air within the tyre, so the platelets form a plug which helps keep blood within the circulatory system. Injury to a blood vessel usually exposes its collagen lining; platelets are attracted to the collagen.

Platelets also contain enzymes and chemicals which play a part in blood coagulation and a powerful vasoconstrictor agent known as serotonin. When a plug forms and serotonin is released, it causes the arterioles to constrict (become smaller). Since the blood vessels are now smaller, less blood can flow through the vessels so that the blood loss is reduced. The normal range of platelets in the blood is 150 000–450 000/mm^3.

WHAT IS PLASMA?

About 55% (100% − 45%) of the volume of blood is plasma and about 92% of plasma is water. There are some gases dissolved in plasma, and all oxygen and carbon dioxide must pass through the plasma on their way from the red cells to the tissues or *vice versa*. Plasma contains important nutrients like glucose, fatty and amino acids and hormones. In addition, plasma contains waste products like urea and many important inorganic ions such as sodium, potassium, calcium, chloride and bicarbonate (HCO_3^-).

The biggest constituent after water is the plasma protein, which normally weighs from 5 to 8 grams/100 ml of plasma. There are many types of plasma protein, including some enzymes. In some diseases, the cells become damaged and certain enzymes leak out of the tissues into the blood. For example, when heart muscle cells die or are injured, certain enzymes leak out of the cells into the blood. These enzymes are creatine phosphokinase (CPK), serum glutamic oxalacetic transaminase (SGOT) and lactic dehydrogenase (LDH), and their concentrations in the blood can help determine whether or not a myocardial infarction ("heart attack") has taken place, and they can provide some idea as to the size of the infarct.

The bulk of the plasma proteins are, however, usually classified into three distinct groups or fractions: the albumin fraction, the globulin fraction and fibrinogen. Albumin and fibrinogen are made in the liver; thus, if this organ is diseased or damaged it will be reflected in their decreased levels in the plasma.

A. Albumin

Albumin is the smallest of the plasma proteins in size and molecular weight (about 69 000). It makes up 80% of the plasma protein molecules so its chief role is in maintaining the osmotic pressure of the blood. Remember that the plasma is mostly water and it is imperative that the plasma water remains in the circulatory system and does not diffuse into the tissues. If the liver is diseased, as may happen if the individual drinks alcohol to excess, the liver may not be able to synthesize adequate amounts of protein, including albumin. As the albumin concentration decreases, the osmotic pressure of the plasma is reduced so more of the plasma water diffuses out of the circulatory system and into the other tissues.

Albumin also plays an important part in the transporting of many substances which are not very soluble in water and need a vehicle to take them from tissue to tissue; this group of molecules includes many drugs and hormones.

B. The globulins

This is a very diverse group of proteins and can be separated into four groups: the α_1 and α_2 globulins, the β globulins, and the γ globulins. The α_1, α_2 and β globulins are synthesized in the liver; the γ globulins are synthesized by the plasma cells in the lymphoid tissue and lymph.

a. The α_1 and α_2 globulins. This group contains ceruloplasmin (the copper-transporting protein) and haptaglobin (the protein which transports haemoglobin after it has been released from the red cell). Many of the α globulins are increased in inflammation, in tissue-injury and in cancer. The mechanism for this increase is not understood.

b. The β globulins. The two chief proteins in this group are the lipoproteins and transferrin. Just as oil and water don't mix, fats and plasma are not very soluble. Since fats supply a major portion of the energy, there must be a way to transport efficiently the fats in the plasma to the tissues even though the fats are not very soluble. Fat transport is accomplished by the fats binding to the lipoproteins: they are released from the lipoproteins to the tissues which metabolize them.

The other important β globulin is transferrin. This protein transfers iron from the intestine, where it is temporarily stored after absorption, to the liver, where it is stored and channelled into haemoglobin synthesis. Normally, the transferrin in the plasma is about one-third saturated with iron. The amount of transferrin and its per cent saturation change during certain infectious disease states and in iron deficiency.

c. The γ globulins. The γ globulin fraction contains the antibodies discussed in the section on B-lymphocytes. These include IgG, IgE and IgM. There are many commercial preparations of γ globulins available and in the past they have been widely used to prevent infection. Clinical experience of recent years has greatly reduced the number of conditions for which γ globulin therapy is appropriate.

A profile of the plasma proteins may provide some general information on a patient's status, though there are only a few conditions for which it can provide evidence of specific diagnostic importance. The technique used to provide this information is that of zone electrophoresis. This takes advantage of the fact that the proteins are charged particles; like charges repel, opposite charges attract. A very small amount of serum is placed on a strip of paper or cellulose acetate and an electric current is passed through the strip. The proteins will move at rates that are chiefly dependent on their charge. The more negatively charged proteins will move more rapidly than the less negatively charged proteins. The strip may then be stained to show the five groups and permit quantitation. A typical electrophoretic pattern is shown in Figure 4.7.

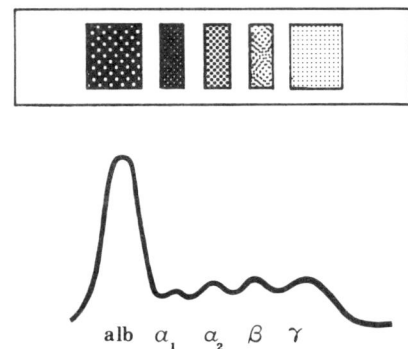

Figure 4.7 Normal electrophoretic strip and scan.

C. Fibrinogen

This protein is very important in the formation of a blood clot.

HOW DOES BLOOD CLOT?

This is a good question, but an equally good question is: why is it that most of the time blood does not clot? If a clot were to form within a blood vessel it could be very harmful, for it might block an artery and thus prevent oxygen from reaching the tissues supplied by that artery.

A clot is a jelly-like mass of cells trapped in a complex net of insoluble fibrin. Fibrin comes from fibrinogen, a protein that is present in plasma. In the final step of clot formation the enzyme, thrombin, splits off some amino acids from the fibrinogen molecule to form fibrin. This change permits the fibrin molecules to link together, to polymerize into long chains of fibrin. Calcium accelerates this polymerization, and other factors increase the strength of these fibrin strands by linking them together.

Thrombin comes from prothrombin, an enzyme circulating in the blood. The formation of thrombin from prothrombin can be triggered by either of two mechanisms:

In the extrinsic clotting pathway, injured tissues release an enzyme and other compounds which are grouped together under the name tissue thromboplastin (III) (see Figure 4.8). Thromboplastin and a plasma protein called convertin (VII) react with Stuart factor (X). Activated Stuart factor and pro-accelerin act as an enzyme to convert prothrombin (II) to thrombin. Calcium ions must be present for Stuart factor to be activated and for prothrombin to be converted to thrombin. In the hospital, the extrinsic clotting pathway is tested by the one-stage prothrombin time. Blood is drawn carefully (so as not injure tissue and release tissue thromboplastin) and calcium ions are removed to prevent clotting. When the test is ready to be run, calcium ions and tissue thromboplastin are added to the plasma and the time until a clot forms is measured. This test is usually called the pro-thrombin time.

In the intrinsic clotting pathway, a clot is formed without tissue injury and without tissue thromboplastin release. The principle is the same as the extrinsic clotting pathway in that there is an effect like a waterfall — one factor activating another, which in turn activates another. It is a more complex pathway, for more factors are involved and it also takes longer. Tissue thromboplastin is not involved. In summary: Activated Hageman factor activates plasma thromboplastin antecedent, PTA (XI), which activates Christmas factor (IX). Activated Christmas factor and antihaemophilic factor (VIII) work together to activate Stuart factor (X). Activated Stuart factor, lipid and proaccelerin (V) all work together to activate prothrombin (II). In the body, Hageman factor can be activated by making contact with the collagen lying beneath the endothelium, as might happen if the blood vessels are injured. Other intrinsic factors can activate Hageman factor, and its importance is not limited to formation of the blood clots. Activated Hageman factor eventually leads to the formation of plasmin from plasminogen. Plasmin attacks and disrupts fibrin causing dissolution of the clot.

In test tubes, the Hageman factor may be activated by glass and a number of other compounds including talc and spider's webs. The intrinsic clotting pathway is measured by adding kaolin, a Hageman factor activator, and calcium ions to calcium-free plasma. The test is called the partial thromboplastin time (PTT) and is the most sensitive and useful test of clot-forming ability. Serum is the clear fluid that would remain in the test tube after the clot has been removed.

A thrombus is a clot or plug in a blood vessel, or one of the chambers of the heart. The clot remains at the point of its formation. An embolus is a clot which forms in one blood vessel and travels in the circulation until it becomes stuck in a smaller blood vessel. Patients who are immobile after surgery are particularly susceptible to emboli formation. Large clots can build up in the leg vein, break loose and block an artery in the lung with very serious consequences for the patient. For example, if an embolus travelled through the arterial system and lodged in one of the small arteries of the brain, the brain tissue supplied by that artery might die for lack of oxygen-carrying blood.

Our knowledge of how to prevent clotting began in the

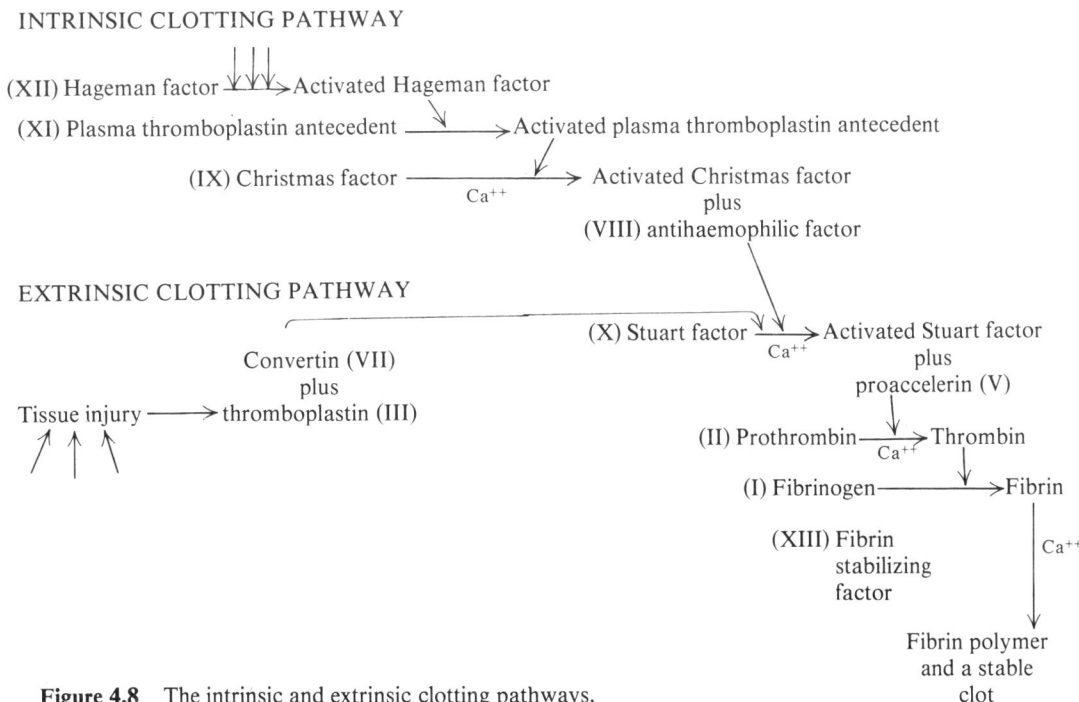

INTRINSIC CLOTTING PATHWAY

(XII) Hageman factor ⟶ Activated Hageman factor

(XI) Plasma thromboplastin antecedent ⟶ Activated plasma thromboplastin antecedent

(IX) Christmas factor ⟶ Activated Christmas factor
Ca^{++} plus
(VIII) antihaemophilic factor

EXTRINSIC CLOTTING PATHWAY

Convertin (VII)
plus
Tissue injury ⟶ thromboplastin (III)

(X) Stuart factor ⟶ Activated Stuart factor
Ca^{++} plus
proaccelerin (V)

(II) Prothrombin ⟶ Thrombin
Ca^{++}

(I) Fibrinogen ⟶ Fibrin

(XIII) Fibrin
stabilizing
factor Ca^{++}

Fibrin polymer
and a stable
clot

Figure 4.8 The intrinsic and extrinsic clotting pathways.

1920s with some farmers whose cattle were dying because they were bleeding to death after cutting themselves on the sharp barbed-wire surrounding their pastures. Scientists became interested as to why the cow blood would not clot. They investigated and learned that a chemical in the improperly-cured hay that the cows ate was responsible; today this chemical is known as dicoumarol. It prevents clotting by interfering with the action of vitamin K. This vitamin is necessary for the synthesis by the liver of several clotting factors including prothrombin. If there is no vitamin K or if its action is blocked by dicoumarol, blood will not clot. Heparin is another anticoagulant and is immediately effective, whereas dicoumarol takes about three days to become effective. Heparin blocks the action of thrombin and prevents prothrombin from being converted to thrombin.

Any compound which binds or removes calcium ions will prevent clotting by inhibiting the conversion of prothrombin to thrombin. Compounds that bind calcium include citrate, oxalate and ethylenediamine tetra-acetic acid (EDTA).

With so many factors involved in the clotting process it is not surprising that defects can arise and that there are patients whose blood does not clot. This can happen for a number of reasons: the clotting factor may not be synthesized at all or it may be synthesized in a non-functional form, or there may be present some antagonists or even antibodies to the factor.

The most famous of the clotting diseases is haemophilia. In classic haemophilia, the antihaemophilic factor which is synthesized is non-functional and the intrinsic clotting pathway cannot be activated. Haemophiliacs will have a long PTT and are threatened by the possibility of serious internal haemorrhage. The disorder is hereditary and usually limited to males. The son of a haemophiliac will neither have the disease nor carry the gene for the disease; however, his daughter will usually not have any symptoms of the disease but will pass it on to 50% of her sons, while 50% of her daughters will be carriers of the disease.

It is interesting to note that haemophiliacs will have a normal bleeding time. The bleeding time is a test that measures the time until a very small cut, most likely of the finger tip, stops bleeding. Haemophiliacs have normal platelet function and the bleeding time test is an indicator of this function.

The bleeding time, prothrombin time and PTT are common clinical tests. They are used as screening tests for suspected blood diseases and are routinely used to test the clotting ability prior to a patient's going to surgery.

WHAT ABOUT TRANSFUSIONS?

There are times when a person cannot increase his rate of red cell synthesis fast enough to keep up with his body's needs. A person who has lost a lot of blood or is very anaemic might need a transfusion, a reception of someone else's blood. Not very long ago, all that was necessary for a transfusion was a donor, someone willing to give his blood to someone else. Sometimes the patient, or the recipient, would improve after the transfusion and some times the transfusion would only add to his or her distress. Today we know more about blood and why certain transfusions were bound to fail.

The red blood cell membrane has a glycoprotein (carbo-

hydrate plus protein) structure called an agglutinogen. The agglutinogen can have two different shapes, and you can imagine that one of them is "A"-shaped and the other is "B"-shaped, though in reality this is not true. With two kinds of agglutinogens, it would be possible to have four different kinds of red cell membranes. Red cell type "A" would have the A agglutinogen on its membrane, type "B" the B agglutinogen, type "AB" would have both the A and the B agglutinogens, while blood type "O" would have no agglutinogen on its membrane.

In the plasma are agglutinins. Agglutinins are specific proteins that react with certain agglutinogens, much like an antigen–antibody reaction. When an agglutinogen and its complementary agglutinin come together the red cells stick to one another and the process is called agglutination. Agglutination should not be confused with coagulation, for in agglutination the cell membrane is destroyed and haemolysis results. There are two types of agglutinins and, therefore, four kinds of plasma. There is the agglutinin which reacts only with the A agglutinin and is called anti-A; and the agglutinin which reacts only with the B agglutinogen and is known as anti-B. Some people have both anti-A and anti-B, while others have neither. Since, normally, blood cells are not haemolyzed, you can deduce that a person does not have agglutinins against his own agglutinogens. This is correct, for it has been shown that a person with a type A cells has anti-B in his plasma, while type B carries anti-A; blood type AB carries no agglutinins, while type O has both anti-A and anti-B agglutinins (see Figure 4.9).

In transfusing blood it is important to ensure that the donor's red cells will not be haemolyzed by the agglutinins in the recipient's plasma. Ideally, this is done by transfusing only identical types of blood. Often, particularly in rural hospitals, it is not possible to match the recipient's blood with an identical type. Should this be the case, it is necessary to give a blood type, the red cells of which will not be agglutinated by the agglutinins in the recipient's plasma — for

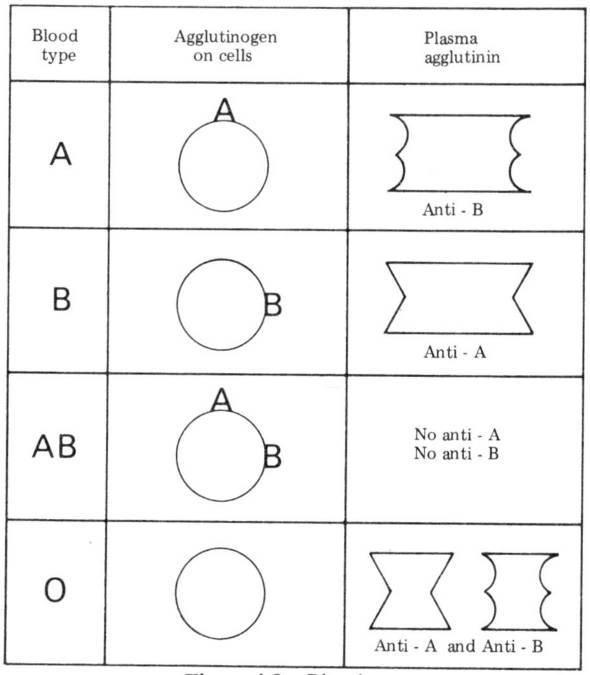

Blood type	Agglutinogen on cells	Plasma agglutinin
A	A	Anti - B
B	B	Anti - A
AB	A B	No anti - A No anti - B
O		Anti - A and Anti - B

Figure 4.9 Blood types.

example, you would never want to give type A to type B or *vice versa*. There is a simple mnemonic for remembering which types can be transfused in an emergency. The rule to remember is that any group can give to the group beneath it or receive from the ones above it (see Figure 4.10). Since O can give to O, A, B and AB it is called the universal donor. AB is called the universal recipient because it can receive from O, A and B.

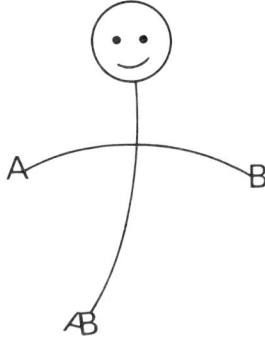

Figure 4.10 Any blood group can give to the blood group beneath it or receive from the blood group above it.

In addition to the A, B, AB and O agglutinogens, there are many other agglutinogens. One group is the Rh series of agglutinogens. The same principle applies to the Rh agglutinogen as to the other groups: if the red cell contains the Rh agglutinogen, the plasma will not contain any Rh factor. People who carry the Rh factor are often said to be Rh-positive or, simply, positive. My blood type is B-positive. This means my red cells contain both the B and Rh agglutinogen while my plasma contains anti-A agglutinin. If a Rh-negative person receives Rh-positive blood he or she will become sensitized and their lymphocytes will produce anti-Rh antibodies. These are not harmful unless a second transfusion of Rh-positive blood is given, which leads to a secondary immune response that will cause agglutination.

Should an Rh-positive man marry a Rh-negative woman it is possible that a Rh-positive child will be conceived. Significant amounts of foetal red cells enter the mother's circulation during parturition. The numbers are such that they can stimulate antibody production or sensitize the mother. During a second pregnancy, the small number of Rh-positive cells which do cross the placenta long before parturition takes place can initiate a secondary immune response in which maternal agglutinins will be synthesized in

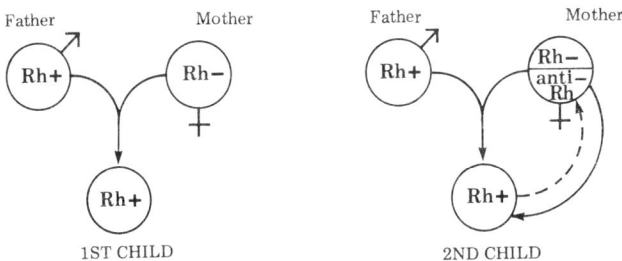

Figure 4.11 The red cells in the second foetus will be destroyed by anti-Rh from the mother, which she synthesizes in response to the Rh positive cells which escaped into her circulation from the first foetus at parturition. If the mother is given anti-Rh immediately after the birth of the first child, it will react with the Rh of the foetal cells and she will not synthesize any anti-Rh of her own.

large amounts and will attack and destroy the foetal red cells. This disease is known as erythroblastosis foetalis. The only way to save the life of the foetus is to give it transfusions of Rh-negative blood. Erythroblastosis foetalis can be prevented if, immediately after the birth of the first Rh-positive child, the mother is given anti-Rh agglutinins. The agglutinins will react with the agglutinogens of the foetal red cells which have escaped into the mother's blood and will destroy them as well as prevent them from initiating any immunological response in the mother. Thus, no anti-Rh will be synthesized and the cells of the second foetus will be safe (see Figure 4.11).

SOME CLINICAL CONSIDERATIONS

Patients in hospital sometimes complain that they feel like pin cushions because they are so often stuck with needles to have blood samples drawn. Much useful information concerning the patient can be ascertained from the blood. Supposing you are helping to take care of a patient who is scheduled to have a major surgical procedure, what sort of information could be obtained from the blood that might prove useful?

Prior to surgery it is necessary to be certain that the patient is not seriously anaemic and has sufficient blood to tolerate the stress of surgery. It would be more than embarrassing if the surgeon were to discover during the operation that the patient had a deficiency of one or more of the clotting factors or had been taking an anti-coagulant. To eliminate these possibilities the prothrombin and partial thromboplastin times can be measured.

Even with the best of surgeons, some patients' blood loss is inevitable and, depending on the surgical procedure, blood loss may be quite significant. To lessen the possibility of the patient's bleeding to death, a sample of blood is drawn prior to surgery and sent to the blood bank to be "typed and crossed". This means that the patient's blood will be typed as to whether or not it is A Rh-positive, B Rh-negative, etc., and it will be cross-matched to blood from a donor. The donor's blood will probably have been treated with citrate to remove the calcium and prevent it from clotting while being stored. The donor's blood is also checked to see that it does not contain certain infectious agents.

It might also be important to know that the patient's electrolytes are in order, i.e. sodium, potassium, chloride and calcium ions are within normal limits. This information would be derived from a blood sample.

Of course, you don't have to be having major surgery to merit an examination of some blood function. An haematocrit is such an inexpensive, simple test to perform that it is part of many screening procedures, and it is always useful to be certain there is no anaemia.

If a person has a fever it may be important to know if there is a leucocytosis and the body is responding to an infection. A look at a blood smear and a differential count could help to rule out a leukaemia and could discriminate between a bacterial infection, which tends to be associated with increased neutrophils, and the lymphocytosis sometimes associated with increased neutrophils, and the lymphocytosis occasionally associated with viral infection.

The above is not exhaustive but may help the sceptical to proceed with their studies in the hope that they actually are of value.

5. The Skeletal System

INTRODUCTION

All too often students beginning the study of the skeletal system are overwhelmed by the anatomy and the task of learning the bones and their often strange-sounding names. Students may lose sight of the fact that bone is a living tissue, with a very active metabolism which is controlled and regulated by hormonal and nutritional factors. One of the best illustrations of the dynamic nature of bone is the fact that they mend and build themselves anew once they have been broken. Although bones can break they are really very strong for their weight, being stronger than most woods and about the strength of cast iron. In addition to supporting the body and protecting certain organs, the bones provide attachment for most voluntary muscles, form a large reservoir of calcium and produce blood cells.

WHAT IS THE STRUCTURE OF BONE?

Bone is a connective tissue and, thus, has cells, fibres and intercellular substance. It differs from cartilage in that it is very vascular and has a great reconstructive capacity when it has been injured. A typical bone has four components (see Figure 5.1).

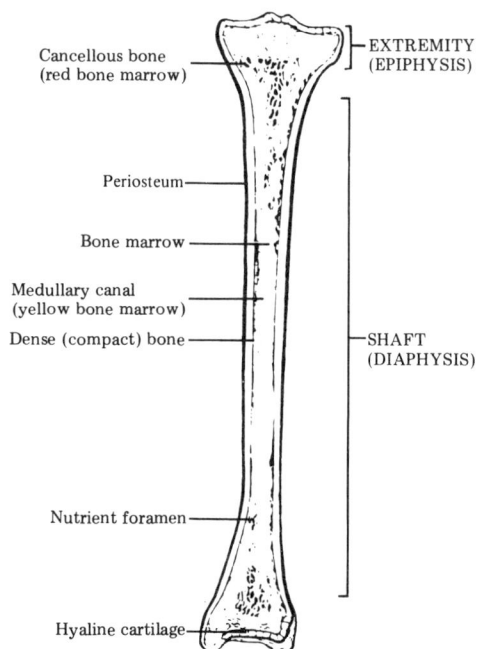

Figure 5.1 Longitudinal section of a typical (long) bone.

A. The periosteum

The periosteum is a membrane covering all bone surfaces except joint surfaces, which are covered with hyaline cartilage. The outermost layer of the periosteum is tough, fibrous and made of dense, collagenous connective tissue through which blood vessels and nerves pass and distribute themselves. The inner layer is loose connective tissue and contains cells involved in the building, maintenance and remodelling of bone. A similar membrane of loose connective tissue, the endosteum, lines the marrow bone cavity and extends into the canal system that is found throughout the hard and cancellous parts of the bone.

There are four types of cells unique to bone. These are:

(1) Osteoprogenitor cells
(2) Osteoblasts
(3) Osteoclasts
(4) Osteocytes

Osteocytes are the principal cells of mature bone and are found in the lacunae of the calcified interstitial substance. Osteoprogenitor cells, osteoblasts and osteoclasts are found within the loose connective tissue of the endosteum, the canal system and periosteum. These cells are discussed in the coming sections. The periosteum serves a protective function, participates in and also limits bone growth and contributes to the attachment of tendons from skeletal muscle.

B. Dense (compact) bone

This is the strongest component of bone and is tough and hard like the ivory of an elephant's tusks. Under the microscope a transverse section of dense bone shows a beautiful series of circles within circles (see Figure 5.2).

In the centre of each circle, running parallel to the long axis of the bone, is the Haversian canal. These canals

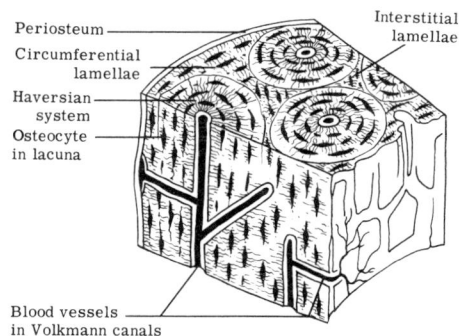

Figure 5.2 Dense (compact) bone.

are named after the anatomist who discovered them and each contains an artery, vein and the nerves which supply them. Intersecting the Haversian canals are the Volkmann canals which pass horizontally through the bone and also contain nerves and blood vessels.

Surrounding each Haversian canal are circularly arranged layers (lamellae). Chemically they are made of mucopolysaccharide and collagen fibres upon which calcium and phosphate ions have combined and initiated the process of crystal formation. A crystal has a symmetric form, a great rigidity and an ability to withstand mechanical stress; this is because of the regular and fixed arrangement of the molecules within it. Many of the crystals in bone are hydroxy-apatite: $3Ca_3(PO_4)_2.Ca(OH)_2$. The arrangement of both the collagen fibres and the crystals which are embedded in the fibres is highly ordered. This double ordering of collagen and crystal is responsible for the great strength of bone tissue. It is possible to dissolve the crystals out of the bone tissue by placing a bone in a dilute acid solution; without the crystals, bone is very flexible.

Bone may also contain other elements beside those mentioned. The strontium isotope (^{90}Sr), which is released during some atomic explosions, is absorbed by the body and has a very harmful effect on bone and will cause malignant degeneration of the tissue. Lead is sometimes eaten by children in flakes of leaded paint, or consumed in foods stored in lead-lined containers, or breathed in the air from paint vapours, or can be inhaled in the fumes arising from combustion of petrol which contains lead. The lead can be absorbed into the bone crystal and accumulate there until a fever or an increase in metabolic activity releases it into the blood. Lead poisoning has different forms and affects many tissues but the central nervous system is often more seriously affected.

Circularly arranged within the lamellae are lacunae or small cavities which contain osteocytes. Originally osteocytes were osteoblasts which formed collagen and released enzymes, including the enzyme, alkaline phosphatase, which induced the precipitation of calcium and phosphate upon the collagen. As crystal formation increases, the osteoblasts become less active and become osteocytes. The long, slender processes of the osteocytes project into the canaliculi, which are small channels connecting with the larger Haversian canals. Pictures taken through an electron microscope show that the osteocytes in neighbouring lacunae make contact with one another at the ends of their slender processes. This helps to explain how stimuli or events taking place at the outer surface of the bone can influence distant osteocytes.

Osteocytes can, in response to hormonal stimulation, change their metabolic activity and release enzymes which break down bone; this leads to a release of calcium ions from the bone into the blood. It is possible that an osteocyte might become an osteoclast. These osteoclasts are cells which are able to release enzymes, such as collagenase and acid phosphatase, which can break down collagen, dissolve crystal and release calcium ions. Nutrients from the Haversian canals reach the osteocytes via the canaliculi; inasmuch as the canaliculi are small and relatively inefficient transport systems, an osteocyte must be no more than a fraction of a millimetre away from an Haversian canal if it is to receive sufficient nutrients and survive.

C. Cancellous bone

Chemically this is similar to dense bone but it has a very different, somewhat spongy appearance. This is because the Haversian system is much less ordered if not as dense. Some cancellous bone receives its nutrients from blood vessels which branch before entering it. Cancellous bone also contains marrow.

D. Bone marrow

In the adult two kinds of marrow are found, red marrow and yellow marrow. Red marrow is found in the meshes of cancellous bone. It contains a supporting network of reticular fibres, and parent and stem cells which develop and differentiate into various blood cells. (The Chapter on the blood should be consulted for details on the control of blood cell formation.) Red marrow is also found in the long tubular medullary cavity of bones in the foetus.

In many bones this red marrow ceases to produce cells and becomes infiltrated with adipose tissue which gives it a yellowish colour. This changeover takes place slowly from childhood to maturity; however, the cavities of the sternum, rib bones, vertebrae and skull resist this process and continue to manufacture blood cells throughout life.

E. Cells in bone and their control

It is necessary to know how certain cells function in bone if you are to get a better understanding of how bone is formed, remodelled and participates in calcium homeostasis.

Osteoprogenitor cells are found in the inner loose connective tissue of the periosteum, the endosteum, the Haversian and Volkmann canals and in the cartilage of the epiphyseal plate of growing bones. Osteoprogenitor cells give rise to osteoclasts, osteoblasts and osteocytes. Osteoclasts are essentially bone-destroying cells, and osteoblasts are essentially bone-forming cells. Surprisingly, although osteoclasts and osteoblasts have different functions, it is possible for osteoclasts to become osteoblasts, and osteoblasts to become osteocytes and possibly even osteoclasts.

The conversion of these cell types and their subsequent actions are strongly influenced by two hormones; parathyroid hormone (PTH) which is produced by the parathyroid gland, and calcitonin (CT) which is produced by the "C" cells of the thyroid gland and also by the thymus gland. PTH seems to stimulate the conversion of progenitor cells to osteoclasts. The hormone also seems to stimulate the osteoclasts to release hydrolytic enzymes from their lysosomes and produce an acid environment by synthesizing lactic and citric acids. PTH can also stimulate osteolytic activity in osteocytes. The net effects of PTH on bone are to promote the resorption (breakdown) of bone and, by doing so, raise the blood calcium ion concentration. PTH has other effects outside bone and can influence the conversion of vitamin D to a more potent form, which then increases calcium absorption by the digestive tract, and PTH can promote phosphate excretion by the kidneys.

CT seems to be able to promote bone formation by inhibiting the osteolytic activity of osteocytes, promoting the conversion of osteoclasts to osteoblasts, and stimulating osteoblasts to greater activity. By its actions on bone, CT is able to lower the level of calcium ion in the blood. CT is particularly important in infants and children who consume milk and other calcium-containing foods and who must deposit this calcium in bone mineral.

In a typical 70 kg adult, 1 kg of mass would be calcium; 99% of this calcium is in bone. Calcium is lost in the urine and faeces, so about 1 gram of calcium a day is required for an adult to stay in calcium balance. CT, PTH and other hormones function to keep the calcium ion in the blood within normal limits, and to keep in balance the continuous bone-forming–bone-destroying processes.

Other aspects of calcium metabolism are discussed in the Chapter on the endocrine system.

Bones may also be classified according to their shape:

a. Long bones. The majority of bones in the skeleton are long bones. Each bone has an elongated shaft (diaphysis) with enlarged endings called epiphyses (see Figure 5.1). The shaft or the diaphysis surrounds the medullary cavity and is made of dense bone, while the epiphyses have a thin layer of dense bone which covers the cancellous bone. Blood vessels which supply the shaft and some of the epiphyses enter the bone through an opening called the nutrient foramen. The bones of the limbs are long bones.

b. Short bones. These bones are found in the wrist and ankle and are box-like in shape. They do not have a shaft and consist of a small amount of cancellous bone covered with dense bone.

c. Flat bones. The skull bones are examples of flat bones. They have a layer of cancellous bone sandwiched between two layers of dense bone. In some of the skull bones part of the cancellous bone is absorbed and hollow sinuses are formed.

d. Irregular bones. The shape of these bones cannot be described simply, for it is so variable. Like other bones they consist of dense bone which surrounds cancellous bone. The vertebrae are examples of irregular bones.

e. Sesamoid bones. These bones might be considered irregular bones because of their shape, yet they are given a separate classification, for they develop from and within tendons. The patella (knee cap) is an example of a sesamoid bone.

HOW DOES BONE DEVELOP?

Bone development is influenced by many factors. Genetic inheritance plays a role as evidenced by the fact that tall parents generally have tall children. Nutritional factors are important, for malnutrition can hinder a child's growth. Vitamins C and D are important and there must be adequate calcium and phosphate in the diet. The amount of fluoride ion may be important as well. Growth hormone, somatomedin, PTH, thyroid hormone, CT, insulin, androgens, oestrogens and glucocorticoids are among the hormones which influence growth processes.

Ossification (bone formation) begins with pre-existing connective tissue and proceeds by one of two possible mechanisms:

a. Endochondral ossification. In the foetus, hyaline cartilage models of the bones are formed in the sites which

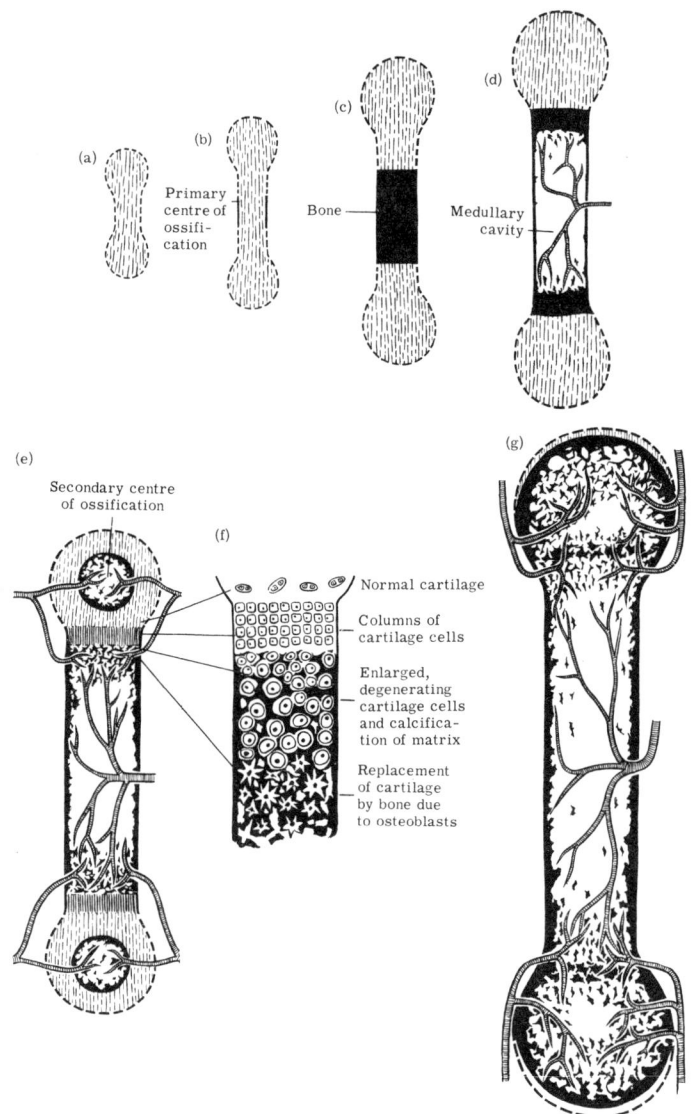

Figure 5.3 Cartilaginous (endochondral) ossification of a typical long bone. (a) Cartilaginous model (about 6–7 weeks of foetal life). (b) Primary centre of ossification round shaft (about 8 weeks of foetal life). (c) Ossification spreading in shaft. (d) Formation of medullary cavity and vascularization of shaft (before birth). (e) Vascularization of end bones (epiphysis) and commencing ossification of epiphysis (secondary centres of ossification); separation of shaft from epiphysis by cartilaginous epiphyseal plate (growth plate). (f) Details of growth plate. (g) Adult bone showing disappearance of growth plates (fusion of epiphyses with shaft) at 16–18 years.

will later be occupied by mature bone (see Figure 5.3). After the 2nd month of foetal life, the cartilage within the diaphysis becomes calcified and begins to break down. This degenerating cartilage is invaded by capillaries and other cells, including osteoblasts from the periosteum which surrounds the cartilaginous model. The osteoblasts secrete collagen, and alkaline phosphatase activity helps cause ion precipitation and initiate crystal formation. From this primary centre, ossification spreads upward and downward towards each epiphysis. After birth the epiphyses are vascularized and the process repeats itself so that each epiphysis is ossified, except for the cartilage which remains on the surface and articulates with other bones. A zone of cartilage, called the epiphyseal plate, remains between each epiphysis and the diaphysis and continues to grow. Growth continues at the epiphyseal plate and is responsible for much of the longitudinal growth of bones which takes place over the first two decades of life. Ultimately, when the areas of spreading ossification in the diaphysis and epiphyses meet, further growth in length is impossible; this is called closure of the epiphyses.

Growth in the width of long bones takes place by intramembranous ossification and involves osteoblasts of the periosteum. While the bone is formed on the outside, bone resorption (breakdown) takes place on the inside in the medullary canal as a result of osteoclast activity. As bone is laid down superficially it is removed internally so that the width of the bone and the medullary canal increases but the actual thickness of the dense bone remains the same (see Figure 5.4). This correlates with the histology which shows that osteoblasts predominate in the periosteum and osteoclasts predominate in the endosteum. Hormonal deficiencies or excesses can upset the remodelling process. In a healthy adult, bone resorption and bone formation occur at approximately the same rate, although with advanced age there is a decrease in the quantity of bone tissue. This is called osteopenia.

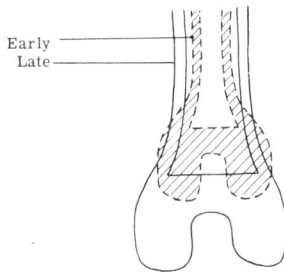

Figure 5.4 Modelling of lower end of femur during growth in length and width.

b. *Intramembranous ossification*. This process occurs on the surface of bones formed by endochondral ossification, and is also entirely responsible for the formation of bones in the vault of the skull which covers the brain and also parts of the facial skeleton. It is not preceded by cartilage formation. Instead, in those places where the bone is to develop, a membrane of loose connective tissue is first formed. Cells within this membrane differentiate and become osteoblasts. These cells multiply, secrete collagen and alkaline phosphatase and the collagen becomes calcified and ossified. This ossified tissue replaces the original membrane. This process is not completed at birth but has advanced far enough so that adjacent bones are separated by a strip of connective tissue called a suture because of its resemblance to stitches (sutures). Where more than two cranial bones approach each other there will be a large area of connective tissue between them and this is referred to as a fontanelle. (These will be discussed in more detail later in this Chapter.)

Growth processes continue in the infant skull so room is made for the rapidly growing brain. Much of the bone formed on the inner surface is destroyed by osteoclasts while new bone is formed on the outer surface by osteoblasts from the periosteum; this permits the skull to enlarge as the brain expands.

SOME DEFINITIONS

There are many specific terms associated with bones in addition to their names. All bones are not straight and smooth structures but have many irregularities where they articulate with one another, have attachments for muscles or openings for the passage of nerves and blood vessels. It is necessary to know these terms to understand the descriptions of the bones which follow:

Articulation — a joint (union) between two bones.
Border — the edge (ridge) which separates two surfaces of a bone.
Facet — a small and usually flat articulating surface.
Foramen (foramina) — an opening or hole in a bone.
Fossa (fossae) — depression or notch.
Meatus — a tube-shaped cavity within a bone.

The projections from bones have many names. Where they form a joint they are smooth, whereas they are rough if they serve to attach muscles. The size of the rough projection will depend on the number of muscles attached and the force of their contraction.

Articular projections (smooth)
Condyle — a smooth oval-shaped projection.
Head — a smooth rounded projection.

Non-articular projections (rough)
Process — a projection.
Tubercle — a small projection.
Tuberosity — a larger projection.
Trochanter — still larger projection.

WHAT IS THE ANATOMY OF THE SKELETAL SYSTEM?

The skeletal system is composed of about 200 bones which make up the living framework of the body. It may be divided into the axial skeleton and the appendicular skeleton. The axial skeleton includes the skull, vertebrae, ribs and sternum. The appendicular skeleton refers to those bones which are attached or appended to the axial skeleton and includes the limb bones and pectoral and pelvic girdles. In anatomic usage the upper extremity refers to the pectoral girdle and upper limb, while the lower extremity refers to the pelvic girdle and lower limb.

In learning the bones you can be helped by the text and descriptions, but actually seeing and examining the bones or models of them is by far the best method of learning. Another useful technique is to make simple sketches of the bones and list the bones they articulate with.

THE AXIAL SKELETON

A. The Skull

The skull or bony framework of the head rests upon the upper or cephalic end of the vertebral column and has two divisions, the cranium and the face. In the adult the skull bones are firmly united except for the lower jaw (mandible), whose motion is easily demonstrated by yawning or chewing.

a. The cranium

The cranium is a box-like structure which supports and protects the brain. The dome-shaped roof of the cranium is called the vault, while the floor is called the base of the skull. The vault is also called the skull cap or calvaria (calvarium is incorrect).

The cranium consists of eight bones (see Figure 5.5):

1 Frontal
2 Parietal
1 Occipital
2 Temporal
1 Sphenoid
1 Ethmoid

(1) *The frontal bone* forms the forehead and the upper part of the orbit of the eye. Above each orbit is a ridge to which the facial muscles used in raising the eyebrows are attached. Above the nose and between the two layers of dense bone are the frontal sinuses. Developmentally the frontal bone is formed from two parts which are separated by the single frontal suture. By the eighth year a single bone has been formed and the frontal suture has disappeared. In the adult other sutures remain, the largest being the two coronal sutures which separate the two parietal bones from the frontal bone. The frontal bone also forms immovable joints with the sphenoid, zygomatic, lachrymal, nasal and ethmoid bones.

(2) *The parietal bones* form the largest part of the side walls and part of the roof of the cranium. The parietal bones articulate with each other in the midline by the sagittal suture; anteriorly with the frontal bone via the coronal suture, posteriorly with the occipital bone via the lambdoid suture and laterally with the temporal bones via the squamous suture.

(3) *The occipital bone* is a flat bone which forms part of the back and the base of the skull (see Figures 5.5 and 5.6). It articulates with the parietal bone via the lambdoid suture and also with the temporal and sphenoid bones. The bone curves down and inward; in this inner cavity rests the hindbrain. On the outer surface is the occipital protuberance to which the muscles involved in raising and lowering the head attach. Two condyles project downward on each side of the bone

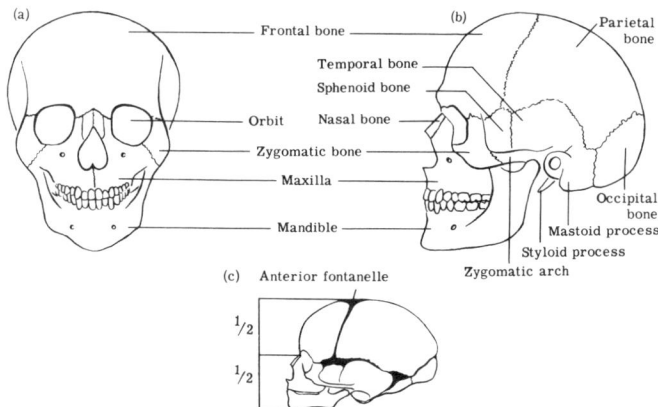

Figure 5.6　Base of the skull. (a) Inferior view. (b) Superior view.

and articulate with the atlas, the first bone of the vertebral column. The joint formed by the occipital articular condyles and the atlas is a hinge joint which is involved in nodding the head. Beside each condyle is the hypoglossal canal through which cranial nerve XII (the hypoglossal) leaves the skull to innervate the tongue. Between the two occipital articular condyles is the foramen magnum through which the spinal cord, nerves, ligaments and blood vessels pass to and from the brain.

The word occipital is derived from the Latin word *occipio* meaning I begin. The occipital bones are the first part of the skull to emerge from the birth canal during normal childbirth.

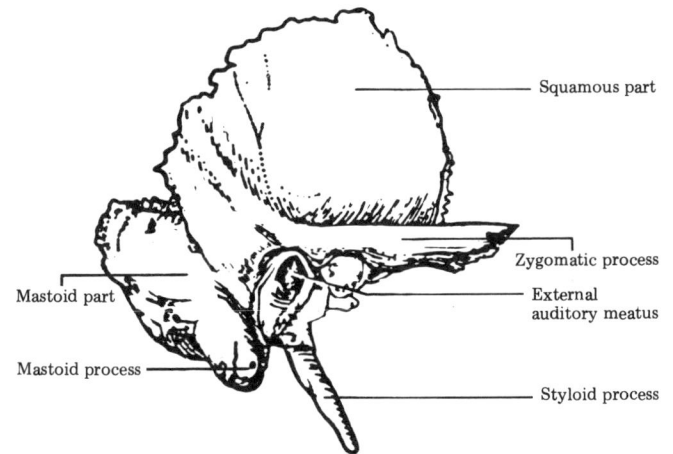

Figure 5.7　The temporal bone.

(4) *The temporal bones* form the lower sides of the skull (see Figure 5.7). Each temporal bone can be described as having four parts:

(i) The squamous part is a fan-shaped portion which articulates with the parietal bone above at the squamous suture and anteriorly with the sphenoid bone. The zygomatic process projects forward from the squamous part to meet the zygomatic bone and so completes the zygomatic arch.

(ii) The mastoid part lies below and behind the squamous part. You can feel the mastoid process of the mastoid bone if you place your hand behind your ear. The mastoid bone contains small air spaces communicating with the middle ear. These air spaces are lined with mucous membrane and may become infected. The sternocleidomastoid muscle attaches to the mastoid process and is important in turning the head either to the right or to the left and also flexion.

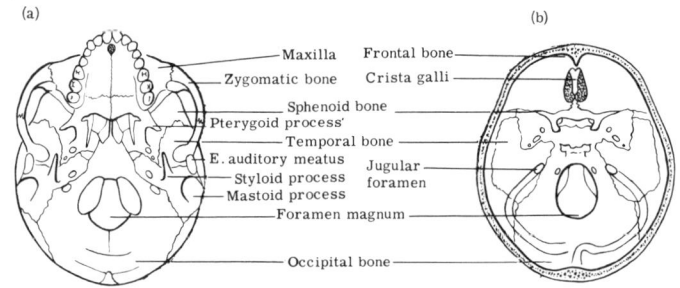

Figure 5.5　The bones of the skull. (a) Anterior view. (b) Side view. (c) Proportions.

(iii) The styloid process is a long thin bone which curves downward and forward from near the mastoid process. The styloid process serves as an attachment for the styloglossus, stylopharyngeus and stylohyoid muscles which move the tongue, pharynx and hyoid bone respectively.

(iv) The petrous portion of the temporal bone is not seen from a lateral view of the skull, for it is deep within the base of the skull. Each petrous bone contains either the right or left inner ear. The posterior portion of the petrous bone contains an opening, the internal auditory (acoustic) meatus, through which cranial nerves VIII (auditory) and VII (facial) leave the cranial cavity. The jugular foramen is a large opening situated between the lateral part of the occipital bone and petrous portion of the temporal bone. Cranial nerves IX (glossopharyngeal), X (vagus) and XI (spinal accessory) leave through this opening.

The word temporal is derived from the Latin word *tempus* meaning time. With time, grey hairs usually first appear in the area over the temporal bone.

(5) *The single sphenoid bone* is an irregular, wedge-shaped bone which lies in the centre of the base of the skull and is not visible from the outside. It has a central body and two wings, and is said to resemble the shape of a bat (see Figure 5.6). On the upper surface of the body is a small depression called the sella turcica (hypophyseal fossa) in which the pituitary gland sits. In the anterior medial part of the bone are four openings — two on either side. The round opening is the foramen rotundum and through it passes the maxillary branch of cranial nerve V (trigeminal). The mandibular branch of cranial nerve V passes through the foramen ovale. The superior portion of the bone contains the optic foramen through which cranial nerve II (optic) and the ophthalmic artery pass on their way to the eye. The sphenoid articulates with the frontal, temporal, parietal, ethmoid, zygomatic, vomer, palatine and occipital bones. (There are twelve altogether — four single, four paired.)

(6) *The ethmoid bone* is a box-shaped bone which occupies the anterior portion of the base of the skull. The roof of the ethmoid bone forms the cribriform plate, which is behind the frontal bone between the two orbits; the cribriform plate is perforated and through it pass fibres of the olfactory nerve fibres carrying smell information to the brain. Perpendicular to, and suspended from, the cribriform plate is the perpendicular plate. The perpendicular plate projects downward from the roof and forms the upper part of the nasal septum which separates the right and left nasal cavities. The side wall of each ethmoid bone contains projections which extend into the nasal cavities; the upper projection is the superior nasal concha, while the one beneath it is the middle concha. There is an inferior nasal concha below the middle concha which is a separate bone and is classified with the bones of the face. The structure of the nasal cavity will be covered after completing the bones of the face, and there are additional details in the Chapter on the respiratory system. Because of its shape and position, the ethmoid bone contributes to the formation of the base of the skull, the orbital cavity, the nasal septum and the walls of the nasal cavity. Both the sphenoid and the ethmoid bones contain sinuses.

There is a considerable amount of ossification of the skull after birth so that the bones of the child are closely knit.

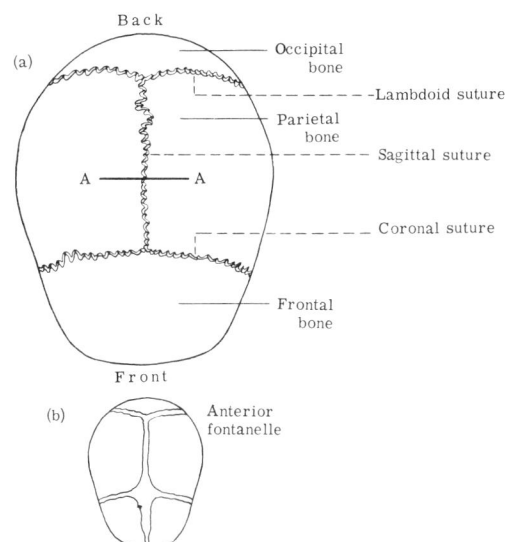

Figure 5.8 The sutures of the skull. (a) An adult skull. (b) A child's skull.

Before this takes place some bones are separated by large areas of membrane called fontanelles (see Figure 5.8). The largest of these fontanelles is the anterior fontanelle, which is located in the junction of the sagittal, coronal and frontal sutures. It is diamond-shaped, about 3 cm long and is a "soft spot" beneath which the brain or blood vessels may easily be injured or ruptured. The first sign of increased pressure within the infant's cranium is a bulging anterior fortanelle. Pressure will increase in meningitis when the meninges, membranes covering the brain, become infected. In infants, a bulging fontanelle may indicate meningitis, though other conditions can be associated with increased intracranial pressure. Conversely, when the pressure within the cranium is reduced, as happens when an infant is dehydrated, the anterior fontanelle becomes sunken. The gradual process of closure of the anterior fontanelles is usually completed after a year and a half of life; however, there is considerable variation, and closure can take place within 3–27 months. The posterior fontanelle is formed by the junction of the sagittal and lambdoid sutures and is closed by 4 months after birth. There are also two antero-lateral fontanelles and two postero-lateral fontanelles.

b. The face

The 14 bones which make up the face (see Figure 5.5) are:

2 Zygomatic bones
2 Maxillary bones
2 Nasal bones
2 Lachrymal bones
1 Vomer
2 Inferior conchae
2 Palatine bones
1 Mandible.

(1) *The zygoma (zygomatic) bone* forms the hard prominence of the cheek. It also forms part of the floor and lateral walls of the orbital cavity, a structure that in the living person contains the eye. Posteriorly the zygoma articulates with the zygomatic process of the temporal bone to complete

the zygomatic arch. Medially it articulates with the maxilla (the upper jaw bone).

(2) *The maxillary bones* are two irregular bones which unite to form the upper jaw bone; the upper set of teeth are contained in the alveolar cavity which is found in a projection from the maxillae. Behind the teeth the maxillae form part of the roof of the mouth (which is also part of the floor of the nasal cavities). If you feel the roof of your mouth you can feel how hard the front part of it is; this is called the hard palate. Each maxilla also contains an air sinus lined with mucous membrane which opens into the nasal cavities (see Figure 5.9). The maxillae articulate with the zygomatic, lachrymal, frontal and nasal bones. The two nasal bones unite anteriorly to form the bridge of the nose articulating superiorly with the frontal bone and laterally with the maxillae.

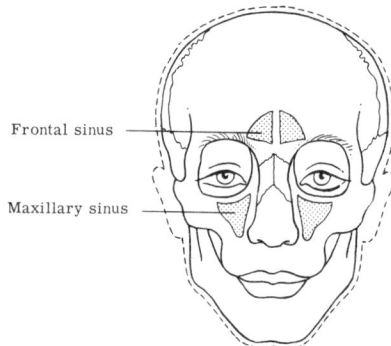

Figure 5.9 Position of the frontal and maxillary air sinuses.

(3) *The lachrymal bones* are small and flat and form part of the medial wall of the orbit; each articulates anteriorly with the maxillae and posteriorly with the ethmoid bone of the cranium. Each bone has a small foramen which contains the naso-lachrymal duct. Fluid continually washes over the eyes and passes through this duct into the nasal cavities where it is ultimately absorbed. We become conscious of tear formation when the rate of formation is greater than the amount which can be absorbed into the naso-lachrymal duct and the tears start to run down the cheek.

(4) *The nasal bones* lie between the frontal processes of the maxillae and join each other medially. They are small flat bones forming most of the lateral and superior surfaces of the bridge of the nose. They articulate superiorly with the frontal bone; their inferior borders are attached to nasal cartilages (see Figure 5.10).

(5) *The vomer* is a small bone that projects upward from the middle of the hard palate; it gets its name because of its supposed resemblance to an old-fashioned plough. The vomer articulates with the perpendicular plate of the ethmoid bone and thus contributes to the medial wall of the nasal septum. The septal cartilage joins with both the vomer and the perpendicular plate of the ethmoid bone to complete the medial wall of the nasal cavity. The medial wall of the nasal cavity is also the septum of the nose and is formed from the septal cartilage, the vomer and the perpendicular plate of the ethmoid bone.

(6) *The inferior conchae* contribute to the lateral walls of the nasal cavity. Each concha is a long scroll-shaped bone which projects into the nasal cavity. The inferior concha is located below the middle concha.

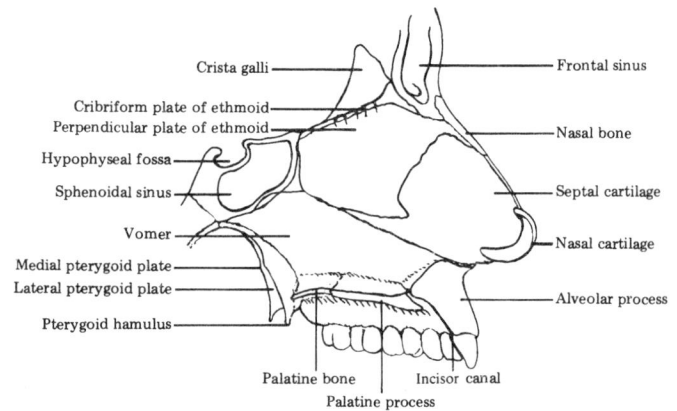

Figure 5.10 The nose.

(7) *The palatine bones* are two "L"-shaped bones; each palatine bone has a horizontal plate and a perpendicular plate. The two horizontal palatine plates unite to form a posterior part of the hard palate; while the two perpendicular plates project upward from the hard palate to contribute to the formation of the lateral walls of the nasal cavity.

The structure of the nasal cavities can be reviewed. Think of a box which has a divider in the middle, and openings in the front and the back. The divider is the nasal septum which separates the right and left nasal cavities. The roof of the box is formed from nasal cartilage and (going front to back) from the following bones: nasal, frontal, cribriform plate of the ethmoid bone and part of the sphenoid. The floor is formed from the maxillae and horizontal plates of the palatine bones. The two lateral walls are uneven. Two conchae from the ethmoid bone project into the cavity as does the large inferior concha. The lateral wall is formed from the ethmoid bone and the two inferior conchae. The maxilla and lachrymal bones contribute to the anterior portion of the lateral wall, while the perpendicular plates of the palatine bones and the sphenoid bone contribute to the posterior portion of it. Air enters the nasal cavity through the nostrils. Air leaves the nasal cavity via the posterior nares through which the air enters into the nasopharynx.

(8) *The mandible* is the lower jaw bone and is the only movable bone of the skull (with the exception of the middle ear bones, discussed in the Chapter on the eye and the ear). The mandible is the largest, strongest bone of the face and is formed from a "U"-shaped body and a pair of rami (see Figure 5.11). The external surface has a faint median ridge which marks the point of fusion of the two halves of the mandible at the symphysis menti. (Menti is derived from the Latin words *mens*, *mentis*, which mean mind. People deep in thought often support their head by resting their jaw on their hand.) There are two mental foramina for passage of the inferior dental nerves and blood vessels. The upper border of the mandible is termed the alveolar part and contains sockets which anchor the teeth. (Teeth are discussed in the Chapter on the digestive system.) One ramus projects upward from each end of the mandible at an angle averaging 120°. The curved upper edge of the ramus forms the mandibular notch, while the lateral surface provides insertion for the masseter muscle, an important muscle used in chewing. The condyloid

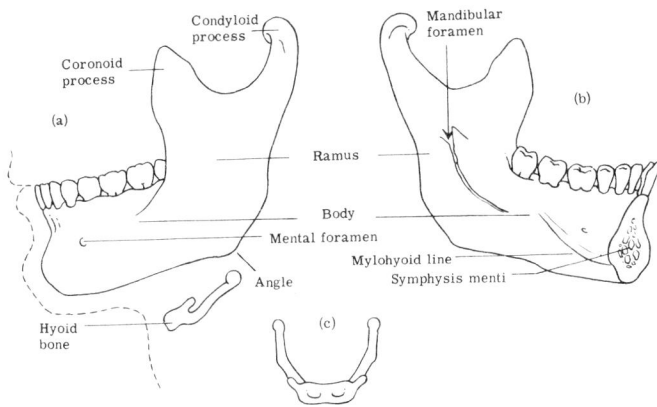

Figure 5.11 The mandible. (a) Outside view. (b) Inside view. (c) Hyoid bone.

(condilar) process forms the head and neck of the mandible; the head articulates with the temporal bone to form the temporo-mandibular joint. The coronoid process receives the insertion of the temporalis muscle and other ligaments. The temporalis, masseter and pterygoid muscles are important in chewing and help elevate the mandible at rest.

The hyoid bone is not a bone of the skull but is often described with the skull. This is an isolated "C"-shaped bone lying above the larynx (voice box) and below the mandible in the soft tissues of the neck (see Figure 5.11c). It does not articulate with any bones but is connected by ligaments and muscles to the styloid process of the temporal bone. It also gives attachment to the muscles of the base of the tongue.

Before going to the vertebral column it would be a good idea to review some of the bones by studying the bones which make up the orbit. The orbit contains the eye and its nerves. muscles, blood vessels and connective tissues. Part of the frontal bone and the small wing of the sphenoid bone form the roof. The base of the orbit is formed by part of the maxilla, the orbital process of the zygomatic bone and, to a lesser extent, by part of the palatine bone. The vertical, medial wall of the orbit is formed from parts of the sphenoid, ethmoid and maxillary bones and also the lachrymal bone. The large wing of the sphenoid bone and the orbital process of the zygomatic bone contribute to the orbit's lateral wall. In the posterior part of the orbit, above the great wing of the sphenoid bone is the superior orbital fissure. Through this wide opening pass cranial nerve III (occulo-motor), IV (trochlear), VI (abducent) and the ophthalmic branch of V (trigeminal). Cranial nerves III, IV and VI supply the muscles of the eye, while the ophthalmic division of cranial nerve V carries general sensory information from the face and eye.

B. Vertebral column

The vertebral column is composed of 33 irregular bones called vertebrae and functions to protect the spinal cord which passes through it within the vertebral canal. The column supports the skull and also gives attachment to the shoulder girdle and upper limbs, the ribs and the pelvic girdle and lower limbs. The shape of the column depends on the age of the individual. The foetus grows within the uterus with its

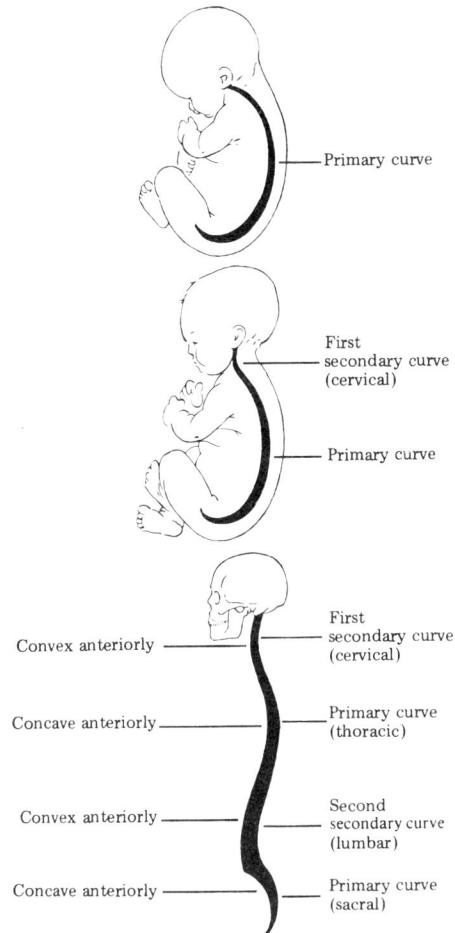

Figure 5.12 Development of the vertebral column.

head and knees flexed so that they almost touch; the foetal position results in the primary curve of the spinal cord. Several months after parturition (birth) the infant begins to maintain his head in an upright position and the first secondary curve is formed. Still later as the infant begins to walk the second secondary curve develops (see Figure 5.12). The primary curves in the adult are described as being concave anteriorly and the secondary curves are convex anteriorly. There are:

7 Cervical vertebrae
12 Thoracic vertebrae
5 Lumbar vertebrae
5 Sacral vertebrae
4 Coccygeal vertebrae

The 5 sacral vertebrae become fused together to form the wedge-shaped bone called the sacrum and the 4 coccygeal vertebrae become fused together to form the triangular-shaped coccyx. The coccyx is at the tail-end or caudal-end of the vertebral column and articulates with the sacrum (see Figure 5.13).

Movements between the separate vertebrae are restricted but movements of the column as a whole are more extensive. These include bending sideways (lateral flexion) and turning around (rotation). The greatest amount of movement is in the cranial and lumbar regions. Each vertebra has a disc-shaped body and an arch which surrounds the neural canal. The

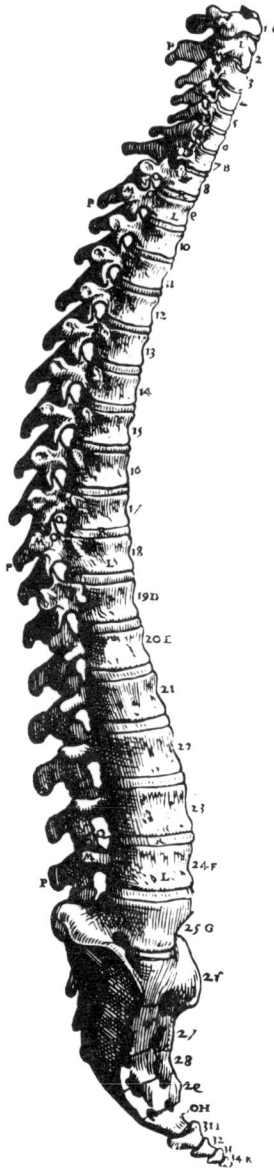

Figure 5.13 The vertebral column from Versalius' *De Humani Corporis Fabrica* (Concerning the Structure of the Human Body).

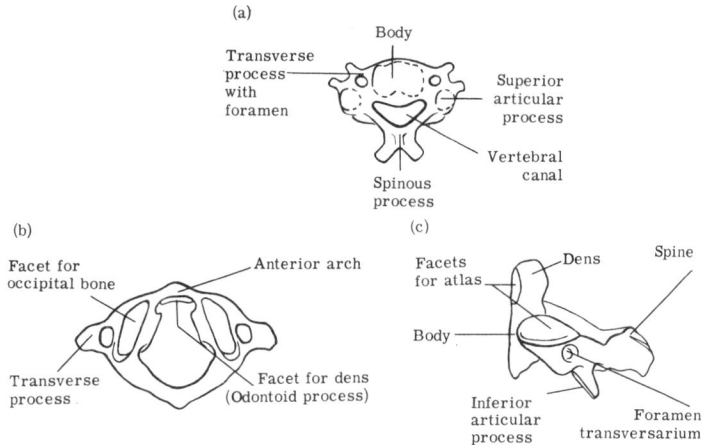

Figure 5.14 Cervical vertebrae. (a) Superior view. (b) Atlas — superior view. (c) Axis — side view.

process has a foramen for passage of the vertebral arteries which help supply blood to the brain. The spinous process is "V"-shaped to permit passage of ligaments and muscle attachments.

The first cervical vertebra is called the atlas, the second is the axis, and the remainder are called by position in the numerical order — 3rd to 8th. The atlas and axis are not typical cervical vertebrae however (see Figure 5.14b and c). The atlas is essentially a ring of bone surrounding the spinal cord for it has no body or spinous processes. The superior surface of the atlas has two facets which articulate with the occipital condyles of the skull. These are the joints by which the head nods. The dens or odontoid process of the axis projects upward from the axis into the anterior part of the neural canal of the atlas; it is separated from the spinal cord by a transverse ligament. Rotation of the head takes place at this joint.

b. The thoracic vertebrae. These are larger than the cervical vertebrae and are 12 in number. Their bodies are heart-shaped and the spinous processes project downwards as well as posteriorly (see Figure 5.15); those of the middle four are nearly vertical. The transverse processes become shorter although the size of the body increases as you descend towards the 12th thoracic vertebra. The body has four facets for rib articulation, two above and two below on both sides. The transverse processes of the first ten thoracic vertebrae also articulate with the ribs.

c. The lumbar vertebrae. These five bones are the largest single vertebrae and support the most weight. Their bodies are kidney-shaped and do not have any articulations for the ribs. The vertebral canal is small and triangular, while the spinous processes are large and horizontal (see Figure 5.16).

d. The sacrum. The bodies of the five sacral vertebrae begin to fuse with one another after the 17th year. In the

bodies are separated from one another by thick pads of fibrocartilage called the intervertebral discs. Each arch has three rough processes for the attachment of muscles and ligaments. The two laminae of the arch unite with the two pedicles of the body; at each junction a transverse process protrudes laterally. At the union of the two lamina a spinous process projects posteriorly. (A laminectomy is a surgical procedure in which parts of the lamina are removed to reduce pressure on the spinal cord resulting from injury or disease.) Only the superior and inferior surfaces of the neural arch and the articular processes articulate with the vertebrae above and below. On the bottom of each arch are notches which permit the spinal nerves to enter and leave the vertebral canal.

a. The cervical vertebrae. These are the smallest of the vertebrae and also differ from the others for they are oblong in shape, the longest axis being right-to-left instead of back-to-front (see Figure 5.14a). In addition, each transverse

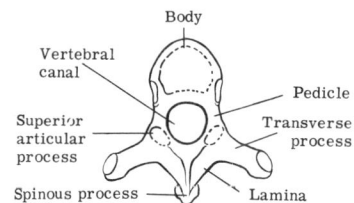

Figure 5.15 Thoracic vertebra — superior view.

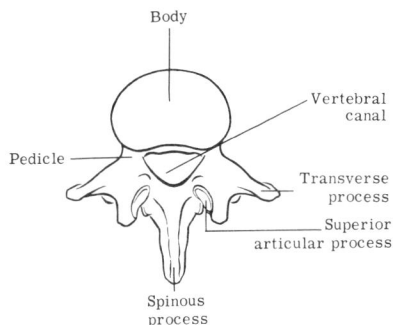

Figure 5.16 Lumbar vertebra — superior view.

adult, the sacrum is a single triangular-shaped bone. The neural canal continues into the sacrum and the spinal nerves leave through foramina in the sacrum. Each side of the sacrum articulates with the ilium of the innominate bone to form the sacro-iliac joints. The sacrum and the innominate bone form the pelvic girdle. Superiorly the sacrum articulates on the 5th lumbar vertebra and inferiorly with the coccyx (see Figure 5.17).

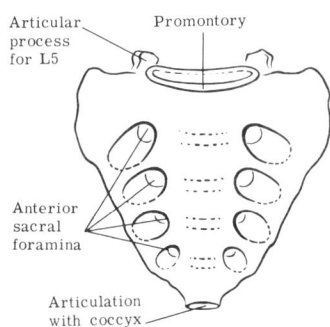

Figure 5.17 Sacrum — anterior view.

e. The coccyx. The coccyx consists of the caudal four small vertebrae which become fused in the adult. The joint between the sacrum and the coccyx is slightly moveable.

f. Ligaments of the vertebral column. These are strong bands of fibrous connective tissue which bind the vertebrae together although their bodies are separated by connective tissues. The anterior ligament extends the whole length of the vertebral column and is firmly attached to the anterior surface of the body of each vertebra, thus helping to hold it in place. The posterior longitudinal ligament lies within the vertebral canal and also extends the whole length of the column. The anterior and posterior ligaments thus keep the vertebrae from putting pressure on the delicate spinal cord. Other ligaments connect the laminae of adjacent vertebrae together (see Figure 5.18).

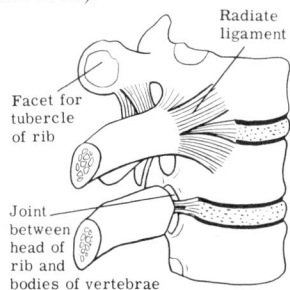

Figure 5.18 Articulations of the posterior end of the rib with the vertebrae.

C. The thorax

The thorax (chest cavity) is formed posteriorly by the thoracic vertebrae, anteriorly by the sternum (breast bone) and the remainder of the circumference by the ribs (see Figure 5.19).

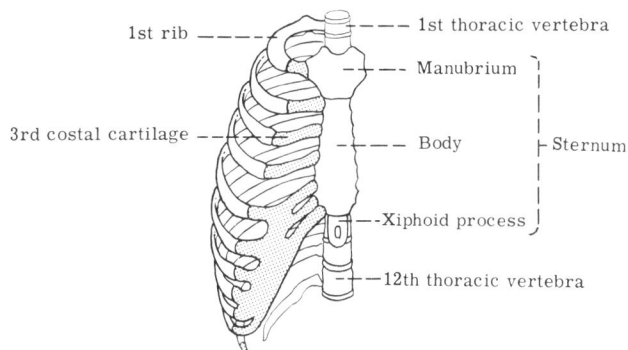

Figure 5.19 The thorax.

a. The sternum is a flat dagger-shaped bone easily felt beneath the skin in the middle of the chest. The sternum articulates with the costal cartilages and has three parts:

(1) The uppermost part is the manubrium; on its upper lateral surfaces are the clavicular notches by which the sternum articulates with the clavicles. Below these are facets for articulation with the 1st rib. The 2nd rib attaches at the junction of the manubrium and the body at the sternal angle.

(2) The body of the sternum is long, narrow and serves as the attachment for the 3rd, 4th, 5th and 6th ribs while the 7th attaches to the junction of the body and xiphoid process.

(3) The xiphoid process is a small triangular-shaped tip of the sternum which usually does not completely ossify. A part of the diaphragm, the fibres of the linea alba, and fibres of the rectus abdominalis muscles are all attached to the xiphoid process.

b. The ribs are 12 pairs of flat, curved bones which pass forward and downward from their articulations with the thoracic vertebrae. Ribs are classified as either true ribs or false ribs. The first seven ribs are considered to be true ribs because they are attached directly to the sternum by means of hyaline cartilages known as costal cartilages. The 8th to the 12th ribs are considered false ribs for they do not attach directly to the sternum. The 8th, 9th and 10th ribs each fuse with the costal cartilage of the rib above them. The 11th and 12th ribs do not fuse with the costal cartilage of any rib and extend only partly around the circumference of the thorax. About 1 in 20 people has a 13th rib.

A typical rib has a head, neck and shaft (see Figure 5.20). The heads articulate with the costal facets of the vertebrae.

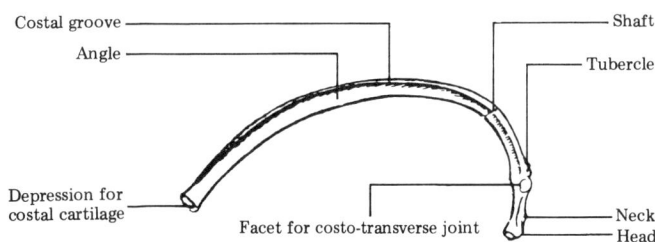

Figure 5.20 A rib.

During inspiration, all the ribs except the 1st are lifted upward at this joint. The neck is a narrow portion of bone immediately anterior to the head and has a facet for articulation with the transverse process of the corresponding thoracic vertebrae. The shaft is curved and twisted. Hyaline cartilage attaches the hollowed-out end of the shaft to the sternum. In a living individual, the space between the ribs is filled with the external and internal intercostal muscles.

THE APPENDICULAR SKELETON

A. The upper extremity

The upper extremity is composed of the shoulder girdle, the upper arm, the forearm, the carpus (wrist), the metacarpals and the phalanges (fingers). The shoulder girdle, formed by the clavicle and scapula, attaches the upper arm to the trunk. The humerus forms the upper arm and the radius and ulna form the forearm. Eight carpal bones form the wrist and the metacarpal bones form the palm of the hand. The phalanges form the digits: each finger has three phalanges while the thumb has two phalanges, making a total of 14 bones (see Figure 5.21).

a. The shoulder girdle.
(1) The clavicle (collar bone) is a somewhat "S"-shaped, long bone. It forms the anterior part of the shoulder girdle and some muscles of the arm and neck are attached to it (see Figure 5.21). The rounded medial extremity articulates with the manubrium of the sternum and the lateral end articulates with the scapula. The clavicle is one of the most commonly broken bones, most commonly as the result of a fall.
(2) The scapula is a flat, triangular-shaped bone which forms the posterior part of the shoulder girdle. The scapula lies over the ribs but does not articulate with them for it is separated from them and held in place by muscles (see Figure 5.21). The anterior surface is concave which enables it to fit more closely over the ribs and is called the subscapular fossa. The posterior convex surface has a ridge of bone called the spine of the scapula which ends laterally in the acromion process that overhangs the shoulder joint and articulates with the clavicle at the acromio-clavicular joint. Because the scapula is not attached to the ribs it can move forward as the upper limbs are brought together, or backward as the upper limbs are stretched behind the body. It also rotates as you raise your hand high above your head. Both the acromion process and the more medial coracoid process serve to attach muscles. At the intersection of the superior and lateral borders of the scapula is a shallow, pear-shaped cavity called the glenoid cavity; this articulates with the humerus to form the shoulder joint. Because each scapula lies flat against the posterior wall, it is seldom fractured.
b. The upper arm. The humerus is a long bone and is the longest bone in the upper limb; it extends from the shoulder joint to the elbow (see Figure 5.21). The upper extremity of the humerus articulates with the glenoid cavity, is hemispherical, covered with hyaline cartilage and is referred to as the head of the humerus. A slight groove surrounds the head as it joins the shaft and the groove is called the anatomical neck of the humerus. Lateral to the head are the greater and the lesser tuberosities to which muscles attach. Below the

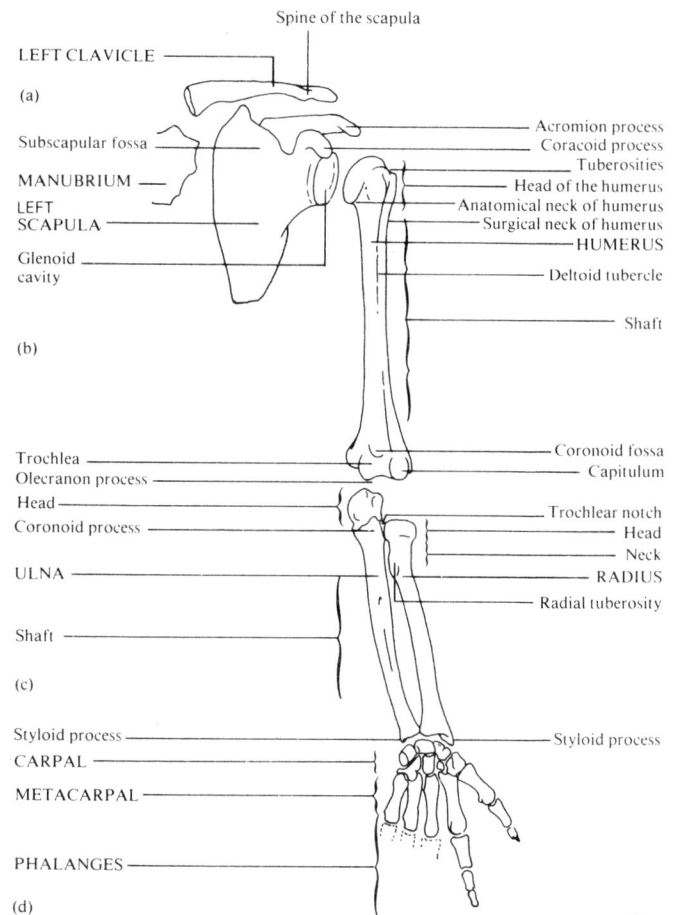

Figure 5.21   The upper extremity.

tuberosities the shaft narrows and the area is called the surgical neck of the humerus, as this is the most common site for fractures of the humerus. Midway in the shaft is found the deltoid tubercle which gives insertion to the deltoid muscle. The flat distal end has two articular surfaces, the lateral capitulum and the medial, pulley-shaped trochlea for articulation with the radius and ulna respectively. Above the articular surfaces on the posterior surface is the olecranon fossa and on the anterior surface is the coronoid fossa.
c. The forearm.
(1) The ulna is longer than the radius (see Figure 5.21). The proximal end of the ulna contains the trochlear notch which is "C"-shaped and articulates with the trochlea of the humerus. Overhanging this notch is the beak-like olecranon process which forms the point of the elbow. When the forearm or elbow is extended the olecranon process of the ulna fits into the olecranon fossa of the humerus. From beneath the trochlear notch projects the coronoid process. This fits into the coronoid fossa of the humerus when the arm is flexed. The head of the radius articulates with the lateral surface of the coronoid notch. The triangular-shaped shaft has a rough ridge for attachment of muscles and fibrous interosseous membrane which separates the radius from the ulna. The shaft expands slightly to form the head of the ulna and on the medial side of the bone is the styloid process which proceeds from the ulna and serves as an attachment for the ligaments of the wrist joint.
(2) The radius is the outer lateral bone of the forearm (see

Figure 5.21). Like the ulna it is a long bone which has a shaft and two extremities. The button-shaped head of the bone has a small depression for articulation with the capitulum of the humerus while the side of the head articulates with the radial notch of the ulna. The angular ligament holds the radius against the ulna. The radius has a narrow neck which joins the head to the shaft. On the medial surface just below the neck is the radial tuberosity to which the biceps brachii muscle attaches. The shaft has a sharp interosseous ridge which faces the ulna and is attached to it by the interosseous membrane. The distal end of the radius articulates with the carpal bones of the wrist. The styloid process projects from the lateral surface of the distal end and can easily be felt at the base of the thumb.

Both the radius and the ulna are commonly fractured. Elderly people (whose bones are more brittle) often fall upon their outstretched hands and fracture the radius a few centimetres above the wrist; this is called Colle's fracture. The styloid process of the ulna is also broken off in hard falls.

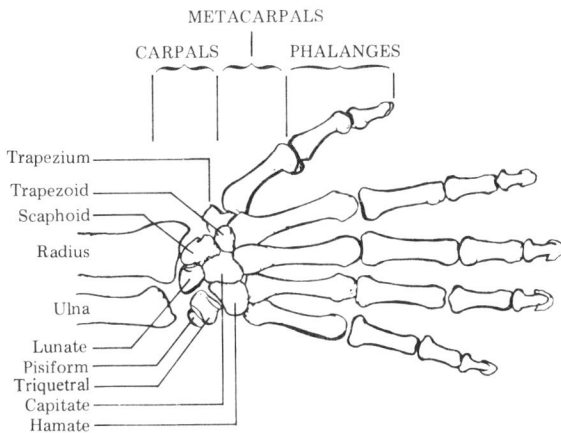

Figure 5.22 The wrist and hand — anterior view of the left wrist and hand.

d. The carpus (*wrist*). There are eight irregular bones which make up the wrist. These are arranged in two rows (see Figure 5.22). Beginning medially and proceeding laterally they are:

1st row (Proximal)	*2nd row* (Distal)
scaphoid	trapezium
lunate	trapezoid
triquetral	capitate
pisiform	hamate

The scaphoid and lunate bones articulate with the lower end of the radius and help hold it in place.

e. The metacarpals are five small long bones which form the palm of the hand. The proximal ends articulate with the carpal bones and the distal ends articulate with the phalanges to form the knuckles.

f. Each finger has three phalanges while the thumb has only two. The phalanges are small long bones.

B. The lower extremity

The lower extremity contains 31 bones and consists of the following (see Figure 5.23):

1 Innominate bone
1 Femur
1 Tibia
1 Fibula
1 Patella
7 Tarsal bones
5 Metatarsal bones
14 Phalanges.

The pelvic girdle consists of two innominate bones and the sacrum.

a. The innominate bone. The innominate (hip) bone is formed from three separate bones which unite to form a single bone in the adult. The bones that ultimately unite to form the irregular hip bone are the ilium, the pubis and the ischium (see Figure 5.23). The ilium is the broad flat uppermost part of the bone. The iliac crest surrounds the bone and gives attachment to the abdominal muscles. Anteriorly the crest forms the anterior superior and anterior inferior iliac spines. There are also posterior superior and posterior inferior iliac spines. The surface between the two posterior iliac spines of each bone articulates with the sacrum to form the sacro-iliac joint. The pubis is the lower front part of the innominate bone. It is square-shaped and the anterior part articulates with the anterior part of the pubis of the other hip bone to form the symphysis pubis which is a slightly-moveable joint. The ischium is the thickest part of the innominate bone and is its lower posterior part. The ischial tuberosity supports the trunk of the body when sitting and also serves as an attachment for the hamstring muscles. The three bones unite with one another to form the deep cup-shaped acetabulum with which the head of the femur articulates to form the hip joint. Below the acetabulum and

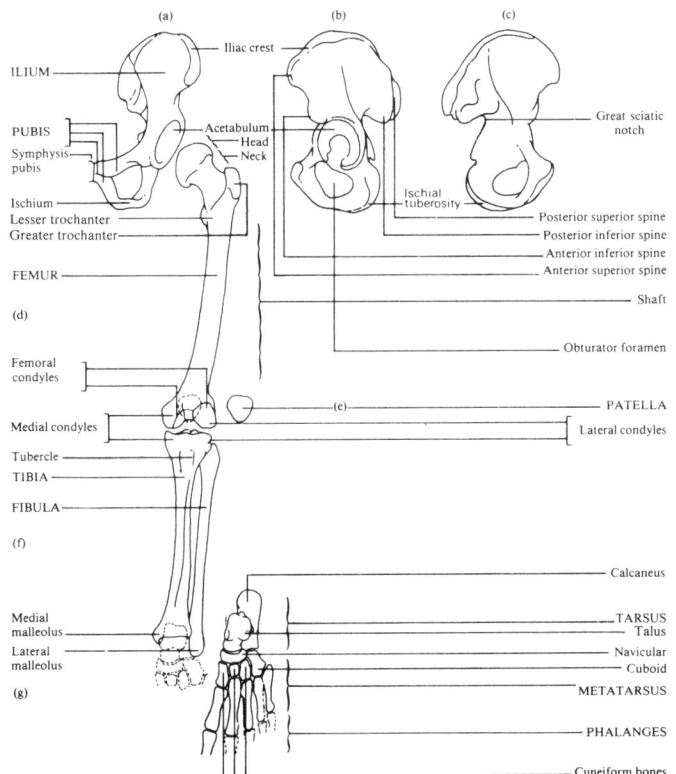

Figure 5.23 The lower extremity.

bounded by the ischium is the large oval-shaped obturator foramen through which blood vessels, lymphatics and nerves pass to and from the thigh. Above and behind the acetabulum is the great sciatic notch through which the sciatic nerve and blood vessels pass down the back of the thigh and leg.

The pelvic girdle is formed from the innominate bones which articulate anteriorly at the symphysis pubis, posteriorly at the sacro-iliac joint. The pelvis itself is sometimes divided into a false pelvis and a true pelvis. The false pelvis forms part of the abdominal cavity and is that part of the abdominal cavity which is above a line drawn between the symphysis pubis and the upper end of the sacrum and which is bounded by the two iliac bones. The true pelvis is below this plane, is bounded by ischium and pubis on the sides and front and the sacrum behind, and forms the long canal through which the foetus passes during childbirth. In Latin the word *pelvis* means basin. The shape of the "basin" is slightly different in males and females as is illustrated in Figure 5.24, which shows how the female pelvis is roomier. Although the female pelvis may contain more room than the male, the female bones themselves are lighter and smaller.

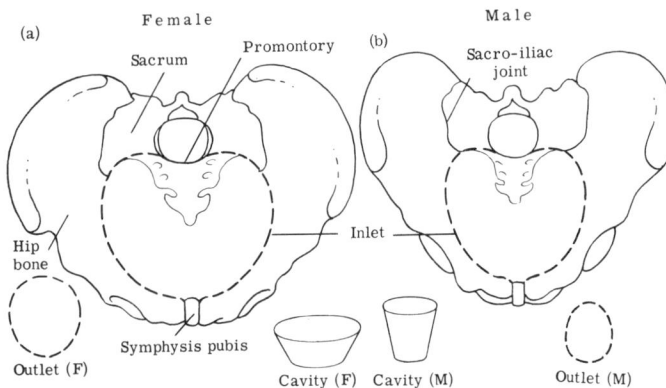

Figure 5.24   The pelvis. (a) Female pelvis. (b) Male pelvis.

b. The thigh. The thigh is formed by the femur, which is the longest and strongest bone in the body (see Figure 5.23). The femur is a long bone with two extremities and a shaft. The upper extremity consists of a head, neck and the greater and lesser trochanters. The head is round and is found at the end of a long neck. The head fits into the acetabulum and contains a small notch which gives attachment to the ligamentum teres that runs from the head of the femur to the base of the acetabulum. The neck is at an angle to the shaft. The greater and lesser trochanters are found where the neck joins the shaft and these two large prominences serve to attach muscles. The greater trochanter is on the lateral side and can easily be felt beneath the skin. The shaft of the femur is smooth and arched forward, like the curve of a bow. On the upper two thirds of the posterior surface of the femur there is a well-marked ridge called the linea aspera (rough line) to which many muscles attach. In the lower third of the femur the linea aspera divides in two, and a smaller ridge goes to each of the two femoral condyles of the lower extremity. The triangular area between these two ridges is called the popliteal surface of the femur. The lower extremity consists of the medial and lateral condyles which are separated by the intercondylar fossa and are covered with cartilage which

forms a surface for articulation with the knee cap (patella). The two condyles articulate with the condyles of the tibia to form the knee joint. Above the medial condyle is a small tubercle, the adductor tubercle, to which part of the adductor magnus muscle is attached. The neck of the femur is susceptible to fractures, often as a result of a fall; fractures here are particularly common in the elderly.

c. The patella. This is a triangular-shaped sesamoid bone which develops in the tendon of the quadriceps femoris muscle (see Figure 5.23). The anterior surface is rough while the posterior surface is smooth and articulates with the patellar surface of the femur. The tip of the patella points downward and from this point the patellar ligament travels downward to the tubercle of the tibia. The patella functions to ease the movement of the tendon over the knee joint as the leg moves.

d. The leg. In correct anatomic usage the leg refers to the tibia and the fibula and its associated soft tissue (see Figure 5.23).

(1) The tibia is medial, the longer of the two bones and is also known as the shin bone; it has a shaft and two extremities. The upper extremity is broad and has two condyles and two shallow depressions for articulation in which the condyles of the femur fit to form the knee joint. Between the two sockets is a rough spine to which the two cruciate ligaments attach. The patellar tendon attaches to the tubercle of the tibia on the front of the bone. The lateral condyle has a facet which articulates with the head of the fibula at the superior tibio-fibular joint. The shaft of the tibia is triangular in shape; the anterior surface is very prominent, is called the crest of the tibia and forms the shin. The lower extremity of the tibia is smooth and flat where it articulates with the talus to form the ankle joint. The medial surface of the lower extremity contains a prominent downward projecting process called the medial malleolus which helps in the formation of the ankle joint.

(2) The fibula is a slender long bone which lies parallel and lateral to the tibia. The upper extremity forms the head which articulates with the lateral condyle of the tibia but it does not enter into the formation of the knee joint. The shaft is embedded in the muscles of the leg to which it gives attachments; between the shaft of the two bones is an interosseous membrane. The lower extremity also has a projection called the lateral malleolus. It is similar to the medial malleolus of the tibia in that it gives attachment to ligaments.

e. The ankle, heel and instep. These structures are formed by the tarsus which consists of seven short bones (see Figure 5.23). The tarsal bones include the following seven bones:

(1) The talus supports the tibia and is held between the lateral and the medial malleolus, forming the ankle joint. The talus is sometimes called the ankle bone.

(2) The calcaneus is sometimes called the os calcis (the heel bone) and is the largest bone of the foot. Superiorly it articulates with the talus and posteriorly transmits the weight of the body to the ground. The calcaneus is a rough bone to which many muscles that move the ankle joint are attached; they are attached by means of the Achilles tendon.

(3) The navicular (scaphoid) bone is a disc-shaped bone which was thought to resemble a ship by the early anatomists.

(4) The cuboid is at the lateral aspect of the foot between the calcaneus and the metatarsals.

(5–7) The three wedge-shaped cuneiform bones are arranged in a row and articulate proximally with the three other tarsal bones and distally with the five metatarsals. The navicular, cuboid and cuneiform bones form the instep.

f. The metatarsals are five long bones which form the greater part of the dorsum of the foot. Proximally they articulate with the tarsal bones and distally with the phalanges. They are not individually named but are numbered; the 1st metatarsal is the most medial and the 5th is the most lateral.

g. The 14 phalanges in each foot make up the toes. They are arranged in a manner similar to that of the fingers of the hand. The big toe has two phalanges, while the four smaller toes each have three phalanges.

h. The arches of the foot and their support. The foot is not simply a weight-bearing structure but also plays an important role in walking, running and jumping, activities in which the body's weight is shifted. The arches of the foot give some flexibility to the bones of the foot so that it is adapted to perform these functions. Four arches are present in the foot: two longitudinal arches (heel-to-toe) and two transverse arches (lateral-to-medial). The highest arch is the medial longitudinal, which is formed by the calcaneus, the talus, which is at the summit of the arch, the navicular, the three cuneiform bones and the heads of the three medial metatarsals. The lateral longitudinal arch is less pronounced and is formed by the calcaneus, cuboid and two outer metatarsal bones. The transverse tarsal arch is formed by the tarsal bones. The transverse metatarsal arch is formed by the metatarsal bones. The latter arch is small and almost in contact with the ground when standing but becomes more prominent when the foot is at rest. The arches are formed or "held up" by the close arrangement of the bones, and the arrangement of muscles which tie to the top of the arch, tie to the base of the arch and form a sling under the summit of the arch. The strong ligaments of the foot also help to maintain the arch.

Should the arches not be maintained and fall, a "flat foot" results. While the arches are falling the foot is painful because of the rearrangement of the bones and the pressure on nerves. When the process is completed the resulting flat foot is not necessarily painful but it is not well adapted to bear the stresses and strains the foot is subject to. Policemen, postmen, nurses and other individuals who walk and stand during work are more likely to suffer from falling arches than more sedentary individuals.

WHY DO BONES BREAK AND HOW ARE FRACTURES REPAIRED?

A fracture is a break in the continuity of a bone. Fractures are classified according to the type of break in the bone. In a simple (closed) fracture the bone breaks but does not protrude through the skin. A compound fracture is when the bone protrudes through the skin and makes contact with the air. In a comminuted fracture the bone is broken into several pieces, while in an impacted fracture one end of the bone is driven into the other, resulting in breakage. An incomplete fracture occurs when the bone is cracked or fissured on only one side and merely bent on the other; sometimes this type of fracture is called a greenstick fracture.

A bone will break when the force applied to it is greater than the bone can withstand. There are certain metabolic conditions which can weaken bones. Osteoporosis is a chronic disease of the elderly in which there is a decrease in bone mass and an increased likelihood of fractures. Decreased bone mass means that there is a loss of both mineral and protein matrix components. The cause of osteoporosis is not completely known, but the essential problem is that bone breakdown proceeds faster than bone formation. Reduced amounts of oestrogens and other hormonal and nutrient factors may contribute to this imbalance between bone breakdown and bone formation. Calcium deficiencies or a failure to absorb sufficient calcium may be an important factor. Calcium absorption requires vitamin D. The diets of the elderly are often low in both vitamin D and calcium. A common symptom of osteoporosis is low back pain. The weakened weight-bearing joints are compressed and may press on the spinal nerves. Immobilization also leads to osteoporosis, for bone, like muscle, needs action if it is to remain healthy. There are some forces however, most frequently encountered during falls, which even the healthiest of bones cannot withstand.

When a bone breaks, the muscles and other soft tissues surrounding the bone are also injured. Frequently the muscles go into spasm and pull on the broken bone parts, causing the ends to overlap. If the injured person moves or is moved carelessly these sharp ends might do further damage to nerves, blood vessels and other tissues.

Two basic processes are involved in the repair of a fracture: bone resorption and bone formation. Bone resorption begins by the activation of osteoclasts and the death of osteocytes due to lack of adequate circulation. Blood that has been lost from the injured tissues surrounds the injured bone and it clots. A loose fibrin network forms the first bridge which unites the broken ends and serves as a scaffold for the subsequent repair processes. Granulocytes and macrophages are drawn to the site and remove some of the debris. Cells similar to fibroblasts become active and collagen is deposited. Up to this point the process is similar to the repair of a wound in the soft tissues. Osteoprogenitor cells are recruited and all bone-forming cells are activated. These cells form a cartilaginous sleeve called the callus. The callus usually exists for only a few weeks, for its cartilage becomes calcified and undergoes changes similar to those observed in endochondral ossification. The cancellous bone that is formed may then be replaced by dense or compact bone. A plaster cast helps keep the proper alignment between the bones while the callus is being formed and the fracture heals.

Mention must be made of osteomalacia, a disease in which there is a reduction only in the mineral content of the bone, and the bones are more likely to bend than break — in contrast to osteoporosis, in which both the protein matrix and the minerals are reduced. Rickets is a childhood form of osteomalacia and is most often due to a vitamin D deficiency.

6. The Joints or Articulations

INTRODUCTION

A joint or an articulation is the site at which two or more bones come together. You might be able to get some insight into the problem of keeping bones together by trying a simple experiment. Take two pencils and try to find some way to keep them together. You could try to keep them together by using glue or paste or epoxy resin. One of these will fix the two pencils together but no motion can take place. You could take another approach and tie the pencils together using elastic or a rubber band. Here the "joint" would be movable but if force were applied the pencils would come apart. Unlike pencils, bones are living tissue, must support considerable weight, withstand considerable strain and last for the life of the individual.

Studying the joints also enables you to revise some of the skeletal anatomy and prepares the way for the study of the muscles. Before proceeding however, it is necessary to give some definitions.

SOME DEFINITIONS

We describe motion in a variety of ways. Skipping, running, bending-over backward and waltzing are examples. In clinical work it is necessary to be much more specific about individual movements (see Figure 6.1).

Flexion means bending; usually the motion is directed forward, but in the case of the knee and foot, the motion is directed posteriorly. Bending of the head on the neck, bending the forearm at the elbow and backward bending of the leg at the knee are all examples of flexion.

Extension is the opposite of flexion and refers to straightening or backward motion. Looking up to see the stars, bending the trunk backward at the hip and straightening the upper limb are all examples of extension.

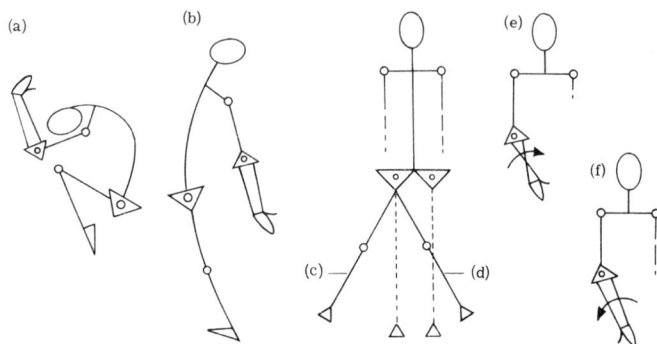

Figure 6.1 Individual movements. (a) Flexion. (b) Extension. (c) Abduction. (d) Adduction. (e) Pronation. (f) Supination.

Adduction refers to movement towards the midline. When you move your right leg to the left you are adducting the lower limb. In the hand and foot the terms adduction and abduction refer to movement toward and away from the midline of the part.

When you shake hands with someone you first flex your arm by bringing it forward, then you flex the forearm by bending it at the elbow. Next you adduct the upper limb until you reach the other person's hand. When you have finished shaking hands you abduct the upper limb, extend the forearm and extend the arm. These actions return the upper limb to its original position.

Rotation is movement around the long axis of a part. When you turn your head to the right or to the left you are rotating your head.

Circumduction refers to the movement of a limb in a circle and is thus a combination of flexion, extension, adduction and abduction. When you bowl a cricket ball (overarm) you are circumducting your arm.

Pronation refers to the turning of the hand so that the palm is down, or facing posteriorly.

Supination refers to the turning of the hand so the palm is upward or facing anteriorly. When you move your upper limb to receive change you supinate the hand.

WHAT ARE THE DIFFERENT TYPES OF JOINTS?

There are three basic types of joints: fibrous, cartilaginous and synovial.

A. Fibrous joints

The sutures of the skull are examples of fibrous joints (see Figure 5.8). The flat bones of the skull develop from separate centres of ossification. As the edges of the bone ossify, the amount of cartilage between the bones is reduced, so ultimately only a narrow band of fibrous connective tissue joins the bones. In the infant some movement is possible at the fontanelles because of the large amount of connective tissue which separates the bones; during childbirth the bones are even pushed over one another. The teeth are held in their sockets by fibrous tissue and the articulating surfaces of the tibia and fibula are also held together by fibrous tissue (see Figure 6.2).

B. Cartilaginous joints

These are classified as either primary or secondary cartilaginous joints (see Figure 6.3).

62

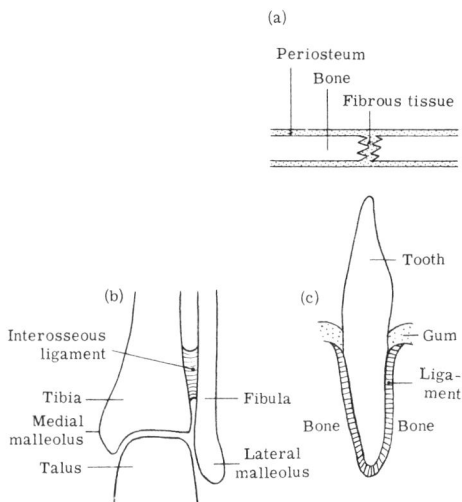

Figure 6.2 Fibrous joints. (a) Section through sutures of the skull. (b) Joints between the lower ends of the tibia and the fibula. (c) Articulation of a tooth with a jaw.

a. Primary cartilaginous joints. In these joints two bones are joined together by hyaline cartilage. This type of joint is seen in the adult at the junction of the first rib and the manubrium of the sternum. They are more common in the growing child however. In growing long bones the epiphysis is joined to the diaphysis by hyaline cartilage. This cartilage gradually becomes completely ossified and the growth of the bone stops.

b. Secondary cartilaginous joints. In these joints the ends of the bone are covered with hyaline cartilage but this cartilage does not unite the bones. Instead, the hyaline cartilage ends are separated from one another by a disc of fibrocartilage. These joints are slightly moveable and are found in the midline of the body. They are found in three locations:

(1) The first joint between the manubrium and the body of the sternum.

(2) The bodies of the vertebrae are capped with hyaline cartilage and connected to one another by fibrocartilage and dense fibrous tissue which is arranged to form a ring around the joint. Only a little movement is possible at these joints because the vertebrae can only compress the intervertebral discs to a limited extent. These small movements do accumulate, so that there is more movement of the column as a whole than is possible between the individual vertebrae.

(3) The anterior ends of the two pubic bones articulate with one another by means of a cartilaginous joint and also

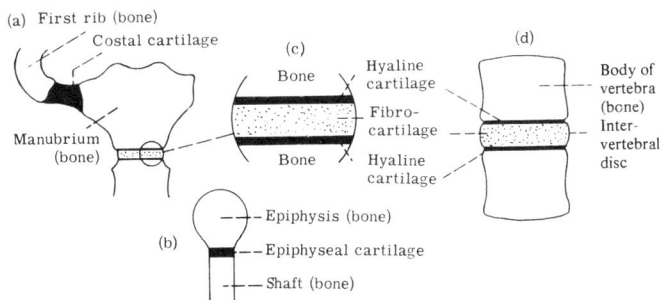

Figure 6.3 Cartilaginous joints. (a) Primary. (b) Secondary. (c) Section through the joint. (d) Detail of the joint.

ligaments which surround the cartilage and run from bone to bone. Because of the endocrine changes which take place during pregnancy the ligaments become weakened and the ends of the pubic bones may be absorbed. This makes it easier for the two pubic bones to pull apart and facilitate childbirth but often causes the woman to have a feeling of instability when walking. The ligaments and bones are restored after childbirth.

C. Synovial joints

These joints are not as strong as cartilaginous joints but are freely moveable. The shape of the joint determines which motions can take place, so there is some variation in the structure of the various joints (see Figure 6.4). The end of each bone is covered by a layer of cartilage called articular cartilage; this is typical hyaline cartilage and has no nerves, blood vessels or lymphatics. The bones are held together by a joint capsule which has two layers.

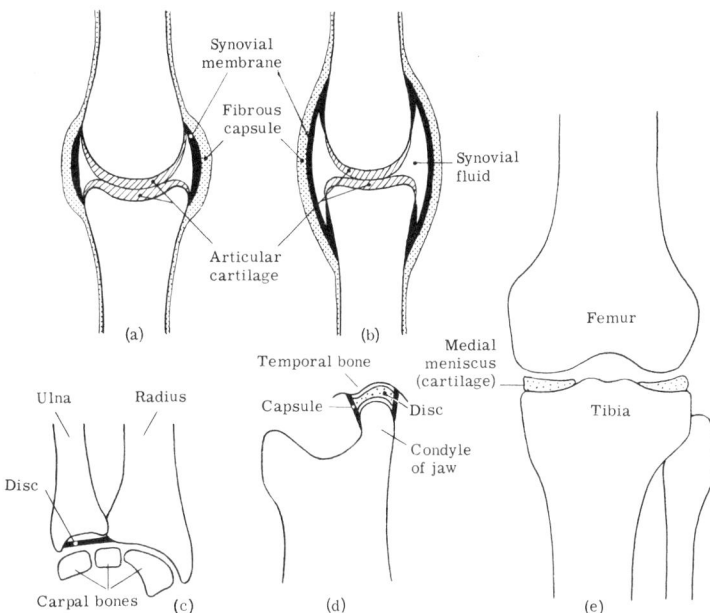

Figure 6.4 Synovial joints. (a) Section through the joint. (b) Section through a joint in which the fibrous capsule is attached beyond the articular cartilage. (c) Wrist. (d) Mandibular and (e) Knee joints showing intra-articular fibrocartilaginous discs (menisci in the knee joint).

The outer layer is called the fibrous capsule and is composed of sheets of collagen fibres; it is not very elastic so it contributes to the strength and stability of the joint. The fibrous capsule is continuous with the periosteum.

The inner layer of the joint capsule is the synovial membrane which is chiefly formed from loose connective tissue. The synovial membrane has a very rich supply of nerves, blood vessels and lymphatics. The membrane forms the synovial fluid which fills the synovial cavity. This thick fluid lubricates the joint so that friction between the two articular cartilages is reduced and also nourishes the cartilage which has no blood supply of its own.

Within the capsule of some synovial joints are cartilaginous discs (menisci) or tendons. These structures often give stability to the joint and reduce pressure and friction on the articular cartilages during movement.

Synovial fluid deserves extra attention because of its unique importance. An examination of synovial fluid in joint and connective tissue disease is comparable to the analysis of urine in a patient with kidney disease. Essentially, synovial fluid is a filtrate of plasma into which the synovial membrane has secreted hyaluronic acid. This compound gives the synovial fluid the texture and thickness of egg white. The fluid is clear and has a light yellowish tinge. There are proteins present, between 1.5–2.5 g/dl, but there is no fibrinogen, so normal synovial fluid does not clot unless acid is added to it. In healthy joints there is relatively little fluid — 3 ml or so in a knee joint. The volume decreases with age but can increase in many diseases.

In normal synovial fluid there are less than 200 white blood cells per mm^3, and less than 25% of these will be polymorphonuclear leukocytes (polymorphs). If there is a septic arthritis and the joint is inflamed and infected with bacteria or fungi, then the number of white blood cells can increase to as high as 100 000/mm^3, and more than 90% of them will be polymorphs. Changes in the number of cells and changes in the content of the fluid are noted in other inflammatory diseases of the joints.

A bursa is a fibrous sac which is lined with synovial membrane and contains synovial fluid. Bursae are located outside joints, between the muscle tendon and the bone or between muscles. They function to reduce friction between these structures.

Synovial joints are classified according to the shape of the articular surfaces and the movements which are possible.

a. Ball and socket joints. These are the most freely moveable of all joints and capable of flexion, extension, abduction, adduction, rotation and circumduction. Structurally they consist of a hemispherical head which fits into a cup-shaped socket. The shoulder joint and the hip joints are ball and socket joints.

b. Hinge joints permit movement in one plane only, thus, only flexion and extension can take place at a hinge joint. Examples of hinge joints include the elbow, knee and ankle joints. The joint between the occipital bone and the atlas of the vertebral column is a hinge joint as are the interphalangeal joints of the fingers and the toes.

c. Gliding joints. In this type of joint the articular surfaces are relatively flat and the surfaces glide over one another during movement. Movement may take place in all directions at a gliding joint, but the extent of the movement is usually quite limited. The joints between the carpal bones and also between the tarsal bones are gliding joints. The sterno-clavicular joint and the acromio-clavicular joint are also gliding joints.

d. Pivot joints. These joints allow movement around one axis only — that is rotation. The joint between the odontoid process of the axis and the atlas permits rotation of the head (see Figure 6.5a). The superior and inferior radio-ulnar joints permit the radius to rotate about the ulna.

e. Condyloid joints. This joint is basically a hinge joint which also permits some lateral movement. Structurally it consists of two convex surfaces which fit into two concave surfaces. The temporo-mandibular joint is a hinge joint; you can easily raise and lower your jaw but side-to-side

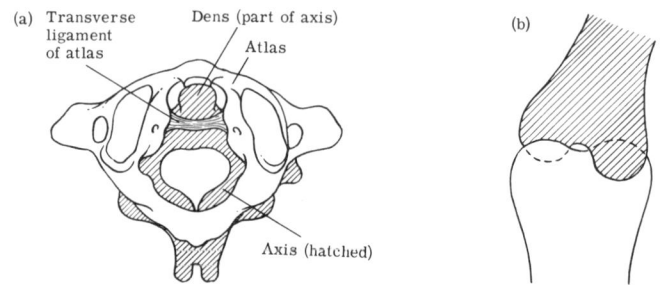

Figure 6.5 Synovial joints. (a) Pivot joint. (b) Saddle joint.

movement is much more restricted. The articulation of the radius with the carpal bones and the metacarpo-phalangeal joints are condyloid joints.

f. Saddle joints. Each bone in a saddle joint has one concave surface and one convex surface and the opposite-shaped surfaces fit in with one another. The joint between the metacarpal bone of the thumb and the trapezium is saddle-shaped, and limited movement in all three axes is permitted (see Figure 6.5b).

WHAT IS THE STRUCTURE OF THE PRINCIPAL JOINTS OF THE BODY?

A. The shoulder joint

This is a ball and socket joint and is the most freely moveable in the body. The round head of the humerus fits into the glenoid cavity of the scapula (see Figure 6.6). The surfaces of the cavity and the head of the humerus are lined with hyaline cartilage.

The glenoid cavity has a rim of fibrocartilage called the glenoid labrum which goes around the rim of the cavity; this deepens the cavity and adds to the stability of the joint without restricting movement. Within the capsule is also found the long tendon of the biceps muscle. This tendon lies in the bicipital groove of the humerus and runs through the joint cavity before attaching itself to the scapula and thus helps to keep the articular surface in position. The capsular ligaments which run from the scapula to the head of the humerus are loose fitting so movement is not restricted.

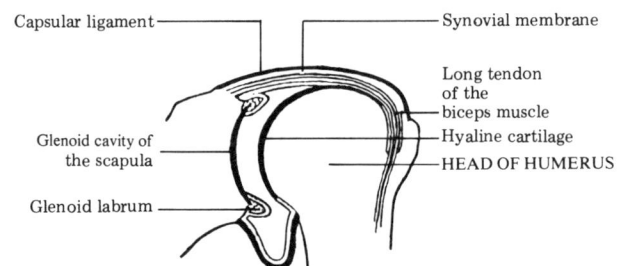

Figure 6.6 The shoulder joint.

B. The elbow joint

This is a hinge joint formed by the articulation of the trochlea and capitulum of the humerus with the trochlear notch of the ulna and the head of the radius (see Figure 6.7). Since this is a hinge joint, flexion and extension of the forearm are the only possible motions.

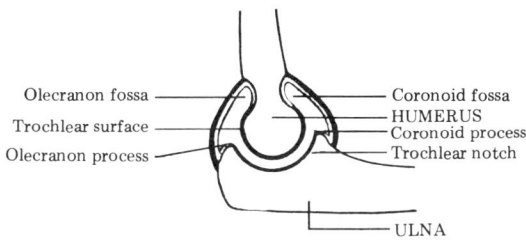

Figure 6.7 The elbow joint.

C. The superior and inferior radio-ulnar joints

The superior radio-ulnar joint is within the joint capsule of the elbow. The head of the radius articulates with the radial notch on the lateral side of the proximal extremity of the ulna. The two bones are held together by the annular ligament. This ligament is outside the joint capsule, surrounds the head of the radius and is attached to the anterior and posterior margins of the radial notch of the ulna. The inferior radio-ulnar joint is between the distal end of the radius and the head of the ulna (see Figure 6.8a). The two bones are held together by ligaments. Both the superior and inferior are pivot joints so the movement is rotatory: pronation and supination of the forearm.

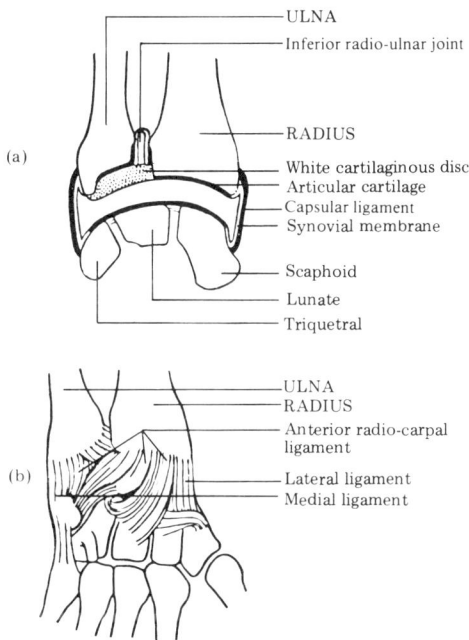

Figure 6.8 The wrist joint. (a) The structures of the joint — anterior view. (b) The supporting ligaments.

D. The wrist joint.

This joint is a condyloid joint formed by the distal end of the radius and the proximal ends of the triquetral, lunate and scaphoid bones. A disc of white fibrous cartilage separates the joint cavity from the ulna and also articulates with the carpal bones of the wrist. The medial, lateral and anterior radio-carpal ligaments attach to the joint capsule (see Figure 6.8b). The wrist can bend forward (flexion), backward (extension), towards the radial side (abduction) or towards the ulnar side (adduction) or some combination of these movements.

E. The hip joint

If the essential feature of the shoulder joint is mobility, the essential feature of the hip joint is its stability. This is particularly important, for the hip joint bears the body weight when we are standing and is subject to a great deal of strain, especially in activities like jumping. The hip joint is similar to the shoulder joint in that it is a ball and socket joint and that the cup-shaped acetabulum is rimmed, like the glenoid cavity, with fibrocartilage which gives the joint added stability. Within the capsule there is a ligament which grows out of the head of the femur and inserts below the rim of the acetabulum (see Figure 6.9). It is called the round ligament (the ligamentum teres) and contains a blood vessel which distributes blood to the head of the femur. The chief support of the joint comes from three extracapsular ligaments. The ilio-femoral ligament is a "Y"-shaped ligament going from the ilium of the innominate (hip) bone to the femur. The pubo-femoral ligament passes below the ilio-femoral ligament, between the pubis and the femur. The ischio-femoral ligament passes from the ischium to the posterior surface of the femur. Because it is a ball and socket joint, a great amount of movement is possible. This includes bending the thigh upward towards the trunk (flexion), movement of the thigh backwards (extension), adduction, abduction, circumduction and rotation.

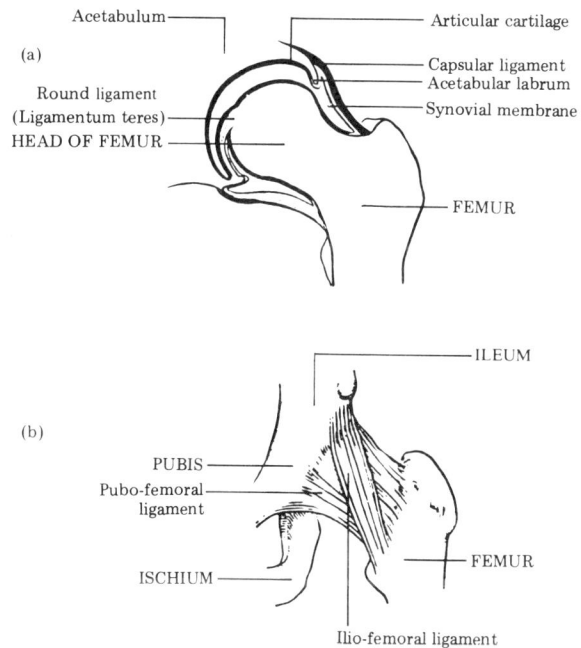

Figure 6.9 The hip joint. (a) The structures inside the joint. (b) The supporting ligaments.

F. The knee joint

This is the largest joint in the body and is formed from the condyles of the lower extremity of the femur, the condyles of the upper extremity of the tibia and the posterior surface of the patella (see Figure 6.10). It is a hinge joint and permits flexion and extension. The fibrous capsule encloses the joint on the posterior, medial and lateral surfaces. The anterior part of the capsule is formed by the tendon of the quadriceps

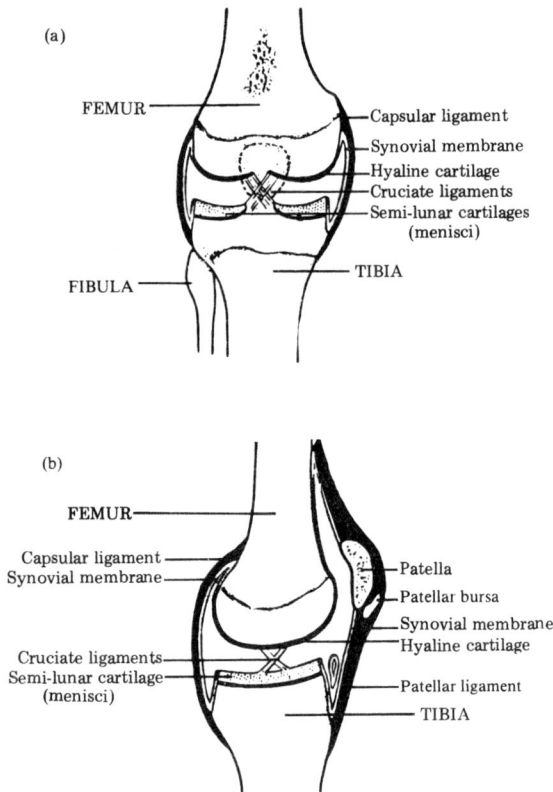

Figure 6.10   The knee joint. (a) The intracapsular structures — anterior view. (b) The position of the patella — lateral view.

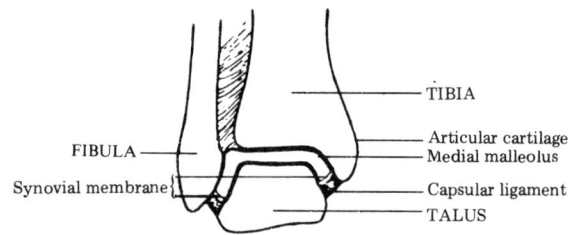

Figure 6.11   The ankle joint — anterior view.

femoris muscle which contains the patella. Beyond or distal to the patella the ligament is known as the patellar ligament and it attaches to the upper end of the tibia. Within the joint are the cruciate ligaments which are attached above to the intercondylar notch and below to the upper surface of the tibia. These ligaments get their name from the fact that they are arranged so that they cross over each other (the Latin word meaning cross is *crux, crucis*). They bind the bones more firmly together helping to limit movement at the joint. Within the joint are semi-lunar cartilages (menisci) which lie on top of the articular condyles of the tibia; these also have some stabilizing effect on the joint.

Pads of fat and numerous bursae are found within the capsule and help to reduce friction. Bursae are also found outside the capsule between the skin and the tendon. If the bursae should become infected, enlarged or inflamed the condition is called bursitis. Those who kneel for long periods are susceptible to this condition so it is also known as "house maid's knee". Bursitis is not limited to the knee however.

G. The ankle joint

This joint is formed by the lateral malleolus of the fibula, the distal end of the tibia and its malleolus, all of which articulate with the talus of the foot (see Figure 6.11). It is a hinge joint, so flexion and extension are possible. Extension of the foot by moving it upwards is also referred to as dorsiflexion, while flexion of the foot by pointing it downwards is called plantar flexion. There are no major intracapsular structures within the capsular ligament which surrounds the joint. This

ligament is given additional support by four other ligaments; the anterior, posterior, lateral and medial ligaments. (The medial ligament is also called the deltoid ligament.) These ligaments may be sprained or torn and the bones may be forced out of their natural positions (dislocated). Pain and swelling follows, so the ankle should have ice or cold water applied to it, then be firmly bandaged. An X-ray is often desirable because one of the malleoli or one of the tarsal bones may have been fractured.

WHAT IS ARTHRITIS?

While nearly everyone knows somebody with arthritis, not everyone knows what arthritis is. Arthritis simply means inflammation of the joints and really does not define a specific disease process. Arthritis is a common condition: in Switzerland, for example, it is estimated to be responsible for about 16% of all absences from work.

As mentioned before, bacteria can infect a joint and can cause it to become inflamed. Apart from bacteria, certain viruses, fungi and even parasites can cause arthritis. Other diseases that are not primarily joint diseases can also cause it. A person with haemophilia may bleed into a joint: if the bleeding is chronic, the synovial membrane becomes inflamed and enlarged, and articular cartilage can be destroyed.

Gout is a metabolic disorder in which uric acid levels in the blood are high and in which sodium urate crystals are formed in the synovial fluid. The crystals initiate an inflammatory response in the synovial membrane which is extremely painful. One patient with an attack of gouty arthritis said that his big toe was so very sensitive that the pressure of a bedsheet caused him excruciating pain (Gout is a genetic, metabolic disorder and is not caused, as is sometimes said, by laziness or high living.)

In common usage, rheumatism refers to pain or stiffness in the joints or muscles. It should not be confused with rheumatoid arthritis. The latter is a chronic systemic disease with exacerbations and remissions and is of unknown cause, and although other parts of the body may be affected, the predominant pathology is in the inflamed synovial membranes. Early in the course of the disease a single joint may be stiff, but with time the disease tends to be bilaterally symmetrical and affects several joints. These joints may become inflamed, painful, tender and swollen with the overlying skin being hot and erythematous (reddish) in colour. The initial cause of this inflammation is not known but a virus and/or disordered immune response is suspected. Lymphocytes and polymorphs accumulate in the inflamed joint. The synovial membrane hypertrophies; the fibroblasts proliferate; collagen is laid down and a dense connective tissue pannus is formed. The pannus fills the joint space and may eventually enlarge still more; the pannus covers and destroys articular cartilage. Treatment of the disease often involves rest, aspirin (salicylates) or other drugs which reduce the inflammation. Surgery may be necesary to replace a destroyed joint.

Osteoarthritis is not primarily an inflammatory disease of the joint but a degenerative one. The term degenerative joint disease (DJD) is being used more frequently as a replacement for osteoarthritis. The cause of DJD is most often the wear and tear of age — 90% of the population over 40 is affected or shows some signs of DJD. In DJD there is some erosion, flaking and ulceration in the articular cartilage. This leads to some secondary inflammation of the synovial membrane. Involvement of the knee is a common source of disability in DJD. In obese people, the weight-bearing joints are particularly affected, and treatment should be directed at reducing weight. Anti-inflammatory drugs may be useful in DJD.

There are other causes of arthritis and there are diseases other than those mentioned that are associated with arthritis. It is impossible to overstress the importance of physical and occupational therapists for persons with crippling arthritis. If a joint is stiff, painful or hurts when it is moved, a patient may be quite reluctant to move it. If the patient does not move the joint, his or her bones and muscles will weaken and atrophy, and movement will be made even more difficult. A vicious circle begins and can lead to further crippling.

Healthy people perform so many complex activities without thinking, we tend to be unaware how difficult these actions can be if limited in movement by joint disease. Buttoning buttons, putting keys in locks and turning on water taps are extremely difficult for the person with deformed hands, and walking and climbing stairs may not be easy for the person with hip or lower limb disease. With help, education and appropriate aids, the person with arthritis can make significant strides and either overcome or bypass some of the hardships and handicaps of disease.

7. The Muscular System

INTRODUCTION

Life moves. Even when standing still, the individual's muscular system is still important and still working. The mere act of standing up requires considerable muscular effort to overcome the force of gravity and the work of the respiratory muscles continues from the first breath of life to the last.

There are more than 400 muscles within the human body and this great number permits an infinite variety of human activities. These include the incredibly complicated movements of lips and tongue which produce speech and the amazing feats of human endurance such as climbing mountains and running a mile under 4 minutes.

Skeletal muscle is strengthened by exercise, weakened by lack of use and is subject to a number of diseases. Our knowledge of muscle and its physiology has increased dramatically in recent years. The electron microscope has provided evidence which makes possible an understanding of contraction at the molecular level. Regardless of all these new developments, the gross anatomy of the muscular system remains unchanged.

WHAT IS THE STRUCTURE OF MUSCLE?

Muscle is one of the four basic tissues. There are three types of muscle: skeletal, cardiac and smooth. Although all three muscle types have certain common properties, there are distinct anatomical and physiological differences. In this section, skeletal muscle will be considered in detail.

Skeletal muscle is also called voluntary muscle because it is under control of the will. This means that under most conditions we have control over our skeletal muscles — we can choose to clap our hands or sit on them. When an action has been "willed" or decided upon, impulses are relayed from the brain to motor neurones. Impulses travel down the axons of the motor neurones and cause a chemical signal to be sent to the appropriate muscles. This chemical signal causes impulses to be generated and travel over the muscle cells, stimulating the muscles to contract.

A muscle is made up of many cells known as muscle fibres, which are specifically adapted for contraction and conductivity (see Figure 7.1). A muscle fibre is a long, thin cell surrounded by a membrane (called the sarcolemma) with one or more nuclei, mitochondria and specialized structures called myofilaments (myofibrils). Each cell contains many thousands of these thread-like myofilaments. Myofilaments are special contractile protein structures and are either one of two kinds, myosin or actin.

Myosin is a thick, complex protein containing an enzyme, adenosine triphosphatase (ATPase), which is able to release

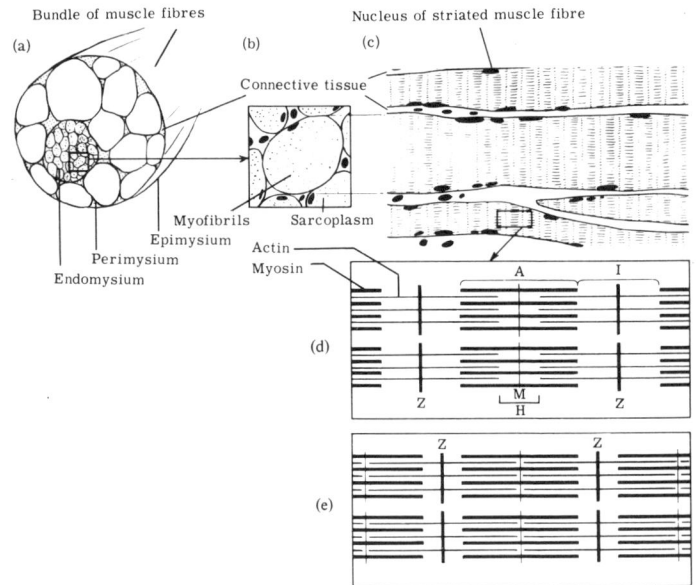

Figure 7.1 Muscle structure. (a) Transverse section of whole striated muscle. (b) Transverse section of single muscle fibre. (c) Longitudinal section of single muscle fibre. (d, e) Diagrams of electron microscope appearances of (d) uncontracted and (e) contracted myofibrils.

energy by breaking down ATP to ADP. There are at regular intervals short projections from the myosin myofilament. These specialized protein projections angle towards the surrounding actin myofilaments and are the essential parts of the bridges or temporary linkages connecting the myosin and actin myofilaments during the process of contraction.

The actin myofilaments are much thinner than the myosin myofilaments. In addition to the protein, actin, they contain two other proteins. Tropomyosin is coiled around the actin molecules. At regular intervals on the tropomyosin another protein called troponin is bound to the tropomyosin. Troponin is a protein that has a greater affinity for binding calcium ions. It is thought that the contraction of a muscle occurs when the calcium ions bind to the troponin molecules and form a linkage with the myosin projections. More will be said about this later in the section dealing with the mechanism of contraction. The actin myofilaments are attached to the Z line. The Z line is really an inward projection of the sarcolemma. There is a series of vesicles and tubules surrounding the myofibrils which is called the sarcoplasmic reticulum. The sarcoplasmic reticulum is the muscle's communication and transport system. It is generally agreed that one of the first steps in contraction is the release of calcium ions from vesicles in the sarcoplasmic reticulum. For the muscle to relax, calcium ions must be pumped back from the troponin to the vesicles within the sarcoplasmic reticulum, and this process requires ATP for energy.

To understand contraction, however, you must understand the arrangement of the myosin and actin filaments (see Figure 7.1d and e). There are six actin myofilaments for each myosin myofilament, and each actin myofilament is attached to the Z line. The distance between the two Z lines is referred to as the sarcomere. The space on either side of the Z line contains only the thin actin filaments and is called the I band. The area next to the I bands contains actin filaments which overlap thick myosin filaments, and in its most central areas, only myosin. This area between the I bands which contains myosin is called the A band. Because the myofilaments in a cell are placed in a regular and repetitive order, parallel to and in register with one another, the whole cell will show the striations resulting from the alternating A and I bands.

Bundles of muscle fibres are wrapped in a delicate layer of capillary-containing connective tissue called the endomysium and groups of muscle bundles are wrapped in a stronger connective tissue membrane called the perimysium (see Figure 7.1a). The tough outermost sheath of connective tissue which surrounds the entire muscle is called the epimysium. This tough connective tissue helps protect the muscle from bacterial invasion and infection. It should be noted that the words endomysium, perimysium and epimysium are terms derived from microscopic observation. In gross dissection or during surgical procedures the word fascia is most frequently used to refer to the connective tissue surrounding muscle. Fascia also lies beneath the skin and covers various organs of the body.

Most skeletal muscles are attached to the bones or skin by means of tendons. The connective tissue of the endomysium, perimysium and epimysium is continuous with the connective tissue of the tendon which attaches directly to bone or skin. These attachments are very strong and can withstand great force, although they may be torn or pulled away from the bone or muscle or cut in an accident. A thin, flat tendon that occasionally covers a muscle or connects it to the structure it moves is called an aponeurosis.

WHAT IS THE ANATOMY OF THE SKELETAL MUSCULAR SYSTEM?

In the human there are more than 400 skeletal muscles so it is not possible to list or describe them all here. Most descriptions of skeletal muscles state that one end of the muscle is the origin and the other end is the insertion. These terms refer to the fact that when a muscle contracts and shortens, one of its attachments usually remains fixed and the other end moves towards the fixed end. The fixed end of the muscle is called the origin while the movable end is termed the insertion. These terms are not always accurate, for in some cases both ends of the muscle will shorten or the insertion will remain fixed and the origin will move. After each description the prime action caused by contraction of the muscle is listed. Attention should be called, however, to the fact that most movements do not involve contractions of

single muscles but co-ordinated actions of muscle groups. Muscles working together to produce a single movement are called synergists. Antagonists are muscles which oppose that movement. Smooth, graceful movements result from the combined actions of groups of synergists and other groups of antagonists working together.

Muscles frequently receive their name from the Latin word or its derivative which describes their shape, position and movement produced or the structure with which the muscles are associated or attached. The body is a symmetrical structure and most muscles are represented on both the right and left sides of the body. When the text refers, for example, to the gastrocnemius muscle of the leg, it should be understood that there are two gastrocnemii, one on each leg.

A. The muscle of facial expression and mastication

The chief muscles associated with facial expression are the occipito-frontalis, the orbicularis oculi, the orbicularis oris and the buccinator (see Figure 7.2). These muscles do not have to lift the heavy loads that other muscles of the body do but they are capable of producing an infinite variety of facial expressions. They do not have the strong tendons other muscles have but generally have their origin on fascia or facial bones and insert into the skin by thin and isolated strands of connective tissue. There is also a great deal of difference in the size, shape and strength of the facial muscles.

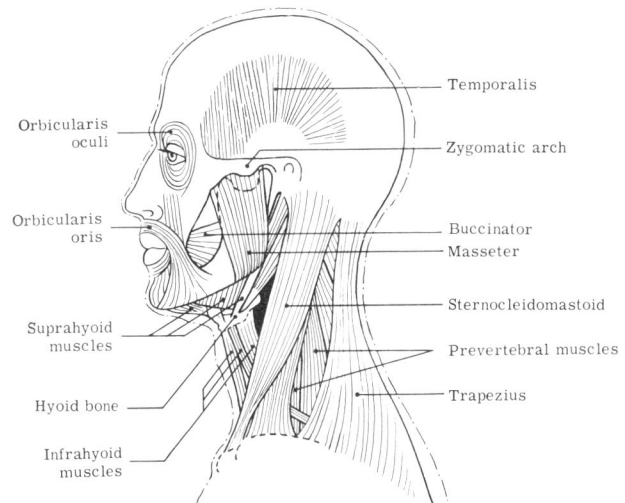

Figure 7.2 The muscles of the head and neck.

The muscles of mastication are the masseter, the temporalis and pterygoid muscles. The word mastication comes from the Latin word *masticare* meaning to chew and refers to the movement of the lower jaw at the temporo-mandibular joint. These movements tear, grind and chew food.

a. The occipito-frontalis muscle. The posterior part of this muscle lies over the occipital bone while the anterior part, the frontalis, lies over the frontal bone in the forehead. The two parts are connected to the sheet of fibrous connective tissue covering the vault of the skull (the aponeurosis). The occipito-frontalis arises in the skin at the root of the nose and along the eyebrows; contraction of this muscle causes raising of the eyebrows and "wrinkling" of the forehead.

b. The orbicularis oculi. This thin muscle surrounds the orbit of the eye and is the sphincter muscle of the eyelid. Fibres of this muscle are responsible for blinking and for closing the eyes in sleep. The antagonist of the orbicularis oculi is the levator palpebrae superioris, which raises the eyelid and exposes the front of the eye bulb. Contraction of the circular fibres draws the eyelids tightly shut and draws the skin of the temple, forehead and cheek towards the midline.

c. The orbicularis oris. This muscle surrounds the mouth and also receives fibres from other facial muscles. It closes the lips and can protrude (pucker) the lips in whistling and kissing.

d. The buccinator. This muscle makes up the main part of the cheek between the maxilla and the mandible. It draws the corner of the mouth laterally and helps push food between the teeth. It is also involved in whistling and is important in blowing certain musical instruments such as the trumpet.

The facial muscles on each side of the face are supplied by either the right or left facial nerve. If the facial nerve on one side is injured or diseased the muscles on the corresponding side of the face become paralyzed. In a condition known as Bell's palsy the facial nerve is diseased and the patient's facial movements are greatly restricted.

e. The masseter. This powerful muscle extends from the zygomatic arch to the angle of ramus of the lower jaw or mandible. Its action is to raise forcefully the lower jaw; the masseter can be palpated if you clench your teeth.

f. The temporalis. This fan-shaped muscle covers the squamous portion of the temporal bone and passes downwards beneath the zygomatic arch and is inserted on the coronoid process of the mandible. Its action is to elevate the mandible at rest.

g. Pterygoid muscles. There are two pterygoid muscles (pterygoid means wing-shaped). The internal and external pterygoid muscles run from the greater wing of the sphenoid bone to the medial surface of the mandible and thus

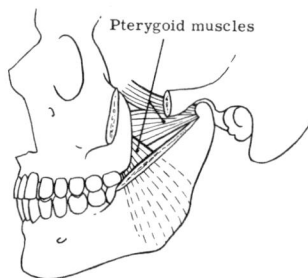

Figure 7.3 The muscles of the face.

contribute to the formation of the mouth (see Figure 7.3). The internal pterygoid assists in closing the jaws while the external pterygoid helps to open the jaws.

(The muscles of mastication are innervated by the mandibular branch of cranial nerve V (the trigeminal).)

B. The muscles of the neck

These muscles are responsible for flexing the head and turning it from side to side. The two most important muscles are the sternocleidomastoid and the trapezius (see Figure

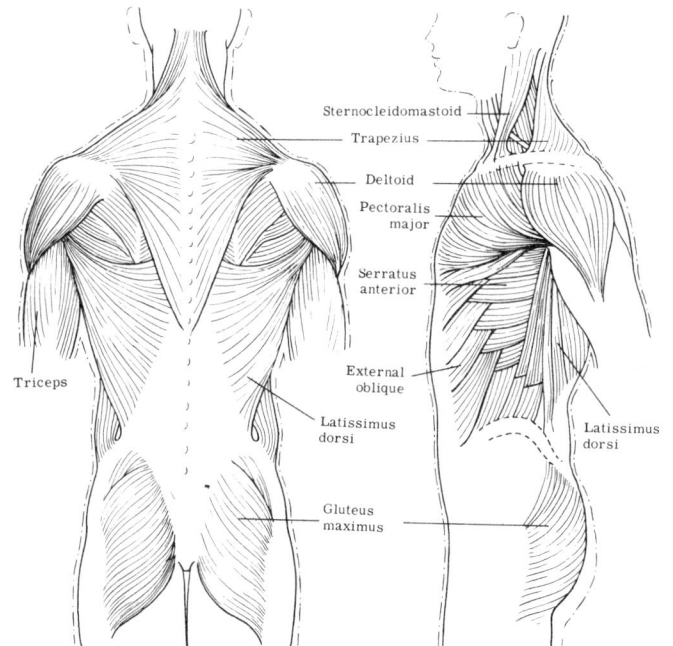

Figure 7.4 Superficial muscles of the back, neck and trunk.

7.4). The neck also contains an intricate series of muscles which raise and lower the larynx. You can easily demonstrate this by gently placing your fingers on the hard thyroid cartilage (Adam's apple) in the front of the neck and then swallowing. Other neck muscles attach to the hyoid bone. The tongue is attached to the hyoid bone and these neck muscles thus help position the tongue.

a. The sternocleidomastoid. This muscle arises from the sternum and clavicle and passes at an angle to the mastoid process of the temporal bone. When the right and left sternocleidomastoids contract together they flex the head toward the chest or draw the sternum and clavicle upwards. This happens when the normal muscles of respiration are not functioning properly and breathing must be maintained by the accessory muscles of respiration. If one sternocleidomastoid acts alone, the head is turned towards the opposite side of the body and tilts the chin slightly upward. Thus, contraction of the right sternocleidomastoid will pull the head to the left. (Accessory nerve XI.)

b. The trapezius. This muscle is triangular-shaped and is responsible for the sloping ridge of the neck. The broad base of the triangle is the origin of the muscle. The uppermost attachment is to the occipital protuberance of the skull; it continues in the midline of the back to the 12th thoracic vertebra. The muscle has a continuous insertion on two bones: the lateral third of the clavicle, and the acromion process and spine of the scapula (see Figure 7.4). When the uppermost parts of both muscles contract they pull the head backwards. When both the middle and lower parts contract they pull the shoulders backwards, or "square" them. Injury to the trapezius results in drooping or stooped shoulders. The muscle's action in relation to movement of the shoulder will be discussed in the section on the muscles which join the upper limb to the thorax and move the shoulder joint. (Spinal accessory nerve and 3rd and 4th cervical nerves.)

C. The muscles of the back

These muscles are responsible for movements of the trunk and participate in the movement of the head and limbs. They also have postural and synergistic functions. You can demonstrate this by placing both hands, palms down, over your lower back and then walking. You can feel the contractions on alternate sides as the weight of the body is shifted from foot to foot. The main muscles of the back and posterior abdominal wall are (a) the sacrospinalis muscle, (b) the latissimus dorsi, (c) the quadratus lumborum, (d) the psoas and (e) the iliacus.

a. The sacrospinalis muscle. The sacrospinalis is not a single muscle but a group of muscles which run parallel and lateral to the vertebral column (see Figure 7.4). Some fibres have their origin in the iliac crest and insert into the lowest ribs and vertebrae. Other fibres begin in the lower vertebrae and insert on higher vertebrae, or the occipital bone.

These muscles extend the trunk and the head. Looking up to see the stars involves contractions of the sacrospinalis. (Posterior primary divisions of spinal nerves.)

b. The latissimus dorsi. This large, superficial, triangular-shaped muscle arises from the spines of the lower thoracic vertebrae and from fascia attached to the spines of the lumbar and sacral vertebrae and to the iliac crest. It passes obliquely around the side of the trunk and then continues upward to insert into the front of the humerus (see Figure 7.4). (Its action on the arm and shoulder girdle will be discussed in a subsequent section.) The latissimus dorsi, by virtue of its attachment to the ribs, can serve as an accessory muscle of respiration and assists during expiration. You can feel the latissimus dorsi contract if you place your hand on your thorax, several centimetres below the axilla and cough. (Thoracodorsal nerve.)

c. The quadratus lumborum. This wide muscle is attached to the posterior part of the iliac crest and passes upward to the lowest rib and the transverse processes of the lumbar vertebrae. The quadratus lumborum is thought to play a role

in inspiration by holding the bottom rib steady and thereby aiding the diaphragm. If the muscle on only one side contracts, it will cause lateral flexion of the lumbar region of the trunk. (12th thorax and 1st lumbar nerves.)

d. The psoas. The psoas joins the axial skeleton and the lower extremity. It arises from the lumbar vertebrae and passes across the bones of the false pelvis and enters the thigh beneath the inguinal ligament to be inserted into the lesser trochanter of the femur (see Figure 7.5). When both feet are on the ground it flexes the trunk. It flexes the thigh and advances the limb when walking. (Branches from the lumbar plexus.)

e. The iliacus. This triangular-shaped muscle arises from the inner crest of the iliac fossa of the innominate (hip) bone and inserts into the tendon of the psoas muscle (see Figure 7.5). Its actions are similar to the psoas. Some authorities consider the iliacus and the psoas to be a single muscle, the iliopsoas. (Femoral nerve.)

D. The anterior abdominal wall

The contents of the abdominal cavity are protected anteriorly by the muscular abdominal wall. This consists of the rectus abdominis, the external oblique, the internal oblique, the transversus abdominis and the aponeuroses of these muscles. These muscles are arranged in sheets and can adapt to the changes imposed by pregnancy or increased deposition of fat; the muscles thin out and the nerves and blood vessels lengthen. Most surgical approaches to the abdominal cavity require cutting of these muscles.

The abdominal wall is divided into right and left halves by the linea alba (white line) which consists of tough fibrous connective tissue (see Figure 7.6). The navel (umbilicus) penetrates the linea alba just below its midline. The umbilical arteries and veins pass through this opening carrying wastes and nutrients to and from the mother via the placenta.

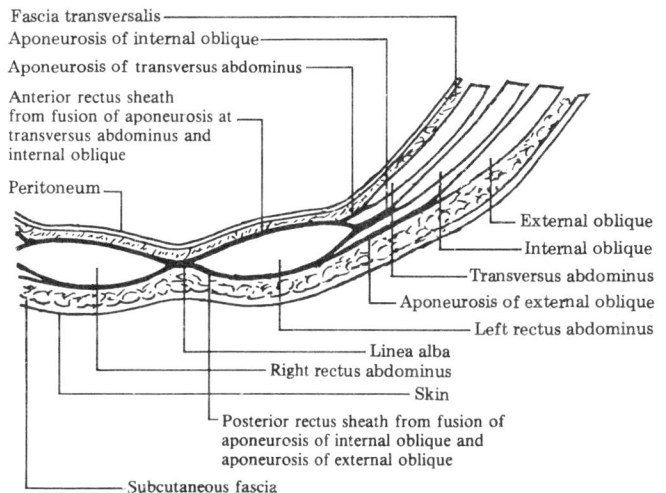

Figure 7.6 Planes of fascia and muscle in cross-section.

a. The rectus abdominis. This long and thin muscle is the most superficial of the four muscles. It is attached above the xiphoid process of the sternum and below to the pubic crest and the symphysis pubis. The muscle is surrounded by a connective tissue sheath formed from the aponeuroses of the other muscles of the anterior abdominal wall; the

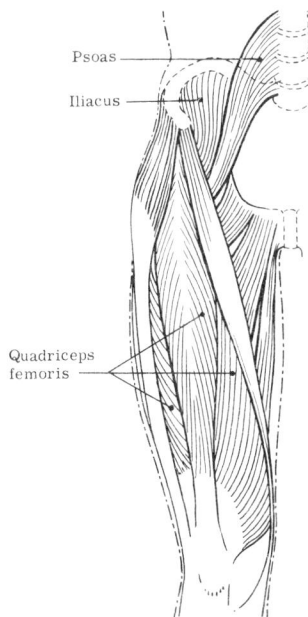

Figure 7.5 Muscles on the front of the hip and thigh.

aponeuroses meet in the midline to form the linea alba (see Figure 7.7). The rectus abdominis flexes the trunk and compresses the abdominal viscera. When you bend over to touch your toes you are contracting the rectus abdominis. (Intercostal nerve.)

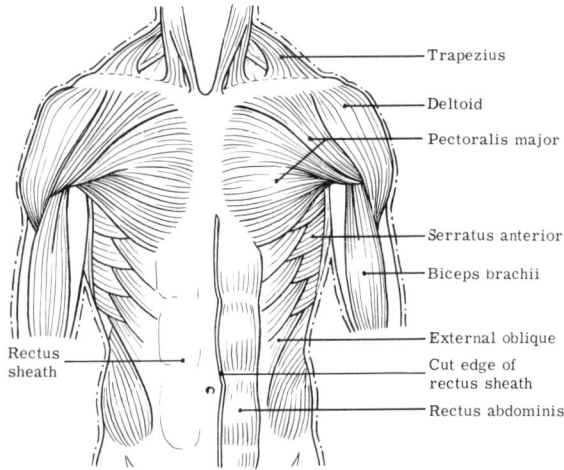

Figure 7.7 The muscles of the front of the trunk.

b. The external oblique. This is the most superficial and largest of the three muscles lateral to the rectus abdominis (see Figure 7.7). It arises from the lower eight ribs and travels downward and medially to be inserted into the iliac crest and rectus sheath by an aponeurosis. This aponeurosis is important because it contains a small opening, the superficial inguinal ring. The inguinal ring is above the inguinal ligament. This ligament is the lowermost part of the aponeurosis and runs from the anterior iliac spine to the pubic tubercle. (Intercostal nerve.)

c. The internal oblique. This muscle lies beneath the external oblique and its fibres take origin from the crest of the ilium and pass upward and medially to insert into the lower ribs and by an aponeurosis to the linea alba. When the external oblique and internal oblique of one side contract, the trunk will bend to that side, that is, either to the right or to the left. (Intercostal nerve.)

d. The transversus abdominis. This is the deepest of the three muscles. It takes origin in the lowest ribs and the iliac crest, and its fibres run more or less horizontally to insert into the linea alba by means of an aponeurosis. Beneath the fascia of the transversus abdominis is another layer of fascia called the fascia transversalis which contains a slit-like opening called the deep inguinal ligament ring. Simultaneous contraction of the internal and external obliques and the transversus abdominis can lead to a great increase in pressure within the abdomen. These muscles thus play a role in vomiting, defaecation, forceful expiration, micturition and parturition. (Intercostal nerve.)

An abdominal hernia is the protrusion of some internal body structure through the body wall. An umbilical hernia is a type of abdominal hernia in which part of the intestines protrude through the abdominal wall at the umbilicus; the protruding intestine is covered with skin and subcutaneous tissue. Most hernias occur in men and can be classified under the term groin (inguinal) hernia. (The groin is the lowest part of the abdominal wall, near its junction with the upper part of

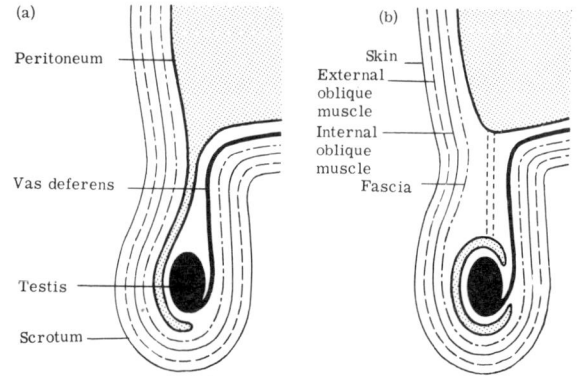

Figure 7.8 (a) Layers of the abdominal wall passing down into the scrotum together with the testis and peritoneum. (b) The disappearance of peritoneum between the inguinal wall and testis.

the thigh.) In many inguinal hernias, some part of the intestines follows the route used by the testes in descending into the scrotum. It leaves the abdomen via the deep inguinal ligament ring, passes obliquely through the abdominal wall and exits via the superficial inguinal ligament ring (see Figure 7.8). Other inguinal hernias are caused by a defect in the transverse fascia of the lower abdominal wall. Women, too, can have hernias but the route taken by the intestines does differ from the route of the most common male hernia.

If the structures protruding through the abdominal wall cannot be returned to their proper domain, the hernia is said to be incarcerated. The risks of an incarcerated hernia include intestinal obstruction and reduction of blood supply to the intestine. Correction of the hernia by surgery can prevent these complications.

E. The muscles of the pelvis

The levator ani and the coccygeus are the muscles of the pelvis which, with the fascias, contribute to the formation of the pelvic floor (see Figure 7.9). This is really the lowest part of the body wall and is important in supporting the abdominal viscera.

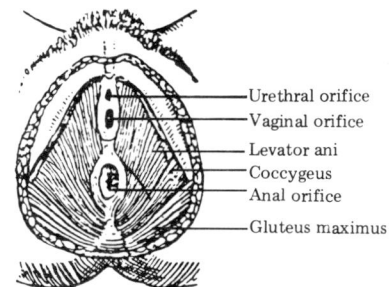

Figure 7.9 The muscles of the pelvic floor.

a. The levator ani. This muscle runs almost horizontally in the pelvis, taking its origin chiefly from the anterolateral wall of the true pelvis and running backward to insert on a raphe (seam) of connective tissue which connects to the levator ani from the other side. The anterior part of the muscle is separated from its mate by a genital hiatus through which the urethra, vagina and anal canal pass in the female, and the urethra and anal canal pass in the male. Contraction of the levator ani supports and raises the pelvic contents and is of importance in micturition and defaecation. Parts of this muscle may be torn during parturition. (Branches of pudendal nerve.)

b. The coccygeus. This small muscle originates in the ischial spine and passes behind the levator ani to insert on the coccyx. It also supports the pelvic viscera. (Branches of pudendal nerve.)

F. The muscles of the thoracic cage related to respiration

Breathing requires muscular work. Expansion of the thorax causes the lungs to enlarge and the pressure within them to fall. This permits environmental air to enter into the lungs. The external and internal intercostal muscles and the diaphragm are chiefly responsible for expanding the chest during a normal quiet inspiration. Expiration is a more passive phenomenon requiring little or no muscular effort. As the thorax returns to its resting volume, pressure within the lungs increases and air leaves the lungs. The internal intercostal muscles play some part in a quiet expiration. During more forceful respiration like that experienced during exercise, many other muscles participate in both inspiration and expiration.

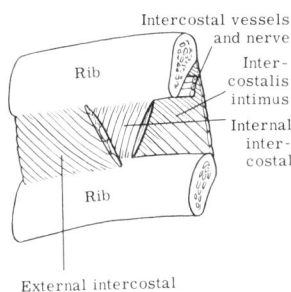

Figure 7.10   The external and internal intercostal muscles.

a. The external intercostal muscles. There are 11 pairs of these muscles which occupy the 11 spaces between the 12 ribs. The muscles pass downward and forward, beginning on the inferior edge of the rib above and passing to the superior edge of the rib below (see Figure 7.10). When these muscles contract they lift the ribs upward and outward so that the thorax enlarges in a front-to-back plane and a side-to-side plane. The easiest way to demonstrate this is to watch your chest as you take a big breath. During expiration these muscles gradually reduce their activity so the ribs are gradually lowered back to their rest position (see Figure 7.11). (Intercostal nerve.)

b. The diaphragm. This dome-shaped muscle with a tendinous centre separates the thoracic and abdominal cavities and is the most important respiratory muscle. Fibres originate from the circumference of the trunk and insert into a central aponeurosis. Anteriorly the fibres originate from the posterior surface of the xiphoid process, laterally from the lower ribs and posteriorly from two fibrous bands (crura), which are in turn attached to the right and left aspects of the first three lumbar vertebrae. There are three major openings within the diaphragm: the aortic opening, through which the aorta passes carrying blood to nourish the abdominal

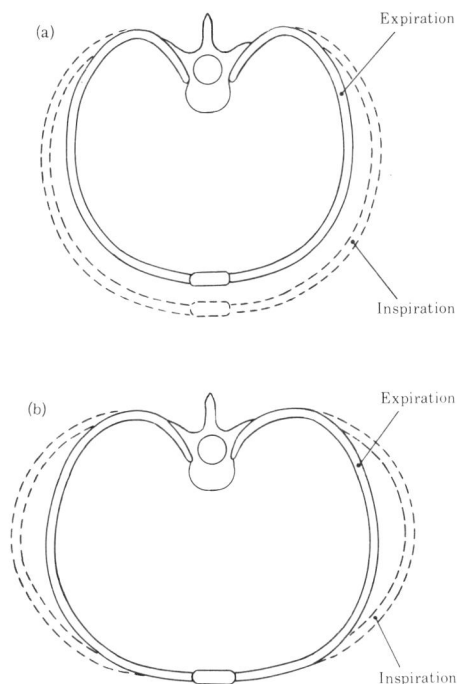

Figure 7.11   Movements in the thoracic wall during breathing. (a) The upper part, showing increase in the transverse and anteroposterior diameters. (b) The lower part, showing increase only in the transverse diameter.

structures and lower limbs; the opening for the inferior vena cava, which carries venous blood from the abdomen and lower limbs back to the heart; and the oesophageal opening, through which the oesophagus carries food and fluids to the stomach (see Figure 7.12). The diaphragm is innervated by the right and left phrenic nerves. Injury to these nerves can cause paralysis of the diaphragm and seriously interfere with, if not stop, normal respiration. In quiet breathing, contraction of the diaphragm causes it to descend slightly more than 1 cm. This increases abdominal pressure and reduces thoracic pressure. If the diaphragm does not develop properly, is weak, or is subject to some kind of stress so that an abdominal structure passes through it and enters the thoracic cavity, a diaphragmatic hernia results. (Phrenic nerve.)

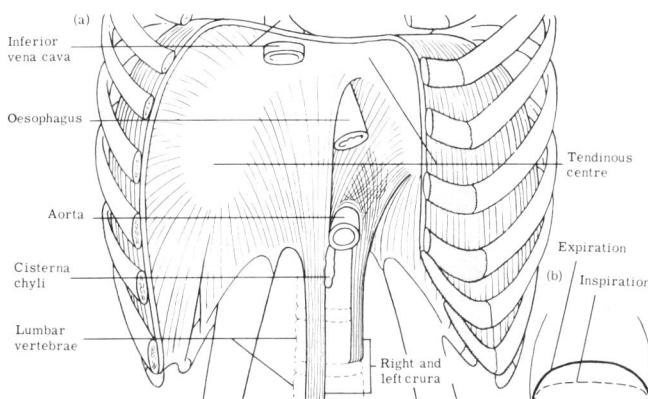

Figure 7.12   The diaphragm. (a) The front is partly removed to show the structures which pass through it. (b) Movements in the diaphragm during breathing.

c. The internal intercostal muscles. There are 11 pairs of these muscles which lie between the ribs beneath the outermost external intercostal muscles (see Figure 7.10). These muscles pass downward and backward. There is evidence that some parts of the internal intercostals contract during inspiration. (Intercostal nerve.)

None of the intercostal muscles can be said to be responsible for a quiet expiration, for this is a passive phenomenon in which the lungs and thorax return to their rest positions by virtue of their elastic properties.

G. Muscles which join the upper limb to the thorax and move the shoulder joint.

The shoulder joint is a ball and socket joint and has the greatest range of movement of any joint within the body. The movements possible at this joint are adduction, abduction, flexion, extension, circumduction and rotation. This great range is possible because the scapula itself is mobile and can accompany movements of the shoulder joint, and also because the fit of the head of the humerus into the glenoid cavity and its surrounding capsule is not tight. The stability of the joint depends largely upon the surrounding muscle tissue and, thus, the humerus can be forced out of its socket in dislocation of the shoulder joint. The following muscles are included in this section: (a) the pectoralis major (b) the serratus anterior (c) the latissimus dorsi (d) the teres major (e) the trapezius and (f) the deltoid (see Figure 7.4).

a. The pectoralis major. This muscle is thick, large and triangular in shape. The base of the triangle is formed by the origin of the muscle from the anterior surface of the sternum, clavicle and first six costal cartilages and from the aponeurosis of the external oblique of the abdomen. The muscle forms a large part of the anterior wall of the axilla ("armpit") as it tapers to form the tip of the triangle which inserts into the bicipital groove of the humerus (see Figure 7.4). The action of this muscle is to flex and adduct the arm forward and toward the midline of the body. It is important in actions like throwing, shovelling and shaking hands. (Medial and lateral anterior thoracic nerves.)

b. The serratus anterior. This is another large muscle which has eight separate origins from the outer surface of the upper eight ribs and inserts into the vertebral border of the scapula (see Figure 7.4). The muscle pulls the inferior angle of the scapula forward and laterally. This movement of the scapula is important in abduction of the arm and elevation of the arm above the horizontal. (Long thoracic nerve.)

c. The latissimus dorsi. This muscle takes origin from the vertebrae and passes upward over the thorax to insert in the bicipital groove of the humerus (see Figure 7.4). (The muscle is described more fully in the Section on the muscles of the back.) The muscle is a forceful extensor of the arm and can also adduct and rotate the arm medially. The down-stroke motion of the arm as used in swimming is an example of the use of this muscle. (Thoracodorsal nerve.)

d. The teres major. This muscle and the latissimus dorsi contribute to the formation of the posterior wall of the axilla. The origin of the teres major is on the inferior angle of the scapula and its insertion is on the lesser tubercle of the humerus. The muscle acts with the latissimus dorsi in extending and adducting the arm. (Lower subscapular nerve.)

e. The trapezius. This muscle takes origin in the midline of the back and neck and inserts into the clavicle and scapula (see Figure 7.4) as described in the Section on the muscles of the neck. Movement of the shoulder joint is usually accompanied by movement of the shoulder girdle; this movement gives greater freedom to movement of the arm. The trapezius helps to rotate the scapula by drawing the lateral angle of the scapula laterally and medially. This action causes the socket for the head of the humerus to look upward and thus increase the extent to which the arm may be abducted. Contraction of the trapezius and rotation of the scapula is important when you raise your hand or reach for something on a high shelf. (Spinal accessory nerve.)

f. The deltoid. This muscle is sometimes called the shoulder-pad muscle because it is superficially located, is thick and is responsible for the characteristic roundness of the shoulder. The muscle has a wide origin. Anteriorly it begins on the lateral third of the clavicle and posteriorly from the crest of the spine of the scapula, with a medial group of fibres beginning on the lateral border of the acromion process of the clavicle (see Figures 7.4 and 7.13a). When all three parts of the muscle contract the arm is abducted or elevated in the plane of the scapula. Contractions of the clavicular (anterior) part of the deltoid flex the arm and rotate it medially. The middle part of the muscle abducts the arm in the plane of the scapula while the spinous (posterior) part extends the arm. The deltoid also has a stabilizing action on the joint, especially in those actions which involve horizontal motion such as writing on a blackboard. (Axillary nerve.)

H. Muscles of the arm, forearm, hand and fingers

Painting, typing and performing surgery are examples of incredibly complex, precise and careful movements. We tend to think of them in terms of the talent of the artist, the efficiency of the secretary and the skill of the surgeon. In reality these talents and skills are marvels of muscular contraction and co-ordination. The muscles of the upper limb, unlike the muscles of the back or thorax, have an exceptionally rich nerve supply which permits greater control of the contraction.

The muscles of the arm which move the elbow joint are the biceps, the brachialis and the triceps. The muscles of the forearm which move the superior radio-ulnar joint are the pronator teres and the supinator. The muscles of the forearm which move the wrist joint are the flexor carpi radialis, the flexor carpi ulnaris, the extensor carpi radialis longus and the extensor carpi radialis brevis. The flexor digitorum profundis and the extensor digitorum longus are both located on the forearm and have very long tendons; they move the wrist and the fingers.

The intrinsic muscles of the hand which move the fingers are the thenar group of muscles, the hypothenar muscle group, the lumbrical muscles and the interossei muscles (see Figure 7.13).

a. The biceps brachii. This is one of the most widely known muscles of the body made famous by weight-lifters and beach musclemen who "bulge their biceps" when they flex their well-developed forearms. (Actually contraction of the brachialis helps push the biceps up.) The biceps is the most superficial muscle of the anterior forearm and has two heads,

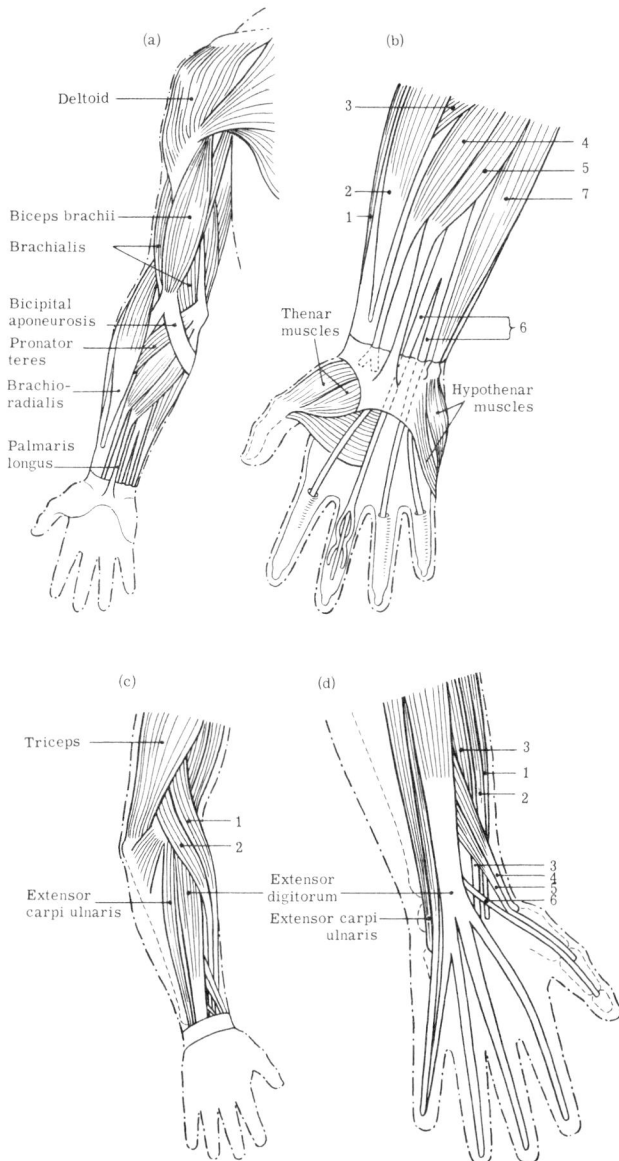

Figure 7.13 The muscles of the upper limb. (a) Front view. (b) The forearm and hand. 1; The extensor carpi radialis longus: 2; The brachio-radialis: 3; The pronator teres: 4; The flexor carpi radialis: 5: The palmaris longus: 6; The flexor digitorum superficialis (sublimis): 7; the flexor carpi ulnaris. (c) The back of the upper limb. (d) Muscles and tendons on the back of the wrist. 1; The brachio-radialis: 2; The extensor carpi radialis longus: 3; The extensor carpi radialis brevis: 4; The abductor pollicis longus: 5; The extensor pollicis brevis: 6; The extensor pollicis longus.

and supination of the forearm. It also gives stability to the shoulder joint and helps in the flexion of the upper arm at the shoulder joint. (Musculocutaneous nerve.)

b. The brachialis. This muscle lies on the anterior aspect of the upper arm beneath and lateral to the biceps. Its origin is from the anterior surface of the shaft of the humerus and its insertion is in the capsule of the elbow joint and the tuberosity of the ulna (see Figure 7.13a). The brachialis assists the biceps in flexing the forearm at the elbow. (Musculocutaneous nerve.)

c. The triceps. This muscle forms the bulk of the back of the arm and has three heads (origins). The long head of the triceps takes origin from the infraglenoid tubercle of the scapula, and the medial and lateral heads take origin from the medial and lateral aspects of the posterior surface of the humerus. The triceps is inserted into the olecranon process of the ulna (see Figure 7.13c). The main action of the triceps is to extend the forearm at the elbow — important in motions like pushing. The muscle also contributes to the extension of the arm. (Radial nerve.)

d. The pronator teres. This long, round, superficial muscle passes downward and laterally across the anterior surface of the forearm. The origin of the muscle is chiefly from the medial epicondyle of the humerus and the insertion is on the lateral surface of the radius (see Figure 7.13a and b). The muscle pronates the forearm, that is, turning the palm backward (posteriorly) or downward. The muscle also assists in flexing the forearm. (Median nerve.)

e. The supinator muscle. As the name states, this muscle supinates the forearm which is really lateral rotation of the forearm so that the palm faces anteriorly. The supinator is a deep muscle which runs across the posterior and lateral aspects of the forearm. The origin of the muscle is from the lateral epicondyle of the humerus and the crest of the ulna. The insertion is in the upper third of the shaft of the radius. (Radial nerve.)

f. The flexor carpi radialis. The origin of this muscle is from the common tendon of the medial epicondyle of the humerus. The muscle crosses over the radius on its anterior surface and its long tendon is inserted into the second and third metacarpal bones of the hand (see Figure 7.13d). The muscle's action is to flex the wrist. (Median nerve.)

g. The flexor carpi ulnaris. This muscle shares part of its origin with the flexor carpi radialis on the common tendon of the medial epicondyle of the humerus. The muscle's second origin is by an aponeurosis from the posterior border of the shaft of the ulna (see Figure 7.13b). The muscle passes beneath the flexor carpi radialis, parallel to the ulna, to insert into the pisiform, hamate and fifth metacarpal bones, and flexes the wrist. It also acts synergistically with the flexor carpi radialis to steady the wrist when the thumb and fingers move. (Ulnar nerve.)

h. The extensor carpi radialis longus and the extensor carpi radialis brevis. These two muscles are superficial muscles of the back of the forearm and have similar actions. The longus and the brevis have their origin on the lateral epicondyle of the humerus. The fibres of the longus insert into the back of the base of the second metacarpal while those of the brevis insert into the bases of the second and third metacarpal (see Figure 7.13d). They work with other muscles either to extend or to abduct the wrist. (Radial nerve.)

or more properly two origins. The short (medial) head of the biceps arises from the coracoid process of the scapula, while the long head derives from a long tendon from the rim of the glenoid cavity and passes through the joint cavity to run in the bicipital groove of the humerus; this tendon is held in this groove by the transverse humeral ligament. The two tendons give rise to two bellies, which soon unite into a single muscle, which then forms a tendon that inserts into the posterior part of the tuberosity of the radius (see Figure 7.13a). Because the muscle has two origins and spans both the shoulder and the elbow joint, its actions are varied. At the elbow joint, contraction of the biceps can bring about flexion *i. The flexor digitorum profundus.* This deep muscle of the forearm has a wide origin from the upper half of the anterior and medial surface of the ulna. It passes through the carpal canal and divides into four tendons which insert on the base of the distal phalanges excluding the thumb. Its action is to flex the fingers and the hand. (Median nerve.)

j. The extensor digitorum longus. This muscle arises from the lateral epicondyle of the humerus and passes over the posterior surface of the forearm. Before crossing the wrist the tendon of the muscle divides into four tendons which ultimately insert into the dorsal surface of each of the phalanges except the thumb (see Figure 7.13c and d). The muscle's action is to extend the wrist and fingers. (Radial nerve.)

There is one movement of the hand that is of the greatest importance to man. It is called opposition and refers to the movement of the thumb across the palm of the hand to make contact with the tips of the other fingers. When you hold a pen you oppose your thumb to your index finger. Many movements of the hand are produced by muscles situated on the forearm and their long tendons. Some movements of the hand, such as the opposition of the thumb, arise from the intrinsic muscles of the hand.

k. The thenar group of muscles. These muscles form a fleshy eminence at the base of the thumb (see Fig. 7.13b). The origin of the thenar muscles is from the scaphoid, trapezium and sesamoid bones, and the flexor retinaculum (the fibrous band that binds the flexor tendons of the five fingers). These muscles insert on the thumb and flex, abduct and adduct the thumb. (Median nerve.)

l. The hypothenar muscle group. This group of muscles form a fleshy eminence at the base of the little finger (see Figure 7.13b). Their origin is from the pisiform and hamate bones and their insertion is on the fifth metacarpus and the proximal phalanx of the little finger. They flex and abduct and oppose the little finger. (Ulnar nerve.)

m. The lumbrical muscles. There are four lumbrical muscles. Their origin is on the tendon of the flexor digitorum profundus and they are inserted into the lateral sides of the proximal phalanges of each finger with the exception of the thumb. The lumbricals flex the fingers although they can work with other muscles and act as extensors at the interphalangeal joints. (Median and ulnar nerves.)

n. The interossei muscles. There are eight interossei muscles, four on the palmar surface of the hand and four on the dorsal surface. Each palmar interosseus arises from a single head from the metacarpal shaft on either the first, second, fourth or fifth fingers. The insertion is on the base of the proximal phalanx of the first, second, fourth and fifth fingers. These muscles adduct the fingers toward a line drawn through the middle finger. The dorsal interossei have more complicated origins and insertion but they are abductors and draw the fingers away from a midline drawn through the third finger. (Ulnar nerve.)

I. Muscles which move the joints of the lower limb

The lower limb, unlike the upper limb, is not usually capable of delicate and specialized movements. The thigh, leg and foot are specialized for support and locomotion. When describing the lower limb it is traditional to include the transitional muscles which attach the thigh to the hip and which are prominent in locomotion.

a. The muscles of the buttocks. The buttock is often called the gluteal region because it is chiefly formed from three overlapping gluteal muscles.

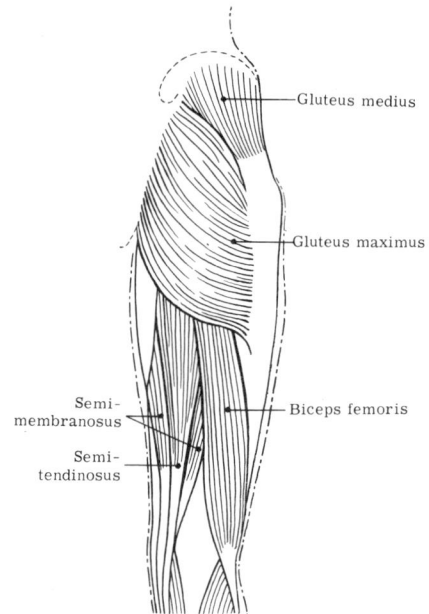

Figure 7.14 The muscles of the back of the hip and thigh.

(1) The most superficial of the three is also the largest and is called the gluteus maximus (see Figure 7.14). It takes origin from the dorsal surfaces of the sacrum, coccyx and ilium and inserts into the gluteal tuberosity of the femur and the fascia lata of the thigh. This muscle is a powerful extensor of the thigh and is used in forceful motions such as running, climbing and also for rising from a sitting position. By acting from a fixed insertion, the muscle can help extend the trunk which is important in extension from a stooped position. This muscle is also used as a site for injections; they are usually given in the upper, lateral quarter of the muscle to avoid large nerves which go to the thigh and leg. (Inferior gluteal nerve.)

(2) The gluteus medius is beneath the gluteus maximus.

(3) The gluteus minimus is the innermost muscle, lying beneath the gluteus medius. Both muscles have their origin on the outer surface of the ilium and insert on the lateral surface of the greater trochanter of the femur. (Superior gluteal nerve.) The muscles function to abduct the thigh and rotate it medially. During walking the two gluteal muscles of the limb that is on the ground tilt the pelvis so that the other limb can swing forward freely.

The muscles which move the thigh include the psoas, the iliacus, the sartorius and the quadriceps femoris. The psoas and iliacus were described on page 71. Their origin is from the lumbar vertebrae and iliac crest respectively. They are inserted into the lesser trochanter of the femur and flex it at the hip.

b. The sartorius. This long, thin muscle arises from the anterior superior spine of the ilium and takes a spiral course over the front of the thigh to insert on the medial surface of the tibia (see Figure 7.5). The chief action of this muscle is to act as a flexor of the thigh and the leg. The name sartorius is derived from the Latin word for tailor (*sartor*). Tailors are traditionally pictured sitting cross-legged on a table covered with their sewing. In this position the thigh is flexed and slightly rotated laterally. The sartorius participates in these motions. It is the longest individual muscle in the body. (Femoral nerve.)

c. The quadriceps femoris (quadriceps muscle). This is one of the body's largest and most powerful muscles and forms the bulk of the fleshy anterior part of the thigh (see Figure 7.5). The muscle has four separate heads or origins and a common insertion. The four heads are (1) the rectus femoris (2) the vastus lateralis (3) the vastus intermedius and (4) the vastus medialis.

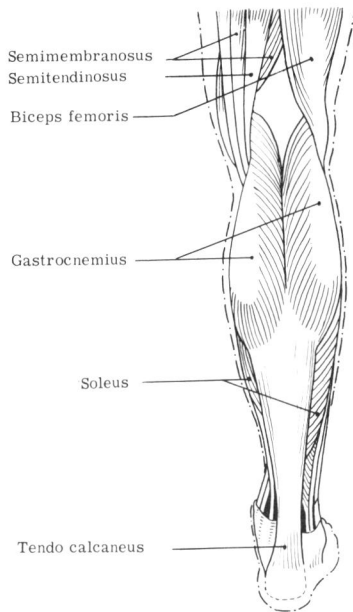

Figure 7.15 Superficial muscles of the back of the leg.

(1) The origin of the rectus femoris is from the anterior inferior iliac spine and from the superior rim of the acetabulum. Part of the tendon of the rectus inserts into the patella while the rest of the tendon continues on the tuberosity of the tibia. That part of the tendon between the patella and the tuberosity of the tibia is known as the patellar ligament. The rectus femoris flexes the thigh at the hip joint and extends the leg; it is sometimes called the kicking muscle because of its role in that action.

(2, 3, 4) The vastus lateralis, the vastus intermedius and the vastus medialis arise from the lateral, central and medial parts of the proximal end of the femur. They insert into the tendon of the rectus femoris at the patella; the force generated by their contraction is transmitted to the tibia via the patellar ligament. The three muscles extend the leg at the knee; they cannot flex the thigh as the rectus femoris can, because they are not attached to the hip. The knee-jerk reflex is triggered by tapping the patellar tendon and stretching the quadriceps femoris; the subsequent contraction of the quadriceps extends the leg at the knee joint — the knee jerk. (Femoral nerve.)

The muscles of the back of the thigh are collectively called the hamstring muscles. These include the biceps femoris, the semimembranosus and the semitendinosus (see Figure 7.15).

d. The biceps femoris. This is a muscle with two heads. The so-called "long head" of the biceps arises from the ischial tuberosity of the femur and the "short head" comes from the shaft of the femur. The insertion of the muscle is on the head of the fibula and its action is to extend the thigh and to flex the leg at the knee joint (see Figure 7.15). (Sciatic nerve.)

e. The semimembranosus. This arises from the ischial tuberosity and it has a complicated set of insertions but the main insertion is on the medial condyle of the tibia (see Figure 7.17). (Sciatic nerve.)

f. The semitendinosus. This muscle has a common origin with the long head of the biceps. The tendon of insertion crosses the semimembranosus muscle and inserts into the fascia of the leg and the upper part of the medial surface of the tibia (see Figure 7.15). Both the semitendinosus and the semimembranosus extend the thigh, flex the leg and are also medial rotators of the leg. (Sciatic nerve.)

The medial surface of the thigh has a group of muscles whose prime action is to adduct the thigh:

g. The adductor muscles. There are four main adductor muscles:

   (1) The adductor longus.
   (2) The adductor brevis.
   (3) The adductor magnus.
   (4) The gracilis.

All these muscles have their origin on the body of the pubis or on the ramus of the pubis. The adductor magnus has an additional origin from the ischial tuberosity. The three adductor muscles have broad insertions on the femur, while the thin gracilis has a narrow insertion in the middle of the tibia.

All four muscles are used in motions in which the thighs are pressed together and also act as stabilizers during flexion and extension of the thigh. (Obturator nerve.)

Like the thigh, the muscles of the leg can be grouped into anterior, lateral and posterior groups. The tendons of these muscles pass over the ankle and insert on the bones of the foot. The anterior group includes the tibialis anterior, the extensor digitorum longus and the extensor hallucis longus (see Figure 7.16); the lateral group includes the peroneus longus and the peroneus brevis. The posterior group includes the gastrocnemius, the soleus, the flexor digitorum longus and the flexor hallucis longus (see Figure 7.17).

h. The tibialis anterior. This muscle arises from the lateral condyle of the tibia and from the upper two-thirds of the shaft of the tibia, and it inserts into cuneiform bone and first metatarsal and it dorsiflexes and inverts the foot (see Figure 7.16). In inversion, the sole of the foot faces inward and the inner border of the foot moves upward and inward. (Anterior tibial nerve.)

i. The extensor digitorum longus and the extensor hallucis longus (see Figure 7.16). These two muscles arise mostly from the shaft of the fibula. The tendon of the extensor digitorum longus divides into four tendons at the ankle and one of these goes to and inserts on each of the four lateral toes; the muscle extends the toes and dorsiflexes the foot. The extensor hallucis longus inserts into the superior surface of the distal phalanx of the big toe; the muscle extends the big toe. (Anterior tibial nerve.)

j. The peroneus longus. Peroneal means pertaining to the fibula or front of the leg. The origin of this muscle is primarily

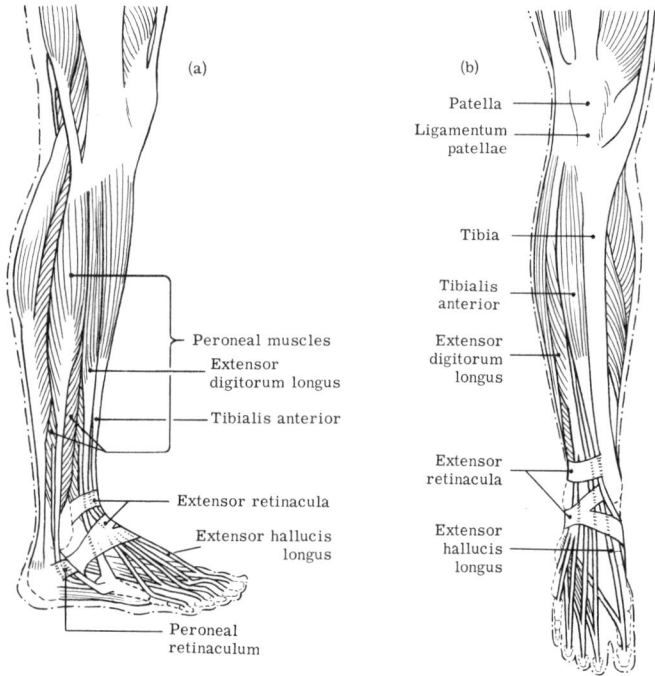

Figure 7.16 The muscles of the leg. (a) The front and outer side. (b) The front of the leg.

from the upper two thirds of the lateral surface of the shaft of the fibula and also from the lateral condyle of the tibia (see Figure 7.16). The tendon of insertion is narrow and curves under the foot, crossing the sole of the foot to insert into the lateral side of the medial cuneiform and in the first metatarsus. The muscle plantar flexes and everts the foot. In eversion the sole of the foot turns outward and the outer border of the foot moves upward and outward. Eversion and inversion of the foot are necessary for walking on uneven surfaces. (Peroneal nerve.)

k. The peroneus brevis. This lies beneath the peroneus longus and arises from the lower, lateral surface of the fibula (see Figure 7.16). The tendon of the muscle inserts into the fifth metatarsal and the muscle everts the foot. (Peroneal nerve.)

l. The gastrocnemius. The back of the leg is often called the calf of the leg. The most superficial of the calf muscles is the gastrocnemius which arises from two heads; one on the medial condyle and the other on the lateral condyle of the femur. The muscle spans the knee and ankle joint and inserts into the calcaneus (heel bone) via the tendocalcaneus (see Figure 7.15). Because the gastrocnemius is a two-joint muscle it can plantar flex the foot and flex the knee if the foot is fully dorsiflexed. These actions are important in walking and running. (Posterior tibial nerve.)

m. The soleus. This thick, flat muscle lies beneath the gastrocnemius (see Figure 7.17). It arises from the upper posterior surface of the fibula and the soleal line of the tibia. Its tendon joins the tendocalcaneus to insert on the calcaneus bone; the muscle plantar flexes the foot. (Posterior tibial nerve.)

In Greek mythology the warrior Achilles was made invulnerable to injury after his mother held him by the heels and dipped him into the river Styx. His heels, however, never touched the miraculous waters and hence, during the battle of Troy, Achilles was killed by an arrow in the heel. The tendocalcaneus is often called the Achilles tendon and in literature a flaw in the hero's character is sometimes referred to as his Achilles heel.

n. The flexor digitorum longus and the flexor hallucis longus. These two muscles lie beneath the soleus. The flexor digitorum longus arises from the middle posterior surface of the tibia and its tendon of insertion divides into four small tendons, each of which inserts into the four lateral toes. The flexor hallucis longus arises from the posterior surface of the lower fibula; its tendon runs across the sole of the foot above the tendon of the flexor digitorum longus and inserts into the

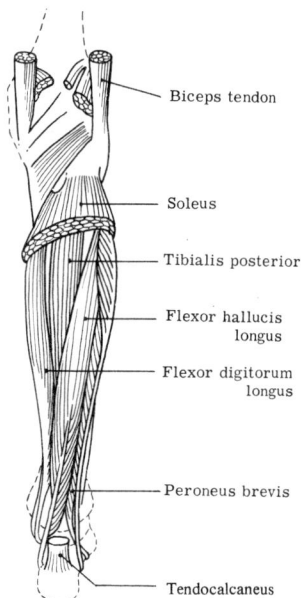

Figure 7.17 Deep muscles of the back of the leg.

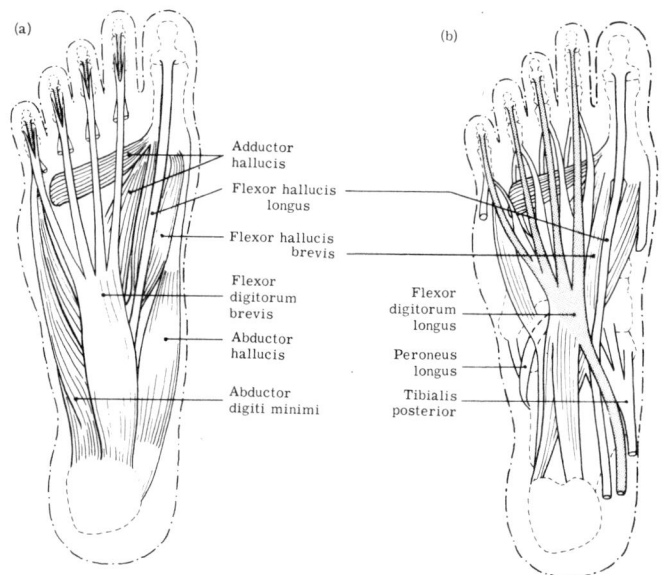

Figure 7.18 The muscles of the sole of the foot. (a) Superficial muscles. (b) Deep muscles.

inferior aspect of the distal phalanx of the big toe. This muscle flexes the distal phalanx of the big toe. (Posterior tibial nerve.)

Figure 7.18 shows the intrinsic muscles of the foot. The pattern of the muscles is similar to that of the hand and their names are indicative of their action. Most of the major movements of the toes are caused by contractions of the muscles of the leg and their long tendons which cross the foot.

WHAT HAPPENS AT A MYONEURAL JUNCTION?

We know that actions are chosen or willed in the brain and that instructions concerning the intended action are sent to the muscles in the form of impulses conducted along nerve fibres. The impulse is a bio-electric event and can be called an action potential. The nerve endings are not in direct contact with the muscles but in "functional contact". This means that, although very small spaces separate the nerve endings and the muscle membrane, the instructions from the nervous system are able to reach and to stimulate the muscle. The impulse is conducted along the axon of the motor neurone but it is not conducted across the space separating the nerve and the muscle. Instead, the impulse causes the end feet of the neurone to release granules containing a chemical called acetylcholine (ACh). ACh diffuses from the end feet of the neurone across the synaptic space to receptors on the surface of the muscle membrane. This chemical acts as a transmitter between the nervous system and skeletal muscles.

Its action on the muscle membrane is not fully understood but ACh does initiate permeability changes in the muscle membrane which cause impulses to be conducted over the muscle cells, which in turn triggers off the contraction. These permeability changes in the muscle membrane permit a flow of ions into and out of the muscle cell and generate a bio-electric current, which depolarizes the muscle membrane and initiates the subsequent contraction. (These currents are discussed in greater detail in the Chapter on the nervous system, in the sections dealing with resting membrane potentials and the neural impulses.)

For ACh to be able to induce another contraction, the muscle membrane must return to its resting state. The process in which the muscle membrane returns to its resting state is called repolarization and involves the movement of ions in and out of the cell so the original or resting ionic environment is achieved.

A single burst of ACh from a nerve ending cannot cause the muscle to remain permanently contracted because an enzyme called acetylcholine esterase (AChE), located near the receptor, splits the ACh molecule into a choline molecule and an acetate molecule. Thus, ACh leaves the nerve ending, makes contact with the receptor on the muscle membrane, initiates the impulse and muscle contraction, then the ACh leaves the receptor and makes contact with the enzyme AChE (see Figure 7.19). This enzyme splits ACh into choline and acetate molecules which do not react with the muscle membrane receptor and therefore cannot cause contraction. Because ACh is rapidly broken down by AChE, ACh must be continuously released by the end feet of the neurone if the muscle is to continue to contract. When

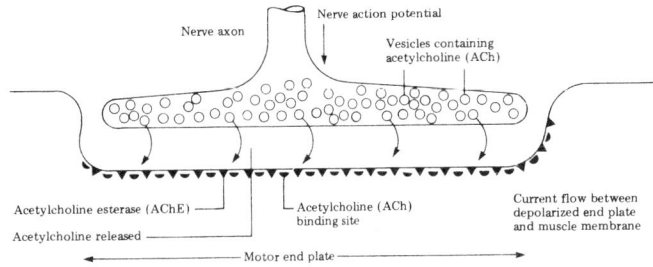

Figure 7.19 Events at a myoneural junction which lead to contraction in the muscle.

the ACh has been broken down by AChE, the muscle relaxes. There are limits to the ability of the nerve ending to synthesize and release ACh.

WHAT DRUGS AFFECT THE MYONEURAL JUNCTION?

Pharmacologists have traditionally shown great interest in the myoneural junction. This is because the chemical events which take place are easier to modify and control than the impulses conducted along the axon of the neurone. Long before pharmacology was an established science, the Indians of the Amazon basin in South America made use of a compound which was named curare and came from plants indigenous to that area. These Indians were hunters and used arrows dipped in compounds containing curare to paralyze and kill game animals. Hundreds of years later investigators found that curare caused paralysis by blocking the ACh receptor sites on the muscle membrane. The lock and key analogy is often used to explain this effect. Many keys can fit into a door lock but only the key with the specific matching fit can turn the lock and open the door. If a key which does not precisely match the lock is inserted into the lock, the door will be prevented from opening. Curare is like the mismatched key in that it fits into the ACh receptor site but cannot initiate muscular contraction. It prevents ACh from making contact with the receptor and therefore causes paralysis of the muscle.

The use of curare has not been limited to South American Indians. Many times it is necessary to temporarily paralyze muscles during surgery so they will be completely relaxed and so no movement can take place. Curare is sometimes used to accomplish this, for curare-caused paralysis is only temporary. Of course any patient receiving curare or an agent having similar effects will have to receive artificial ventilation because of the paralysis of the respiratory muscles.

Certain different drugs act by blocking the enzyme AChE rather than the ACh receptor sites. The disease myaesthenia gravis is characterized by sporadic periods of muscular weakness and the rapid onset of muscular fatigue. The cause of this disease is not known. It may be that there is a defect in the synthesis of transmitter or that there is an abnormality of the receptors so that additional ACh is required. Recent work suggests that myaesthenia gravis may be an immunological disease in that antibodies may be formed which block the ACh receptors. This condition is treated by drugs such as neostigmine which block AChE.

Because AChE cannot function to break down ACh into acetate and choline, ACh will accumulate at the myoneural junction and the additional ACh increases the likelihood of contraction.

Blood plasma contains an enzyme called pseudocholine esterase (pseudoAChE). This enzyme will break down ACh and other molecules having a chemical structure similar to it, but the enzyme is not as efficient as the AChE found in the myoneural junction.

Succinylcholine is similar to ACh. It will "fit" the ACh receptor on the muscle and can cause a depolarization of the muscle membrane as well as a contraction of the muscle. Succinylcholine is not, however, destroyed by the AChE in the myoneural junction. This means that, as long as succinylcholine is occupying the muscle receptor sites, the muscle cannot repolarize. Interruption of the depolarization–repolarization cycle by succinylcholine relaxes and paralyzes the muscle.

Anaesthetists commonly use succinylcholine to relax muscles and prevent them from contracting during surgery. Succinylcholine is broken down by pseudoAChE. For succinylcholine to be effective it must be infused almost continuously at a rate faster than the ability of pseudo-AChE to break it down. Muscle can repolarize and be ready to contract within a few minutes after cessation of the succinylcholine infusion. This gives the anaesthetists a greater degree of control over the relaxation process.

About 1 in 3000 patients lack pseudoAChE and therefore the action of small amounts of succinylcholine will be quite prolonged.

WHAT HAPPENS WHEN A MUSCLE CONTRACTS?

Prior to contraction of the muscle the end feet of the motor neurone release ACh, which diffuses across the synaptic space and makes contact with receptors on the muscle membrane. This initiates permeability changes in the cell and causes impulses to be initiated and conducted over the muscle fibres. These impulses stimulate the muscle to contract, that is, to generate a force, though the exact manner in which the impulse causes contraction is not known.

When a muscle contracts, it pulls on its attachments. There are two kinds of contraction. If you push with all your might against a wall your muscles contract forcefully even though neither the wall nor your arm moves. You can verify this by pushing against a wall, feeling the hardness of your arm muscles and noting how quickly fatigue sets in. These contractions in which there is no motion and the muscle contracts and remains essentially the same length are called isometric contractions. It is interesting to note that lions, in the confines of their zoo cages, maintain their strength by doing isometric exercises — they stretch and simultaneously contract flexors and extensors so that the forces generated balance each other and there is no net movement. Physical therapists have found isometric exercises useful for maintaining muscle tone in patients in wheel-chairs and with limb injuries who cannot perform "typical" exercises. If you bend over only to touch your toes you perform an isotonic exercise, as all movements involve isotonic contractions. The

molecular events taking place in isotonic and isometric contractions are identical.

So many life processes are concerned with growth and expansion that the phenomenon of muscular shortening (contraction) has been uniquely puzzling. Prior to the invention and use of the electron microscope there were nearly as many theories of contraction as there were researchers. Some thought muscles shortened like elastic or rubber-bands; whereas others thought muscles shortened in the manner of a pocket-knife when the blade closes.

Evidence from the electron microscope supports the sliding filament theory which suggests that muscular contraction is analogous to the shortening of a telescope. When a telescope is closed the individual parts of the telescope do not change in length, but the whole telescope shortens as the sections slide over one another and the two ends approach each other. In the contracting muscle the Z bands approach one another but neither the actin nor the myosin molecules shorten. It is thought that as the impulse is conducted over the cell it leads to the release of calcium ions from the sarcoplasmic reticulum, which surrounds the myofibrils. The calcium ions are attracted to calcium-binding sites on the troponin molecules located at regular intervals along the actin myofilaments. In some way the calcium ions trigger and participate in the formation of links or bridges between the actin and myosin filaments. These molecular bridges are able to pull the actin filaments towards the centre of the sarcomere, so the Z bands are drawn closer together (see Figure 7.1).

Mention should be made of the process of muscular relaxation, which is an active physiological process, not simply the cessation of contraction. For muscle to stop contracting, the calcium ions must leave the actin and myosin myofilaments and be transported to, and concentrated by, the sarcoplasmic reticulum storage sites. This process, in which the ions are returned to their storage sites and concentrated, is the opposite of simple diffusion and requires energy. ATP is the source of this energy.

Evidence that relaxation is an active, energy-dependent process comes from rigor mortis (the rigidity of death). Dead muscle tissue is not supple but is cold and stiff. In time the muscle proteins ultimately decay and the remaining muscle tissue permanently relaxes.

WHAT INFLUENCES THE FORCE OF CONTRACTION?

Not only is there an infinite variety of movements but also there are essentially similar motions which may require the generation of varying degrees of contractile force. It takes more muscular effort to pick up a heavy stone and raise it above your head than it does to pick up a feather and raise it in a similar manner. The force of contraction must be proportionate to the required force, otherwise the movement will be inappropriate or inadequate.

A. Muscle length

Muscle length does not refer to the fact that the muscles of the thigh are longer and more powerful than the short muscles of the fingers. Instead, muscle length refers to the length of a muscle as it is stretched or shortened. If you take an elastic or rubber-band, stretch it and release it, the elastic will snap back. Within limits, the greater the stretching force on the rubber-band, the greater the force with which it will snap back. A muscle does contain some elastic connective tissue. When the muscle is stretched, this elastic tissue is pulled taut, and the response of the muscle will be increased.

The amount of stretch placed on a muscle also affects the relationship between the actin and myosin filaments and this too affects the contractile response. You will recall that during a contraction there is some contact established between the thin actin filaments and thick myosin filaments, so that the actin filaments are pulled over the myosin filaments and the Z bands are drawn together (see Figure 7.1). If the muscle is greatly stretched there will be no overlap of actin and myosin filaments; contact between the two filaments cannot be established, so contraction cannot be initiated. When the muscle is not stretched, the thin actin filaments, as well as the myosin filaments, overlap one another, and the efficiency of contraction is reduced (see Figure 7.20).

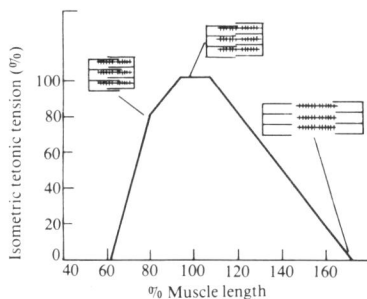

Figure 7.20 Graph showing how isometric tetonic tension varies with muscle length. The efficiency of contraction is reduced when the muscle is greatly extended or contracted.

In the body, most muscles are attached to bones, so the range over which a muscle can be stretched is limited. Nevertheless, this can be an important factor. You instinctively know that it is easier to lift something heavy when your forearms are partially flexed at the elbow than when they are fully extended or straight. When your arms are fully extended the biceps and the brachialis muscles are stretched and the amount of overlap between actin and myosin is less than when the forearms are partially flexed.

B. Number of motor units

In the Section on muscle anatomy it was stated that contraction of a specific muscle produces a specific effect; for example, contraction of the triceps causes extension of the forearm. It should not be inferred from this that all the fibres of a muscle contract every time a muscle contracts. To know why this is so it is necessary to understand the concept of the motor unit.

·A motor neurone is a neurone in the spinal cord which receives instructions from the brain and relays them to skeletal muscle cells, which carry them out by contracting; these instructions are in the form of impulses. A motor unit is made-up of a single motor neurone and all the muscle cells it innervates. If the motor neurone is stimulated and generates impulses, all the muscle cells it innervates will contract.

A fasiculation is a spontaneous contraction of a number of muscle fibres which are all innervated by the same motor neurone. Fasiculations are often visible through the skin and may represent damage to the motor neurone or its axon. Fasiculations are often seen in healthy individuals, particularly in times of stress and fatigue.

If no impulses are generated by the motor neurone, none of the muscle cells it innervates will contract. The number of muscle cells that a single motor neurone innervates is variable. If the muscle is capable of delicate and precise activity, a single motor neurone will innervate only a few cells; while a motor neurone will innervate many cells if the muscle's action is not so precise. The control of the nervous system over a particular muscle increases as the number of muscle cells in the motor unit decreases. Thus, the motor units of the eye and finger muscles have only a few muscle cells for each motor neurone, whereas those of the back muscles have hundreds of cells for each motor neurone.

Inasmuch as all the fibres in a motor unit will contract if the motor neurone is adequately stimulated, the force of muscular contraction will depend on the number of motor units that are activated. If only a few motor units which supply a muscle are activated, the contraction will be weak because only a few muscle cells will contract. When you make a maximal effort you activate all your motor units and all, or nearly all, of the muscle cells in the muscle contract, so the force of contraction is great.

Some insight into the concept of the motor unit can be achieved in experiments using the frog nerve-muscle preparation. Usually, an electric stimulator is applied to the frog's sciatic nerve and the force of contraction in the gastrocnemius is recorded. When single, very weak stimuli are applied to a nerve, no response or contraction is noted and this level of stimulation is called sub-threshold. As the intensity of stimulation is increased, there will come a point when a response is noted; this is referred to as a threshold stimulus. This level of stimulation causes impulses to be generated in a few axons so that all the muscle cells in the motor units supplied by those axons will contract progressively. Increasing the intensity of stimulation above the threshold level will cause more and more axons to generate impulses and more and more muscle cells will be stimulated to contract. There will come a point when all the axons will generate impulses and all the muscle cells within the muscle will contract. The mechanical response of a muscle to a single experimentally-induced stimulus which causes each muscle cell to contract is called a twitch. If the intensity of stimulation is still increased, there will be no increase in the contraction, because all the muscle cells will have been recruited and will contract. This level of stimulation is referred to as supramaximal stimulation.

C. Frequency of stimulation

The time between the application of a stimulus and the development of tension by the muscle is called the latent period. The period of time in which the tension developed by the muscle increases is called the contractile phase and the period in which the muscle tension is reduced is called the relaxation phase. The relaxation phase is longer than the contractile phase.

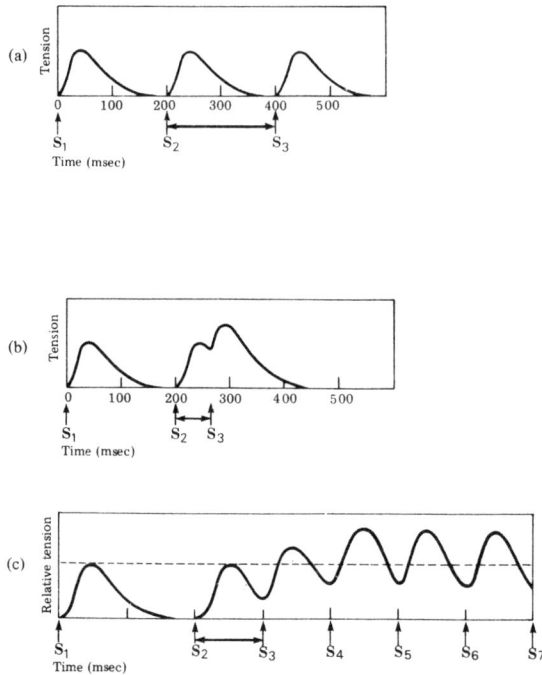

Figure 7.21 Isometric tetanic contraction produced by muscle stimuli compared to a single isometric twitch. (a) 10 stimuli per second. (b) 50 stimuli per second. (c) 100 stimuli per second.

The tension developed by a muscle can be increased by increasing the rate or frequency of stimulation. This is true even though the *intensity* of the stimulus remains the same. For example, a single supramaximal stimulus is given and the response is recorded as shown in Figure 7.21a. Since the stimulus is supramaximal, it will not be possible to increase the strength of contraction by increasing the strength of the stimulus. This is because all the motor units will have discharged. When a second supramaximal is given at S_2, after the muscle has relaxed, the muscle will contract as before. If a stimulus is presented at S_3, 1/10th of a second after the preceding stimulus (see Figure 7.21b), the stimulus will arrive at the muscle before the relaxation phase has been completed. The muscle will begin to contract again and the total tension developed will be greater than that of the preceding contraction. The tension developed by the second contraction is added to the tension remaining from the first contraction. The property of skeletal muscle in which the response to a second stimulus is added to the response to the first stimulus resulting in a greater response is called summation. As the frequency of stimulation increases, the amount of summation and tension increases (see Figure 7.21c). It should be emphasized that the increase in tension is not due to an increased recruitment of muscle fibres but to the fact that the individual fibres are increasing the total amount by which they are shortened. The second stimulus arrives before the relaxation process is completed and the fibre shortens an additional amount. The electron microscope would show that the amount of overlap between the thin actin filaments and the thick myosin filaments has increased and the Z lines are drawn closer together. With intense rapid stimulation it is possible for a muscle to shorten to 40% of its original length.

The response to a low frequency of stimulation in which the tension increases and decreases, but does not reach zero,

is called an unfused tetanus. When the frequency of stimulation is so rapid that the total tension appears constant, the response is called fused tetanus (see Figure 7.22). The ability of a muscle to maintain a state of tetanus depends on many factors. The ability of the nerve endings to synthesize and release ACh is of prime importance. Even if the nervous system is bypassed and the muscle is stimulated directly, there are limits to the muscle's ability to maintain an unfused tetanus. Tetanus can be maintained only as long as there is adequate ATP to provide the energy for this considerable effort. Adequate ATP in turn can be synthesized only if there are adequate nutrients and oxygen.

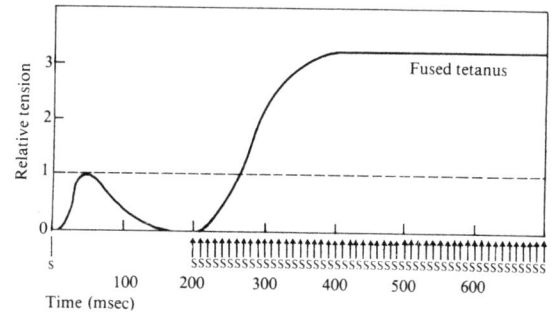

Figure 7.22 Fused tetanus.

Finally, it should be pointed out that the central nervous system can regulate the force of contraction by simultaneously varying the number of motor units called into play and the rate of stimulation. A single neurone can send impulses once a second or hundreds of times per second.

D. Amount of activity

You know from your own observations that people who do physical labour and exercise have better muscular development than people who don't. Bricklayers generally have better muscular development and more strength than physicians. An increase in muscular size is referred to as hypertrophy. When a muscle hypertrophies, new muscle cells are not formed but the existing cells increase in size. This is due to an increase in water and actin and myosin filaments within the cell. These additional filaments increase the amount of work which the muscle is capable of. Hypertrophy in response to exercise is specific. If you lift weights with your right arm and do not use your left arm, only your right arm will hypertrophy. (The mechanism which triggers this additional syntheses of actin and myosin is not known.)

If on the other hand, the muscle is not active, it will weaken and atrophy. Patients who have a limb in a cast, or have some joint disorder which hinders motion, can have significant atrophy in the affected limbs. When a nerve which innervates a muscle is injured or destroyed the muscle will begin to atrophy. It is possible that some regeneration of motor neurone axons may take place to restore the innervation. If there is insufficient regeneration of axons or if the cell bodies of the motor neurones are seriously injured, as sometimes happens in polio, muscular atrophy may be irreversible.

Physical therapists can play a vital role in helping patients regain muscular strength or maintaining muscle tone. For example, some patients with arthritis can remain active and mobile if they follow a prescribed regimen of physical therapy. Failure to do so can lead to muscle weakness which can make walking even more difficult.

E. Disease

Generally, when muscle tissue is diseased it is weak. It is one of the ironies of modern medicine that, although there is much information and understanding of normal muscle physiology, there is comparatively little understanding of muscle diseases. Some of the diseases of muscle tissue such as the muscular dystrophies are inherited diseases. These diseases are characterized by progressive muscle weakness. Children with these diseases may at first have difficulty running and walking, then difficulty in standing and finally difficulty in breathing. These severe diseases are fortunately quite rare. There is little understanding of their basic pathology and at present there is no adequate treatment.

In certain other diseases, muscle weakness can be caused by an enzymatic deficiency. Muscular contraction requires energy which can come only from the metabolism of appropriate substrates. Should an enzyme be lacking or not able to function adequately, muscular function will be impaired. In one type of muscle disease the muscle lacks the enzyme which breaks down glycogen. These muscle cells can function adequately for short periods of time but are unable to perform long or forceful work because the energy stores of the muscle cannot be released and broken down.

Muscle weakness can occur following injury or disease of another system. As mentioned previously, skeletal muscle is completely dependent on the nervous system, so it is always necessary to determine if the muscle weakness originated in the muscle or follows as a consequence of neural trauma or injury. Injury or disease of the circulatory system can also affect muscle function. Finally, nutritional deficiencies and endocrine disorders can have an effect on muscular development and function.

WHAT DOES MUSCLE METABOLIZE?

This topic will be discussed here because muscle has some unique metabolic properties and, as more than 40% of the body is muscle, the substrate which muscle metabolizes or doesn't metabolize can have an effect on the other tissues of the body. (Metabolism will be covered in much greater detail in the Chapter on metabolism and nutrition.)

Muscle receives its energy from the metabolism of fatty acids and glucose and requires amino acids for the maintenance and synthesis of actin and myosin filaments. Insulin increases the uptake of amino acids into muscle cells and is essential if glucose is to be able to cross the muscle cell membrane. If insulin is deficient and glucose cannot enter into muscle cells, the glucose concentration in the blood will increase and the muscle tissue will metabolize fatty acids and their breakdown products.

Some muscle fibres can contract even when oxygen (O_2) levels are low. In the absence of O_2, glucose cannot be oxidized to CO_2 and water. Some fibres can, however, partially break down glucose to lactic acid and derive some energy for the synthesis of ATP from this process. One molecule of glucose will give two molecules of lactic acid in the absence of O_2. This is referred to as *anaerobic* metabolism; *aerobic* metabolism is metabolism in the presence of O_2.

Anaerobic metabolism is much less efficient than aerobic metabolism when it comes to ATP production. Since ATP is necessary for muscular contraction, anaerobic metabolism will not be adequate for long-term muscular effort which requires large energy expenditures. If you do some strenuous exercise or work, the circulatory system will not be able to deliver sufficient O_2 to all the muscle tissue, so some fibres will metabolize anaerobically and lactic acid will accumulate. When you have completed your exercise, the lactic acid which has accumulated will be oxidized, aerobically, to CO_2 and water. This partly explains why you continue to breathe forcefully even though you have stopped your muscular effort. (This topic is covered more fully in the Chapter on metabolism and nutrition.)

In addition to ATP, skeletal muscle has a back-up energy system useful in supplying some energy reserves during strenuous activity. This energy comes from a compound known as phosphocreatine. Phosphocreatine is synthesized from creatine and phosphate and is similar to ATP in that energy is readily usable. In fact, energy from the breakdown of phosphocreatine goes into the synthesis of ATP from ADP and phosphate. This can take place under anaerobic conditions when the muscle has depleted its ATP supply. Later, under aerobic conditions, both ATP and phosphocreatine will be synthesized. The relationship between phosphocreatine and ATP is shown by the equation:

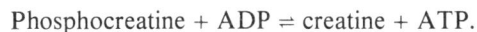

$$\text{Phosphocreatine} + \text{ADP} \rightleftharpoons \text{creatine} + \text{ATP}.$$

As an aside, it might be interesting to point out that in some animals the division of muscle tissue into white meat and dark meat reflects the different metabolic characteristic of muscle fibres. White meat contains muscle fibres rich in glycogen and capable of intense anaerobic activity. Dark meat contains muscle fibres which are capable of prolonged contractions, require higher levels of oxygen and contain myoglobin, a dark pigment which can bind oxygen until it is needed and released to the tissues. In humans, light and dark fibres are mixed, though some muscles may have more light or more dark fibres.

WHAT IS PROPRIOCEPTION?

Previous Sections have considered the way in which muscle tissue responds to instructions sent *from* the nervous system. It is now necessary to consider briefly the information which the joints and muscles send *to* the nervous system. Information from receptors in joints and muscles travels over nerve fibres to the spinal cord. In the spinal cord these fibres may ascend directly to the brain, synapse with a second neurone (which then relays the information), or synapse with a motor neurone whose fibres leave the spinal cord and innervate the muscle. The impulses that reach the brain from the receptors are responsible for the sense of proprioception.

Proprioception is that sense which enables the individual to know the position of the body's parts because of stimuli arising from within those parts. This is such a basic sense that it is often overlooked. You can demonstrate your proprioceptive abilities by first closing your eyes, then extending your arms in front of your body. Now, with your eyes closed, clap your hands, stop, then quickly touch the tip of your nose with the tip of your first finger, then clap your hands again. These actions are quite complicated and with your eyes closed you are completely dependent on proprioceptive information from your muscles and tendons to execute them.

Individuals suffering a proprioceptive disorder might not be able to perform these tasks with their eyes closed. They also have difficulty walking in the dark, for they are unable to see their limbs and, thus, do not know where their limbs are and the limbs' relationship to one another. Another insight into proprioception can be gained by thinking of the problem an artist would have if he or she tried to paint a picture blindfolded. The blindfold would not interfere with the artist's creative imagination nor directly affect the motor neurones in the brain and spinal cord or the muscles; however, to paint, an artist does need sensory information so that he or she can guide the arm and put the brush in the correct place. Even in supposedly simple actions such as walking, proprioceptive information is necessary if individuals are to maintain their balance, move their weight from foot to foot and extend and flex their legs properly.

In recent years, there has been considerable controversy over which receptors were responsible for generating proprioceptive information. It now appears that receptors in both muscles and joints contribute and that receptors in both sites are sensitive to stretch. In muscle tissue the proprioceptors are called muscle spindles (intrafusal fibres or stretch receptors) (see Figure 7.23). A muscle spindle contains 20–30 very thin muscle fibres which are surrounded by a connective tissue sheath and are parallel to, and surrounded by, the striated

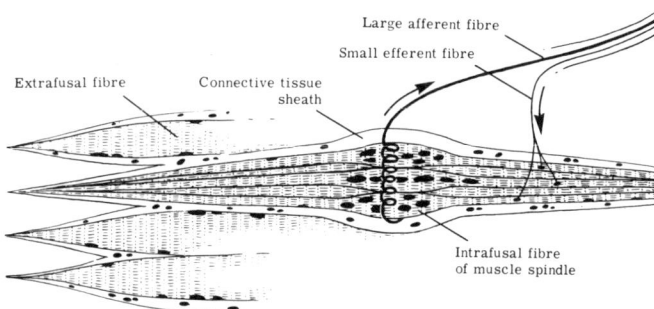

Figure 7.23 Diagram of a muscle spindle, showing the main sensory and motor innervation.

muscle fibres making up the bulk of the muscle. In the middle of the spindle of the cell are the nuclei of the spindle cells. Coiled sensory nerve endings surround the nuclear region and are called the annulospiral endings.

There are other nerve endings on the spindle and elsewhere in the muscle. When the muscle is pulled or stretched the receptors are also stretched and this causes them to generate more impulses. The greater the stretch on the muscle, the greater will be the number of impulses that the muscle spindle generates. Because the muscle spindles are parallel to the muscle fibres, the stretch imposed on the muscle fibres will also be imposed on the muscle spindle. Information on the amount of stretch will be relayed to the brain and spinal cord in the form of impulses generated by the muscle spindle.

There are also nerve endings in the muscle tendons which are sensitive to stretch. It is important to note, however, that the tendon and its receptors will be stretched when the muscle contracts. This is because the tendon, which is located between the bone and the muscle, is in series with the muscle, not parallel to it. Contraction of the muscle increases the tension of the tendon, which causes the receptors in the tendon to increase their rate of discharge.

Now that the anatomy has been discussed, it is necessary to explain the mechanism of proprioception. It might be easiest to explain by using an example. Extend completely one arm in front of you and close your eyes. Now flex the forearm a little at the elbow and stop. As you flex your forearm you are shortening your biceps and stretching your triceps. This will cause a different rate of discharge in the proprioceptors of the biceps and triceps muscles and their tendons. The more the arm is flexed, the more the biceps shortens and the triceps stretches. This means that the rate of discharge of the tendon proprioceptors of the biceps will increase and that of the triceps will be reduced. The muscle spindles of the triceps will also increase their discharge. These impulses from the receptors will go to the spinal cord and travel to the higher centres in the brain (see Figure 7.24). The brain has learned to interpret this increasing discharge from the biceps tendon and decreasing discharge from the triceps

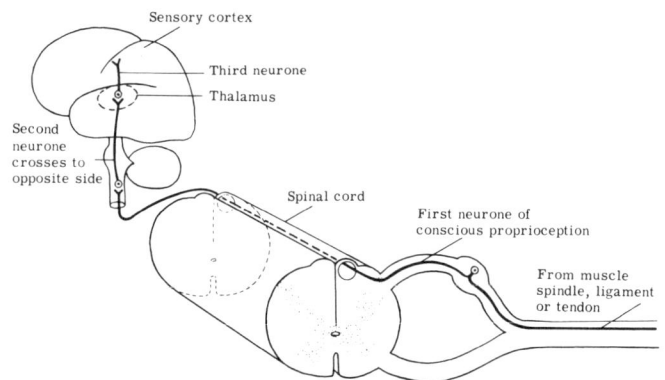

Figure 7.24 The pathway of conscious proprioception from the periphery of the body to the cerebral cortex.

tendon as flexion of the arm. Conversely, as the arm is extended, the triceps contracts and the biceps is stretched. The brain interprets the increased discharge from the triceps tendon and reduced discharge from the biceps tendon as extension of the arm. Though the muscles vary, the principle is the same for the other body parts. Every body position will cause a different stretch of the proprioceptors which will generate a unique proprioceptive input to the brain. The brain will interpret this information and learn the position of the body's parts.

WHAT IS THE KNEE-JERK REFLEX AND HOW DOES IT WORK?

Although reflexes will be discussed in more detail in the Chapter on the nervous system, this is a good place to make some mention of reflexes. A reflex is an involuntary response to a stimulus without conscious participation of the brain.

Posterior median
septum   Connector   Sensory
Posterior   neurone   neurone
horn   From muscle spindle
or ligament or tendon

Central
canal   To muscle fibres
Anterior median   Anterior   Motor neurone
fissure   horn

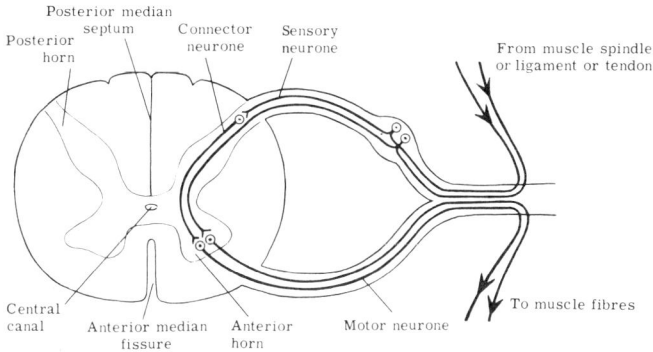

Figure 7.25 Cross-section of the spinal cord and the formation of a spinal nerve, showing the basic neurones of either a monosynaptic or a disynaptic arc.

The knee-jerk reflex is usually demonstrated by tapping on the patellar ligament of an individual who is in the sitting position. The tapping causes the knee to jerk forward. Proof that this is a reflex comes from the observation that the knee jerk will occur in an individual who is paralyzed and cannot move his leg of his own volition.

The explanation of this reflex depends on an understanding of the muscle spindle. When the patellar ligament is tapped the quadriceps muscle is stretched and this simultaneously stretches the muscle spindles in the quadriceps muscle. Some fibres of the muscle spindle enter the spinal cord and synapse directly on the large motor neurones which innervate the quadriceps muscle. These large motor neurones are often called the α motor neurones. The sudden stretching of the spindle generates impulses which simultaneously arrive at the motor neurones, cause them to discharge and stimulate the quadriceps to contract so that the leg kicks out (see Figure 7.25). If either the nerve carrying impulses from the muscle spindles to the spinal cord, or the nerve carrying impulses from the spinal cord to the quadriceps is injured, the reflex will be abolished. Similar reflexes can be demonstrated in the biceps, triceps and gastrocnemius muscles. Hyperactive reflexes may also be indicative of pathology.

If you look again at the diagram of the muscle spindle (Figure 7.23) you will see that the muscular portion of the muscle spindle receives small efferent motor fibres. These fibres are sometimes called the gamma (γ) motor fibres and they arise from small motor neurones in the spinal cord called the γ motor neurones. Impulses from the γ motor neurones stimulate the motor fibres of the muscle spindle to contract. Since these fibres are located above and below the sensory endings in the central nuclear region, their shortening will stretch or increase the tension in the nuclear region and the receptors there will increase their rate of discharge.

Knowing this you can now trace the γ motor loop:

(1) Stimulation of the small γ motor neurones causes contraction of the muscle in the intrafusal fibres.

(2) This contraction stretches the nuclear region, and the annulospinal endings increase their rate of discharge.

(3) Impulses from the muscle spindle receptors travel to the spinal cord over afferent nerve fibres which synapse on the large α motor neurones in the spinal cord.

(4) These neurones increase their rate of discharge to the extrafusal fibres which partially contract, and tension in the muscle increases.

There are thus three ways to cause the muscle to contract: (1) stretch it, (2) stimulate the γ motor neurones, (3) stimulate the α motor neurones. The brain sends impulses to both α and γ motor neurones. This will be covered in much greater detail in the Chapter on the nervous system.

8. The Circulatory (Cardiovascular) System

INTRODUCTION

To gain an introduction to the cardiovascular system it may be useful to take a "journey" around the system. We begin our journey in the heart, in one of its four chambers called the right atrium (see Figure 8.1). Here are blood cells which have returned from many parts of the body, including the brain, muscles, liver and even the heart itself. Suddenly, the thin atrial musculature contracts, forcing the cells into another chamber of the heart beneath the right atrium called the right ventricle. This chamber has thicker muscular walls than the atrium and contains about 150 ml of blood. The doors (valves) through which the cells entered into the ventricle have now shut. The cardiac muscle fibres contract nearly all in unison and the pressure rises. There seems no way out; but now, a different set of valves, the pulmonic (pulmonary) valves, are forced open by the greater pressure within the right ventricle. About 70 ml of blood are forced out and the cells enter the pulmonary artery. The pulmonary artery valves close behind and the going becomes rougher as the cells leave the wide artery and enter the narrow arteriole. The pressure drops and soon the cells enter the capillary; they have to go slowly and in single file because a capillary is only wide enough for a single red cell. All that separates the cells from the air-filled alveolus are two thin epithelial membranes — one belonging to the capillary, the other to the lung. The CO_2 quickly diffuses out of the red cell into the alveolus, while O_2 diffuses into the cell and is picked up by the haemoglobin.

Leaving the pulmonary capillary, the cells travel into the wider venule, then into the pulmonary vein where they meet many other cells that have taken other pathways through different capillaries of the lung. Passing through the left atrium of the heart, they journey on into the left ventricle; the valves which separate the atrium and the ventricle are open because the pressure in the atrium is greater than that of the ventricle. So far the whole trip has taken only a few seconds. More blood enters the ventricle. The atrium contracts, forcing still more blood into the ventricle whose fibres stretch a little because of the increased volume of blood. The valves which have been floating on top of the blood snap shut making a loud noise; the septum, which separates the right and left ventricles, stiffens. The pressure builds up intensely, but there seems to be no escape, for again, all the valves are closed. Although the pressure seems to be many times greater than that in the right ventricle, there does not seem to be any injury to the blood cells because of the smooth endothelial lining on the inner surface of the ventricle. We see that the pressure is so great within the left ventricle that the two mitral valves, which separate the atrium and ventricle, would be forced open and blood would leak into the atrium if it were not for the connective tissue, the chordae tendinae and papillary muscle which hold the valves in place. The pressure increases till suddenly the semilunar valves, which lead out of the ventricle and separate it from the dorsal aorta, are forced open. The cells quickly speed out of the ventricle up the aorta, the largest artery in the body. The aorta has an endothelial lining and behind that is lots of elastin, some smooth muscle and, behind that, collagen fibres. The elastin has been stretched by the sudden input of 70 ml of blood and, as it starts to return to its original size, it is helping to squeeze the cells along. The semilunar valves snap shut as the cells speed smoothly and quietly onwards; the driving pressure falls until there is another beat of the heart, another increase in pressure and another push forward on our journey.

The aorta bends, revealing other branches of the aorta which leave and head upwards to the head and brain. We bypass these and travel instead towards the feet. Some cells leave us, heading for the bronchi and oesophagus before we

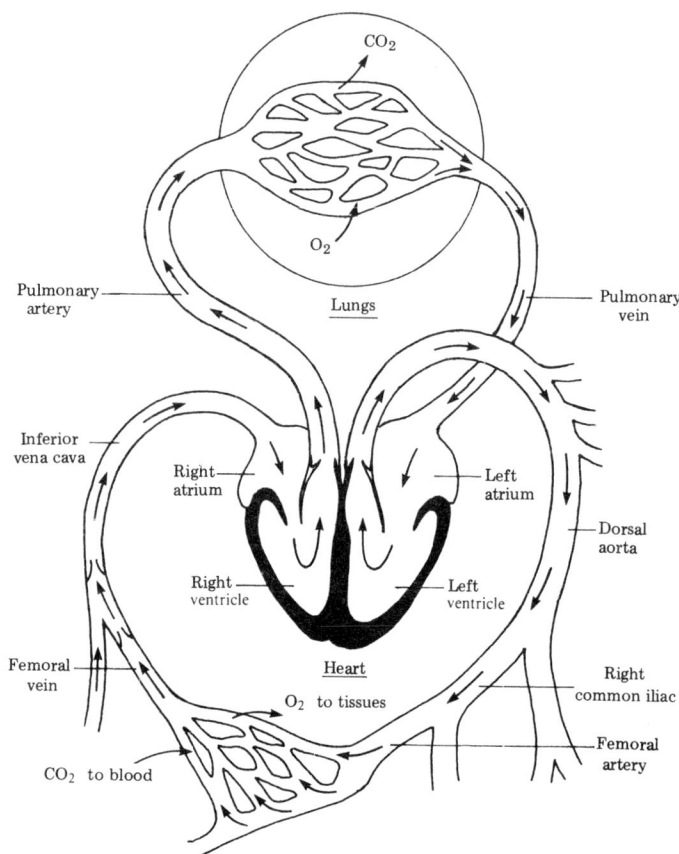

Figure 8.1 The circulatory (cardiovascular) system.

pass through the diaphragm into the abdomen. We cross the abdomen and come to a fork in the aorta.

We bear to the right, choosing the right common iliac artery. Another division and we find ourselves in the narrower external iliac artery which, after it leaves the abdomen, is called the femoral artery, because of its association with the femur bone. This artery becomes the popliteal artery as it passes on the dorsal surface of the leg at the knee joint. It again divides and we take the posterior tibial artery, which supplies the gastrocnemius muscle, among other things, as it continues its journey to the foot.

Entering a narrow arteriole the cells lose much energy because of the resistance and friction it offers. The arteriole is different from the artery, for although it has an endothelial lining, the smooth muscle which surrounds it predominates over the elastin. In some arterioles, the smooth muscle is tightly constricted so that the lumen is very narrow and only small amounts of blood can enter them. The arterioles are short and it does not take long to traverse them, even though the speed and pressure have been greatly reduced from what they were in the arteries. The pressure, too, no longer increases with every beat of the heart but is constant and ensures a steady flow through the open arterioles. At angles to the arterioles are smaller capillaries but most of them seem to have their entrances constricted by smooth muscle, the precapillary sphincter.

This is the most important part of our journey. Again, the capillary is not very wide, so the cells have to proceed one-by-one, cell-by-cell. The capillary itself is very thin, only a single endothelial cell thick. O_2 leaves the haemoglobin and the red cell, diffuses through the plasma and the endothelial cell of the capillary, rapidly crosses the interstitial fluid and enters the working muscle cell. CO_2 traverses the reverse route, some of it ending up on the haemoglobin molecule and helping force off additional O_2. Other CO_2 molecules enter the red cell and combine with water to form H_2CO_3. This acid breaks down into H^+ and HCO_3^-; the H^+ goes to the haemoglobin molecule and most of the HCO_3^- diffuses into the plasma.

Aside from all these changes in the red cell, changes also take place outside the cell in the plasma. Some of the plasma, which carries glucose and other nutrients, diffuses out of the capillary through small pores between the cement of the endothelial cells. This fluid joins the intercellular fluid which bathes and nourishes the cells. It also appears that a few proteins have escaped from the plasma into the inter-cellular fluid. Ultimately, some of the fluid, which leaves the cardiovascular system and joins the intercellular fluid, is returned to the venous system by means of the lymphatics. As we approach the venous half of the capillary, the driving pressure continues to fall and some of the fluid which escaped at the arterial end is now returning to the capillary, being drawn by the osmotic pressure exerted by the plasma proteins which cannot leave the capillary. The returning fluid contains the metabolic waste products of the muscle.

As the cells leave the capillary and enter the wider venule, the speed increases a little although the pressure has again decreased. They enter the short saphenous vein. It is wider than the arteriole although the wall is thinner. It has the same three layers of endothelium, smooth muscle and connective tissue as the arteries do, though the smooth muscle and connective tissue are not well developed. The pressure is insufficient to drive the cells upward from the leg to the heart. There is a pause for a moment inside the vein, then the skeletal muscle surrounding the vein contracts, causing the whole vein to be constricted and the cells squeezed. They pass through two open valves in the vein, which soon close behind them, preventing them from sliding back to where they came from. Another muscular contraction, another squeeze, more progress.

The journey continues in this way from the short saphenous vein to the popliteal vein and then to the femoral vein, which leaves the lower limb under the inguinal ligament where it is called the external iliac vein. This vein soon turns into the inferior vena cava, a huge vessel which receives blood from the veins draining the abdominal wall, the reproductive organs, the kidneys and liver. Another problem arises. In the abdomen, there are no valves in the veins and there does not appear to be any skeletal muscle to surround and squeeze the vein. The human takes a breath. As he inhales, the diaphragm descends, increasing the pressure in the abdomen which squeezes the inferior vena cava. With the expansion of the thorax, the pressure ahead is reduced and the net driving pressure is increased, so the cells now hurry through the diaphragm into the thorax where the inferior vena cava enters the right atrium. So the journey ends.

You are not expected at this point to understand all of the journey, but after you have finished this section, read it again, and hopefully you will understand it better.

The function of the cardiovascular system is to transport oxygen, nutrients, hormones and heat to every cell in the body and to remove CO_2, metabolic wastes and excess heat from every cell in the body. To accomplish this, there is a pump (the heart) to propel the blood, arteries to deliver it, capillaries where exchange between blood and tissues takes place and veins to return the blood. The operation of the circulatory system would be incredibly simple if it were not for the fact that the needs of the cell change. Resting muscle needs relatively little oxygen and, therefore, relatively little blood flow, while exercising muscle needs a great deal more O_2 and must have a greatly increased circulation. Temperature and posture also affect the cardiovascular system and bring about the need for change — it will obviously require greater blood pressure to send blood to your brain when you are standing up than will be needed when you are lying down. Therefore, the cardiovascular system will have to include a means of transport, sensors to determine which areas need additional flow and effectors to bring about these changes. The mechanisms by which these changes are brought about will be discussed in the physiology Section, but first it is necessary to discuss the anatomy.

WHAT IS THE STRUCTURE OF THE HEART?

Your heart is roughly the size of your fist and lies in the thorax behind the sternum between the lungs. It lies at an angle, a little to the left of centre, with the base above and its apex below. The apex lies about 9 cm to the left of the sternum in the 5th intercostal space; the base extends to the 2nd costal cartilage on the left, about 1 cm from the sternum (see Figure 8.2). Knowing the position of the heart is

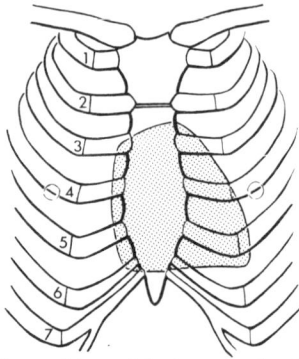

Figure 8.2   The position of the heart in the thoracic cavity.

important when listening to the heart sounds. The heart itself is made up of three different layers:

A. The pericardium

The outermost covering is called the pericardium which is composed of two layers — the outer parietal pericardium and the inner visceral pericardium (see Figure 8.3). The parietal pericardium is continuous with the great blood vessels which enter the heart. At the apex of the heart it connects to the tendon of the diaphragm and this helps to anchor the heart in place. The outer layer of the parietal pericardium is a tough

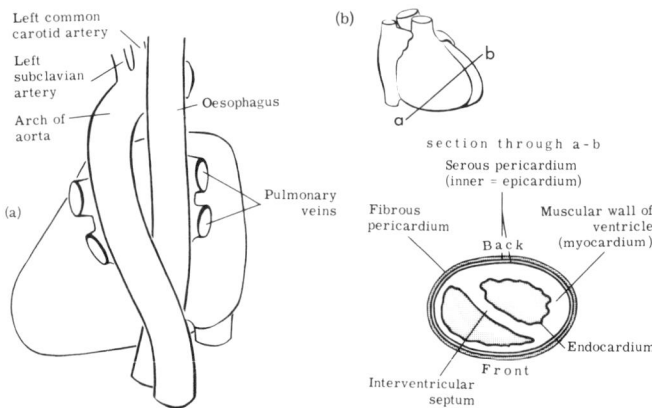

Figure 8.3   (a) The back of the heart showing the position of the aorta and oesophagus. (b) Cross-section through the ventricles, showing the comparative thickness of ventricular walls, oblique interventricular septum and the structure of the heart wall.

layer of thick, fibroelastic connective tissue, while the inner layer is a serous membrane of squamous epithelial cells which secrete a clear watery solution. The outermost layer of the visceral pericardium is also a serous membrane. It rests upon a connective tissue membrane which connects directly to the heart muscle.

There is a small fluid-filled space between the two serous membranes. This fluid reduces the friction generated by the contraction and movement of the heart. The tough connective tissue of the parietal pericardium will not stretch as blood enters the heart, and the ventricles enlarge. The parietal pericardium thus sets a limit on the amount of blood that can enter the heart. In certain pathological conditions too much fluid or blood accumulates in the space between the two serous membranes, and the filling of the heart with blood is impaired. This is called cardiac tamponade and is very serious because, if the heart cannot fill with blood, it cannot pump blood.

B. The myocardium

The myocardium is the muscular and thickest part of the heart wall (see Figure 8.3). It is thickest at the apex and thinnest at the base of the heart. The ventricles, in fact, have three layers of muscle — two spiral layers and one circular layer. This arrangement and the contraction pattern of the heart work so that blood is squeezed upward and out of the heart into the arteries. Go back to the Chapter on the cells and tissues and read again the Section on cardiac muscle.

The heart muscle may become diseased. Lack of adequate protein and/or vitamin B_1 and excessive alcohol can damage heart muscle. The myocardium may also be invaded by adipose tissue as happens in very obese persons. Fat-infiltrated mycardium cannot respond to the increased demands placed on it by certain stresses such as surgery, which helps to explain why very obese patients are poor surgical risks.

Since the myocardial tissue is muscle tissue which is working continuously, it must have oxygen delivered to it all the time. If the arteries which deliver oxygenated blood became blocked or clogged with atherosclerotic plaque, reducing the blood flow so that adequate amounts of oxygen are not delivered, the myocardial cells will die. An infarct is an area of necrosis (cell death) resulting from an obstruction of the circulation to that area. A myocardial infarct refers to death of myocardial muscle cells because of an inadequate arterial blood supply. (In clinical work, the term myocardial infarct is often referred to as an MI.) Although the lay person's use of the words "heart attack" can have many meanings, it most often refers to the immediate effects of a myocardial infarction. If the muscle is not receiving adequate oxygen, the individual may experience pain. The "typical" pain involves the central portion of the chest and the epigastrium. Sometimes this pain is described as a tightness in the chest or a crushing pressure on the chest. In about 25% of the cases, pain radiates to the arms. Because the myocardium must do more work when a person exercises, it will require more oxygen. If the demands of the heart cannot be met, pain results. For this reason chest pain during and after exercise or hard work is a significant symptom and may indicate heart disease or, much more likely, disease of the blood vessels supplying the heart.

C. The endocardium

The innermost layer of the heart is a delicate endothelial layer connected to the myocardium by connective tissue (see Figure 8.3). The endothelium reduces friction and prevents injury to the red cells. The capillaries are endothelial cells, and the endothelium which lines the heart is continuous with the endothelium of the arteries, capillaries and veins.

D. Chambers and valves of the heart

If you were designing a heart, you would have at least two basic problems. You would have to be certain that the oxygenated and unoxygenated blood were never mixed and that blood flow was always unidirectional, from vein to atrium to ventricle to artery and not the reverse. These problems have been solved by having the heart divided into

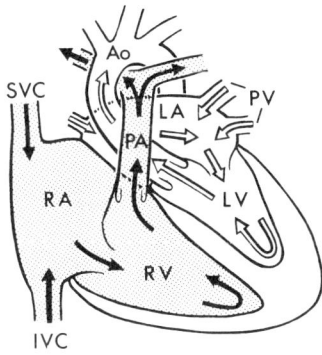

Figure 8.4 The interior of the heart, showing the individual chambers and the circulation of the blood. SVC, superior vena cava; IVC, inferior vena cava; RA, right atrium; RV, right ventricle; PA, pulmonary artery; PV, Pulmonary vein; LA, left atrium; LV, left ventricle; Ao, aorta.

four chambers and having four sets of valves to regulate the direction of flow (see Figure 8.4).

The atria are the recipients of blood; the right atrium receives unoxygenated blood from the superior and inferior vena cavae, while the left atrium receives oxygenated blood from the four pulmonary veins. The right and left atria are separated by a thin muscular septum; the walls of the atria are thin for they only have to pump blood to the ventricles below. The right and left ventricles are separated by the thick interventricular septum (see Figure 8.3). The atrial and ventricular septa separate the heart into the right heart containing venous blood and the left heart containing arterial blood.

The bicuspid and tricuspid valves separate each half of the heart into the upper atria and the lower ventricles; they are sometimes called the auricular–ventricular or the atrio-ventricular valves (A–V valves) (see Figure 8.5a). The valves themselves are folds of epithelium which have been made

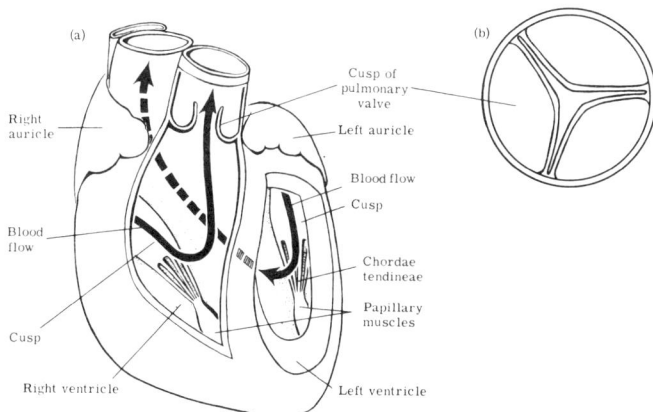

Figure 8.5 (a) The atrio-ventricular valves. (b) The aorta semilunar (tricuspid) valve.

much stronger by a layer of dense connective tissue. They act like a set of doors which can only swing one way. If the A–V valves are open, blood flows from the atria into the ventricles, but after they have swung shut, blood can flow neither from the atria to the ventricles nor from the ventricles back to the atria, for they have completely closed and separated each chamber. The valve between the right atrium and the right

ventricle has three leaflets and is called the tricuspid valve. The valve between the left atrium and the left ventricle has two leaflets and is called the bicuspid valve, though it is sometimes called the mitral valve because the shape of its two leaflets somewhat resembles a bishop's hat, his mitre. You can easily remember the position of the mitral valves if you think of the story of the famous British scientist who had an argument with a bishop over evolution and walked away saying, "The bishop is never right". Attached to the A–V valves are dense cords of connective tissue, the chordae tendinae, which connect to the papillary muscle which attaches to the ventricular septum. This arrangement helps prevent the A–V valves from being forced open by the great pressures generated in ventricular contraction.

There are exit valves which prevent blood from returning to the ventricles after it has been ejected into the arteries. The exit valve between the right ventricle and the beginning of the pulmonary artery is called the pulmonary semilunar valve. The aortic semilunar valve is between the left ventricle and the start of the aorta and like the pulmonary semi-lunar valve has three half-moon shaped leaflets (see Figure 8.5b). After the ventricles have contracted and the pressure within them is greater than that of the arteries the valves are forced open and blood enters the arteries. When the ventricles relax and the pressure in them falls, the valves snap shut and blood cannot flow back into the ventricles.

Injury or disease of the valves can seriously hinder the functioning of the heart. If the semilunar valves become stiff and hard and unable to open easily, the ventricles will have to do more work to force the blood into the arteries. Should the semilunar valves not be able to shut completely, blood will flow backwards from the arteries into the relaxed ventricles. If the A–V valves cannot shut completely, some blood will flow into the atria during ventricular contraction instead of all the blood going into the arteries.

When the health worker places the stethoscope on your chest, he or she is listening to the sounds arising from the heart. The first sound, "lub", is due to the closing of the auricular–ventricular valves and the vibrations caused by ventricular contraction, while the second heart sound, "dub", arises from the closing of the semilunar valves and the vibration of blood within the aortic valves and closure of the pulmonic valves. The aortic valve should always close before the pulmonic valves, and sometimes the second sound is referred to as a "split-second heart sound" because the two components can be heard.

The heart sounds are best learned by listening to them rather than reading about them, but until you do have the opportunity to listen to them, here are some points to learn and keep in mind. If the valves are not competent, that is, if they cannot completely close, blood will flow backwards in the heart and a murmur will result. For example, if the aortic valves are incompetent, aortic valve insufficiency occurs. A high-pitched murmur will begin immediately after the second heart sound and is caused by blood flowing from the aorta back into the left ventricle. There may be insufficiencies of the mitral, tricuspid and pulmonic valves as well as the aortic valves.

Stenosis means narrowing of a duct, canal or opening. In mitral stenosis the mitral valves are diseased so that they cannot completely open. This narrowing increases the turbulence with which the blood flows from the left atrium into the left ventricle. The turbulent blood flow into and within the ventricle causes a low-pitched or rumbling murmur, sometimes said to resemble the roll of a drum. This murmur precedes the first heart sound. The other valves of the heart may become stenotic.

In listening for murmurs, the examiner must determine their timing, the pitch of the sound and how it changes, and the location of the murmur. The pulmonic and tricuspid valves are located near the chest, while the aortic valves are situated deep within the chest, and their sounds are transmitted in the direction of blood flow. The areas in which the closing of the different valves can usually be heard to best advantage are as follows:

(a) Pulmonary valves — over the second left intercostal space.

(b) Aortic valves — over the second right intercostal space.

(c) Tricuspid valves — over the lowest part of the body of the sternum.

(d) Mitral valves — over the fourth or fifth intercostal space in a line with the middle of the left clavicle.

Before listening to the heart it is best to feel the pulsation caused by the contraction of the heart. This is done by placing your hand over the precordium. The precordium is the anterior surface of the chest, closest to the heart. The point of the pulsation which is best felt in adults with healthy hearts is usually over the apex of the heart, in the fifth intercostal space, in a line with the middle of the left clavicle. Disease may cause the pulsation to be displaced.

Rheumatic heart disease is the most common heart disease in school-age children. The heart valves may become inflamed, thickened or destroyed so that they do not open easily or close completely. This happens in about 3% or less of those patients who have severe infections with Group A β-haemolytic bacteria and are not given appropriate treatment. There is a delay of two or more weeks between the onset of the bacterial infection and the beginning of the valvular changes. The exact mechanism of valvular destruction is not understood, but it is thought that the heart tissue and the bacteria have certain antigens in common. When significant amounts of antibody to the bacteria are made, it will cross-react with the common antigen on the heart and initiate the pathological process.

E. Conduction in the heart

Each muscle fibre in the heart is capable of contracting by itself, without stimulation by nerves or chemicals. For the heart to work efficiently, however, the individual cells must work together. The heart muscles must contract in an orderly sequence, as a unit, so that sufficient pressure is generated to force the blood through the arterial system.

Within the heart there is specialized conduction tissue. Its function is to excite the heart muscle and spread this excitation throughout the heart quickly and in an orderly sequence. Because of this conduction tissue, the atria contract before the ventricles (thus ensuring that the ventricle is full when it contracts), and the ventricles contract forcefully as a single unit; there are no weak and random contractions of isolated independent muscle fibres.

The excitation or stimulus to contract begins in the most excitable part of the heart, the sino-atrial (S–A) node, which is found at the entry of the superior vena cava and the beginning of the right atrium. The S–A node is often called the "pacemaker", for it sets the pace or rate of the heart beat. Normally, an adult pacemaker gets excited roughly 70 times a minute. The excitation generated by the pacemaker is bio-electric in nature, an impulse which causes depolarization and contraction of the cardiac muscle. An early investigator compared the spread of excitation over the atria from the pacemaker to the pouring of water over a table. The excitation is more complicated than that, but in essence, the analogy is correct, for the area closest to the pacemaker will be excited first, the area most distant from it will be excited last. The excitation cannot be conducted directly from the atria to the ventricles because they are separated from one another by fibrous connective tissue which acts as a barrier to the spread of excitation. What is needed is a conductive bridge to take the excitation across the connective tissue into the ventricles.

In the lower portion of the right atrium, near the interatrial septum, is found the auricular–ventricular or atrio-ventricular node (A–V node). The A–V node and the fibres which leave from it form the communications network between the atria and the ventricles. When the excitation reaches the A–V node, the node becomes excited and conducts this excitation through the connective tissue to the ventricles via the bundle of His which consists of many thin muscle fibres that are specialized for the conduction of impulses and grouped tightly together in a "bundle". The bundle of His splits in two, with one branch travelling down the right side of the interventricular septum and the other down the left. These branches give rise to the Purkinje fibres, which deliver the impulse into the ventricular muscle (see Figure 8.6). The rate of conduction through the A–V node is slow, but rapid down the bundle

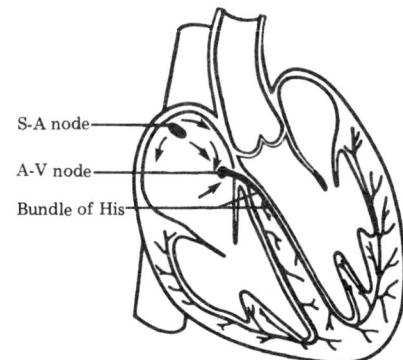

Figure 8.6 The conducting system of the heart.

branches, ensuring that the ventricle receives the stimulus quickly so that all the ventricular muscle will contract at approximately the same time. Should the bundle of His be injured, there will be no bridge between the atria and the ventricles and the ventricles will beat at their own rate, independent of the S—A node and the atrial contractions. If the S—A node should fail to become excited, the A–V node will take over and act as a replacement pacemaker. All these bio-electric events take place over a very short period of time, for the entire cardiac cycle of excitation and contraction has to be completed within one seventieth of a minute.

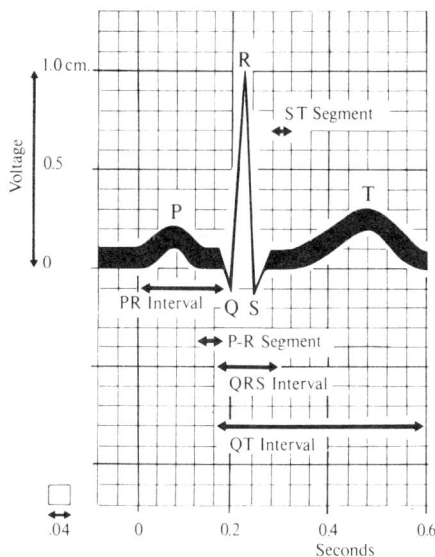

Figure 8.7 A typical electrocardiogram shown on standard recording paper. The distance between each thick line horizontally represents 0.2 seconds at the standard rate of 25 mm/s, and, when correctly standardized, each cm in a vertical direction is equivalent of 10 mV.

It is possible to measure the bio-electric activity of the heart by placing electrodes on the body and connecting them to an instrument known as an electrocardiograph. A typical electrocardiogram is shown in Figure 8.7.

The P wave represents the bio-electric activity in the spread of the impulse over the atria; the time between the beginning of the P wave and the beginning of the QRS complex represents the time it takes for the impulse to travel from the S–A node to the ventricular septum. The QRS complex represents the electrical activity in the ventricle prior to contraction, while the T wave represents the bio-electric activity in the ventricle prior to relaxation.

Interpreting electrocardiograms is like reading a foreign language — it's a learned skill. Electrodes are placed over different parts of the body and each electrode will give a different picture of the bio-electric activity of the heart. The bio-electric events are the same but the electrocardiographic "pictures" are different because the electrodes in different locations will see the bio-electric event from a different anatomical perspective. A horse always looks like a horse, but there is a big difference in photographs taken facing the head of the horse, and those taken facing its rear end. The student should not be overwhelmed by the different leads and the different records the electrocardiogram produces. Even a novice reader of them can get some information from looking at them.

First, always determine the rate of the heart beat. Since the QRS complex precedes ventricular contraction, you can determine the heart rate simply by counting the number of QRS complexes per unit of time.

Next, investigate the rhythm of the heart beat. Determine if the distance between successive QRS complexes is constant or if there is a great deal of variation. There is usually a small variation with respiration. If the heart beat has a regular

rhythm, the distances between QRS complexes will be relatively constant. In the normal heart the rhythm is determined by rate of depolarization of the S–A node. This means that the P wave which precedes atrial contraction should come before the QRS complex and ventricular contraction.

The time between the beginning of the P wave and the beginning of the QRS complex is important, for it represents the time it takes the impulse to travel from the atria to the ventricles. The normal interval between the beginning of the P wave and the beginning of the QRS complex is 0.12–0.21 seconds (see Figure 8.7). An interval longer than 0.21 seconds indicates that there is a defect in conduction to the ventricles, and this delay is called *first* degree heart block (see Figure 8.8a). The usual site of the delay is within the A–V

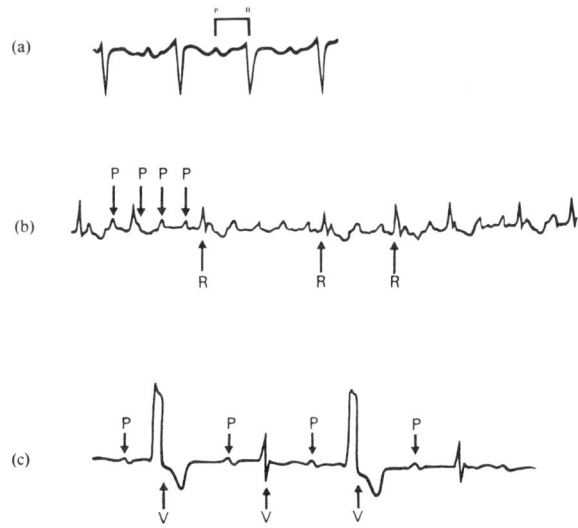

Figure 8.8 Electrocardiograms demonstrating heart rhythm disturbances. (a) First degree heart block. (b) Second degree heart block. (c) Third degree heart block.

node. Sometimes the conduction delay is so great that the S–A node depolarizes and generates a second P wave before the ventricles contract. In *second* degree heart block (see Figure 8.8b), there are more P waves than QRS complexes, because only a fraction of the atrial depolarizations reach the ventricles and excite them. In *third* degree heart block there is no causal relationship between the P wave and the QRS complex (see Figure 8.8c). This is because conduction is so delayed that the ventricle, rather than the S–A node, acts as its own pacemaker and may cause bizarre appearances of QRS complexes. Abnormal QRS complexes will also appear if conduction through either branch of the bundle of His is damaged.

The effect of many rhythm disturbances is variable. One rhythm disturbance which is not compatible with life is ventricular fibrillation. This is really an arrhythmia, as the heart has no rhythm. Instead, different parts of the ventricle contract chaotically and randomly. The irregular twitches of the ventricle are said to resemble a "bag of worms". On an electrocardiogram, ventricular fibrillation is generally easy to recognize because the tracing is totally irregular in appearance, without the repetition of pattern (see Figure 8.9). While the ventricle is fibrillating it is not capable of pumping blood.

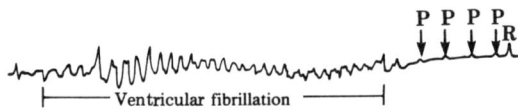

Figure 8.9 Electrocardiogram demonstrating ventricular fibrillation.

This is a true medical emergency requiring immediate action — defibrillation, external cardiac massage, etc. Among the causes of ventricular fibrillation are hypoxia and electrolyte disturbances. Ventricular fibrillation is not an uncommon occurrence after myocardial infarction. This is one of the reasons for developing cardiac units with their elaborate monitoring units, which specialize in the care of patients who have suffered myocardial infarcts.

There is a Swahili proverb, "Heri Kufa macho Kuliko Kufa moyo." (Better the eye should die than the heart.) This is scientific truth, for if the heart stops beating for more than a few minutes, the brain will be deprived of oxygen and will quickly die. Of course the heart itself needs its own oxygen supply if it is to function properly. The heart receives its blood supply from the right and left coronary arteries, which arise from the dorsal aorta just after it leaves the left ventricle (see Figure 8.10).

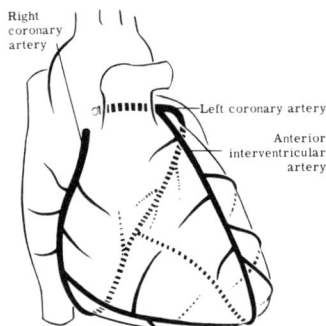

Figure 8.10 The coronary arteries.

The right coronary artery arises from the right side of the aorta and curves around the right ventricle, travelling in the atrio-ventricular groove. The artery and its branches supply the right atrium, right ventricle and posterior portion of the left ventricle. It also supplies the sino-atrial node, the atrio-ventricular node and the bundle of His.

The left coronary artery arises from the left side of the aorta and has two major branches. The left coronary artery travels a short distance in the atrio-ventricular groove and then branches. One branch, the anterior descending branch, descends towards the apex of the heart where it supplies much of the interventricular septum and the anterior part of the left ventricle with blood. The circumflex travels on in the atrio-ventricular groove. It supplies the left atrium and also the lateral portion of the left ventricle, and some of its branches may anastamose with branches of the right coronary artery.

These arteries may become partially or completely blocked with atherosclerotic plaques. These plaques are characterized by a thickening of the innermost part of the artery due to a localized accumulation of lipid and fibrous tissue. They reduce the blood supply to the heart and thus reduce the amount of work that the heart can perform; this may cause

the death of the heart muscle. The formation of these plaques is not fully understood but it is correlated with:

(a) Diets high in animal fats.
(b) Cigarette smoking.
(c) Lack of exercise.

Plaque formation is not limited to coronary arteries however. Thrombi may lodge in the coronary arteries. Coronary thrombosis, in association with atherosclerotic plaques, is a major cause of coronary occlusion.

The veins of the heart accompany the coronary arteries and empty into the coronary sinus which empties its blood into the right atrium.

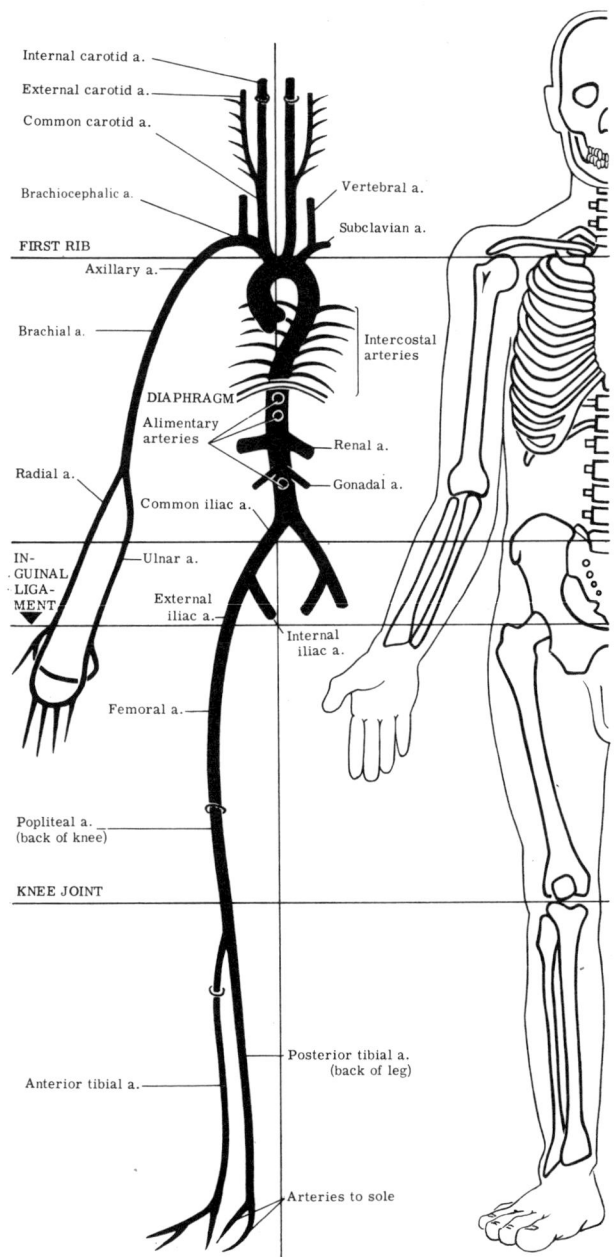

Figure 8.11 The arterial system.

WHAT IS THE ANATOMY OF THE ARTERIES AND THE VEINS?

A. The systemic circulation: the arteries

When blood leaves the left ventricle, it enters the arterial system (see Figure 8.11). The arteries contain an inner lining of endothelial cells, elastic tissue, smooth muscle and a connective tissue covering (see Figure 8.12). The relative amounts of these components change as you proceed away from the heart — the ratio of smooth muscle to connective

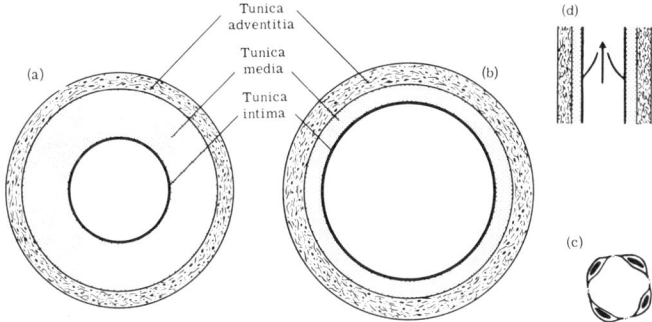

Figure 8.12 The circulatory vessels — transverse sections. (a) Artery. (b) Vein. (c) Capillary. (d) Longitudinal section showing a valve.

tissue is greater in the arterioles than in the aorta, for example. Sometimes the arterial system is called the arterial tree, as it begins with a single trunk, the large aorta, which gives off branches, which in turn give off branches, which become smaller and smaller. The amount of branching is immense, for no cell in the body is farther than 0.7 mm away from a capillary.

Arteries and veins often get their names from the bones or organs which they supply. The route they travel is important too, inasmuch as they must travel where they will not be subjected to the risk of cutting or injury from outside the body, or constriction or bending caused by movement. Generally, arteries take the safest route, on the inner or medial side of the bone where there is only one bone in the limb, or between the bones when there are two bones in the limb. They cross the flexor surfaces where they will be exposed to reduced pressure and less risk of injury.

a. Blood supply to the thorax and abdominal cavity

The aorta is the single artery which leaves the left ventricle. It ascends and arches to the left, quickly giving off the small coronary arteries which supply oxygenated blood to the heart. The next branch is the brachiocephalic, which quickly divides to form the right subclavian (beneath the clavicle) and the right common carotid. Further down, the aorta gives off the left common carotid and, further down, the left subclavian leaves directly from the aorta. The aorta continues caudally, giving off branches to the wall of the thorax and the oesophagus.

After passing through the diaphragm, the artery has a new name, the abdominal aorta (see Figure 8.13). The first arteries to leave the abdominal aorta are the phrenic arteries to the diaphragm. Next to leave is the large coeliac artery; this is sometimes called the coeliac trunk because it is big and soon divides into three branches: the left gastric artery, the common hepatic artery and the splenic artery.

The left gastric artery runs in the lesser curvature of the stomach and helps supply this organ and the end of the oesophagus.

The common hepatic artery usually has five major branches:

(1) The gastroduodenal artery, which branches into: (1a) the retroduodenal artery, which supplies the duodenum; (1b) the right gastroepiploic artery, which runs from right to left in

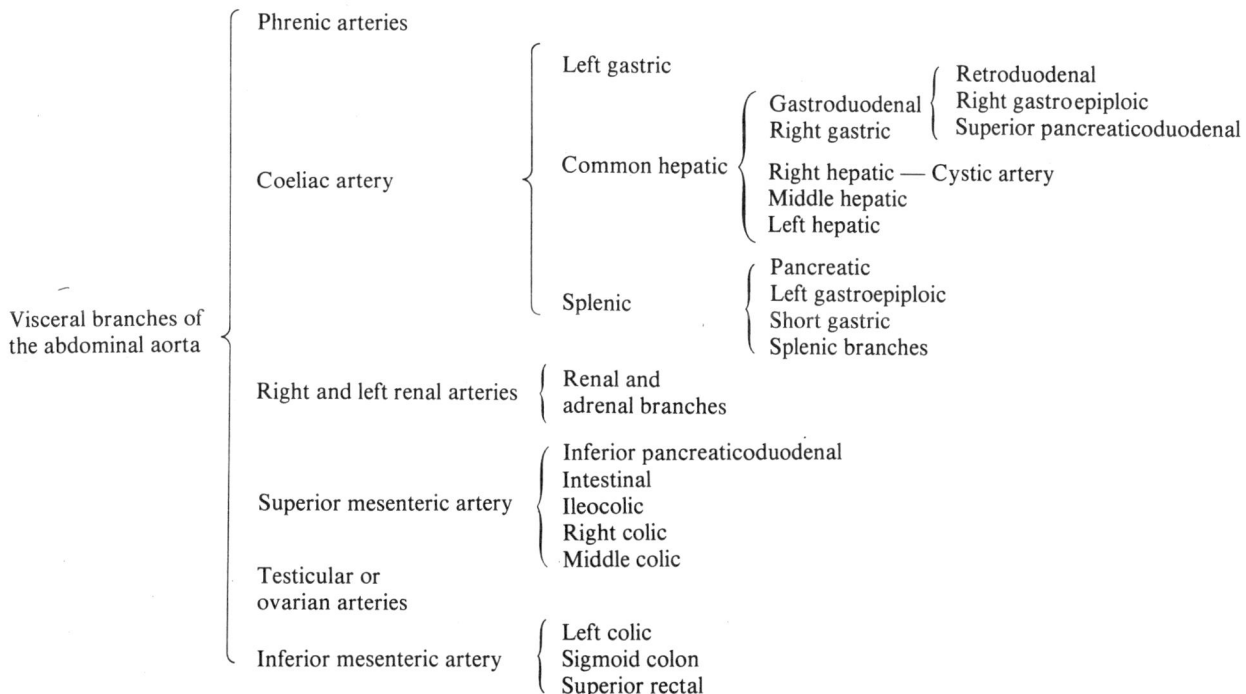

Figure 8.13 The abdominal aorta.

the greater curvature of the stomach and supplies the pylorus and other parts of the stomach; (1c) the superior pancreatico-duodenal artery and supplier of parts of the pancreas.

(2) The right gastric artery, a short branch of the common hepatic artery which runs in the lesser curvature of the stomach and joins the left gastric artery from the coeliac artery.

(3) The right hepatic artery supplies the right lobe of the liver; branches from this artery form the cystic artery which supplies the gall bladder.

(4) The middle hepatic artery supplies the quadrate lobe of the liver.

(5) The left hepatic artery supplies the left lobe of the liver.

The splenic artery is the largest from three branches of the coeliac trunk and it has four major branches. The splenic runs horizontally near the pancreas to reach the spleen.

(1) It gives off several small branches to the pancreas.

(2) Before reaching the spleen it gives off the left gastro-epiploic, which runs in the greater curvature of the stomach and joins the right gastroepiploic.

(3) There are also several short gastric arteries that go from the splenic artery to the stomach.

(4) The splenic artery then divides and supplies the spleen.

Back to the abdominal aorta again. After the single coeliac trunk is given off, the two renal arteries exist, one to each kidney. Branches of these arteries supply the adrenal glands.

Next to leave is the large superior mesenteric artery. This is important because it supplies part of the pancreas and all of the small intestine (except part of the duodenum) and also the caecum, the ascending colon and about half of the transverse colon. The branches of the superior mesenteric artery are named for the structures they supply, and they include:

(1) The inferior pancreaticoduodenal to the pancreas and inferior duodenum.

(2) The intestinal to the jejunum and some of the ileum.

(3) The ileocolic to the terminal parts of the ileum, the appendix, the caecum and the start of the ascending colon.

(4) The right colic to the ascending colon.

(5) The middle colic, which supplies part of the transverse colon.

In the male the two testicular arteries leave the aorta for the gonads after the superior mesenteric; in the female the arteries are the ovarian arteries and supply the ovaries.

The final artery to leave the abdominal aorta is the inferior mesenteric artery, which supplies those parts of the large intestine not supplied by the superior mesenteric artery. The inferior mesenteric artery has three branches:

(1) The left colic, which supplies the descending (left) colon and also joins with the middle colic to complete the supply of the transverse colon.

(2) The sigmoid colon branch, which supplies the sigmoid (pelvic) colon.

(3) The superior rectal, which supplies parts of the rectum.

Many of the names will make more sense when you get to the Chapter on the digestive system.

After giving off the inferior mesenteric artery, the abdominal aorta does not come to a dead end; instead it splits in two, forming the right and left common iliac arteries.

b. Blood supply to the brain.

There are four possible routes to the brain. To visit the brain you have to travel via the carotid arteries or the vertebral arteries. The name "carotid" comes from the Greek word *Karotides* which means "plunging into sleep". The anatomists who named them knew that constriction caused fainting. The right common carotid artery arises from the brachiocephalic artery (which comes from the arch of the aorta). The left common carotid arises directly from the aorta itself. These two arteries travel cranially on either side of the trachea. At the level of the Adam's apple (the thyroid cartilage of the larynx) each common carotid divides into an internal and external carotid artery (see Figure 8.11).

In the angle of the bifurcation is the small carotid body which contains receptors which monitor the partial pressure of oxygen in the arterial blood going to the brain. When they are stimulated they send information to the brain which can increase respiratory movements. The carotid sinus is a spindle-shaped out-pocketing of the internal carotid artery, or of the common and internal carotid arteries near the point of division. The walls of the carotid sinus contain pressorecep-tors (baroreceptors) that report on changes in blood pressure which are mediated by differing amounts of stretch in the walls of the receptor. The information is reported to the vasomotor centre in the medulla of the brain and has importance in the reflex regulation of blood pressure, which will be discussed later. The carotid sinus receptors may have other functions in the control of blood pressure.

The external carotid divides into:

(1) The facial artery — which supplies the face.

(2) The temporal artery — which supplies the side of the head.

(3) The occipital arteries — which supply the back of the head.

The external carotid also sends small branches to the thyroid, pharynx, tongue, maxilla and ear.

The internal carotid enters the skull through the carotid foramen in the side of the head. The internal carotid artery gives off (see Figure 8.14):

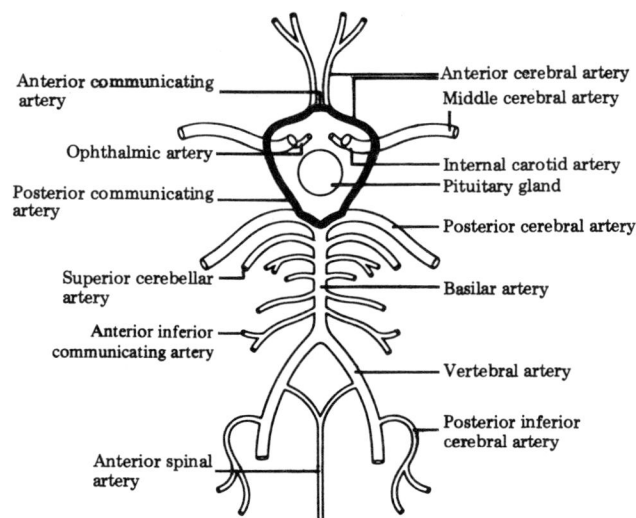

Figure 8.14 The arterial system of the brain, showing the circle of Willis.

(1) The ophthalmic artery to the eye.
(2) The anterior cerebral artery.
(3) The middle cerebral artery.
(4) The posterior communicating artery.

The latter three arteries participate in the formation of the circle of Willis.

The two vertebral arteries arise from the subclavian arteries and head towards the back (dorsal) surface. They go cephalad by passing through the foramen of the transverse processes of the cervical vertebrae and enter into the skull through the foramen magnum. The two vertebral arteries then unite to form the single basilar artery, which shortly divides to form the two posterior cerebral arteries, which also contribute to the circle of Willis.

The circle of Willis is at the base of the brain and is formed from (see Figure 8.14):

(1) The posterior cerebral arteries which arise from the basilar artery.
(2) The anterior cerebral arteries.
(3) The middle cerebral artery.
(4) The posterior communicating arteries which arise from the internal carotid.
(5) The anterior communicating artery which connects the two anterior cerebral arteries.

This arterial circle gives off branches which supply the brain and ensure that, should one of the four major arteries to the brain be blocked, alternative routes of supply will be available.

Atherosclerotic plaques may form in cerebral arteries. The accompanying reduction in blood flow may cause the death of brain tissue supplied by the occluded artery. Plaque formation increases with age. More details on the circulation of the brain will be presented in the Chapter on the nervous system.

c. Blood supply to the upper limb

The right subclavian begins as a branch of the brachio-cephalic, whereas the left subclavian arises directly from the aorta (see Figure 8.11). The subclavian arteries also give off the vertebral arteries and the internal mammary arteries which supply many structures in the thoracic cavity. After the subclavian goes under the clavicle, it becomes the axillary artery, the same artery with a different name.

Upon leaving the axilla it becomes the brachial artery, which runs down the humerus on the medial side of the biceps muscle. This artery is very important for it is normally used in the measuring of blood pressure.

Past the bend of the elbow, the brachial artery divides into the radial and ulnar arteries. The radial artery passes down the outside of the limb to the wrist, where it lies superficially. This artery is often used for taking the pulse to determine the heart rate. The radial artery continues around the base of the thumb and enters the palm of the hand where it contributes to the deep palmar arch and the superficial palmar arches. The ulnar artery runs down the inner side of the wrist where it is joined to the radial artery by means of the deep and superficial palmar arches. The palmar arteries give off the digital arteries which supply the fingers. It should be pointed out that the larger arteries give off many small arteries to the limb as they pass by.

d. Blood supply to the lower limb

The special supply to the lower limb begins with the common iliac arteries which are formed from the division of the abdominal aorta. The common iliac passes in front of the sacro-iliac joints, where it divides into the internal and external iliac arteries. The internal iliac artery supplies blood to the pelvis while the external iliac crosses the groin and goes down the inside of the thigh where it becomes the femoral artery because of its association with the femur.

The femoral artery gives off many branches which supply the thigh muscle as it passes dorsally to the back of the knee where it becomes the popliteal artery.

The popliteal artery crosses the popliteal space and divides into the anterior and posterior tibial arteries. The anterior tibial artery passes between the tibia and the fibula as it runs down the leg; it passes over the ankle and becomes the dorsalis pedis artery which supplies the dorsal part of the foot. The posterior tibial runs down the back of the leg, crosses the ankle on the inner or medial side and forms the plantar arch, which supplies the sole of the foot. Part of the physical examination most often involves palpation of the pulses in the dorsalis pedis and posterior tibial arteries. The presences and quality of the pulses in these arteries give a crude but valid indication of the flow within the lower limbs.

B. The systemic circulation: the veins

After traversing the capillaries, blood returns via the veins (see Figure 8.15). The veins or venules near the capillaries are small but they get much larger and fewer in number as they approach the heart. Although the veins have thinner walls than the arteries because they contain less smooth muscle and elastic and fibrous tissues, they are wider than the arteries and contain more than twice the blood found in the arteries (see Figure 8.12). At any instant, more than 70% of the blood is found in the veins. For this reason the venous system can act as a blood reservoir or storage centre. The venous pressure is less than the arterial pressure, the blood moves more slowly and the veins of the limbs contain valves which prevent the backflow of blood.

There are two main types of veins:

(1) The superficial veins.
(2) The deep veins.

The superficial veins run in the fatty tissue beneath the skin. If you let your hand hang freely at your side, you can usually see the superficial veins in the back of the hand fill with blood. The superficial veins empty into the deep veins. The deep veins accompany the main arteries and often have the same name as that of the artery.

a. Blood return from the brain and thoracic cavity

Blood is returned from the brain by special channels inside the skull known as sinuses. The sinuses are made of endothelium and dura mater — the tough outer connective tissue covering of the brain. The largest of these sinuses is the superior sagittal sinus, which drains the blood from the superior part of the brain and lies in the middle of the brain between the two cerebral hemispheres (see Figure 8.16). The superior sagittal sinus divides into the two transverse sinuses draining the back of the brain. The inner parts of the brain

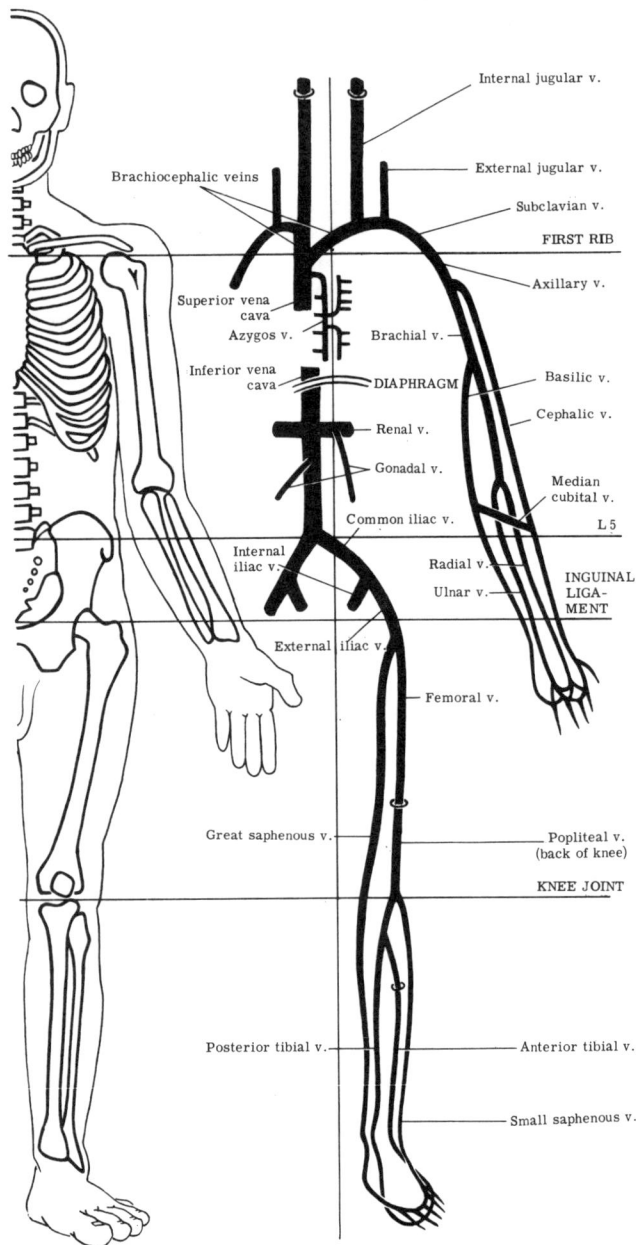

Figure 8.15   The venous system.

cava and from there into the right atrium. The superior vena cava is the final common vein for blood returning from the brain, upper limbs and thoracic cavity.

b. Blood return from the upper limb

The deep veins drain the inner part of the limb, accompany the arteries and have similar names. They are:

(1) The digital veins.
(2) The deep and superficial palmar arches.
(3) The ulnar and radial veins.
(4) The brachial veins.
(5) The axillary vein.
(6) The subclavian vein.

The superficial veins are important as these veins are used in giving intravenous infusions and blood transfusions and for withdrawing blood samples. The superficial veins begin in the hand and form three veins which run up the forearm:

(1) The cephalic vein.
(2) The median vein.
(3) The basilic vein.

In the upper arm, the median joins the basilic and then both the cephalic and the basilic enter the axillary.

As the median vein approaches the forearm it becomes the median cubital vein. Often, instead of simply joining the basilic, it forms a "Y"; one branch draining into the basilic, the other draining into the cephalic (see Figure 8.15). Sometimes the median cubital is a separate vein connecting

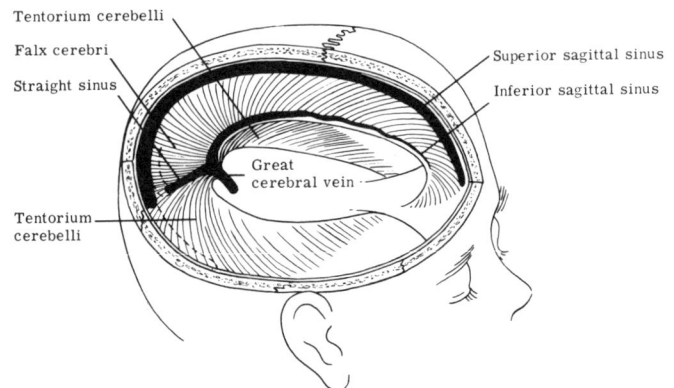

Figure 8.16   Sagittal and horizontal section through the right half of the skull and brain, showing the venous system of the brain.

the cephalic and basilic veins. The median cubital and its branches are frequently used as the site for venipuncture. There is considerable variation in the superficial veins, as all people who draw blood are well aware.

The axillary vein becomes the subclavian and the subclavian becomes the branchiocephalic after the internal jugular has emptied into it. The right and left brachiocephalic veins come together forming the superior vena cava, which enters the right atrium.

c. Venous return from the lower limb

Blood returning from the lower limb follows the same pattern as that from the upper limb — there are deep and superficial veins.

The deep veins which accompany the arteries are:

(1) The digital veins.
(2) The plantar venous arch.

return blood via the inferior sagittal sinus and the straight sinuses, which empty into the transverse sinuses. The two transverse sinuses join the two internal jugular veins accompanying the internal and common carotid arteries.

Blood from the face is collected by the superficial veins, which also join the internal jugular vein. The internal jugulars run downward in the neck, pass behind the clavicle and join with the subclavian veins to form the brachiocephalic veins (see Figure 8.15). The two brachiocephalic veins unite to form the superior vena cava, which empties into the right atrium of the heart.

Blood from the thoracic cavity is also returned via the superior vena cava. The bronchial veins from the lungs, the oesophageal veins from the oesophagus and the intercostal veins from the thoracic musculature all unite to form the azygos vein. The azygos vein empties into the superior vena

(3) The anterior and posterior tibial veins.
(4) The popliteal vein.
(5) The femoral vein.

The femoral vein goes up the thigh, crosses the groin and becomes the external iliac vein. The external iliac joins with the internal iliac returning blood from the pelvis and becomes the common iliac. The right and left common iliac veins join and form the inferior vena cava, which travels up the posterior abdominal wall to the right of the abdominal aorta. It passes through the diaphragm and enters into the right atrium of the heart.

The chief superficial veins are the short saphenous vein and the long saphenous vein. The short saphenous vein is formed from the union of many small vessels which drain the dorsum of the foot. It ascends on the outer side of the instep and goes along the back of the leg to the popliteal space where it joins the popliteal vein. The long saphenous vein arises on the inside of the instep, runs up the medial surface of the leg and joins the femoral vein. It is the longest vein in the body.

d. Venous return from the pelvic and abdominal cavities

The internal pelvic area is drained by the internal iliac vein. The internal iliac joins the external iliac carrying blood from the leg and together they form the common iliac vein. The two common iliac veins unite to form the inferior vena cava. As the inferior vena cava ascends towards the heart it receives:

(1) Either the ovarian or testicular veins.
(2) The right and left renal veins.
(3) The right suprarenal vein from the adrenal gland (the left suprarenal vein drains into the left renal vein).
(4) The hepatic vein.

The inferior vena cava penetrates the diaphragm and enters the heart.

e. The portal circulation

Perhaps you noticed that not all the abdominal organs were mentioned. What happens to the blood from the intestinal tract if it does not enter directly into the inferior vena cava? To answer this question, you should remember that blood leaving the intestines will be low in oxygen but rich in nutrients, particularly amino acids and glucose. Instead of being returned directly to the heart, after which the nutrients would be sent throughout the body, the blood from the intestine goes first to the liver.

In the liver the nutrients are stored, used for energy, or converted to other nutrients before being released into the blood via the hepatic vein (see Figure 8.17).

The inferior mesenteric vein drains blood from the rectum and part of the large intestine; it joins the splenic vein which drains the spleen and pancreas. The superior mesenteric vein drains the small intestine and part of the large intestine. In general the areas drained by the inferior and superior mesenteric veins parallel the supply of the inferior and superior mesenteric arteries. The superior mesenteric vein and the splenic vein unite to make the hepatic portal vein.

The gastric vein from the stomach enters the hepatic portal vein. Altogether, about 1200 ml of blood/minute enter the liver via the hepatic portal vein. The hepatic portal vein splits in two and these in turn divide and keep dividing so that the

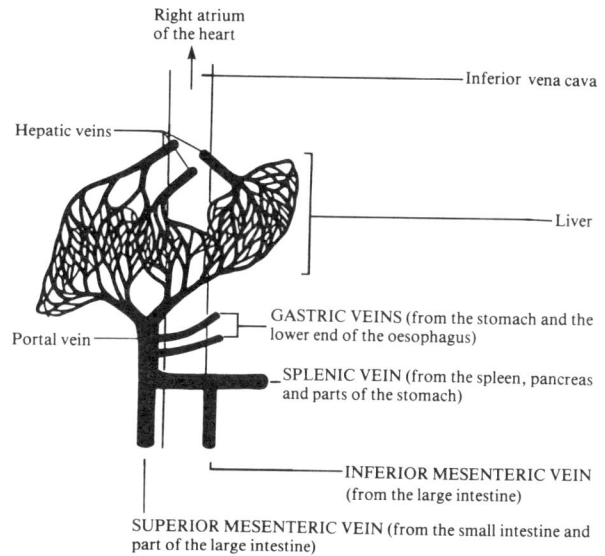

Figure 8.17   The portal circulation.

entire liver is supplied with blood. These vessels empty into sinuses or spaces surrounded by columns of hepatic cells which take up the products of digestion. Blood from the hepatic artery also enters the sinuses providing oxygen to the liver cells. After the blood passes through the sinuses, it enters into venules and ultimately passes into the hepatic veins. The two hepatic veins empty into the inferior vena cava and, from there, blood is returned to the right atrium.

In certain liver diseases such as cirrhosis, the architecture of the liver changes and may become fibrotic. This hinders the flow of blood through the liver and sometimes results in a back up of blood in the veins and an increase in the return of blood to the heart via alternate channels.

C. The pulmonary circulation

The pulmonary circulation comprises the circulation of the blood through the lungs, beginning with the right ventricle and ending with the left atrium (see Figure 8.18).

The pulmonary artery leaves the right ventricle, passes

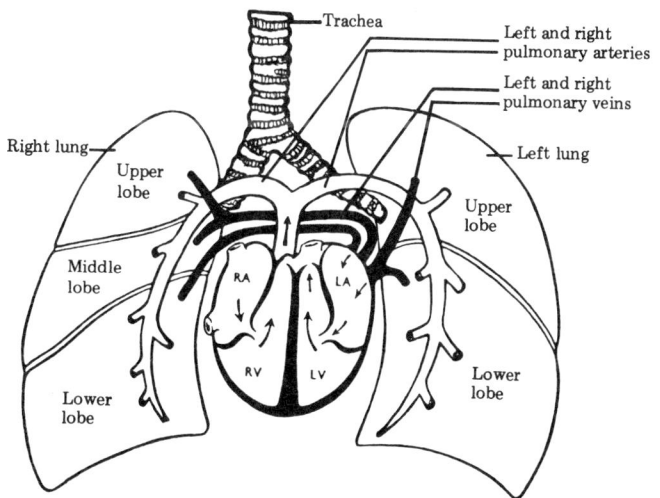

Figure 8.18   The pulmonary circulation.

upward and splits into a left and right pulmonary artery. The left pulmonary artery divides into two branches: one branch goes to the upper lobe of the left lung while the other branch goes to the lower lobe. The right pulmonary artery has three branches, with one branch each to the upper, middle and lower lobes. These arteries divide to form smaller arteries, arterioles and capillaries. In the capillaries, CO_2 diffuses out of the blood into the alveoli while O_2 diffuses into the blood.

The oxygenated blood passes into the venules which unite to form larger veins. The veins from each lobe form a single vein. As there are three right and two left lobes, there are a total of five pulmonary veins. Often the veins from the right upper and right middle lobe join to form a single vein so that four pulmonary veins enter the left atrium of the heart. Pulmonary veins do not have valves.

The trip through the pulmonary circulation is much shorter than the one through the systemic circulation, but it is equally important. If the lungs are not adequately perfused with blood and are not adequately ventilated with air, there cannot be sufficient exchange of gases necessary to maintain life. The pulmonary circulation does differ from the systemic circulation in that it is a low pressure, low resistance system. The pulmonary vessels are generally thinner and more distensible, containing more elastin and less smooth muscle.

More details on flow in the lungs are presented in the Chapter on the respiratory system.

A BRIEF REVIEW OF PHYSICS

Before considering the physiology of the cardiovascular system, it would be good to review some of the basic physics that applies:

A. Pressure

The first concept is that of pressure, or force per unit area. You know that if you push against the wall with your hand, you are exerting a pressure against it; the harder you push, the greater the pressure. Conversely, imagine the wall is going

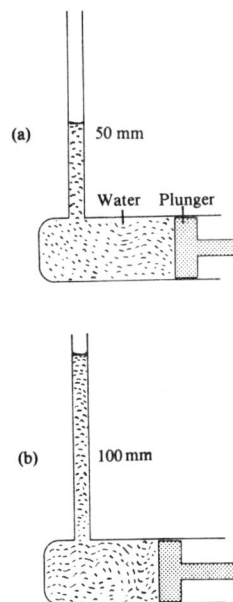

Figure 8.19   The concept of pressure.

to fall and you have to hold it up. The heavier the wall, the more pressure you will have to exert to keep it from falling. But how do we define this pressure? What units do we use to specify its magnitude?

Pressure within the cardiovascular system is usually given in millimetres of mercury (mmHg). A column of mercury is contained within an instrument known as a sphygmomanometer. As the pressure in the piston increases, the height of the column of mercury will also increase. If the height of the mercury is 50 mm and the pressure is doubled, the column will rise to 100 mm (see Figure 8.19). But why is mercury used instead of something ordinary like water? Water could be used, of course, but water is much lighter than mercury. If you had two identical cups and filled one with mercury and the other with water, the mercury cup would weigh 13.6 times as much; and it would take 13.6 times more force to hold the mercury-containing cup than the water one. If you were to put water in a sphygmomanometer, the apparatus which have to be at least 13.6 times as tall as the one with mercury. The same pressure which can force the mercury column to 50 mm would force the water to 680 mm (68.0 cm).

B. Flow

Flow is movement of a fluid. Let us consider some of the factors that can affect flow in a simple tube:

(1) For fluid to flow through a tube, there has to be a pressure difference between the two ends A and B of the tube. If the pressure at both A and B is 100 mmHg, no flow will occur because there is no pressure difference.

(2) Flow will always go from the direction of high pressure to that of low pressure. If the pressure at A is 60 mmHg and at B is 30 mmHg, the fluid must go from A to B and cannot possibly go from B to A.

(3) The greater the pressure, the greater the flow. Assume that the pressure at A is 100 mmHg, at B is 50 mmHg and that 500 ml flow out of the tube in 1 minute. If the pressure at A is increased to 150 mmHg while B stays at 50, the volume of flow will double to 1000 ml. If the pressure at A goes to 1150 mmHg and at B goes to 1050 mmHg, 1000 ml will still flow because there has been no change in the pressure difference between A and B.

(4) The single most important factor in determining the outflow from the tube will be the radius of the tube. To illustrate this point, assume that we have three tubes of the same length and material (see Figure 8.20). Tube 1 is the same tube we have been using in the previous examples. Tube 2 has a radius twice the size of tube 1, and tube 3 has a radius $\frac{1}{2}$ the size of tube 1. The pressure at the "A ends" of the three tubes is 100 mmHg and at the "B ends" is 50 mmHg. In 1 minute, 500 ml of fluid will flow through tube 1, 8000 ml through tube 2 and 31.25 ml through tube 3. This can be proved mathematically and demonstrated quite easily. Although the radius of tube 2 is twice the size of tube 1, 16 times as much fluid will leave in 1 minute, and $\frac{1}{16}$th as much fluid will leave tube 3, although it is only $\frac{1}{2}$ as wide as tube 1.

The great French scientist, Poiseuille, determined that flow through a tube depends on the radius to the fourth power (r^4, the radius multiplied by itself four times). This means that little changes in the size of the tube can have great effects on

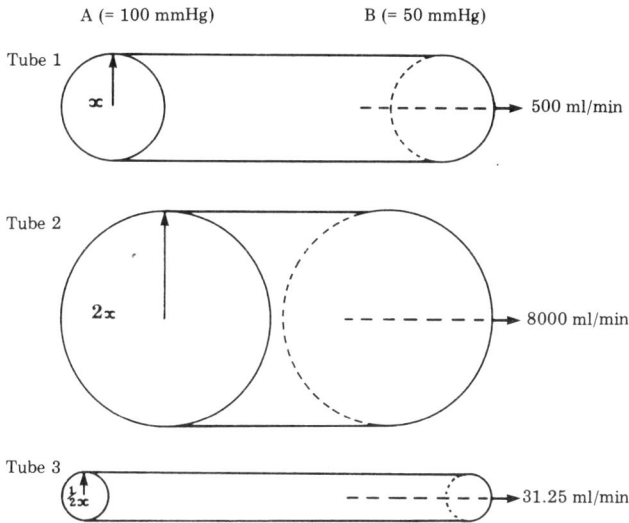

A (= 100 mmHg)   B (= 50 mmHg)

Tube 1

x

→ 500 ml/min

Tube 2

2x

→ 8000 ml/min

Tube 3

½x

→ 31.25 ml/min

Figure 8.20 The relationship between the radius of a tube and the volume of the flow.

the flow through that tube. This is because a big tube cannot only contain more fluid but will also have less resistance to flow. Resistance is the difficulty of flow because of the friction between the fluid molecules themselves and the friction between the fluid and the walls of the tube.

(5) In all previous examples we have been using the same fluid. The volume of flow will also depend on the nature of fluid used. Assume we have our original tube with a pressure of 100 mmHg at A and 50 mmHg at B and a flow of 500 ml in 1 minute. Now we keep the same conditions but substitute a solution of honey and water in place of the original solution; we find that 100 ml leave the tube in 1 minute. Honey has a greater resistance to flow than most other liquids. This internal resistance to flow is known as viscosity.

Let us build onto our simple tube and concern ourselves with the pressure rather than the flow (see Figure 8.21):

Fluid enters a rubber bulb (B) at A; when the bulb is squeezed, a pressure is generated and forces the fluid through a rubber tube towards C. D is a valve which can be adjusted and regulates the opening of the tube. We want to look at the system and ask ourselves what will determine the pressure in the system. Basically, the pressure will be the product of the flow times the resistance ($P = F \times R$). The flow through the system will be determined by the volume of fluid put into the system. If there is no fluid in the system, obviously there will not be any pressure. If the rubber bulb is squeezed frequently, more fluid will be put into the system, the flow will increase and the pressure will increase.

The force with which the bulb is squeezed will also have an effect. The more forcefully it is squeezed, the more fluid will

enter the system and the greater will be the pressure. The chief factor in determining the resistance will be the position of the valve. If the valve is all the way up, the resistance will be quite low; however, if the valve is partially blocking the tube and reducing its radius so that only a little fluid can pass through, there will be a great increase in the resistance and the pressure will increase.

Another factor that will influence the pressure will be the distensibility of the tubing (the ability of the tubing to stretch and expand as fluid enters it). If the tubing is very distensible and easily expands as fluid enters it, the pressure will not increase as much as it would if the tube were rigid.

Of course, the pressure will also depend on where it is measured. If you measure it close to the bulb it will be higher than if you measure it far away. Energy is lost because of the frictional resistance.

The purpose of presenting the model is to lay a foundation for the study of arterial blood pressure. In the model the formula for pressure is:

$$Pressure = Flow \times Resistance.$$

In the cardiovascular system the "formula" for the average (mean) arterial blood pressure is:

Average (mean) arterial blood pressure = Cardiac output × Resistance.

Pressure expresses a relationship between a container and its contents. Arterial blood pressure also expresses a relationship between a container and its contents. The container is the arterial system and its content is the blood within the arteries. Blood is put into the arteries by the heart. Cardiac output is a term which describes the flow of blood out of the heart into the arteries. Resistance is a complex term but here it can be used for the difficulty with which blood flows through the arteries and leaves the arteries to enter the capillaries. The volume of blood in the arteries depends then on the rate which blood from the heart enters the arteries and the rate which the blood leaves the arterioles to enter the capillaries. The cardiovascular system is not a simple pump and open tube as described in the model; it is a complex circuit. Blood leaves the capillaries and is returned to the heart by the veins. If less blood is returned to the heart, less blood can be pumped out of the heart into the arteries. Thus everything is inter-related. Nevertheless, it is good to keep this simple overview in mind as you study the various factors which affect cardiac output and resistance and, therefore, determine arterial blood pressure.

HOW DOES THE HEART FUNCTION?

The principles that apply in the model apply, of course, to the cardiovascular system as well. In the cardiovascular system the heart is the pump, the arteries are the distensible tubes and the arterioles are analogous to the valve which can increase or decrease the resistance and thus control the volume of blood which enters the tissues. Let us look at the heart now.

A. The cardiac cycle

We have established the anatomy of the heart and the specialized conduction pathway in it. Because of the

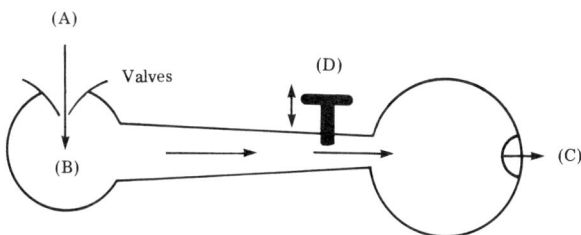

(A)

Valves

(D)

(B)

(C)

Figure 8.21 Factors affecting fluid flow.

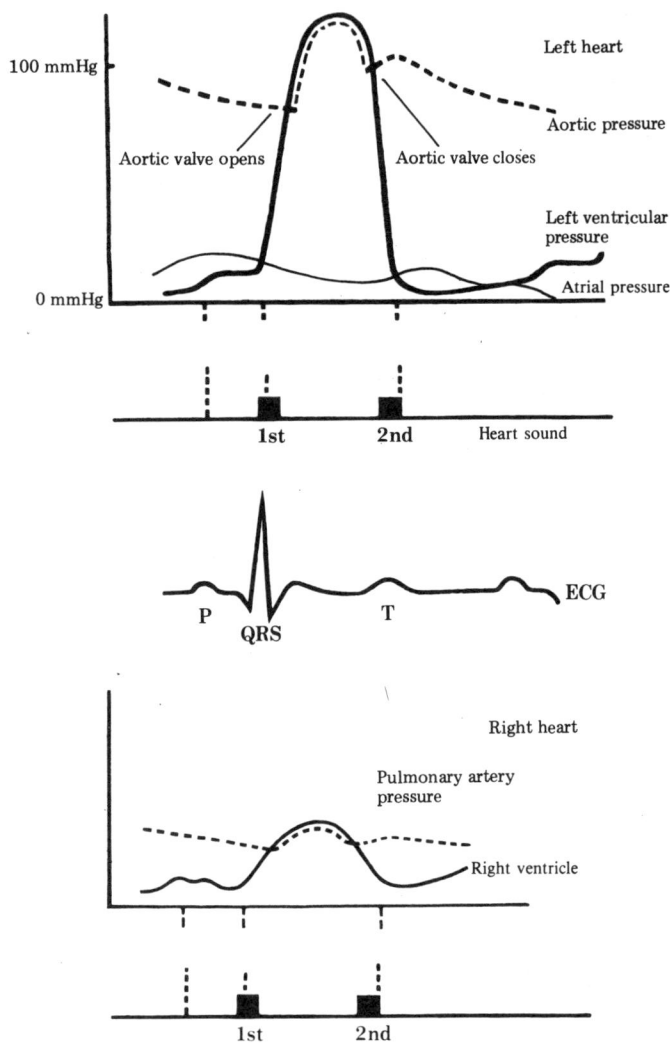

Figure 8.22 The main events of the cardiac cycle for the left side of the heart.

organized spread of excitation, there is an orderly sequence of contraction known as the cardiac cycle (see Figure 8.22):

(1) The atria contract and force some more blood into the ventricles.

(2) The atrio-ventricular valves close, causing the first heart sound, and ventricles begin to contract. Inasmuch as both the A–V valves and the aortic and pulmonic valves are closed, blood can neither enter nor leave the ventricles. Because the volume in the ventricles is constant and the ventricles are contracting, this part of the cycle is referred to as the isovolumetric ventricular contraction phase of the cardiac cycle. Pressure in the ventricles increases dramatically during the phase of isovolumetric ventricular contraction.

(3) When pressure in the ventricles exceeds pressure in the aorta and pulmonary arteries, the aortic and pulmonary valves are forced to open. Blood leaves the ventricles and enters the arterial system; this is known as the ejection phase of the cardiac cycle.

(4) As blood leaves the ventricles, pressure within them falls. Pressure in the aortic and pulmonary arteries exceeds that in the ventricles, and the aortic and pulmonary valves

snap shut causing the second heart sound. When the aortic and pulmonary valves are closed, all the heart valves are now closed and blood can neither enter nor leave the ventricles. This is referred to as the isovolumetric relaxation phase of the cardiac cycle.

(5) Blood entering the atria causes the pressure inside the atria to exceed that in the ventricles; the mitral and tricuspid valves open and the cardiac cycle is ready to begin again.

The time between the closing of the A–V valves and the closing of the aortic and pulmonary valves is known as systole. The remaining time, from the closing of the aortic and pulmonic valves to the closing of the mitral and tricuspid valves, is known as diastole. Throughout most of systole the heart is contracting, while the muscle is relaxed throughout most of diastole (see Figure 8.22).

It should be pointed out that the biggest increase in ventricular volume follows the opening of the A–V valves; the time immediately after their opening is known as the rapid ventricular filling phase.

Sometimes the inflow of blood into the ventricles, and the vibration of blood within the ventricles, give rise to the third heart sound. This sound can be heard in children, and is heard in adults when the left ventricle is failing and when there is a large volume of blood in the ventricle, prior to opening of the A–V valves.

There is only a small increase in ventricular volume following atrial contraction.

B. Cardiac output

The cardiac output is the volume of blood that leaves each ventricle in 1 minute and it is extremely important, for it states how much blood leaves the ventricle and enters the arterial system in 1 minute. (Under most circumstances, the outputs of the right and left ventricles are equal — the cardiac output refers to the output from each ventricle and not the total of the two outputs.)

The cardiac output will be a product of two factors: the heart rate (the number of times that the heart beats in 1 minute), and the stroke volume (the amount of blood to be ejected from the heart with each beat). If the heart rate is 70 beats/min and the stroke volume is 70 ml/beat then the cardiac output will be:

70 beats/min × 70 ml/beat = 4900 ml/min (4.9 litres/min)

Anything that affects either heart rate or stroke volume will affect the cardiac output. Cardiac output is also important because of its relationship to the arterial blood pressure. In the cardiovascular system the relationship which defines arterial pressure is:

Arterial pressure = Cardiac output × Resistance.

Thus, if resistance remains constant, arterial pressure will increase with an increase in cardiac output and decrease with a decrease in cardiac output.

a. Heart rate

Heart rate is controlled by the autonomic nervous system which has two divisions: the parasympathetic nervous system and the sympathetic nervous system. The parasympathetic nervous system is represented by fibres from the vagus nerve and acts as a brake on the heart, causing its rate of beating to slow down. The vagus nerve goes to both the S–A node and the A–V node. When it is stimulated, it releases acetylcholine from its endings which reduces the excitability of the pacemaker and slows conduction through the A–V node. The sympathetic fibres also go to the S–A node. When they are stimulated, their nerve endings release noradrenaline, which accelerates the heart rate. Both the sympathetic and parasympathetic arc tonically active, that is, they continually send impulses to the heart. However, the parasympathetic impulses seem to dominate, for if the vagus nerve is injured or prevented from sending impulses, the heart rate speeds up. Adrenaline, a hormone released by the adrenal medulla during times of stress or excitement, also increases heart rate. Excessive amounts of hormone from the thyroid gland increase heart rate.

Heart rate slows during sleep and increases during exercise or as the result of disease. In general, heart rates of less than 60 beats/min are referred to as bradycardia. Tachycardia is the term often used to refer to heart rates greater than 100 beats/min. During exercise, heart rates can increase to 150 beats/min as a result of sympathetic stimulation.

Because all parts of the heart occasionally have an inherent spontaneous rhythmicity, parts of the atria other than the S–A node may depolarize first and then generate impulses. These sites of depolarization are referred to as ectopic foci. There may be so many ectopic foci that the atrial muscle does not contract in an orderly manner, so the individual fibres contract independently in a random manner. This is called atrial fibrillation. The response of the ventricle to atrial fibrillation is variable and depends on how many impulses from the atria are conducted through the A–V node. Atrial fibrillation may or may not significantly reduce cardiac output. Embolism may be a complication of atrial fibrillation. Blood stagnates in the atria, and this stagnation fosters the development of thrombi, which may embolize to the pulmonary or systemic circulation.

Ectopic foci may arise in the ventricle and may be dangerous if they lead to ventricular fibrillation. Coronary thrombosis can cause ventricular fibrillation, and so can metabolic abnormalities as well as excessive amounts of adrenaline, particularly in patients who are anaesthetized.

Ventricular fibrillation is not compatible with life because the randomly contracting ventricular fibres cannot generate sufficient force to pump significant amounts of blood from the ventricles.

Sometimes ventricular fibrillation is preceded by ventricular flutter. This is when a single ectopic focus in the ventricle fires at a rate of 200–300 times/min, a fast rate that is dangerous, and, moreover, the ventricles do not have adequate time to fill with blood.

b. Stroke volume (see Figure 8.23)

The volume of blood to leave the ventricle with each beat is primarily dependent on the volume of blood in the ventricle before the contraction starts. Within limits, the greater the volume of blood in the ventricle before contraction, the greater the volume to be ejected. The increased blood within the heart stretches the muscle fibres and affects their geometry so that they can contract more efficiently. This relationship between the volume of blood in the ventricle, the

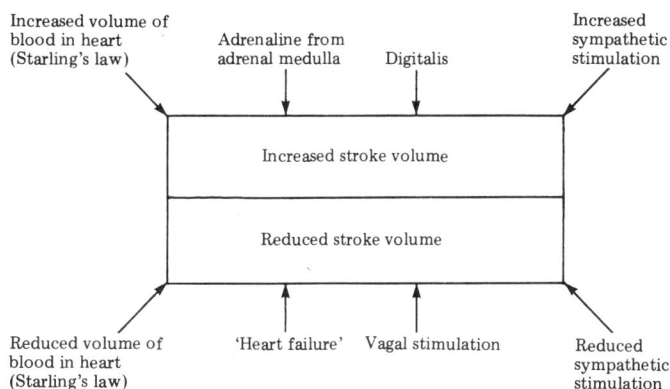

Figure 8.23 Factors affecting stroke volume.

stretch of the muscle fibres and the stroke volume is known as Starling's law of the heart.

Figure 8.24 demonstrates this relationship. As the ventricles cannot store large volumes of blood the heart must pump more blood if additional blood is returned to it. An example might help illustrate this properly. Blood is constantly being returned to the heart and is pumped out of the heart with every beat. If the heart rate is slowed, there will be more time between beats and thus more blood in the heart before each beat, because the heart has had an increased time to fill. Since there is more blood in the heart before it beats, there will be more stretch of the ventricular muscle and more blood will be pumped out of the heart with each beat. (This does not necessarily mean an increased cardiac output. If the heart rate goes from 70 to 50 beats/min, the stroke volume may go from 70 to 98 ml, so the cardiac output will still be 4.9 litres/min.)

It is possible that such an excessive amount of blood may enter the heart that the ventricles cannot compensate for this greatly increased stretch and will then work at reduced efficiency and pump out less blood. The mechanism described by Starling's law ensures that the output of the right and left ventricles will be equal. If, for example, the right ventricle were suddenly to increase its output, there would be an increased volume of blood entering the left ventricle from the lungs. This would cause an increased output from the left ventricle; if the left ventricle did not increase its output, blood would soon accumulate in the lungs. In certain pathological conditions either the right or left ventricle may be damaged and the ventricle may not be able to "obey" Starling's law. This may lead to a backing up of blood into the lungs, the veins or both, which can have very serious consequences.

Look at Figure 8.24 carefully. In a normal heart beat there may be 150 ml of blood within the left ventricle before it contracts (A). The volume of blood ejected in one beat may be 75 ml (A'). If the amount of blood returned to the heart is increased, the amount ejected (stroke volume) will also increase. If 300 ml is returned to the heart (B), about 150 ml will be pumped out (B'). Should there be still more blood returned to the heart, e.g. an increase to 400 ml (C), the stroke volume will fall to (C') — about 100 ml; the large volume has stretched the heart muscle to such an extent that the efficiency has been reduced.

You will often hear the term "heart failure" or congestive heart failure in your clinical work. Heart failure is a condition rather than a specific disease; it refers to the fact that the heart is failing or not fully meeting the needs of other organs for blood. There are many causes of heart failure including diseases of the valves or pericardium and hypertension.

Heart failure also results if the myocardium is diseased; this can happen with infection or nutritional deficiency, but most commonly happens if the blood flow to the myocardium through the coronary arteries is reduced because of atherosclerotic plaque. This causes changes in the myocardium, so the myocardial cells work less efficiently. This reduced efficiency means that the Starling curve of Figure 8.24a will not be valid and that the heart will be working on a different, less efficient Starling curve, as shown in Figure 8.24b.

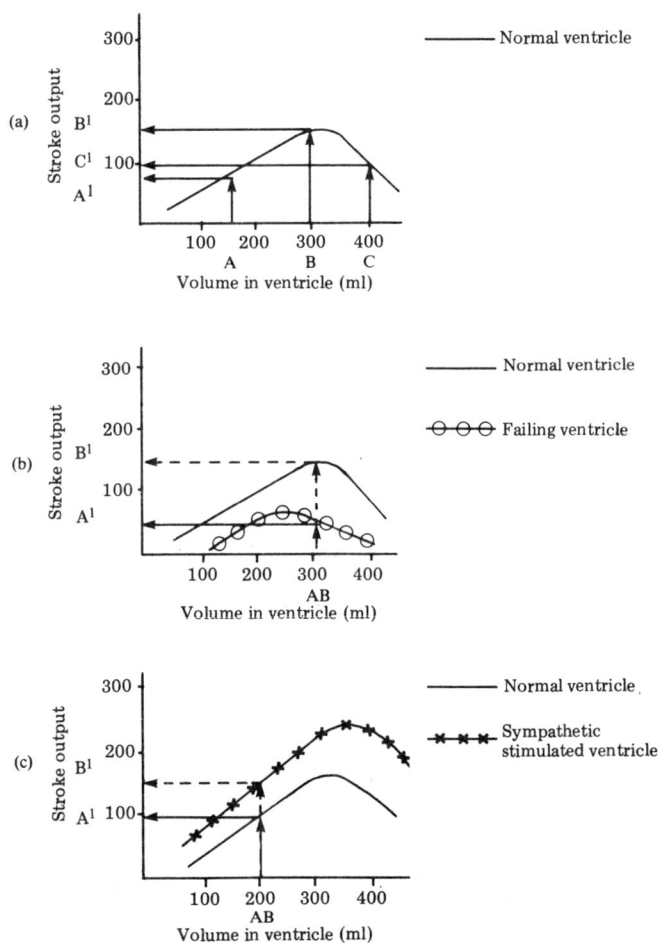

Figure 8.24 The efficiency of the heart. Starling's law of the heart.

As the muscle is working inefficiently and not able to pump out as much as it normally would, more blood will be retained in the heart. This additional volume may cause the heart to be operating on the descending limb of the Starling curve. The extra volume also changes the internal geometry of the heart so that the ventricle must do additional work to pump out the same volume of blood. The heart does more work and requires more energy to pump out 70 ml of blood when there are 300 ml in the ventricle than it does to pump out 70 ml when there are only 150 ml in the ventricle.

Figure 8.24b compares the normal and the failing heart. If both ventricles have 300 ml of blood within them (AB), the healthy heart will eject 150 ml (B'), while the failing heart will have a stroke output of only 50 ml (A'). You can see that a failing heart will not be able to meet the strain caused by exercise and strenuous activities when increased volumes of blood are returned to the heart and must be pumped out to meet the greater demands of the body.

Some of the consequences of ventricular failure include a backing up of blood into the lungs, thereby interfering with respiration and failure to adequately perfuse the kidneys with blood. As a result of reduced kidney perfusion, more fluid is retained within the cardiovascular system, the plasma volume is increased and more of a work load is placed upon the failing heart.

In the Chapter on skeletal muscle some of the ways in which the strength of contraction could be increased were discussed. You can vary the strength of skeletal muscle contraction simply by increasing or decreasing the number of motor units called into play. If you are lifting a light weight, only a few motor units will be activated and only a few muscle fibres will contract. If you are lifting a heavy weight, more motor units will be activated, and more muscle fibres will contract. This mechanism is not available to the heart, for the heart behaves as a single motor unit. Yet, the heart must make great adjustments, increasing or decreasing the force of its contractions. The heart cannot activate more motor units (as in skeletal muscle), but the efficiency or strength of the contraction process can be dramatically increased. The efficiency of ventricular contraction can change in response to sympathetic stimulation or to changes in hormonal and ionic environment. These stimuli presumably increase the ions and energy-providing substrates necessary for a strong contraction.

Drugs such as digitalis and its derivatives can also cause a more efficient, forceful contraction. In exercise, stress or excitement there is an increased sympathetic stimulation to the heart, some of it going directly to the ventricles. The postganglionic sympathetic nerve fibres release noradrenaline, and this chemical affects the myocardial muscle cells so that they contract more forcefully and pump more blood out of the ventricle. Adrenaline from the adrenal medulla and drugs like digitalis can also be used to increase the strength of contraction.

Figure 8.24c illustrates this relationship. If two identical ventricles each have 150 ml of blood in them (AB), the ventricle with sympathetic stimulation will have a stroke output of 125 ml (B'), while the control (normal) will eject 75 ml. This mechanism is extremely important in conditions when the heart must work more efficiently and eject more blood to meet the increased demands made by the body. The increased efficiency of the ventricles following sympathetic stimulation, adrenaline, or certain drugs is often referred to as an increase in contractility. There is some evidence that acetylcholine and vagal stimulation can reduce contractility.

The blood plasma provides the nutrient and ionic environment that nourishes and bathes the heart. The heart can metabolize many substrates including glucose, lactic acid, fatty acids and ketone bodies. The concentration of some plasma ions seems to be more important than the nutrients metabolized by the heart. The heart is uniquely sensitive to the levels of potassium and calcium in the blood. Increases in plasma potassium may reduce contractility or even stop the heart from beating. Cardiac arrest from hyperkalaemia may occur when the plasma potassium reaches levels of 7–10 mEq/l. When patients are in heart failure, they are sometimes given a diuretic to reduce the volume in the circulatory system and digitalis to increase the strength of the heart beat. Some diuretics cause an increased loss of potassium in the urine. The combination of digitalis and low potassium can cause abnormal heart beats and arrhythmias (irregular rates of contraction). High levels of potassium or an alkaline pH can also cause arrhythmias. Increased levels of calcium can stop the heart in mid-contraction. Digitalis also sensitizes the heart to increases in the plasma calcium level.

WHAT IS RESISTANCE AND WHAT AFFECTS RESISTANCE?

Resistance, we said, is the difficulty a fluid has in flowing. Difficulty is caused by the friction between the fluid and the walls of the vessel, and the friction between the molecules themselves. Perhaps an analogy might help establish the concept. Suppose 1000 students had to leave a school on fire-drill. What factors will determine how fast all the students can leave the building? If there are few exits and they are long and narrow, it will take a much longer time than if there were many wide exits going directly outside. (Remember that the width of the exit will be of extreme importance.) Students will have a more difficult time if they have to go through a single exit — resistance will be greater. The way the students behave will also have some affect on the time it takes. If the students co-operate among themselves and leave in an orderly manner, they will all exit more quickly than if there is pushing, fighting and turbulence causing more internal resistance.

(1) *Overall arrangement.* Now that we have some idea of resistance, let us look at resistance in the cardiovascular system. Resistance will depend on the overall arrangement of the vessels, whether they are many or few, and what their radii are. The greatest resistance within the cardiovascular system is found in the arterioles; here the pressure drop is the greatest. True, the capillaries are narrower than the arterioles, but there are so many more capillaries than arterioles that together they offer less resistance. To use again our school analogy, there would be less overall resistance if each student had his or her own exit than there would be if there were fewer but wider exits.

(2) *The radius.* The resistance of the arterioles can change. If the smooth muscle which surrounds the arterioles contracts and squeezes the arteriole so that its lumen becomes smaller (and its radius less), there would be an increase in resistance. As a result of this, there will be considerably less flow through the arteriole. If the smooth muscle relaxes, the arteriole gets bigger, resistance is reduced and flow increases. A 16% increase in the radius of the arteriole can result in the doubling of flow through it.

The radius of the arteriole is not only important in regulating the flow of blood through the arteriole into the tissue but is also extremely important in determining what the blood pressure is. If the arterioles are constricted, blood will enter the capillaries more slowly and more blood will be retained between the arterioles and the heart. Because of the increased amount of blood in the arteries and the increased resistance to flow, there will be an increase in arterial blood pressure. By the same reasoning, when the arterioles dilate and resistance falls, blood leaves the arteries and enters the capillaries more rapidly. Because of the reduced volume in the arteries, and the reduced resistance to flow from the arteries to the capillaries, arterial blood pressure will fall. Thus arterial blood pressure varies directly, as does the resistance.

(3) *Elasticity.* The elasticity of the arteries will also have an effect on the resistance. If the arteries can stretch with each input of blood, there will be less resistance than if the arteries are stiff and rigid. In arteriosclerosis (hardening of the arteries), there will be an increase in resistance and blood pressure.

This point deserves some emphasis because arteriosclerosis is a common disease of the elderly. With age, the arteries lose some of their elasticity, become thickened and hard. Calcium accumulates in these arteries and they become almost like egg-shells. They will not be able to expand or stretch with each new input of blood. Since volume does not significantly change, this means that the same volume of blood is going into an arterial system which has become more rigid and less able to expand. This loss of elasticity leads to an increased resistance and increases the work the heart must do in pumping an adequate supply of blood to the tissues.

(4) *Viscosity.* The viscosity of the blood will also have a small effect on the resistance. If there is a high haematocrit, resistance will also be increased.

Perhaps at this point resistance can be defined again, though in a different way. First, you should recall the formula for average (mean) arterial blood pressure:

Average (mean) arterial blood pressure = Cardiac output × Resistance.

Simply by re-arranging the formula we can come to a definition of resistance:

Resistance = Average (mean) arterial blood pressure/Cardiac output.

This will make more sense to you by the end of the Chapter.

WHAT CONTROLS RESISTANCE IN THE CARDIOVASCULAR SYSTEM AND HOW DOES RESISTANCE CHANGE?

Changes in resistance are brought about by changes in the arterioles which can constrict or dilate, increase or decrease resistance, and increase or decrease the flow of blood to the tissues they serve. The ability to change the volume of blood flowing to a particular tissue is extremely important. During exercise, skeletal muscle needs greater blood flow and the internal organs can use less. When the weather is cold, your body conserves heat by shifting blood from the skin to the internal organs. When you have been lying down and suddenly stand up, there has to be generalized increase in resistance to ensure sufficient pressure to perfuse the brain. All these changes are effected through changes in the arteriolar resistance. Again, resistance is of importance because of its relationship to arterial blood pressure. Should cardiac output remain constant, arterial blood pressure will increase with an increase in resistance and fall with a decrease in resistance.

There are six sets of factors which control resistance.

a. Sympathetic vasoconstrictor tone. The arterioles of all skeletal muscles and organs, with the exception of the brain and heart, have a rich supply of nerve fibres from the sympathetic nervous system. The endings of these fibres release a chemical called noradrenaline, which causes the smooth muscle in the arterioles to contract. The greater the number of sympathetic impulses, the greater the amount of noradrenaline that will be released, causing more constriction of the arterioles. If there is little sympathetic stimulation, there will be little noradrenaline released and the arterioles will dilate, permitting increased blood flow. The number of sympathetic impulses (the sympathetic tone) thus sets the resistance. Some sympathetic fibres also travel to the veins. When they are stimulated, the veins constrict and force more blood into the arterial side of the system.

But where do these sympathetic impulses come from? In the lower part of the brain known as the medulla, there is a group of neurones which make up the vasomotor centre. These neurones send their axons varying distances down the spinal cord. The axons descend and synapse with neurones at different levels of the spinal cord. These second-order neurones send their axons outside the spinal cord and travel a short distance from the spinal cord, where they synapse with neurones in the sympathetic chain ganglia. Neurones in the ganglia send their axons to the smooth muscle of the arterioles or venules. (Sympathetic fibres also go to other structures including the heart.)

The vasomotor centre is always active, but its activity can increase or decrease. Should the vasomotor centre become very active, there will be an increase in arteriolar resistance and an increase in arterial blood pressure (see Figure 8.25). Should the vasomotor centre be injured or the spinal cord severed, there will be a drastic drop in arteriolar resistance and the arterial blood pressure because the sympathetic pathway has been interrupted. The vasomotor centre can be stimulated by low levels of O_2, high levels of CO_2 or strong emotions.

The vasomotor centre receives information from many parts of the brain and other parts of the nervous system. The hypothalamus (a structure in the diencephalon of the brain which sends many fibres to the vasomotor centre) is an important regulating centre for temperature regulation, and also for thirst, hunger and emotional expression among other functions. The vasomotor centre can also respond to chemical changes in the blood which perfuses it. Because of the sensitivity of the vasomotor centre and the great amount of information it receives from different sources, it can respond appropriately and set the vasoconstrictor tone in different parts of the body to meet the needs of the entire body. The importance of the vasomotor centre and the vasoconstrictor tone cannot be overemphasized. The vasomotor tone sets and adjusts the resistance of the cardiovascular system and is therefore of prime importance in the normal maintenance of arterial pressure and its reflex regulation.

b. Sympathetic vasodilator fibres. These fibres are much fewer in number than the vasoconstrictor fibres and only go to the arterioles of skeletal muscle. These fibres do not have their origin in the vasomotor centre and do not release

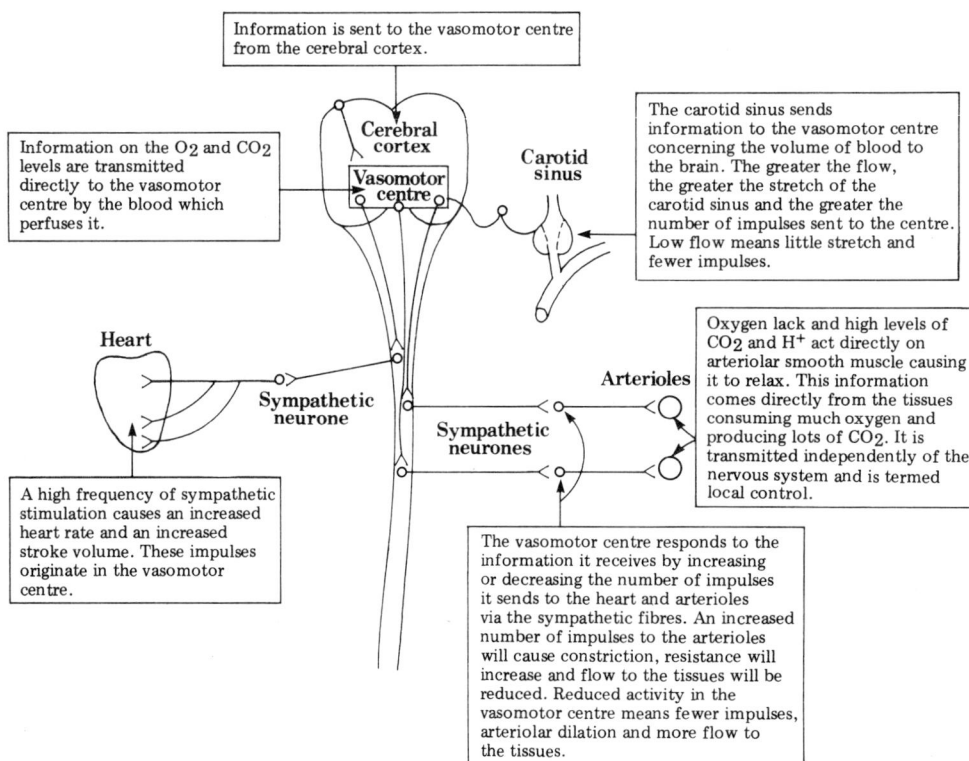

Figure 8.25 The vasomotor centre and its role in blood pressure regulation.

noradrenaline; they do, however, release acetylcholine, which acts on the smooth muscle causing it to relax and the arteriole to dilate. Thus, when the sympathetic vasodilator fibres are stimulated, the skeletal muscle receives an increased blood flow.

c. Local controlling factors. Arterioles have controls that are independent of the nervous system. When an organ or skeletal muscle increases its activity, there is an increase in its metabolic rate and an increased O_2 consumption and CO_2 production. Reduced amounts of O_2 and increased amounts of CO_2 have a direct action on the arterioles, causing them to dilate. This is important because it provides a way in which O_2 and nutrients can be delivered to those tissues which have the greatest need for them. It is a regulatory mechanism that can act independently of the nervous system. A simple experiment can demonstrate this.

If you were to reduce the flow of arterial blood to the hand by placing a tight cuff around the arm for a few minutes and then quickly releasing the cuff, your hand would become warmer and slightly redder indicating an increased blood flow. O_2 lack and CO_2 build-up caused by closure of the brachial artery make the arterioles dilate. When the tourniquet is released, increased amounts of blood flow through the tissues. This phenomenon is known as reactive hyperaemia.

Hydrogen ions and other metabolic products also stimulate the arterioles to relax. Histamine, a compound released when tissues are injured or irritated, is a very powerful vasodilator.

d. Hormones. Adrenaline from the adrenal glands causes constriction of many of the arterioles which lead to the skin and internal viscera, and at the same time causes the arterioles going to skeletal muscle to dilate. This hormone is released in times of fear or stress. It works with the sympathetic vasoconstrictor and vasodilator fibres to bring about a shifting of blood from the skin and viscera to the skeletal muscle. Blood will always take the path of least resistance. If the arterioles of the viscera are constricted while those of the skeletal muscle are dilated, blood will take the low resistance pathway and travel through the wide-open skeletal muscle arterioles. This redistribution of blood is part of the "flight-or-fight" response in which the body prepares itself to respond to emergency situations at the expense of continuing processes like digestion and urine formation. If you are taking flight or are standing your ground and fighting, your skeletal muscles are very active and need much greater amounts of oxygen, the circulatory system will respond accordingly.

The mechanism by which adrenaline and noradrenaline have their diverse effects is discussed several times in this text. More discussion of adrenaline, noradrenaline, α and β receptors is presented in this Chapter in the Section on drugs (*Section f*), and again in the Chapter on the nervous system in the Section dealing with drugs and the autonomic nervous system.

Other hormones are also involved. Adrenal steroids from the adrenal gland are necessary for the normal functioning of arteriolar smooth muscle, and excessive thyroid hormone can increase the effect of noradrenaline and cause vasoconstriction. The most powerful vasoconstrictor is a hormone called angiotensin. Its role in normal arteriolar function is not yet known but it may be important in some endocrine disturbances causing high blood pressure. More will be said about these and other hormones in the Chapter on the endocrine system.

e. Reflex control of resistance. The cardiovascular system will have to make adjustments that are independent of metabolic changes. Perhaps the best indication of this would be the changes that take place when you have been lying down and then suddenly stand up; gravity causes blood to "pool" in the lower limbs. Cardiac output will be reduced, the volume of blood travelling to the brain is decreased and the carotid sinus gets smaller. The vasomotor centre is informed of this change in brain blood supply; this information comes in the form of fewer impulses from the carotid sinus whose walls are stretched to a lesser extent. The number of impulses from the carotid sinus is roughly proportional to the volume of blood in the sinus and the stretch of its walls. When the volume of blood in the sinus is reduced, the stretch in its walls and the receptors they contain are also reduced. Fewer impulses are sent from the receptors in the carotid sinus to the vasomotor centre. The centre reacts to this information by increasing its activity and sending more impulses through the sympathetic fibres to the arterioles of blood vessels going to skeletal muscle and viscera. Constriction of these arterioles brings about an increase in resistance.

Some impulses will also travel to the veins, stimulating them to constrict a little and force more blood into the arterial side of the system. There will be fewer impulses sent down the vagal nerves, more impulses sent down the sympathetic fibres to the heart; heart rate will increase. The net effect of this increased cardiac output and resistance in the vessels of the skeletal muscles and viscera is a rise in blood pressure and an increased flow of blood to the brain. Conversely, increased stretch of the carotid sinus wall will increase the number of impulses generated by the receptor. The vasomotor centre receives this information and responds to it. The sympathetic vasoconstrictor tone to the arterioles is reduced and the arterioles dilate. The heart rate is slowed and the blood pressure drops.

There are also baroreceptors located within the arch of the aorta. Much less is known about their function, though they are thought to function in a manner similar to that of the receptors in the carotid sinus.

This should emphasize again the importance of the vasomotor centre, for it is continuously active, sending impulses to the arterioles and adjusting the resistance of the system. It functions in reflex regulations receiving information from the carotid sinus and other receptors in the arterial system and heart. The centre processes the information and responds to it by either increasing or decreasing the number of impulses to the arterioles, causing either constriction or vasodilation. The centre also influences the heart and its rate through the sympathetic nerves and the vagus nerves. It is sometimes possible to slow the heart rate by gently massaging the carotid sinus; this mimics the effects of stretching the walls of the carotid sinus.

A problem. A distinguished physician and physiologist tells the following story. Once there was a banker who wore very tight and stiffly starched collars. He was in good health and felt fine except for a brief period in the morning and evening when he drove to, and returned from, work. He would come to a busy road junction, stop his car and turn his head to the right and then to the left to make sure no traffic was approaching. At this point he would feel dizzy, light-headed and would nearly faint. After a minute or two he would feel fine and be able to drive on. Why did the doctor prescribe open-collar shirts for his patient?

f. Drugs. Because of the importance of keeping blood pressure within normal limits, there has been an intensive search for drugs that will either raise or lower arterial blood pressure. Inasmuch as the average arterial blood pressure is the product of cardiac output and resistance, drugs can influence blood pressure either by influencing cardiac output or by affecting the resistance. Since resistance is centred in the arterioles, arterial blood pressure can be raised by constricting the arterioles and reduced by lowering the resistance and dilating the arterioles.

To understand how some drugs affect the arterioles and cause them either to constrict or to dilate, it is necessary to know something about α (alpha) and β (beta) receptors. α and β receptors are found on the smooth muscle of the arterioles. The distribution of α and β receptors is variable. The arterioles supplying some organs may have both α and β receptors or a predominance of one type of receptor or the other.

For a molecule to stimulate either an α or a β receptor it must first fit into the receptor to interact with it. This is similar to the relationship a hormone must have with its receptor if it is to have an effect. When a molecule stimulates an α receptor, the smooth muscle contracts and the arteriole narrows. The opposite action occurs when a β receptor of an arteriole is stimulated, for β-receptor stimulation causes the smooth muscle to relax and the arteriole to dilate.

Molecules that stimulate α receptors are referred to as α agonists; molecules that stimulate β receptors are β agonists. Noradrenaline is an α agonist and therefore causes vasoconstriction. In fact, much of the sympathetic vasoconstrictor tone in the arterioles is due to stimulation of the α receptors by noradrenaline from the sympathetic nerve endings. Phenylephrine is a drug that acts as an α agonist. Another drug, isoprenaline (isoproterenol), is a β agonist and can increase blood flow to structures having β receptors. Noradrenaline usually has only a slight effect on β receptors.

Adrenaline is the chief hormone manufactured in the medulla of the adrenal gland. The molecular structure of adrenaline is similar to noradrenaline but not identical. This molecular difference has significant consequences. Adrenaline is able to stimulate α and β receptors and is thus both an α and β agonist. Adrenaline can thus cause both vasoconstriction and vasodilation (see Table below).

The effect of adrenaline on an organ's blood flow will depend on the number and the kind of receptors present in the organ's arterioles. The arterioles of the skin, intestines and kidneys are richly supplied with α receptors, whereas skeletal muscle has a preponderance of β receptors. This means that adrenaline can reduce flow through the skin, intestines and kidneys by acting as in α antogonists and increase flow through skeletal muscle by acting as a β agonist.

Some molecules can bind to α or β receptors and prevent their agonists from stimulating them. In a sense they are analogous to a key that fits into a lock but is not the proper key and therefore can't turn the lock. As long as the wrong key is in the lock, the correct key can't enter the lock and therefore can't turn the lock. Drugs that prevent α or β agonists from stimulating α or β receptors are called blockers (antagonists). Phenoxybenzamine is an α blocker and can prevent noradrenaline from stimulating the α receptors. Isoprenaline and adrenaline cannot stimulate the β receptors in the presence of propranolol, which is a β blocker.

Noradrenaline, adrenaline, and α and β receptors all amplify the ability of the sympathetic nervous system to distribute selectively blood flow to the different tissues. α and β agonists and antagonists are powerful pharmacological tools for raising or lowering blood pressure and for maintaining or redistributing the flow of blood.

Arterioles are not the exclusive site for receptors. The heart contains β receptors and will respond to β agonists with an increased rate and more forceful contraction. β blockers will slow the heart rate and reduce the force of contraction.

In addition to α and β receptors, there appear to be receptors for a chemical called dopamine. Less is known about dopamine and its receptors than other receptors, but we know that dopamine can constrict or dilate certain arterioles; the effect appears to depend on the concentration of dopamine.

At times, it might seem that receptors, their agonists and antagonists are all insignificant. This is not really true. Manipulation of receptors by drugs or hormones has made possible the treatment of hypertension, and often permits life to be sustained in circulatory shock when there is inadequate tissue perfusion.

ARTERIAL BLOOD PRESSURE: HOW IS IT TAKEN AND WHAT DOES IT MEAN?

Arterial blood pressure is an indication of the state of the heart and of the flow going to the tissues. A normal arterial blood pressure suggests, but does not prove, that there is a sufficient volume of blood being pumped by the heart to perfuse adequately all the tissues. From your study of the previous Sections you should have a good idea of the factors which can influence blood pressure. If there is inadequate blood volume and/or blood pressure to perfuse the tissues, the tissues may die or become damaged by hypoxia. Abnormally increased blood pressure (hypertension) has many important consequences and is discussed at the end of this Section.

Receptor	Physiological agonist	Effect	Pharmacological agonist	Pharmacological antagonist
α	noradrenaline adrenaline	constriction constriction	phenylephrine	phenoxybenzamine
β	adrenaline	dilation	isoprenaline	propranolol

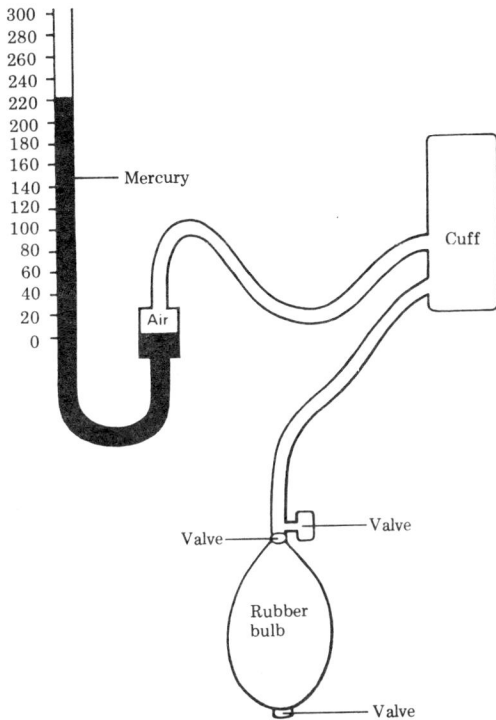

Figure 8.26 The sphygmomanometer.

For the sake of convenience, blood pressure is measured indirectly in the brachial artery with a sphygmomanometer, though it is possible to use other methods and different arteries. The sphygmomanometer consists of an inflatable rubber cuff with a tube which goes from the cuff to a column of mercury (see Figure 8.26). Pressure in the cuff is registered by the height of a column of mercury; the greater the pressure the higher the mercury.

The cuff, positioned above the elbow, is inflated to such a pressure that the brachial artery is completely closed and no blood can flow through it. A stethoscope is placed at the bend of the elbow over the brachial artery. No sound can be heard, for no blood is flowing through the artery. The air in the cuff is allowed to escape slowly, reducing the pressure in the cuff. When the pressure in the brachial artery is just slightly greater than that in the cuff, a jet of blood will spurt through the small opening in the vessel with every beat of the heart, making a sharp tapping sound which can be heard with the stethoscope. At this instant, the level of the mercury is read, and this is called the *systolic* blood pressure; it represents the highest pressure in the artery.

As more air escapes, the cuff pressure falls, blood flow through the artery increases and the sound changes. But if the cuff pressure is at any one time slightly above the lowest pressure in the artery, the vessel will close and the sounds will be distinctly separated. As the cuff pressure falls still more and flow in the artery becomes continuous between heart beats, the sounds will run together and become muffled. The mercury level is read at this instant, and this is called *diastolic* pressure; it represents the lowest pressure in the artery.

With further reductions in cuff pressure, flow becomes smooth and non-turbulent, so no sounds will be heard.

Some precautions should be taken when taking blood pressure:

(1) The cuff should always be at the level of the heart so the effects of gravity are ruled out. If the measurement is made with the cuff at a level above the heart, the true pressure will be greater than recorded. If the cuff is at a level below the heart, the true pressure will be less than the measured pressure.

(2) The width of the cuff is important. It should be wide for people with obese arms, and narrow for children and people with small arms, otherwise the brachial artery will not be compressed.

(3) The subject should be relaxed; fear, stress and pain will cause elevated readings.

(4) Remember it is far better to be unable to get a measurement than to report a false or inaccurate one. At times it may be quite difficult to hear the sounds. If you cannot get a reading after two or three attempts ask someone else to try.

(5) When you take the patient's blood pressure for the first time, it is not a bad idea to take the pressure in both right and left arms. You usually assume that it is the same in both arms, but occasionally you may be surprised, for there are individuals with significant differences.

(6) When you inflate the cuff, you should inflate it to a pressure a little greater than that necessary to cause the artery to be completely closed during systole. You can reliably estimate this pressure by palpating the radial pulse in the arm in which the pressure is being measured. When you inflate the cuff to a pressure that keeps the brachial artery closed during systole, the pulse in the radial artery will disappear. Let the air out of the cuff slowly. The pulse in the radial artery will reappear when the pressure in the cuff is slightly less than the systolic pressure.

Normal blood pressure is often said to be 120 mmHg/80 mmHg. It is, of course, more complicated than that. Blood pressure tends to increase with age and men have higher blood pressures than women. Some average values taken from 250 000 healthy individuals are recorded below:

Age	Systolic	Diastolic	Pulse pressure
Newborn	80	46	34
10 years	103	70	33
20 years	120	80	40
40 years	126	84	42
60 years	135	89	46

Pulse pressure represents the difference between systolic and diastolic pressure. There is an increase in pulse pressure with either an increase in stroke volume or a reduction in the distensibility of the arteries. Setting limits on abnormal pressure is difficult. As a general rule, for a young adult a systolic pressure greater than 145 or a diastolic pressure greater than 90 is considered excessive and indicates *hyper*tension. A systolic blood pressure below 105 indicates *hypo*tension.

Hypotension is a relatively rare disease, while hypertension is a common disease, too common. Most hypertension is called "essential hypertension"; the cause of essential hypertension is not known. It is, however, known that hypertension is an expression of arteriolar disease. The arterioles are excessively constricted and diastolic blood pressure is elevated. What causes this constriction is not known. Excessive sympathetic stimulation, hormones especially angiotensin, altered kidney function, unknown factors or some combinations of this list have been suggested as causes. Hypertension is a serious disease and if it is not treated it can shorten the life span.

People with hypertension have an increased incidence of strokes (cerebral infarcts). Kidney disease is more common in hypertensive patients; this is thought to be caused by the reduced blood flow through the constricted renal arterioles. Heart failure is also more common in patients with hypertension, as the heart has to do more work to pump blood into a system with higher resistance.

Hypertension is often a "silent disease" during its early stages. This means that many people who have hypertension do not know they have it. Often these people are young, appear healthy and say they "feel fine". You usually cannot tell when your blood pressure is elevated and are not conscious of the damage it is doing. This is one reason why the taking of blood pressure is very important. The time to treat hypertension is generally as soon as it is diagnosed, and the first step in diagnosing hypertension is measuring blood pressure. Again, untreated hypertension can lead to serious disability and may shorten a patient's life.

At this point it might be good to revise and take a look at the problems dealing with blood pressure and its regulation.

You will recall the following relationship:

Average (mean) arterial blood pressure = Cardiac output × Resistance.

It might be useful to keep that relationship in mind while studying the following examples:

(1) Haemorrhage means loss of blood. If a person cuts an artery or a large vein and suddenly loses a lot of blood, there will be an immediate fall in both systolic and diastolic pressure and also in cardiac output. This occurs simply because there is less blood in the system and therefore less blood to pump.

The fall in cardiac output results in a reduced flow of blood through the carotid sinus. This change is recognized by the carotid sinus and fewer impulses are sent to the vasomotor centre. The centre responds to this information and increases sympathetic stimulation to the heart and sympathetic vasoconstrictor tone to many of the arterioles. Blood flow through the kidneys, spleen and skin is significantly reduced. Sympathetic stimulation to the heart increases both the heart rate and stroke volume. The latter effect is accomplished by shifting to a different, higher Starling curve — contractility is increased. There is also some constriction of the veins, so some blood is shifted from the venous to the arterial circulation.

A patient who has suffered a haemorrhage is lying flat in bed. His heart rate is 85 beats/min, and blood pressure is 115/85. The patient is helped to his feet so he can stand up; he complains of feeling dizzy and light-headed. While he is standing his heart rate increases to 110 beats/min and his blood pressure becomes 100/90. The patient is helped back into bed and after several minutes the heart rate is back to 85

beats/min, the blood pressure is 115/85 and the patient reports he no longer feels dizzy.

When the patient first stands up, there is a pooling of blood in the lower extremities and a fall in cardiac output that is detected by the carotid sinus. The carotid sinus through its reflex connection informs the vasomotor centre, which causes increases in vasoconstriction, heart rate and stroke output. In the case of this person who has haemorrhaged, these compensatory chages are not adequate to make up for both loss of blood by haemorrhage and the pooling of blood in the veins. Consequently, when he stands up he becomes hypotensive and feels dizzy because of the diminished flow to the brain.

In addition to the acute changes which take place after haemorrhage, there are other metabolic and endocrine changes which eventually lead to increased red cell and plasma protein production, and ultimately a return to normal blood volume and composition. Some haemorrhages, however, are so severe that the body cannot compensate for them.

(2) A patient makes his first visit to the hospital and becomes very frightened by the atmosphere that to him is strange. His vasomotor centre becomes much more active and there is a greatly increased sympathetic discharge. The adrenal medulla releases adrenaline. The arterioles of the skin and viscera are narrowed, so resistance is increased. (There will be some dilation of the arterioles in skeletal muscle and blood flow into muscle will be increased.) The stroke volume and heart rate will both increase, putting more blood into the arterial system. Since the heart is putting increased volumes of blood into the arteries and there is less time between beats for this blood to enter the capillaries, there will be an increase in both systolic and diastolic pressure. The increase in diastolic pressure will probably be greater than the systolic increase, so pulse pressure may be reduced.

(3) An aged patient is suffering from arteriosclerosis. His arteries have become hard and pipe-like and have thus lost their elasticity. Although his cardiac output is normal, his arteries have lost much of their ability to expand and receive the stroke output. The sudden injection of blood into the rigid arteries causes a rapidly rising and very high systolic pressure and an increase in pulse pressure. Because of the increased resistance of the arteries, the amount of work the heart must perform to maintain adequate perfusion is also greatly increased. This intensifies the stress placed upon the heart.

(4) Two students are learning to take blood pressure. They are both in their late 20's and have no physical complaints or known diseases. One student's blood pressure is found to be 142/98. Similar readings are obtained several different times. The student then has a complete history, physical examination and appropriate laboratory examinations. A diagnosis of essential hypertension is made. The student is given a diuretic and his blood pressure goes to 120/80 and stays at that level as long as he takes the diuretic every day.

Diuretics work at the kidneys and increase urine output. This increased amount of urine is initially put out at the expense of the plasma volume. The reduction in plasma volume leads to a reduction in stroke output and consequently to a lowering of blood pressure. Some of the diuretics used in hypertension are also thought to have an action on the arterioles as well as on the kidneys.

Drugs other than diuretics are used in the treatment of hypertension. The choice of the drug depends on the seriousness of the hypertension and other medical conditions. Some drugs interfere with the synthesis of noradrenaline from the sympathetic nerve endings, while other drugs are α blockers and cause vasodilation by antagonizing the action of noradrenaline on the α receptors. Some drugs act directly on the arterioles and cause them to dilate. Other drugs appear to work in the brain and seem to depress the activity of the vasomotor centre. Some of the newer drugs block the β receptors of the heart. This lowers pressure by slowing the heart rate and reducing the stroke volume by making the heart work on a lower, less efficient Starling curve.

In addition to drugs, the reduction of dietary intake of salt may be useful if not absolutely necessary in treating hypertension.

WHAT IS THE PULSE?

With every beat of the heart, about 70 ml of blood are pushed into the aorta. The sudden input causes the aorta to stretch to make room for the additional blood. The wave of expansion (the pulse wave) begins at the aorta and travels to all the other arteries far faster than the blood within the vessels.

The pulse is commonly taken by placing the three middle fingers over the radial artery. Many examiners simultaneously palpate the pulse in both arms to see if there is any difference between the pulse in the right and left arms. In another technique the patient's arm is slightly flexed. The brachial artery is palpated with the thumb of one hand, the radial artery with the middle fingers of the other hand.

The pulse indicates the rate of the heart beat. By taking the pulse, you can also determine the rhythm of the heart beat — whether it is regular (1..2..3..4..5..) or irregular (1 2 .... 3 4 .... 5). The quality is also important. If the heart is beating forcefully, the pulse will be strong. A weak heart beat produces only a small pulse wave which is difficult to detect. "Average" pulse rates are:

Newborn	130–150 beats/min
Child	80–90 beats/min
Adult	60–80 beats/min

Since the pulse indicates the heart rate, those factors which influence the heart rate will influence the pulse. If there is an increased sympathetic discharge or a decreased vagal discharge, both heart rate and pulse will be similarly increased.

Many cardiologists feel that the quality of the pulse is best appreciated by palpating the carotid arteries. Three fingers are used and the artery is gently palpated medial to the sternocleidomastoid muscle, just below the angle of the jaw. One artery is palpated at a time. The pulse may also be palpated in the posterior tibial and dorsalis pedis arteries of the foot.

Along with palpation of the arteries, listening to them can be done. Normally, flow through arteries is silent when ausculated with a stethoscope. If the arteries are partially obstructed, flow through the artery will be turbulent and a murmur or "bruit" will be heard over the artery.

WHAT ARE THE CAPILLARIES AND HOW DO THEY WORK?

Capillaries have their entrance at angles to the arterioles. Their entrance is guarded by short out-croppings of smooth muscle from the arterioles, which can contract or relax, and thus open or close the capillaries depending on the needs of the tissues they serve. Many capillaries are normally closed, particularly in resting skeletal muscle and, as a result, only about 5% of the blood is in the capillaries at any one time.

A capillary is really a tube made of simple endothelial cells and is only one cell thick (see Figures 8.12 and 8.27). The cells adhere to one another by means of intercellular cement which seems to have pores (holes) in it.

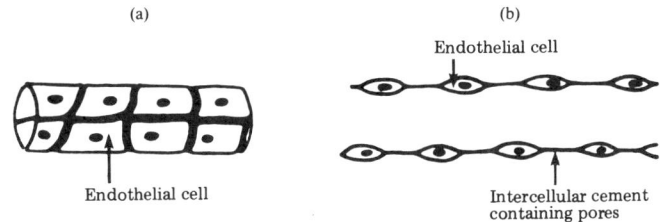

Figure 8.27 The capillaries. (a) The capillary wall. (b) Longitudinal section.

Water, oxygen and carbon dioxide can readily diffuse through the cells because of their great solubility. Most other substances have to travel through the intercellular pores. Glucose, fatty acids, amino acids and other nutrients will be swept along with the fluid that leaves the capillary, passes through the pores and enters the intercellular (interstitial) fluid. The concentration of many of these substances will be greater in the intercellular fluid than in the cell so they can diffuse into the cell. End products of cell metabolism will have different gradients and will travel from cell to intercellular fluid to blood. To explain this process better it is necessary to discuss the forces acting in the capillary.

The pressure within the capillary at the end closest to the arterioles is about 30–35 mmHg; the pressure at the end closest to the vein is about 15–10 mmHg. (Sometimes these pressures are called hydrostatic pressures.) The pressure falls from the arteriolar end of the capillary to the venous end because of the great frictional resistance that the blood encounters as it travels through the narrow capillary. Throughout the capillaries there are pores between the endothelial cells. At the arteriolar end of the capillary a filtrate will be formed and will enter the intercellular fluid. Nutrients, ions and small molecules will be carried in the plasma as it flows through the pores into the intercellular fluid. Cells, large proteins and other molecules that are too big to pass through the pores will stay within the capillaries.

If plasma is filtered at the capillary and leaves the circulation for the intercellular fluid, what will prevent all the plasma from being filtered and leaving the circulatory system? Since the blood or hydrostatic pressure at both ends of the capillary is greater than zero, it will act in the direction of forcing fluid out of the capillary.

What prevents all the fluid from leaving and forces its return to the capillary? The answer is osmotic pressure. At the capillary, we have the three necessary ingredients for an osmotic system:

(1) A semi-permeable membrane: the capillary wall itself.

(2) Free-moving molecules: water ions and other molecules which can cross the membrane.

(3) Osmotically active molecules: the large plasma proteins which cannot cross the capillary wall.

Since the large plasma proteins are within the capillary and cannot enter the intercellular fluid, they will act to draw fluid into the capillary. Measurements of the pressure exerted by the plasma proteins shows it to be approximately 25 mmHg.

Let us analyze what happens at the arteriolar and venous ends (see Figure 8.28). At the arteriolar end, the outward capillary pressure will be about 35 mmHg, while the inward osmotic pressure will be 25 mmHg. The net force (35 mmHg

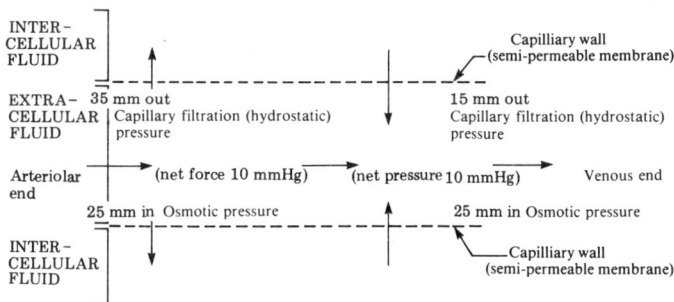

Figure 8.28 Movement of fluid out of and into the capillary.

out − 25 mmHg in = 10 mmHg out) will be directed outward and will be equal to 10 mmHg. Since the net force is outward, toward the intercellular fluid, a filtrate will be formed. The capillary pressure will fall because of the friction, coming close to 15 mmHg at its end, before the venule begins. The osmotic pressure remains unchanged and will be equal to 25 mmHg in, while the capillary pressure will be 15 mmHg out; the net pressure (25 mmHg in − 15 mmHg out = 10 mmHg in) will be 10 mmHg, and is directed from the intercellular fluid into the capillary. So the filtrate will be reabsorbed and fluid will move into the capillary. You can see that there is a balance of forces acting at the capillary (filtration pressure v. osmotic pressure) which forces fluid out at one end and draws it back at the other. If this balance is disturbed, there can be an excess of either filtration or reabsorption. Let us look at some examples and see what happens when this balance is upset.

(1) In certain liver diseases, or as a result of inadequate levels of protein in the diet, the ability of the liver to synthesize plasma proteins, particularly albumin, is reduced. In some renal diseases protein may be lost in the urine. There will be fewer plasma proteins in the blood and thus the osmotic pressure of the blood will be reduced. Reduction of osmotic pressure will lessen the force which causes reabsorption, and cause the tissues to swell. The swelling caused by an accumulation of fluid in the tissue space is called oedema.

(2) When there has been a great haemorrhage, arterial blood pressure falls and the arterioles constrict causing the filtration pressure at the capillary to be reduced. Since the loss of blood will not affect the protein concentration, the balance of forces will be shifted in favour of reabsorption and

intercellular fluid will move into the circulation increasing blood volume.

(3) When capillaries are injured or lose their integrity, they can no longer act as a semi-permeable membrane. Many of the large proteins can cross the capillary and the reabsorption is reduced resulting in oedema. The capillaries can be injured as a result of burns, bacterial toxins, histamine or dietary deficiency, particularly vitamin C.

(4) Should there be an increase in venous pressure, it will be reflected back to the venous end of the capillary. This will result in an effective filtration pressure at both ends of the capillary, and fluid will leave the circulation. People who must stand all day often have oedematous ankles as a result of the increased venous pressure in their legs.

If the right ventricle of the heart cannot pump blood into the lungs, blood will accumulate in the veins, venous pressure will increase and there will be an increase in filtration pressure at the venous end of the capillary as fluid leaves the circulation and accumulates within the cells and in the intercellular fluid. This fluid accumulation can be so great that a pitting oedema results. If the examiner sticks his or her thumb into the skin of a patient, against a bony surface such as the subcutaneous aspect of the tibia, fibula or sacrum, then removes the thumb, an impression of the thumb (a pit) will remain. It is estimated that more than 4 litres of fluid must enter the tissues before a pitting oedema occurs.

Many students have a tendency to confuse an increase in *arterial* blood pressure, with an increase in pressure at the capillary. If an arteriole constricts there will be an increase in resistance and an increase in arterial blood pressure, but the blood which travels through the constricted arteriole will encounter more frictional resistance and lose pressure energy so that the filtration pressure in the capillary will be reduced. (Because of the reduction in radius of the arteriole, the volume of blood flowing through the capillary will also be decreased.) When the arteriole dilates there is less friction and loss of energy, so pressure within the capillary increases. Furthermore, it appears that the smooth muscle of some arterioles has an intrinsic mechanism by which it contracts if high blood pressure stretches and increases the tension within it; the arterial muscle relaxes if arterial pressure falls. This intrinsic regulation is not clearly understood yet but appears to work in some circumstances to maintain a constant flow within the capillary.

It is important to note that the arterial and capillary filtration pressures in the pulmonary circulation are much less than in the systemic circulation. This is chiefly because the thinner right ventricle generates much less pressure than the thicker left ventricle. The plasma osmotic pressure is, of course, the same in both the pulmonary and systemic circulations, for there is no change in the concentration of the plasma proteins.

There is some controversy as to the actual measurement of forces in and around the pulmonary capillaries. There are forces favouring filtration and forces favouring reabsorption.

If much more fluid is filtered than can be reabsorbed, pulmonary oedema will result. Fluid leaves the pulmonary capillaries and enters the alveoli. This is extremely serious, as the fluid in the alveoli severely hinders the diffusion of oxygen from the alveoli into the blood. In effect, the individual may "drown" in his or her own fluid. This may happen if the left ventricle cannot be pumped adequately. Blood will back up into the lungs and the increased blood volume causes an increase in the pulmonary capillary pressure. (Circulation in the lungs is discussed again in the Chapter on the respiratory system.)

As an introduction to the next section you might recall the tender sad love story of the two red blood cells who met in a capillary, but loved in vein.

WHAT ARE THE VEINS AND HOW DO THEY FUNCTION?

The veins are the last segment in the return journey to the heart. Like the arteries, the veins consist of an inner endothelial tissue, elastic tissue, smooth muscle and fibrous covering. They are larger than the arteries but are considerably thinner and contain valves. Because they are bigger than the arteries they contain more blood than the arteries; about two-thirds of the total blood volume is in the veins at any one time.

The venous valves are made of endothelial and connective tissue, are found in the limbs, and function to prevent the backflow of blood. When the skeletal muscles which surround the veins contract, the valves are forced open and blood goes through (see Figure 8.29). As the muscles relax and the valves close, blood is prevented from going

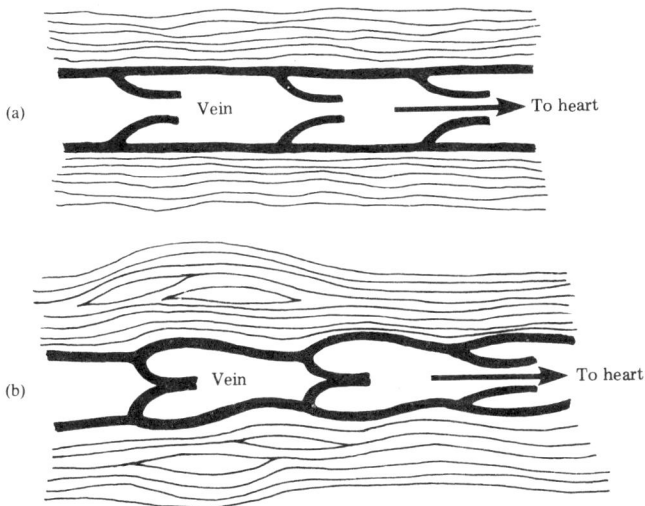

Figure 8.29 Skeletal muscle action on venous valves in the control of blood flow to the heart. (a) Muscle relaxes. (b) Muscle contracts.

backwards. If the valves are injured or degenerate, blood can flow backwards and venous return is hindered. This condition is known as varicose veins. Varicose veins are usually found in the lower limbs, where the veins become full and very prominent.

The veins, like arterioles, are equipped with a sympathetic nerve supply which can constrict the veins. This decrease in size does not affect the resistance as much as it reduces the volume of blood stored in the veins. When there is sympathetic stimulation to the veins, they constrict, forcing blood into the arterial side of the circulation; this often happens after haemorrhage. Pressure in the veins is lower

than in the capillaries and is thus the lowest of all parts of the system. The valves thus assist in the return of blood and help overcome the force of gravity.

Should the skeletal muscle be paralyzed or were the individual to remain completely still, blood would pool in the veins, venous return to the heart would be greatly reduced and the individual would faint. This often happens to soldiers forced to stand still at full attention for a long time. By fainting and lying flat the person is reducing the influence of gravity on blood flow and making it easier for blood to return to the heart and be pumped to the brain. To help understand the force of gravity, simply recall how much easier it is to push a car a given distance than it is to lift that car over the same distance.

There are, however, times when gravity can have practical and therapeutic uses. Suppose, for instance, an individual has gone into pulmonary oedema because of left ventricular failure. The ventricle is at a disadvantage and is working on the descending part of the Starling curve because of the excessive volume of blood in the ventricle. Because the left ventricle cannot pump adequately, the blood "backs up" into the left atrium and lungs. This leads to oedema in the lungs due to increased pulmonary capillary and venous pressure. This problem of pulmonary oedema differs from that of a person who has fainted because of inadequate return of venous blood to the heart. In this case, the individual is in pulmonary oedema because there is more blood in the left ventricle than the left ventricle can pump out. Fluid is entering the alveoli of the lungs because of the increased volume of blood in the left ventricle and the lungs. The return of venous blood to the heart exceeds the capability of the left ventricle to pump the blood into the arterial system. To help reduce the return of venous blood to the heart, the head of the patient's bed is often elevated. This causes a pooling of some blood in the abdomen and extremities and reduces the return of venous blood to the over-loaded heart. Sometimes tourniquets are applied to the extremities. The force of the tourniquets is such that it constricts many of the veins but none of the arteries. Blood enters the extremities as before, but its venous return is slowed. This is useful in that since more blood is retained in the extremities, the volume of blood returned to the heart is decreased and excessive blood does not accumulate in the left ventricle and lungs.

There is a relationship between cardiac output and pressure in the veins. As cardiac output increases, pressure in the veins decreases; a decrease in cardiac output causes an increase in venous pressure. This relationship may become more apparent to you if you think of the heart as a pump, pumping blood from the veins into the arteries. If the ventricles are diseased or failing, less blood will be pumped into the arteries and more blood will accumulate in the veins. As the veins are larger and more distensible than the arteries, they are more able to accept this additional blood, and the pressure change in the veins will be relatively small. Although the change in venous pressure is small, the increased pressure can be transmitted back to the capillaries and lead to oedema. If only the left ventricle is failing, the oedema will first occur in the lungs, whereas if only the right ventricle is failing, the oedema will occur in the other tissues.

In most cases of heart disease or failure, both ventricles are affected. It should be noted that in heart failure several factors contribute to the formation of oedema. The reduction of blood flow through the kidneys and the associated endocrine changes lead to increased salt and water reabsorption by the kidneys. This increases the plasma volume and may make the oedema worse. This will be more clear to you after you have studied the Chapters on the endocrine and urinary systems.

In contrast to arterial pressure, venous pressure may be measured directly by inserting a hollow, saline-filled needle into an arm vein. The needle is connected to a tube which is connected to a saline-filled manometer. The pressure in the vein will be transmitted to the manometer and the height of the saline will represent the pressure in the vein. Saline is used instead of mercury because it is less dense than mercury and venous pressure is much less than arterial pressure. An "average" venous pressure in the antecubital vein of a supine subject may be about 9 cm of saline or 7 mmHg.

Often the pressure in the antecubital vein is not the best reflection of venous pressure throughout the body. To get a better indication of pressure, a small catheter is inserted into the vein and threaded through the veins to near the right atrium of the heart. The catheter is connected to tubing, which is in turn connected to the manometer. The pressure it records is called central venous pressure.

A simpler, indirect estimate of central venous pressure can be obtained by using the jugular veins as manometers and considering those veins to be tubes connected to the right atrium and containing blood rather than saline. The patient's head and shoulders are raised 45° and the jugular veins are examined for signs of venous distension. When the patient's head is elevated to 45° or more, any distension of the external jugular veins indicates an abnormal elevation of venous pressure. A rough estimate of the central venous pressure is made by measuring the vertical distance in centimetres from the sternal angle to the uppermost level of distension of the right external jugular vein. The sternal angle

is used as a reference point, as it is about 5 cm above the mid-point of the right atrium of the heart.

Before leaving the venous system, certain other terms should be mentioned. *Phlebitis* means inflammation of a vein. If a vein becomes inflamed, a thrombosis is likely to form without the vein. The word, *thrombophlebitis*, indicates thrombosis and inflammation of a vein.

Venous stasis refers to slow or negligible blood flow in the veins. This condition occurs in patients who are at complete bed rest. The lack of muscular activity, particularly in the legs of the patient who is resting in bed, gives rise to venous stasis. Venous stasis is likely to cause thrombophlebitis and is probably the major cause of the thrombophlebitis which develops after surgery or childbirth. Prevention of venous stasis is one reason why post-surgical patients are encouraged to walk or move their legs soon after surgery rather than remain almost motionless in bed. The muscular contraction squeezes the veins, reduces venous stasis and thus decreases the chances of thrombophlebitis developing.

The development of thrombophlebitis in one of the deep veins of an extremity can have serious consequences. Because of the interference with venous flow, oedema will develop and the extremity may become swollen and tender. Deep thrombophlebitis also gives rise to the possibility of a pulmonary embolus. Part of the thrombus comes adrift from the vein, embolizes, travels through the large veins, right atrium, right ventricle and gets stuck in one or more of the pulmonary arteries. The clot interferes with blood flow through the lung and this affects the exchange of O_2 and CO_2 in the lungs supplied by the obstructed pulmonary artery.

At this point, you can reflect on how much you have learned. Inflammation, blood clot formation and circulatory anatomy should be familiar to you now. Pulmonary embolism and its significance will mean more to you after you have studied the Chapter on the respiratory system.

9. The Lymphatic System and Lymph

INTRODUCTION

Lymph is a fluid, like blood, containing cells and protein. The lymphatic system is part of the immune system, as both the cells and the structure of the lymphatic system are important components of the structural, humoral and cellular defences of the body. The lymphatic system could also be considered as an adjunct to the circulatory system. Lymph is formed from fluid that has left the circulatory system at the capillaries. It is returned to the circulatory system via two vessels which drain into the venous system.

To start thinking about the lymphatic system you might think of the lymphatic system functioning as a one-way transport system. It returns the extracellular fluid, which has left the circulatory system at the capillaries, back to the circulatory system. The lymphatic system begins with the lymph capillaries located in the interstitial spaces between the capillaries and the cells.

The lymph capillaries unite to form larger vessels which unite again and again until there are only two large lymphatic vessels. Each vessel empties into the venous system at the junction of the jugular and subclavian veins, one on each side of the neck (see Figure 9.1). It is estimated that from 2 to 4 litres of lymph enter the venous system within 24 hours. Lymphatic capillaries are found throughout the body with the exception of the brain and possibly bone tissue. They are particularly abundant in the dermis of the skin and the mucous membrane of the digestive and respiratory systems. Lymph is similar to blood plasma except that it contains less protein than plasma and more lymphocytes and monocytes.

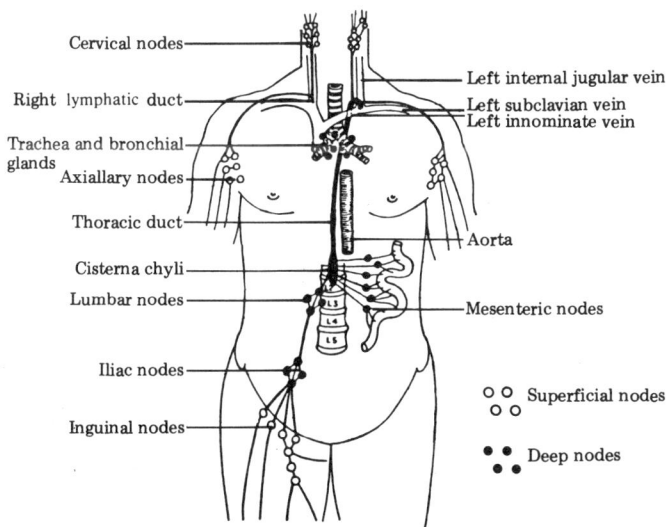

Cervical nodes
Right lymphatic duct
Trachea and bronchial glands
Axillary nodes
Thoracic duct
Cisterna chyli
Lumbar nodes
Iliac nodes
Inguinal nodes

Left internal jugular vein
Left subclavian vein
Left innominate vein

Aorta

Mesenteric nodes

o o Superficial nodes
o o

● ● Deep nodes
● ●

Figure 9.1   The lymph glands and the thoracic ducts.

Situated in the course of the lymph vessels are pea-sized nodes covered with connective tissue and made of lymphatic and reticular tissue.

WHAT IS THE ANATOMY OF THE LYMPHATIC SYSTEM?

A. Lymphatic vessels

The lymphatic capillaries begin in the interstitial spaces. These capillaries are very permeable, even to large molecules. Evidence for their permeability comes from the fact that injections into muscle or skin are absorbed by the lymph capillaries and travel via the lymphatics to the circulatory system, which distributes the medicine throughout the entire body. Special lymph capillaries found in the villi of the small intestine are called lacteals and they absorb fat. The lymph capillaries unite to form large vessels which, though smaller than veins, are similar in structure. The lymph vessels carrying lymph from the lower limbs, the pelvis and abdominal cavities unite to form the large sac-like structure called the cisterna chyli, an elongated ovoid structure about 5 cm in length and lying behind and to the right of the aorta at about the level of the 1st and 2nd lumbar vertebrae (see Figure 9.1). The cisterna chyli narrows and gives rise to the thoracic duct, passes upwards through the aortic opening in the diaphragm, ascends to the root of the neck, turns and empties into the left brachiocephalic vein (see Figure 9.2). There is frequent variation as to where the thoracic duct enters; it usually is in the brachiocephalic vein or somewhere else near the junction of the left jugular and subclavian veins. The thoracic duct also receives tributaries carrying lymph from the left side of the thorax, the left side of the head and neck and the left upper limb.

The right lymphatic duct is little more than 1 cm long and empties into the left brachiocephalic vein (see Figure 9.2). The right lymphatic duct has tributaries which carry lymph from the right side of the thorax, the right side of the head and neck and the right upper limb. All the lymph which does not return via the right lymphatic duct returns via the thoracic duct. Thus, most lymph returns via the thoracic duct.

The lymph vessels contain valves, and lymph is pumped through the lymphatics to the venous system in a manner similar to that of the flow of blood in the veins. Conditions that increase the out-pouring of fluid from the capillaries into the interstitial space will increase the flow of lymph. Lymph formation and flow will increase if there is an increased capillary pressure or capillary flow, or if the capillaries are injured and rendered more permeable. Lymph flow increases when muscles increase their activity.

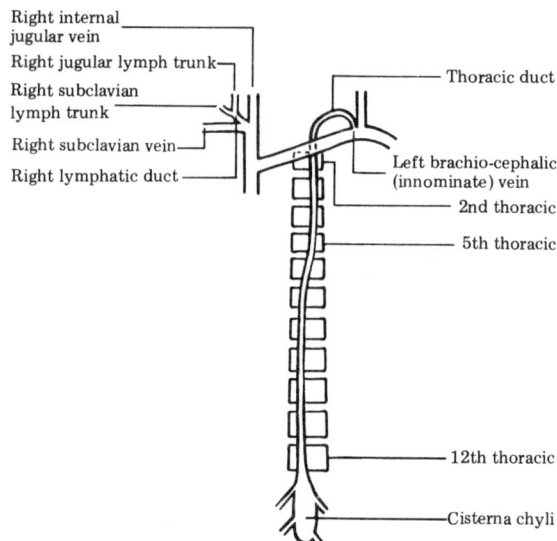

Figure 9.2   The lymphatic system and the thoracic duct.

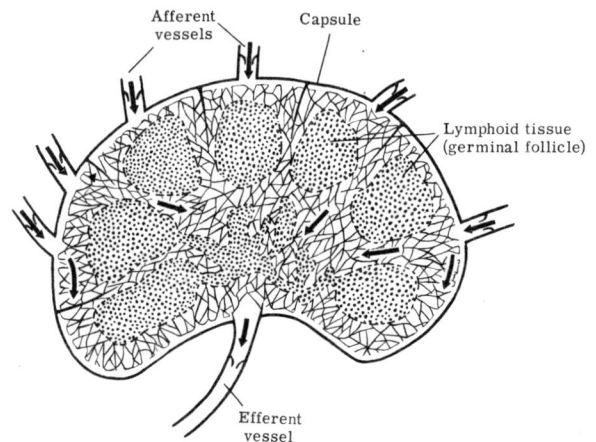

Figure 9.3   The structure of a lymph node.

Obstruction of the lymph vessels can have serious consequences. If the flow of lymph is stopped, pressure behind the obstruction will increase and oedema will result. This is called lymphoedema. The lymphatics may be obstructed by tumours, scars, surgical removal of the lymph nodes or the fibrosis which sometimes follows x-ray therapy and repeated infection.

In tropical parts of the world, lymphoedema and elephantitis are caused by worms (filarial parasites). The larvae of the parasites penetrate into the skin as a result of mosquito bites. The larvae develop and migrate to the lymph vessels, in particular those of the lower limbs and external genitalia. When the worms die, they initiate a severe inflammatory reaction causing a scarring and fibrosis of the lymph vessels, so that they are obstructed. The lymphoedema causes proliferation of the fibrous connective tissue and thickening of the epidermis. The lower limbs and the scrotum may become immense, hence the name elephantitis.

B. Lymph nodes

These nodes are variable in size. They atrophy in old age and often increase in response to infection or other diseases. Lymph enters the lymph nodes through the afferent lymphatic vessels, percolates through the outer cortex and inner medulla and leaves the node via the efferent lymphatic vessels (see Figure 9.3). The node is surrounded by a capsule of fibrous tissue, which sends projections into the cortex of the node. Between these projections of connective tissue are densely packed lymphocytes, which may surround a germinal centre of lymphoblasts and rapidly dividing lymphocytes. The germinal nodes increase in size and activity in response to antigenic stimulation. The medulla consists of lymph sinuses, formed by loose connective tissues and containing scattered lymphocytes and monocytes. Each lymph node also has its own blood supply; arteries enter with the afferent lymph vessels and veins leave with the efferent lymphatic vessels.

Lymphocytes can leave the blood circulation in the post-capillary venule to enter the lymph node. The lymphocytes

found in the lymph node are both the T- and B-lymphocytes; those which are dependent on the lymphoid tissue of the gut (B-lymphocytes) and produce antibody, and those dependent on the thymus (T-lymphocytes) which participate in cell-mediated immunity.

The lymph node has two functions: (a) to act as a filter and (b) to produce lymphocytes and participate in the immune response.

a. Filtration. The lymph node acts as a filter by preventing bacteria from gaining access to the blood stream. If the bacteria or foreign particles overcome the barriers of the skin and mucous membranes they will most likely be trapped in the lymph node. In one experiment, bacteria were injected into an afferent lymph capillary and 99% of them were trapped in the node. Viruses and most macromolecules are too small to be stopped by the lymph nodes. For example, a subcutaneous injection of insulin will be absorbed into the lymph capillaries, pass through the lymph nodes and eventually enter the circulation.

b. Immunological response. If a bacteria, virus or any other foreign agent enters the lymph node and is recognized as being foreign (not belonging to the body), an immunological response will be initiated in the node. The germinal centres in the cortex will respond to the antigenic stimulus, expand and produce more lymphocytes. Lymphocytes will differentiate into plasma cells and antigen production will increase. If bacteria or certain other microbial agents are present, T-lymphocytes may proliferate, macrophages will be attracted to the node and phagocytosis will begin.

The net effect of these changes may lead to a swelling and inflammation of the nodes. Some examples help illustrate this. If you cut your toe and it becomes infected, the infecting agent may travel from lymph capillaries of the toe to the lymph nodes in the groin, which may become inflamed and swollen. If you receive an immunization in your right arm, the immunizing agent will travel to the lymph nodes in the axilla of the right arm, where an immunological response, which includes the production of antibody, will occur. Cancer cells may also travel in lymph channels to the lymph nodes, where they may proliferate and cause the node to hypertrophy. Lymphocytes are also produced within the bone marrow and spleen.

Study of the lymphocytes has been complicated by the fact

that they can leave the cardiovascular system to enter the lymph nodes and then return to the cardiovascular system via the thoracic or right subclavian ducts. There is also considerable migration of lymphocytes during foetal development. The life span of lymphocytes is not known. Some live for hours, while others apparently survive for years. Much more is yet to be discovered concerning the lymphocytes, their development and survival.

C. The spleen

The spleen is a very vascular organ found in the left hypochondrium region. It averages 12 cm long, lies against the diaphragm and 9th, 10th and 11th ribs on the left side. The spleen averages 7 cm in breadth and 200 grams in weight. The organ is almost completely covered with peritoneum. The spleen receives its blood supply from the splenic artery, and blood leaves the spleen via the splenic vein which goes to the hepatic portal vein (see Figure 9.4). Beneath the peritoneum, the organ is covered with a capsule made of collagen, elastin and some smooth muscle fibres; it is pierced by the renal artery and the renal vein.

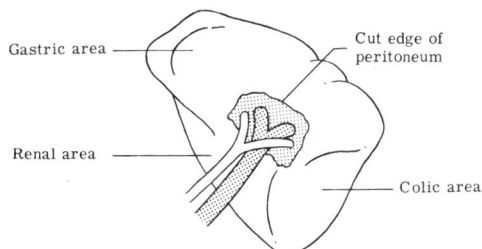

Figure 9.4 Areas of the spleen.

The interior of the spleen is made up of white pulp and red pulp. The white pulp refers to a dense collection of lymphocytes surrounding the arterioles of the splenic artery. The white pulp may form germinal centres for the production of lymphocytes which takes place after adequate antigenic stimulation. The red pulp surrounds the white pulp and contains a complex network of reticular fibres and endothelial-lined sinusoids containing macrophages, histocytes and lymphocytes. Red pulp gets its name because it contains large numbers of red blood cells. These red blood cells are filtered after leaving the capillary bed of the spleen. Old red blood cells are trapped in the red pulp and destroyed. Haemoglobin loses its iron and the haemoglobin is converted into bilirubin; the plasma levels of bilirubin increase when there is increased destruction of red blood cells, though there are other causes of increased bilirubin levels. Bacteria and some other micro-organisms which have overcome the barriers of the skin, mucous membranes or lymph nodes will also be trapped in the red pulp of the spleen. The spleen has very many macrophages. Healthy red blood cells will be returned to the circulation via the splenic vein.

Sometimes the spleen becomes hyperactive, destroys healthy red blood cells and causes anaemia. This may be treated by removing the spleen, for it is not an essential organ. Because the spleen is such a vascular organ, large volumes of blood can be lost into the peritoneal cavity if it is injured.

In bacteraemia, when large numbers of bacteria are present in the blood, or in the case of other diseases like malaria, the spleen will respond to the antigenic stimuli provided by the pathogens and it may become so enlarged that it can be easily felt or palpated during a physical examination. In malaria-infested areas of the tropics it is possible that an infected man's spleen can be ruptured simply by his being hit in the area of the spleen.

D. The thymus

The thymus, named because of its supposed resemblance to the leaves of the thyme plant, is a flat, ribbed organ found behind the sternum in the mediastinum above the arch of the aorta. It has a connective tissue capsule which surrounds two main lobes, each lobe being subdivided into many smaller lobules. The outer portion of the lobules contains densely packed lymphoid tissue with many lymphocytes, while the medulla contains epithelial cells and a few lymphocytes and connective tissue. It is an unusual organ, for it actually begins to become smaller during the early teens. The function of the thymus is not well understood.

In experiments using mice, the thymus gland was removed at birth. These animals had a reduced number of circulating lymphocytes and an impaired ability to fight infections. Sometimes, though rarely, human infants are born without a thymus and these infants likewise have a reduced ability to combat infections, particularly those caused by viruses and fungi. There is evidence that the thymus does process lymphocytes which participate in cell-mediated immunity. These thymus-processed T-lymphocytes are thought to release chemicals which attract, activate and keep macrophages at the site of invasion by microbial agents, or in the presence of foreign tissue. The T-lymphocytes and the activated "angry" macrophages defend the body against infection and may participate in the body's rejection of transplanted tissue. Other evidence indicates that the thymus produces a hormone that influences the T-lymphocytes in peripheral lymphoid tissue. Additional work is now being undertaken to discover the way in which the thymus affects the lymphocyte's ability to distinguish between those tissues which are of the body and those which are foreign to it. The thymus itself is protected from making contact with most antigens because of special adaptations of its capillary membranes. Thus, the thymus, unlike the spleen or lymph nodes, will not become enlarged, even under the most intense antigenic stimulation.

WHAT IS THE FUNCTION OF THE LYMPHATIC SYSTEM AND ASSOCIATED STRUCTURES?

By now, most of the functions of the lymphatic system should be clear. For the sake of review and order, they are listed below.

(1) Lymph is a capillary filtrate. Fluid and proteins which were filtered at the capillaries, but not reabsorbed back into the blood circulation, are absorbed into the lymph capillaries. From the lymph capillaries, the lymph is returned to either of the subclavian veins via the lymphatic vessels.

(2) The lacteals, specialized lymph capillaries in the small intestine, transport digested fat to the large lymph vessels via the cisterna chyli.

(3) The lymph nodes participate in the body's defence by acting as filters so that bacteria and other large micro-organisms cannot gain access to the blood stream. The nodes are also essential centres of lymphocyte production and of the immune response to foreign material, including phagocytosis and antibody production.

(4) The spleen removes worn-out cells from the blood and also filters out certain micro-organisms which may have gained access to the blood. The spleen also contains lymphoid tissue that participates in the immune response of the body.

(5) The thymus is very important in the foetus as a production and processing centre for T-lymphocytes which participate in cell-mediated immunity. It is thought that the thymus produces a hormone which is important for the maintenance of peripheral lymphoid tissues. During its development, the thymus is an organ that may be crucial in determining the lymphocytes' ability to distinguish between the "self" and the "non-self". The function of the thymus in the adult is uncertain.

(6) There are other functions of the lymphatic system which have not yet been determined. In some ways, lymph flow helps in maintaining tissues. When, for instance, the lymphatics of the heart, kidney or lungs are blocked, degenerative changes are seen in these organs.

During the physical examination of the patient, the examiner customarily tries to palpate any enlarged lymph nodes. Particular attention is paid to the lymph nodes in the axilla, those behind and around the mastoid process, the jugular nodes which follow the sternocleidomastoid muscle in the neck and those in the thigh and groin which lie along the inguinal ligament and accompany the saphenous vein.

Enlargement of the nodes may be a response to any one of a number of infectious agents. Infection is not, however, the only cause of enlarged lymph nodes. Many tumours can spread to the nodes and grow there. In addition, the tissues of the lymph node can itself give rise to tumours. Hodgkin's disease is a special type of malignant lymphoma. Often, the first sign of Hodgkin's disease is a painless, swollen lymph node in the neck.

During an examination of the abdomen, an enlarged spleen may be felt. This may be caused by some malignant or infectious process. The lymph nodes and/or the spleen may become enlarged in processes which are neither malignant nor infectious.

10. The Respiratory System

INTRODUCTION

Perhaps no act is more associated with life than breathing, yet we take breathing and the air around us very much for granted. Breathing and respiration are often used synonymously, although this is not strictly correct. Respiration has two meanings: internal respiration refers to the *consumption* of oxygen (O_2) by cells and to the *production* of carbon dioxide (CO_2) as a result of metabolism; external respiration refers to the *transport* of O_2 into the lungs and the *removal* of CO_2 from them. In this Chapter, respiration will be used to mean external respiration, breathing. The respiratory system refers to those structures which function in the exchange of gases between the environment and the individual, and which bring air into and out of the body. In the body, external and internal respiration are linked together by the blood in the circulatory system which carries the gases. For air to be moved in and out of the body, muscles must also contract and so the neuromuscular system plays a role in respiration.

REVIEW OF PHYSICS

There are three states of matter: solid, liquid and gas. A solid will not readily change its shape, while a liquid will assume the shape of the container it is placed in. A gas assumes the size and shape of its container; it fills it completely. If you place $\frac{1}{2}$ litre of liquid in a 1 litre container, the liquid can never fill the container. No matter how little gas you place in the 1 litre flask, the gas molecules will distribute themselves equally throughout the container from top to bottom.

Gases exert a pressure caused by the collisions of the gas molecules with each other and with objects in their presence. The more collisions, the greater the pressure will be. The units of pressure are commonly millimetres of mercury (mmHg) or centimetres of water (cmH_2O). If the temperature and amount of gas in a container is constant, the pressure will vary inversely with the volume of the container, the bigger the volume, the lower the pressure. Assume you have a closed tube and cylinder of gas at a pressure of 10 mmHg (see Figure 10.1). If the piston is moved to "A" so that the volume is reduced by half, the pressure will double to 20 mmHg. If the piston is moved to "C" so that the original volume is doubled, the pressure will fall to 5 mmHg; this is because the molecules occupy more space and the number of molecular collisions (per square unit of surface area) has therefore fallen.

The second important point to remember is that, just as water must always run downhill, gas molecules must always

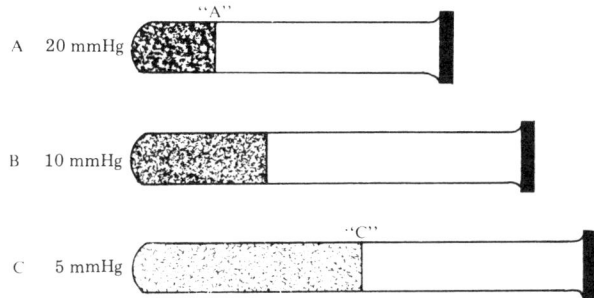

Figure 10.1 The relationship between the volume and the pressure of a gas.

diffuse from areas of high concentration to areas of low concentration in an attempt to equalize concentration differences. Suppose you have two different gasses "A" and "B" in two identical containers separated by barrier "C" (see Figure 10.2). Container A has a pressure of 20 mmHg, while container B has a pressure of 10 mmHg. The pressure in A is twice that in B because there are twice as many molecules in A as in B. (The temperature in containers A and B is the same.) When the barrier between the two containers is removed, each gas will move from areas of high

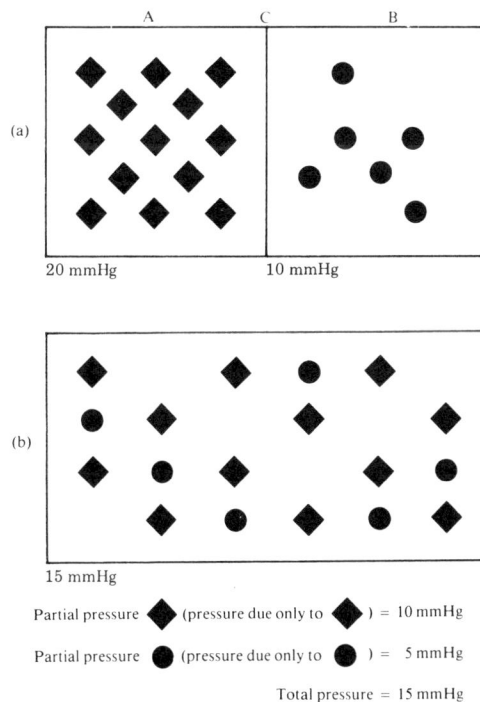

Figure 10.2 The diffusion of gases.

117

concentration to areas of low concentration. In time, an equilibrium will be established so the gases will be equally distributed throughout the single chamber. The total pressure will be 15 mmHg. Since the volume occupied by each gas is doubled, the pressure caused by each gas is halved. Therefore:

$$20 \text{ mmHg}/2 + 10 \text{ mmHg}/2 = 15 \text{ mmHg}.$$

The partial pressure of gas A or the pressure caused exclusively by gas A will be 10 mmHg. this follows because the total pressure is 15 mmHg, and 2/3 of the molecules in the single chambers are gas A molecules.

$$2/3 \times 15 \text{ mmHg} = 10 \text{ mmHg}.$$

The partial pressure of gas B is 5 mmHg.

Sometimes pressure is expressed in units known as the *torr* rather than in mmHg. One torr equals 1 mmHg under standard conditions; 1 torr also equals 1.36 cm of water, as mercury is about 13.6 times as dense as water.

WHAT IS THE AIR?

Air is our most precious resource. Man can live for days without water, but only minutes without air. Water can be purified and transported, but today there is no economical way of transporting clean air to where it is needed. This is particularly unfortunate because the air in some cities has become so polluted that breathing it can be hazardous to one's health. Recent years have witnessed the rapid development and popularization of the science of ecology, that branch of biology which studies the relationships between man, plants, animals and their environment. The air illustrates the important ecological principle of the dependence of life on other forms of life and particularly how human life depends on other forms of life. Oxygen comes from green plants, which take in CO_2 from the air and water from the soil, and synthesize sugar or starch from water and CO_2 by using energy from the sun in a process known as photosynthesis (building by means of light). A chemical reaction for the plants could be written:

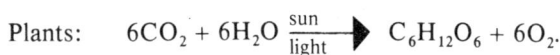

Plants: $6CO_2 + 6H_2O \xrightarrow[\text{light}]{\text{sun}} C_6H_{12}O_6 + 6O_2.$

Man and other animals produce, as a result of their metabolism, CO_2 and water. An equation for man and animals could be written:

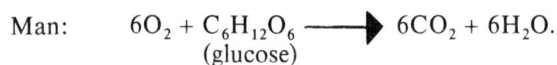

Man: $6O_2 + C_6H_{12}O_6 \longrightarrow 6CO_2 + 6H_2O.$
                   (glucose)

Man, animals and plants work in different ways, yet somehow work together. People need other people, need plants, animals, clean air and water. The earth and all its creatures need to be reverenced. Ultimately disrespect for them is disrespect for oneself, as everything is so interrelated and interdependent.

Air belongs exclusively to the earth. The air around the earth extends upward from its surface for a distance of about 20 miles. The density of air gradually decreases so there is considerably less air at a distance of 4 miles away and breathing becomes difficult. All this air has a weight and exerts a very significant pressure, for at sea level it is sufficient to force a column of mercury 760 mmHg high, or a

column of water nearly 10 metres high. (Remember mercury is 13.6 times as dense as water.) This pressure, which drives a column of mercury 760 mm high, is equal to one atmosphere of pressure. There is a very simple way to demonstrate atmospheric pressure. Take a glass and immerse it upside down in a dish of water until all the air has left the glass. Then slowly lift the glass upwards and watch the water rise within it (see Figure 10.3). As you go higher above sea level, the

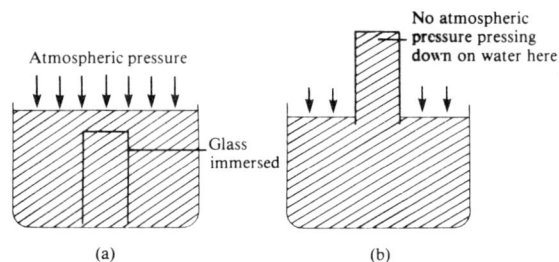

Figure 10.3   Diagram to demonstrate the existence of atmospheric pressure.

amount of air pressing down on you from above is diminished; at 18 000 feet (5486.4 metres) above sea level, the pressure is approximately 380 mmHg.

But what actually is the composition of the air? Air is 79% nitrogen and nearly 21% oxygen. Although carbon dioxide and other gases make up less than 1%, they can be extremely important. These percentages all refer to dry air or air that has had all the water vapour removed. The air we breathe usually has a little water vapour in it, about 1%, although this changes with the weather. More water vapour is added to the inspired air as it makes its way through the respiratory system.

WHAT IS THE ANATOMY OF THE RESPIRATORY SYSTEM?

The respiratory system consists of the following structures: (A) the nasal cavities, (B) the nasopharynx, (C) the oropharynx, (D) the larynx, (E) the trachea, (F) the bronchi, (G) the bronchioles and (H) the alveoli. (Structures A–F are structures leading to the lungs, while structures G and H are within the lungs.)

A. The nasal cavities

The detailed anatomy of the nasal cavities was presented in the Chapter on the skeletal system in the Section on the bones of the skull. A simplified view of the cavities is presented here.

The right and left nasal cavities are separated by the nasal septum (see Figure 10.4a). The openings to the nasal cavities are the nostrils. The anterior walls of the cavities are formed by the nasal bones and cartilage covered with skin. Posterior to the nose, the roof is formed by the base of the skull; the floor by the hard and soft palate. The lateral walls are formed by parts of the maxillary bones and the superior, middle and inferior nasal conchae (see Figure 10.4b). The posterior walls are formed by the wall of the pharynx.

Air sinuses are cavities (hollow spaces) within the bones. The frontal, ethmoid, sphenoid and maxillary bones all have sinuses which empty into the nasal cavities (see Figure 5.10). The openings of the ethmoidal sinuses are between the

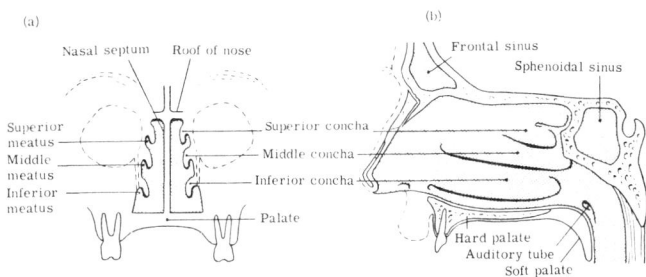

Figure 10.4 The nasal cavity. (a) Coronal section. (b) Lateral wall of the nasal cavity.

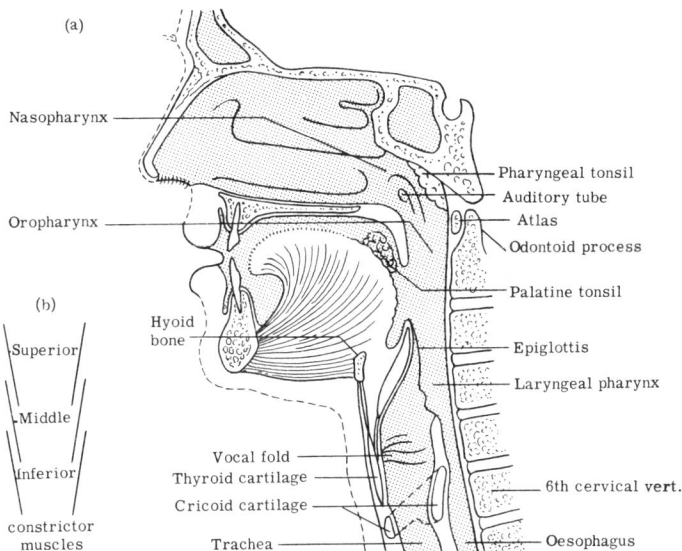

Figure 10.5 (a) Cross-section through the head and neck, showing the different parts of the pharynx and larynx. (b) The arrangement of the constrictor muscles of the pharynx.

superior and middle nasal conchae, and the maxillary sinuses on either lateral wall. The frontal and sphenoidal sinuses open into the roof of the nasal cavity (see Figure 10.4b). The sinuses are lined with a mucous membrane which is similar to that which lines the rest of the nasal cavity. The mucus they produce drains into the nasal cavity. It has been suggested that blowing the nose increases the drainage of mucus from the sinuses into the nasal cavity. Nasal infection which occurs during a "head cold" may spread to the lining of the sinuses, causing sinusitis.

Most of the nasal cavity is lined with ciliated epithelium and mucus-secreting cells. As the air passes over this lining, bacteria, dirt, dust particles, etc., get stuck in the mucus, which is moved by the beating of the cilia to the back of the pharynx where it can be swallowed. The three nasal conchae increase the surface area of the nasal cavities and make it more likely that the air will come into contact with the epithelium and be filtered.

The air passing over these surfaces is also warmed, and water vapour from the cells is added to it. Moisture is added to the air throughout the respiratory tract. You can "see" the water vapour if you breathe into a glass and note the condensation of the water vapour in the glass. In an adult, about 150–200 ml of water from the respiratory tract leave the body every day through the exhaled air. The epithelium also contains olfactory cells which are the sense receptors for the sense of smell. In addition to warming, moisturizing and filtering the air, and being the location for the olfactory receptors, the nose helps in voice production by acting as a resonance structure. Try speaking with your nostrils pinched together and note the difference in the sound of your voice.

B. The nasopharynx

This cavity lies behind the nasal cavities and is lined with the same mucous membrane. It is continuous with the pharynx and lies above the soft palate. On the posterior wall of the nasopharynx is a small mass of lymphoid tissue known as the pharyngeal tonsil (see Figure 10.5). This tissue often becomes infected and enlarged in children and this condition is known as adenoids. Because of their strategic position, adenoids can often block the respiratory passageway and force the individual to breathe through the mouth rather than through the nose. Breathing only through the mouth is harmful, for it can affect facial bone development in children and reduce the moisturization and filtration of the air. Since the pharyngeal

tonsil often becomes infected, the adenoids are removed. The nasopharynx also receives the opening of the pharyngotympanic tube that serves as a connection with the middle ear. This pharyngotympanic tube is also called the Eustachian tube (the auditory tube). Its function will be described in the Chapter on the ear.

C. The oropharynx

The oropharynx is a common passageway for both food, fluid and air (see Figure 10.6). It lies behind the mouth below the soft palate and extends caudad to the level of the 2nd cervical vertebra (see Figure 10.5). The palatine tonsils are found within the oropharynx; they will be discussed later along with digestion. The oropharynx branches into two parts — the larynx and the laryngopharynx which becomes the oesophagus and will be discussed in the Chapter on the digestive system.

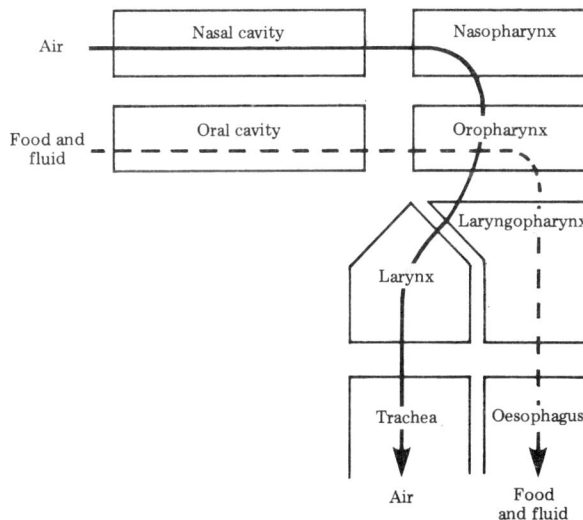

Figure 10.6 An outline of the food and air passages in the pharynx and larynx.

D. The larynx

This structure connects the oropharynx with the trachea and is composed of several irregularly-shaped cartilages. If you place your hand on your neck and feel the hard prominence, you are actually feeling the thyroid cartilage of the larynx (see Figure 10.7). This is often called the Adam's apple. The epiglottis is a leaf-shaped fibro-elastic cartilage attached to the thyroid cartilage and projecting upward between the base of the tongue and the opening of the larynx.

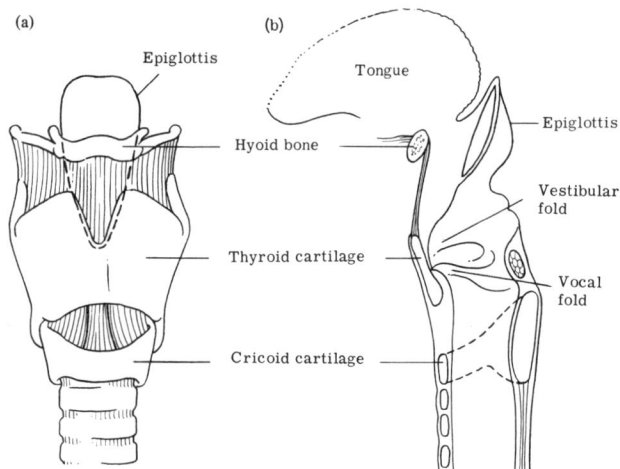

Figure 10.7 The larynx. (a) The skeleton. (b) Sagittal section.

Place your hand on the thyroid cartilage, hold your your head back and swallow. You will feel your larynx brought upward and forward towards the epiglottis. This motion causes the lumen of the larynx to be closed and thus helps to prevent food and fluid from entering the trachea, where they could interfere with air movement and gas exchange. The lumen is always open except when you swallow or when you close your glottis as happens prior to a cough. This means that there is an open passageway for air movement at all times, except when you swallow food or fluid which might enter the air passageway, and just prior to a cough, when air is expelled from the lungs.

The thyroid cartilage is directly above the circular cricoid cartilage, and the two arytenoid cartilages rest upon the cricoid cartilages (see Figure 10.7).

Between the two arytenoid cartilages and the thyroid cartilage are two fibro-elastic bands known as vocal cords (see Figure 10.8). The movement of air from the lungs can force the vocal cords to vibrate and sound to be produced. The pitch of the voice, whether it is high or low, depends on the length and tension of the vocal cords. Men have lower-pitched voices than women because their vocal cords are longer. The individual can raise the pitch of his voice by contracting the muscle around the arytenoid cartilages and increasing the tension on the vocal cords. The loudness of the sound produced depends on the force of the expired air.

E. The trachea

This structure is continuous with the larynx and extends about 10 cm before it divides into two bronchi (see Figure 10.9). The trachea should lie in the midline of the neck; it may be pushed to one side by a tumour, enlarged lymph nodes or an enlarged thyroid gland.

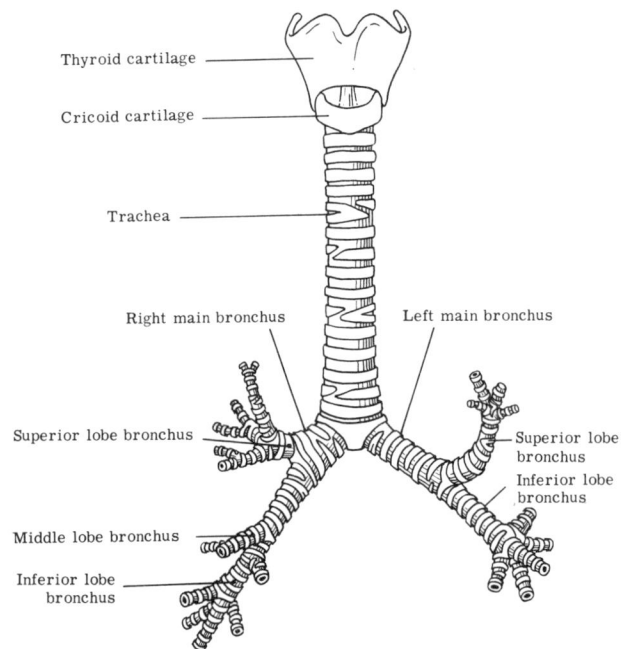

Figure 10.9 The trachea, main bronchi, lobar bronchi and segmental bronchi.

Like most of the larynx, the trachea is lined with a mucous membrane which contains pseudo-stratified ciliated epithelium. There are mucus-producing, goblet cells interspersed in this epithelium, and beneath the epithelium there are mucus-producing glands. The mucus lines the trachea and is often called a mucous blanket.

The cilia beat 600–1000 times a minute, pushing the mucus and trapped particles into the oropharynx where they can be swallowed. The importance of these cilia and their beating cannot be overstated. You breathe in more than 9000 litres of air a day and it must be filtered to remove the dirt and bacteria. If the secretion and removal of mucus is interfered with, mucus and the entrapped dirt and bacteria will continue their movement into the alveoli, where they may initiate disease processes.

The outer surface of the trachea is a wrapping of fibrous tissue which surrounds "C"-shaped bands of hyaline cartilage and some smooth muscle, which completes the circle. These 16–20 cartilage bands prevent the trachea from collapsing and blocking air flow. The muscular portion of the trachea lies over the oesophagus and stretches a little as food passes

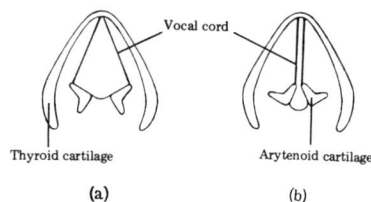

Figure 10.8 The vocal cords. (a) At rest. (b) When used for speaking.

down it, so that food movement down the oesophagus is not blocked.

An endotracheal intubation is a procedure in which a tube is passed through either the nose or mouth into the trachea. A tracheostomy is a surgical procedure making an artificial opening in the trachea, into which a tube may then be inserted. If the patient is unable to bring up his or her secretions they may be suctioned out with a tube or, if the patient cannot swallow properly, the trachea is blocked off above the opening so that food and fluid cannot enter the lungs. The most important function of the endotracheal or tracheostomy tube is, however, to maintain an open air passage to the lungs. In some cases a mechanical ventilator may be attached to the tube to breathe forcefully for the patient. It is essential that a seal exist between the tracheostomy or endotracheal tube and the trachea, otherwise the air will not enter the lungs. A tracheostomy or endotracheal tube may permit bacteria to bypass the anatomical and physiological barriers that normally prevent them from entering the trachea. Strict care must be taken so as not to facilitate infection.

F. The bronchi

The trachea divides into two primary bronchi (see Figure 10.9). These bronchi enter the lungs where they divide into small bronchial tubes, which divide and divide again before giving rise to the narrower bronchioles. The left bronchus is closer to the horizontal plane than the right, so that foreign objects which enter the trachea are more likely to fall into the more vertical right bronchus.

The bronchi are like the trachea in that they are lined with pseudo-stratified ciliated epithelium interspersed with a few goblet cells. Beneath the epithelium there are mucus-producing glands which open into the lumen by means of ducts. The goblet cells can increase in number and the mucus-producing glands can hypertrophy in response to irritants in the air. Cigarette smoke contains numerous irritants which cause these glands to hypertrophy and increase their mucus production. The irritants and the hot temperature of the cigarette smoke also interfere with the ability of the cilia to clear (remove) the mucus from the trachea and bronchi. Ciliary action normally pushes the mucus blanket towards the mouth.

The accumulation of mucus is significant because the mucus can drain into the lower airways, obstruct them and thereby interfere with the exchange of gases. Since the mucus that is retained may contain bacteria, respiratory infections are more common among smokers. Coughing is a mechanism whereby the body attempts to remove this mucus from the lungs. Strictly defined, bronchitis is a condition characterized by chronic cough and excessive sputum production which lasts for at least 3 months of the year for 2 or more successive years. Sputum is the matter which is ejected from the lungs, bronchi and trachea through the mouth. Haemoptysis is the coughing up of blood-stained sputum, or just blood. Sputum may contain bacteria or cells which have diagnostic importance.

Smoking brings up the subject of lung cancer. Lung cancer is 4–10 times more common in smokers than in non smokers. Most cancers that arise in the lungs originate in the epithelial cells of the bronchi. Irritation of this bronchial mucosa by cigarette smoke, environmental pollutants or industrial commodities, such as asbestos, play a prominent role in tumour initiation. The cure rate for lung cancer is very poor; the majority of patients with lung cancer are dead within 5 years after its detection. This is because the cancer is usually not detected until late in the stage of the disease, and the tumour has had time to spread (metastasize) to other parts of the body. (Tumours from other parts of the body sometimes metastasize to the lungs.) Some signs of a lung tumour include cough, difficulty in breathing (dyspnoea) and haemoptysis. As other respiratory diseases share these signs, specific diagnostic tests such as bronchoscopy, cytological examination of the sputum and biopsy of the tumour are needed to confirm the diagnosis of cancer.

G. The bronchioles

The bronchioles are continuations of the bronchial tubes (see Figure 10.10). They have a smaller internal diameter than the bronchial tubes and their histological appearance changes as they lead away from the tubes. The cartilaginous rings of the bronchi gradually disappear leaving a continuous ring of smooth muscles in the smaller bronchioles. The pseudo-stratified ciliated epithelium gives way to flat cuboidal cells. There are no mucous glands and the number of goblet cells decreases.

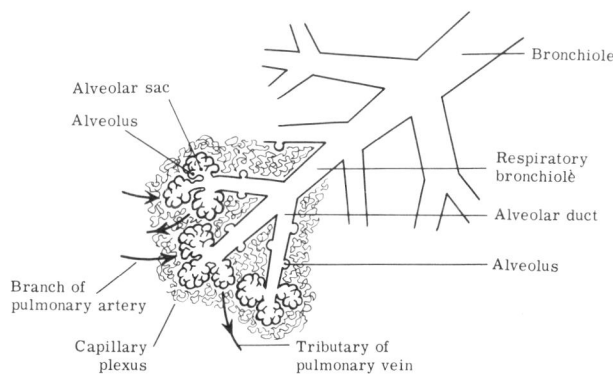

Figure 10.10 Terminal divisions of the respiratory passages.

The smooth muscles of the bronchioles are supplied with β receptors, and sympathetic and parasympathetic nerves, as are the trachea and bronchi as well. In contrast to the arterioles, sympathetic stimulation of the smooth muscle of the trachea bronchi and bronchioles causes the muscle to relax and the bronchioles to dilate. Parasympathetic stimulation constricts the bronchioles, while stimulation of the β receptors by adrenaline or related molecules dilates them.

The resistance to airflow in and out of the lungs is affected by the amount of contraction of the smooth muscle in the bronchi and bronchioles. The narrowing of the airways due to contraction of the smooth muscle can be very severe in those parts of the bronchi and bronchioles where there is little or no cartilage to maintain the open structure of the airway.

Asthma is a common respiratory disease in which the smooth muscle of the respiratory tract occasionally goes into spasm. This increases airway resistance and makes breathing difficult. Some cases are due to an allergic response, whereas others can be precipitated by respiratory irritants, infection or emotional factors. Many of the drugs used in treating asthma are β antagonists which cause the bronchioles to dilate. Patients with asthma should also be well hydrated as this thins the mucus and makes it easier to be cleared. If the mucus is not removed, it can form plugs which will fill the bronchioles and block the movement of air.

Mucus is not the only protective component of the respiratory secretions. Immunoglobins are also present. Lymphoid tissue is present in most of the respiratory tract, including the sinuses, and from the nasopharynx through much of the bronchioles. Lymphoid tissue is found in the pharyngeal tonsil, in lymph nodes in the hilum of each lung, or in nodules and smaller lymphoid aggregates that are found in the submucosa of the respiratory tract.

Antibodies belonging to the class IgA are the predominant immunoglobulins found in the respiratory secretions. IgA is of minor importance to the body's immune defence against bacteria but is far more effective in defending against viruses. The folk wisdom has it that "you can't catch the same cold twice". If properly understood, there is truth in the saying. Most colds are caused by viruses. When a cold virus first invades the respiratory mucosa, it provokes an inflammatory response and stimulates secretions. The virus, which is an antigen, will make contact with lymphoid tissue, T- and B-cells, and antibody against the particular virus will be made. After about 10 days, significant quantities of antibody will be present, and you will be protected against that particular virus because of specific antibody against the virus. This antibody includes IgA in the respiratory secretions.

The respiratory bronchioles and the alveolar ducts are the final branchings of the respiratory airways, and they function to distribute the inspired air to the alveoli (see Figure 10.10). The respiratory bronchioles differ from the larger bronchioles in that the former are partially lined with alveoli.

H. The alveoli

The walls of the alveoli form the gas-exchanging surface of the lung (see Figure .10.11). The walls of the alveoli are polygonal and arranged in a manner similar to the cells of a honeycomb, with the lumen of each alveolus opening into the alveolar duct, which is continuous with the respiratory bronchiole. Each alveolus has three major elements: the alveolar epithelium, the interstitium and the capillary endothelium (see Figure 10.10). There are about 300 million alveoli.

The alveolar epithelium has three types of cells. The most common are thin, flattened epithelial cells covering most of the alveolar surface. Other cells called granular pneumocytes are metabolically active and constitute the reserve pool of cells for epithelial cell renewal. These other cells are also thought to be responsible for synthesizing surfactant (see below). The final type of cell is the alveolar macrophage. These cells are believed to be derived from the bone marrow and are the chief defence mechanism against bacteria and particles that have made the long, hazardous journey to the alveolus. There are no ciliated or mucus-producing cells in the alveolar epithelium.

The interstitial tissues between the alveolar epithelium and the capillary endothelium contains tissue fibrils, elastic fibres and fibroblasts. In some areas, the basement membranes of the epithelium and the endothelium are fused together. Lymphatic capillaries do not penetrate into the alveolar wall; they do, however, appear in the interstitial space surrounding the terminal bronchioles and the small arteries and veins. There is some evidence that the capillary endothelium is relatively permeable, and the fluid and proteins which leave the capillaries travel through discrete channels in the interstitium till they reach the lymphatic capillaries where they are reabsorbed. This relationship will be discussed in the Section on pulmonary oedema.

There are also openings in the alveolar walls called the pores of Kohn which connect the lumen of adjacent epithelium. Gas and liquids can move, and infection can spread, through these pores.

The irregular alveolar outpockets greatly increase the surface area of the lungs. To illustrate this, trace the sketches in Figure 10.12. Both (a) and (b) have the same length and width, but (b) has a far greater surface area. This greater surface area provides a large surface for the diffusion of O_2 into the blood and for CO_2 to diffuse out of the blood into the alveoli. The total surface area of the lungs is estimated to be more than 60 square metres. The surface area of the lungs is greater than the surface area of the skin.

The alveoli must expand during inspiration and this, of course, requires muscular work. One of the forces that must be overcome is the surface tension of the lining of the alveoli. Surface tension is the force resulting from the attraction of like molecules for one another. Normally, this surface tension is reduced by a detergent-like chemical called surfactant. Some infants, particularly premature ones, are not able or ready to synthesize surfactant and thus have to work much harder to inflate their lungs with fresh air. If the forces required to inflate the lungs are greater than they can develop, they will not be able to bring sufficient oxygen into their lungs

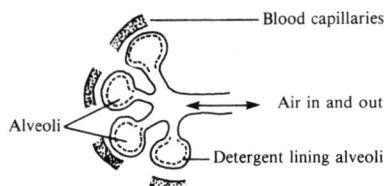

Figure 10.11   Outline of alveolar structure.

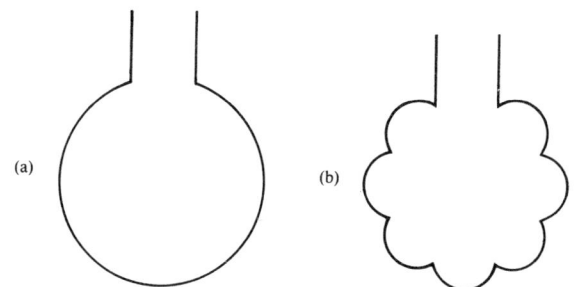

Figure 10.12   Diagram to show the increased area of the lungs by the alveolar pockets.

and will die. Increased difficulty in breathing is known as the respiratory distress syndrome of the newborn and is associated with insufficient surfactant.

I. Gross structure of the lungs

The two cone-shaped lungs lie within the thoracic cavity. The right lung has three lobes, the left but two (see Figure 10.13). The hilum of each lung is where the bronchus, pulmonary artery and veins, enter and leave the lung. The

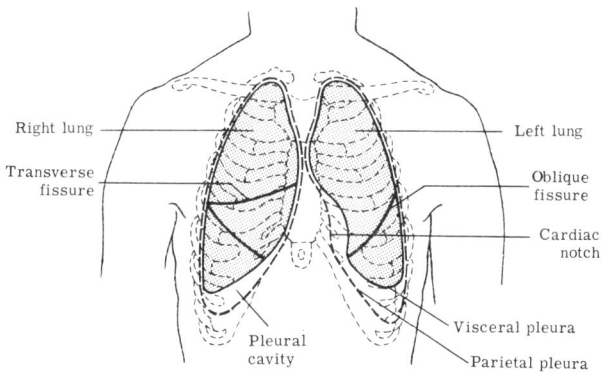

Figure 10.13 Surface markings of the pleurae and lungs.

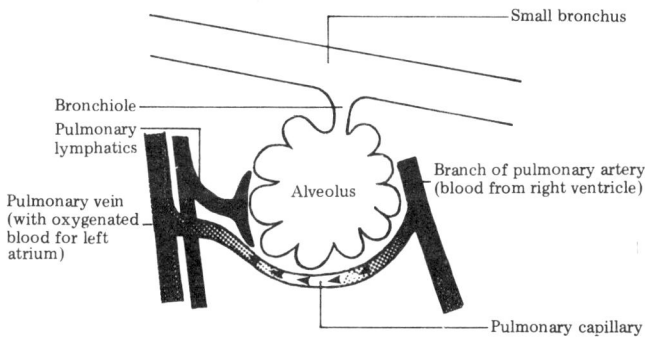

Figure 10.14 Circulatory relationships in the lung.

The lungs are covered with a serous membrane known as the visceral pleura; the walls of the chest cavity are lined with another serous membrane known as the parietal pleura (see Figure 10.13). The fluid secreted by these two serous membranes is responsible for the surface tension which holds the lungs and the chest wall very close together (see Figure 10.15). The fluid is continually produced and continually reabsorbed into the lymphatics. The strength of these surface tension forces can be demonstrated by taking two glass microscope slides, wetting them and placing one on top of the other. The slides will easily slide over one another, but it will take a great deal of effort to pull them apart. Of course, in the body the situation is dynamic and

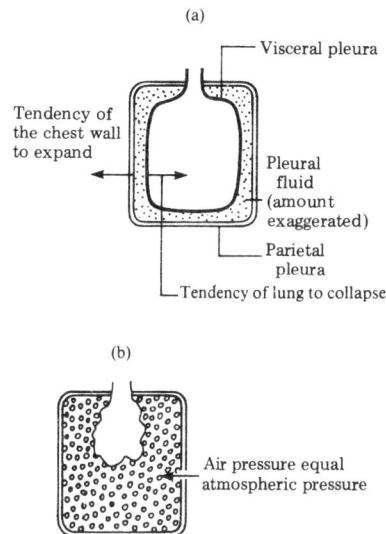

Figure 10.15 Surface-tension forces in the lung. (a) Diagram showing the normal equilibrium between the lung and the chest wall. (Note that the pressure in the intrapleural space is less than atmospheric.) (b) Diagram showing the collapse of the lung and expansion of the chest wall during serious pneumothorax.

more complicated than a layer of water between two glass slides. The small amount of fluid found between the visceral pleura and parietal pleura is called the pleural fluid. Basically, this fluid is a capillary filtrate. To understand the formation of this fluid you should revise, if you don't recall, the forces which operate at the capillary.

The parietal pleura which lines the chest wall has capillaries with pressures in them similar to those throughout the body (previously discussed in the Chapter on the circulatory system). The visceral pleura covers the outer surface of the lungs, and the hydrostatic pressure in its capillaries is considerably less than that found in the parietal pleural capillaries nearby. This is because the blood in the visceral pleural capillaries comes from the pulmonary arteries and right ventricle, rather than the left ventricle and the systemic circulation. As the right ventricle is thinner than the left ventricle and has less muscle mass, it will not be able to generate the contractile force that the left ventricle can (see Figure 10.16). This causes the hydrostatic pressures in the visceral pleural capillaries to be about one-third as great as those in the parietal pleural capillaries. The osmotic pressures in both sets of capillaries will be the same. This means that the forces operating at the two sets of capillaries are such that some of the fluid which is filtered and leaves the parietal pleural capillaries will be absorbed in the visceral pleural capillaries. Thus, the forces which cause this flow of filtrate from parietal to visceral capillaries are responsible for the formation of the pleural fluid and for keeping the visceral pleural surface of the lungs close to the parietal pleural surface of the chest wall. There are also lymphatics present in both the visceral and parietal pleura, which return protein and filtrate to the circulation.

An excess of pleural fluid is called a pleural effusion. A pleural effusion, like oedema, can be caused by anything that upsets the normal balance of forces at the capillaries and the lymphatics. Inflammatory conditions which increase capil-

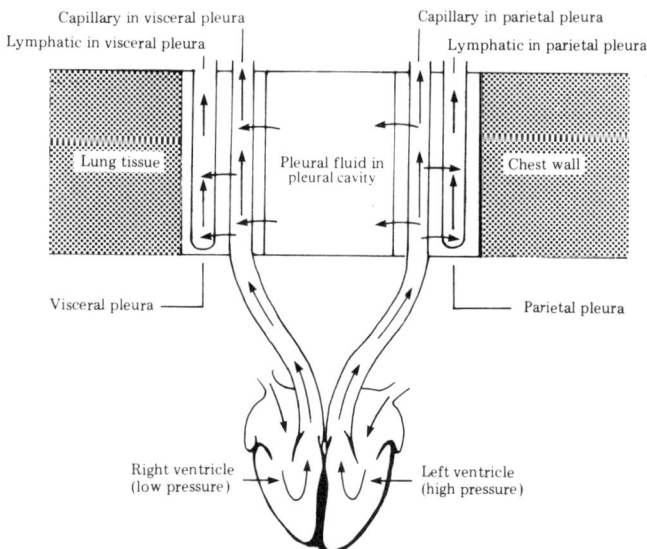

Figure 10.16   Outline of the formation of pleural fluid.

lary permeability, tumours or infections (which block and reduce flow through the lymphatics) and increased pulmonary capillary pressure (such as can occur in heart failure), are among the causes of pleural effusions.

The pleural fluid seal between the lungs and chest wall is important, for it forces the lungs to move, to expand and contract with the movement of the chest wall, and it reduces the friction between the surface of the lungs and the chest wall. Should this seal be broken, as it often is when the chest is punctured, the lungs, or lung, will collapse to a much smaller volume (see Figure 10.15b). The lung tissue is quite elastic so the natural tendency of the lungs is to get smaller, whereas the natural tendency of the chest wall is to get bigger. The lungs and chest wall pull in opposite directions but are held together by fluid forces. The relaxation volume refers to the volume of air in the lungs at the end of a normal expiration and represents the equilibrium point between the lungs favouring collapse and the chest wall forces favouring expansion. Although it is not a true cavity, the potential space between the lungs and the chest wall is referred to as the pleural cavity. Because of the tendency of the lungs to collapse and the chest to expand, the pressure within the potential pleural cavity is less than atmospheric.

WHAT ARE THE RESPIRATORY VOLUMES?

An average person in a typical breath inhales and exhales 500 ml. The volume of air in a typical breath is known as the tidal volume. If you inhale as deeply as you can after taking in a normal breath, this additional air makes up the inspiratory reserve volume. If, after you have exhaled a normal breath, you exhale as much as possible, this volume is known as the expiratory reserve volume.

No matter how hard you try, it is impossible for you to remove all the air from your lungs. The amount of gas which remains in your lungs after a complete forced expiration is the residual volume. It serves a useful purpose, for if you could remove all the air from your lungs, the blood which would pass through them in their airless state would not receive any oxygen. The functional residual capacity is the sum of the residual volume and the expiratory reserve volume.

If you inhale as much as possible then forcefully exhale, the volume exhaled is known as the vital capacity; it includes the tidal volume, the inspiratory reserve volume and the expiratory reserve volume (see Figure 10.17). The sum of the vital capacity and the residual volume equals the total lung capacity. The vital capacity and the rate at which the air is expelled from the lungs are often measured, for they can have clinical significance and can be used in the diagnosis of lung disorders.

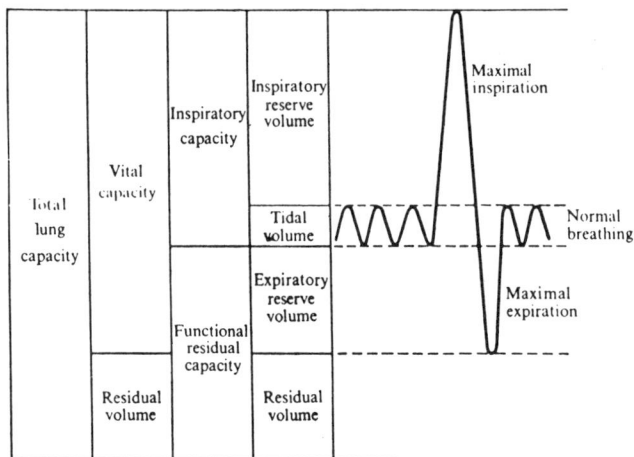

Figure 10.17   The relationship between the various volumes of air in the lungs.

Another useful indicator of respiratory function is the forced expiratory volume in one second (FEV_1). The patient takes a maximal inspiration and then tries to force all the air out of his lungs as rapidly as possible. The volume exhaled in the first second of expiration is recorded as the FEV_1. If the bronchioles are narrowed or the airways are otherwise obstructed, resistance to air flow will be decreased. The patient will take a longer time to force out his air and the FEV_1 will be decreased.

You should not think that all of the 500 ml of air that is taken in during a typical tidal volume ever gets to the alveoli; only about 350 ml do. The remaining air fill what is known as the dead space. This is a misnomer because the tissues of the nose, pharynx, trachea and bronchi are not dead; they just do not exchange gas with the blood. The giraffe provides an illustration of the important concept of dead space. If a giraffe were to take in 1½ litres of air, no air would enter the giraffe's lungs, for it takes more than 1½ litres of air to fill all the dead space in the giraffe's long trachea. The greater the dead space, the greater the volume of air to be inspired. If a patient has a tracheostomy, the dead space is reduced and less air needs to be inspired.

The respiratory rate is the number of breaths per minute (breaths/min). The minute volume is the volume of air inhaled in 1 minute. Alveolar ventilation volume is the volume of air which reaches the alveoli in one minute and is calculated by subtracting the dead space volume from the tidal volume and multiplying the answer by the respiratory rate. Two examples might help:

	Minute volume	Alveolar ventilation volume
Patient A	$500 \times 12 = 6000$ cc	$(500 - 150) \times 12 = 4200$ l/min
Patient B	$250 \times 24 = 6000$ cc	$(250 - 150) \times 24 = 2400$ l/min

Thus, although both patients have the same minute volume, they have very different alveolar ventilation volumes. In fact, it is possible to take so many short breaths that air is never exchanged in the alveoli. This is panting. A dog pants not to obtain O_2 and remove CO_2 but to help regulate his temperature and try to cool himself down.

HOW DOES AIR ENTER AND LEAVE THE LUNGS?

In inspiration, the ribs and sternum are brought upward and outward by the contraction of the external intercostal muscles which lie at an angle between the ribs. The movement of the rib cage has been compared to the upward movement of a bucket handle. The dome-shaped diaphragm contracts and becomes flatter, pressing down upon the abdominal viscera. The result of these two movements is an expansion of the chest from top to bottom and from back to front. (You should consult the Section on the respiratory muscles to revise the anatomy.) Because of the intimate relation between the lungs and the chest, they too must expand with the chest. With an increase in lung size, the pressure within them must fall; there is more room for the air molecules and less chance of a collision. The pressure within the lungs becomes less than atmospheric pressure — the air pressure surrounding the individual is greater than the pressure within the lungs, so the air flows into the lungs until the pressure within the lungs equals the atmospheric pressure.

In expiration, the inspiratory muscles relax and the thorax returns to its original size because of elastic forces and others within the lungs and because of the upward pressure on the diaphragm exerted by the abdominal contents. In expiration, the pressure within the lungs is greater than the atmospheric pressure so air is forced out until the two pressures are equal at the end of expiration and there will be no net flow of air. If the diaphragm and other respiratory muscles are paralyzed, artificial ventilation will be necessary.

Should the chest wall be punctured and the fluid seal between the lungs and chest broken, normal respiration would be impossible and one, or both, lungs might collapse. No matter how great the movement of the diaphragm or chest wall, air would not enter the lungs, for the pressure within the lungs and surrounding the lungs would be atmospheric. It would be somewhat analogous to trying to blow up a balloon which has a hole in it. When a lung collapses because air has entered through a hole in the thorax, the condition is known as pneumothorax (see Figure 10.15). Treatment to restore the lung to its original size should be started as soon as possible, as delay makes re-expansion more difficult. Should the chest wall be open because of a wound, it is necessary to remove any blood and close the wound. Re-expansion of the lung would probably be best accomplished by a chest catheter and water seal drainage. A catheter is introduced into the thorax and immediately connected to a water seal bottle. The end of the tubing is sealed by immersing it a few centimetres below the surface of the water within the bottle. Increasing the suction (negative pressure) within the bottle will increase the drainage of fluid from the thoracic cavity. Most of the gas will be reabsorbed into the blood stream.

In deep breathing, during exercise or in certain diseases, other muscles participate in respiration, including many muscles of the head, neck and shoulders, the chief ones being the scalenes and the sternocleidomastoids during inspiration. Contraction of the abdominal muscles and the internal intercostals helps in forceful expiration. Infants use their abdominal muscles as well.

HOW ARE GASES CARRIED IN THE BLOOD?

Gases diffuse in and out of the pulmonary capillaries. The partial pressure of oxygen in the alveolus is about 100 mmHg. In the venous blood (which enters the lungs via the pulmonary arteries) and in the capillaries, the partial pressure is 40 mmHg. Thus a large diffusion gradient exists.

Oxygen diffuses across the alveolar wall into the plasma within the pulmonary capillaries. This is a critical step. The accumulation of fluid or mucus in the alveolus, or an increase in the connective tissue of the interstitial space, can hinder the diffusion of oxygen and have serious consequences. Normally, however, the alveolar wall is not a diffusion barrier and oxygen quickly crosses it to enter the plasma. Then, most oxygen molecules diffuse out of the plasma, through the red cell membrane to combine with haemoglobin inside the red cells.

Most of the oxygen in the blood is bound to haemoglobin molecules. This process in which oxygen combines with haemoglobin is called oxygenation, not to be confused with oxidation, as no electrons are transferred during oxygenation. The relationship between oxygen and haemoglobin is a casual one, "a handshake between the two molecules", which begins in the lung capillaries and ends in the tissue capillaries where oxygen diffuses into the plasma, then into the extracellular fluid and finally into the tissues.

You should remember that, although thousands of oxygen molecules are contained within each red cell, this oxygen does not contribute to the partial pressure of oxygen in the plasma. The partial pressure of oxygen in the plasma is caused by those oxygen molecules which are dissolved, or are in simple solution, in the watery plasma. This is a small fraction of the total amount of oxygen carried in the blood. Since the tissues consume oxygen, the partial pressure of oxygen in the tissues is less than 40 mmHg, so there will be a diffusion gradient because the partial pressure of oxygen in the arterial blood is about 100 mmHg.

As oxygen leaves the blood, crosses the extracellular fluid and enters the tissues, the partial pressure of oxygen in the venous blood falls to about 40 mmHg. Should the amount of haemoglobin in the blood be reduced, the amount of oxygen that can be carried will also be reduced.

People who are anaemic cannot do strenuous work or exercise without quickly running "out of breath"; the reduced number of red cells or low levels of haemoglobin cannot carry sufficient oxygen to meet the needs of the tissues. It might be well to revise the material on haemoglobin in the Chapter on the blood.

The graph in Figure 10.18 shows the relationship between the pressure of oxygen and the percent (%) saturation of haemoglobin. Sometimes this curve is referred to as the oxygen–haemoglobin dissociation curve. Saturated haemoglobin is haemoglobin that has combined with oxygen to form oxyhaemoglobin. The % saturation (oxyhaemoglobin) curve is sigmoid or "S"-shaped. If the concentration of oxygen in solution in the plasma (the partial pressure of oxygen) is low, the % saturation of haemoglobin (the amount of oxyhaemoglobin) will be low. If the concentration of oxygen in the plasma is high and the partial pressure of oxygen is high, the % saturation will likewise be high. However, as the curve shows, the relationship is not linear.

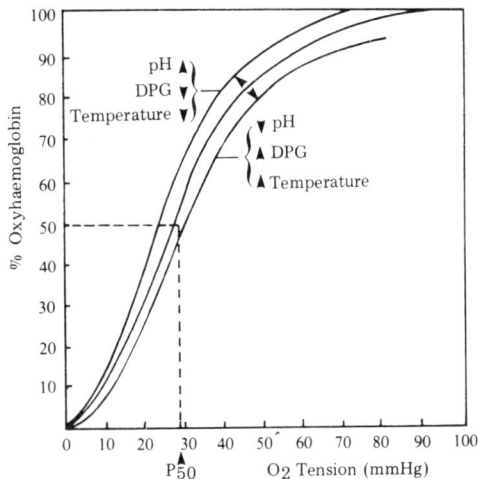

Figure 10.18 Normal oxygen–haemaglobin dissociation curve, showing the effects on oxygen affinity of changes in pH, 2, 3-DPG levels and temperature.

To appreciate the significance of the curve, it might be best to begin by thinking of the situation in the lungs. Because of the high partial pressure of oxygen in the alveoli, the haemoglobin in the blood of the pulmonary capillaries will become almost all saturated with oxygen. When the partial pressure of oxygen is 100 mmHg, the haemoglobin is 97% saturated. As the blood leaves the pulmonary capillaries and moves away from the oxygen-rich alveoli to the oxygen-consuming tissues, the partial pressure of oxygen falls. The amount of oxygen bound to haemoglobin does not, however, fall a like amount. The uppermost part of the curve is flat.

When the partial pressure of oxygen in the plasma falls from 100 to 60 mmHg, the haemoglobin is about 90% saturated. The haemoglobin is still holding on to the oxygen: this facilitates transport of oxygen in the blood and helps ensure that the oxygen will get delivered to where it is needed in the oxygen-consuming tissues.

As the pressure falls below 60 mmHg, the relationship between oxygen and haemoglobin changes. Oxygen is bound less firmly to the haemoglobin molecule and is released more easily. The slope of the curve becomes quite steep. Thus, in the tissue capillaries where the pressure is 40 mmHg or lower, oxygen is readily released and diffuses into the tissues.

Oxygen is loosely bound to haemoglobin all the way down to pressures of 10 mmHg. Below 10 mmHg, the curve flattens and the affinity between oxygen and haemoglobin is released less readily. The partial pressure of oxygen seldom falls this low, with the chief exception of the working muscle tissue when muscle tissue can use all the oxygen that the blood delivers.

The blood returns to the lungs via the veins, heart and

pulmonary arteries. In the pulmonary capillaries the haemoglobin becomes rapidly saturated as the pressure of oxygen increases from 40 to 60 mmHg. The rate of saturation slows as the pressure of oxygen goes from 60 to 100 mmHg or greater. Another way to look at the curve is to realize that normal haemoglobin is 50% saturated with oxygen when the partial pressure of oxygen is about 28 mmHg. The partial pressure of oxygen at which haemoglobin is 50% saturated is referred to as the P_{50}.

The amount of oxygen that haemoglobin can carry is influenced by several factors: the CO_2, pH, temperature and 2,3-diphosphoglycerate. Increases in the amount of CO_2 and hydrogen ion (H^+) reduce the ability of haemoglobin to bind oxygen. In the tissue capillaries, CO_2 and H^+ from the tissues become bound to the haemoglobin. This tends to release additional oxygen so that oxygen will diffuse into the tissues. In the pulmonary capillaries, CO_2 and H^+ leave the haemoglobin molecule so that the ability of haemoglobin to bind oxygen is increased.

Increased temperature also reduces the oxygen-binding ability of haemoglobin. Tissues that are metabolically active release more heat and also require more oxygen. This heat sensitivity of haemoglobin facilitates oxygen delivery to active tissues.

2,3-Diphosphoglycerate (2,3-DPG) is a product of red cell metabolism. It tends to displace oxygen from haemoglobin. The concentration of 2,3-DPG increases in anaemia, which tends to compensate for the reduction in the number of red cells.

Before continuing it is good to recall from the Chapter on the blood the actual amount of oxygen that is transported and used by the tissues. Under standard conditions of temperature and pressure, 1 gram of haemoglobin can bind with about 1.3 ml of oxygen. Since the normal haemoglobin level is about 15 grams/100 ml of blood, there will be about 20 ml of oxygen bound to haemoglobin, and 0.3 ml of oxygen in solution in the plasma if the partial pressure of oxygen is 100 mmHg.

The resting level of oxygen consumption is about 250 ml/min. A little more than 300 ml of CO_2 are produced every minute.

It is possible to measure both the partial pressure of oxygen and CO_2 and the H^+ concentration in a blood sample. This information may be invaluable in that it can indicate if the needs of the tissues for oxygen are being met, and it can provide some clue as to whether the heart and lungs are functioning well enough to exchange gas and circulate blood. The blood sample is usually removed from the artery, often either the brachial, radial or femoral artery, and quickly taken to the laboratory for analysis. Since the arteries are not as superficial as the veins, inserting the needle into them is more difficult and dangerous and also more painful for the patient.

In the Chapter on pH and hydrogen ion concentration more will be said about H^+ concentration, CO_2 and the changes that take place in respiratory disease.

The gas, carbon monoxide (CO), is a poison because it binds very tightly to haemoglobin and takes up all the room normally reserved for oxygen, so that only the small amount of oxygen dissolved in the plasma can be delivered to the tissues. CO is a particularly dangerous gas because the brain is not warned that it is getting inadequate oxygen. This is because the partial pressure of oxygen in the plasma is not affected. When CO combines with haemoglobin, a characteristically bright cherry red colour results. The gas is produced by incomplete combustion of fuel; gas heaters and stoves are potential sources of CO. Smokers and policemen who direct traffic in large cities have less haemoglobin available for oxygen transport because of the small but significant amounts of CO they inhale.

Whenever tissues do not get enough oxygen to meet their needs or are not able to utilize it, the condition is called hypoxia. There can be many different causes of hypoxia:

(1) Anaemic hypoxia can be caused by haemorrhage or anaemia. For sufficient oxygen to be carried to the tissues there must be sufficient haemoglobin.

(2) Hypoxic hypoxia results from an insufficiency of inspired oxygen. Mountain climbers might suffer from this hypoxia.

(3) Stagnant hypoxia occurs when the circulation of blood through the tissues is slowed and oxygen cannot be delivered to the tissues fast enough. Patients in heart failure might suffer from this kind of hypoxia. In stagnant hypoxia, there will be more deoxygenated haemoglobin in the tissue than normal haemoglobin. Deoxygenated blood is bluish in colour. Your veins are transparent and get their blue colour from the deoxygenated blood in them.

(4) Histotoxic hypoxia occurs when cellular or internal respiration enzymes are poisoned. Cyanide is a very powerful respiratory enzyme poison; it is so effective that some countries once used it to execute criminals. Since the tissues receive adequate oxygen but cannot utilize it, histotoxic hypoxia is characterized by a high partial pressure of oxygen in venous as well as arterial blood.

Transportation of CO_2 is a little more complicated. It begins with the production of CO_2 in the cells; the partial pressure of CO_2 is greater in the cells than in the venous blood. Most of the CO_2 diffuses from the tissues to the plasma into the red cells because of the concentration gradient (see Figure 10.19). Within the red cells, CO_2 reacts with H_2O and the enzyme, carbonic anhydrase, to form carbonic acid (H_2CO_3), which dissociates into a hydrogen ion (H^+) and the bicarbonate ion (HCO_3^-).

In the tissue capillaries:

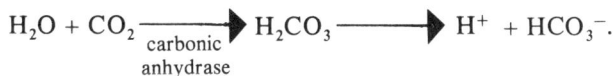

$$H_2O + CO_2 \xrightarrow[\text{carbonic anhydrase}]{} H_2CO_3 \longrightarrow H^+ + HCO_3^-.$$

The hydrogen ion goes to the haemoglobin molecule and helps cause the oxygen to leave for the tissues, while the bicarbonate ion diffuses out of the red cell into the plasma. Some CO_2 will simply combine with the haemoglobin molecule, whereas a very small amount of CO_2 will merely dissolve in the plasma.

In the alveolus, the partial pressure of CO_2 is 40 mmHg compared with 46 mmHg in the venous blood entering the lungs, so a diffusion gradient exists. CO_2 will diffuse out of the plasma into the alveolus where it will be expelled from the body. As the partial pressure of CO_2 in the plasma falls and as oxygen enters the red cell and combines with haemoglobin, the hydrogen ion (H^+) is driven off the haemoglobin molecule and combines with the bicarbonate ion (HCO_3^-);

carbonic acid is formed and this is broken down by the enzyme, carbonic anhydrase, so that CO_2 and H_2O are formed. The CO_2 leaves the cell and ultimately leaves the body:

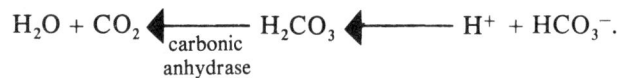

$$H_2O + CO_2 \xleftarrow[\text{carbonic anhydrase}]{} H_2CO_3 \xleftarrow{\hspace{2cm}} H^+ + HCO_3^-.$$

If you were to increase your rate of breathing, you would expel more CO_2 and you would cause this reaction to go faster. As a result, there would be less HCO_3^- in the blood. If you were to reduce your breathing rate, the amount of CO_2 in the blood would increase, which would quickly lead to an increase in the plasma HCO_3^- and H^+. Excessive blood CO_2 levels are called hypercapnoea; low blood CO_2 levels are called hypocapnoea.

When the lungs cannot adequately provide for the exchange of oxygen and CO_2, respiratory failure occurs. This is conventionally defined by arterial blood gas measurements in which the partial pressure of oxygen is less than 50 mmHg and/or the partial pressure of CO_2 is greater than 50 mmHg.

WHAT CONTROLS RESPIRATION?

Respiration is dependent on the control of the contraction of the respiratory muscles. In normal respiration, these are usually the diaphragm and the external intercostals which are innervated by the phrenic and intercostal nerves, respectively. But what controls the rate of discharge of these nerves? And where do the impulses come from? Within the lower part of the brain in the pons and the medulla is a group of neurones that make up the respiratory centre. Impulses which travel to the inspiratory and expiratory muscles originate in neurones there. The neurones of the respiratory centre receive information on the needs of the body and increase or decrease the rate of discharge to the muscles accordingly. The respiratory neurones are spontaneously active but their rate of discharge is regulated by the information they receive. The respiratory centre is influenced by the following (see Figure 10.19).

a. Central chemoreceptors. These receptors are located in the medulla of the brain. They increase their activity in response to increases in arterial CO_2 or H^+. Of course, an increase in arterial CO_2 will lead to an increase in H^+:

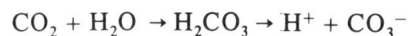

$$CO_2 + H_2O \rightarrow H_2CO_3 \rightarrow H^+ + CO_3^-$$

so a neat separation of the two stimuli is not possible.

If you wilfully choose to stop breathing, CO_2 will not be exhaled and its concentration in the blood will increase. This increase stimulates the chemoreceptors, which in turn strongly stimulate the respiratory neurones and you will be forced to breathe. One way of proving the importance of CO_2 is to hyperventilate — breath frequently and deeply. Hyperventilation will reduce the levels of CO_2. After a period of hyperventilation you will briefly cease breathing until the tissues produce enough CO_2 to return plasma levels to normal values and thus stimulate again the chemoreceptors.

In recent years, evidence has accumulated that there are central chemoreceptors on the surface of the medulla of the brain. The brain and its cavities are bathed in cerebrospinal fluid rather than in blood. The surface medullary receptors

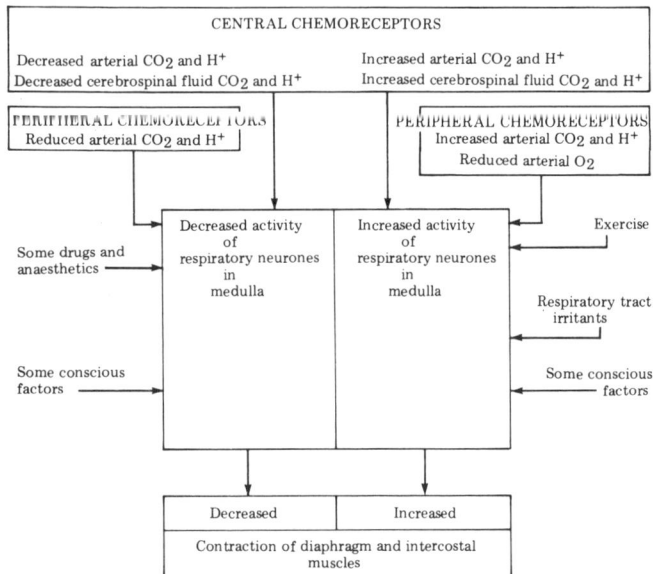

Figure 10.19 Outline of respiratory control.

will stimulate the inspiratory neurones in response to increased CO_2 or H^+ in the cerebrospinal fluid. If CO_2 increases in the blood, CO_2, and ultimately H^+, will increase in the cerebrospinal fluid bathing the brain. The receptor will be stimulated, breathing will be stimulated and the concentration of CO_2 and H^+ will be reduced. These receptors not only regulate respiration but also maintain cerebrospinal fluid H^+ concentration within normal limits. Thus, the surface of the brain is not normally exposed to pH changes caused by CO_2 build-up. The central chemoreceptors do not respond to hypoxia.

b. Peripheral chemoreceptors. These chemoreceptors are located in the carotid body, a small vascular structure near the carotid sinus. Other chemoreceptors are located in the arch of the aorta. Like the central chemoreceptors, these receptors will stimulate the respiratory neurones in response to increased plasma CO_2 and H^+. In contrast to the central chemoreceptors, they will also increase their activity when the partial pressure of oxygen falls. This activity is particularly vital inasmuch as these chemoreceptors are the only source of information that can alert the brain to the danger of hypoxia. If you climb a mountain, your minute volume increases; the reduced amount of oxygen in the air stimulates the peripheral chemoreceptors, which then so stimulate the respiratory neurones that more oxygen is brought into the body.

c. Drugs. Certain drugs and anaesthetics appear to act on the chemoreceptors and, more importantly, on the respiratory neurones themselves, depressing their activity and causing a reduction in the number of impulses to the inspiratory muscles. The newspapers often report that an individual has died from an overdosage of an addictive drug like morphine, heroin or a barbiturate. These drugs have such a powerful action on the inspiratory neurones that they can stop all inspiratory activity, and the individual will die of lack of oxygen because he or she has stopped breathing. Excessive alcohol may be a contributing factor in these deaths. Cessation of breathing is called apnoea.

Some anaesthetics also have an action on the respiratory

centre and tend to depress it. The combination of anaesthesia, muscle relaxants and surgery stress both the cardiovascular and respiratory systems. For this reason respiration is carefully monitored during and after surgery.

Anaesthetised individuals may develop Cheyne–Stokes breathing. This is a cyclic respiratory pattern in which the amplitude of breathing first increases, then decreases, then is followed by a period of apnoea. The cycle continues when the amplitude of breathing increases again. This breathing may also occur in healthy individuals when they ascend to high altitudes or in individuals with heart failure or other diseases. The cause of Cheyne–Stokes breathing is not known.

d. Conscious factors. You can greatly increase your respiratory rate and tidal volume if you consciously choose to. This suggests that the respiratory centre receives impulses from the cerebral cortex, that part of the brain which functions in conscious behaviour. Talking, singing, screaming, whistling all require controlled respiration. You can speak only when you are exhaling. Pain and emotions also affect respiration. We are all familiar with the sigh of relief when we pass an exam, or the sudden gasp that occurs when we are surprised or are injured.

It appears that being conscious of our breathing can affect our respiratory rate; this fact should be considered if you are taking a patient's respiratory rate, since you are possibly changing it if you are making him or her conscious of breathing. Some health professionals take the respiratory rate immediately after they have taken the pulse. They still keep their hand on the patient's radial artery and look at the chest and abdomen, counting the respiratory movements. In this way, the patient is not conscious of the fact that the respiratory rate is being taken.

There are limitations to your ability to control voluntarily your respiration. You cannot choose to hold your breath for more than a few minutes, nor can you perform strenuous exercise or work without increasing your breathing, no matter how much you desire not to do so.

e. Exercise. One way to increase greatly your respiratory rate tidal volume is to exercise. Although you consume more oxygen and produce more CO_2 and H^+ in exercise, the chemical changes are not sufficient to explain the magnitude and swiftness of the respiratory changes. Even if you sit still and just move the fingers of one hand, there is a definite increase in respiration. There are thought to be receptors within the joints and skeletal muscles that increase their rate of discharge when the muscles contract and the limbs move. This increased discharge stimulates the respiratory centre. The rate and depth of the respiratory movements can increase to such an extent that during very strenuous work or exercise, minute volume may exceed 100 l/min. The ability of a patient to exercise can be a real measure of the patient's cardiac and respiratory reserves.

f. Respiratory tract irritants. Should an irritant gain access to the respiratory passageway, the body reflexly tries to get rid of it. If the irritant stimulates the nasal receptors, a sneeze occurs. This is a deep inspiration followed by a strong expiration.

Should the irritant be in the trachea or bronchi, a cough follows. A cough begins with an inspiration after which the glottis closes and the expiratory muscles contract causing great pressure to build up. The glottis opens suddenly and air whizzes out at speeds of 400 mph. The force and speed of this air movement may not only remove the irritant from the respiratory tract, but may also spread it to other individuals. The cough is useful in that it helps remove secretions from the lungs. The mucus brought up in a cough is called sputum and usually includes some mucus from the nasal passages as well as the lungs.

A hiccough results from intermittent spasm in the muscles of the diaphragm. Sometimes hiccoughs are caused by gastric distension in which the stomach presses against the diaphragm. Persistent hiccoughs may be caused by some metabolic conditions, or by tumours or infections which irritate or press upon either the phrenic nerve or the diaphragm. Many times though, the cause (or the cure) of hiccoughs is not known.

Pneumonia is an acute inflammation within the lung tissue and may be caused by bacteria, viruses and even certain parasites, fungi and mycoplasms. The most common pneumonia is caused by pneumococcal bacteria. The presence of the bacteria within the lungs initiates an inflammatory reaction that most often begins in the large bronchi. The inflammation may spread through a single lobe towards the periphery, or spread down the bronchi of several lobes, producing patches of inflammation distributed along the bronchi. The inflammatory process consists of vasodilation of the pulmonary arterioles and capillaries and an outpouring of plasma, fibrin and red and white blood cells in the alveoli and around the respiratory bronchioles and alveolar ducts. The inflamed alveoli are filled with cells and exudate and, therefore, cannot exchange gas. The affected part of the lung is said to be consolidated. In time the exudate and cells are usually resolved and removed.

The significant fact is, however, that the pneumococcal bacteria which causes this inflammation are normal residents of the upper respiratory tracts of many individuals. It has been shown that anywhere from 40 to 70% of the human population are carriers of this virulent bacteria at some time in their lives. Most of the carriers do not get the disease because these bacteria are prevented from getting into the lower airways. Should the body's resistance be reduced by malnutrition or other diseases, the change of getting pneumonia is increased. Intoxication with alcohol or overdosage of drugs reduces the phagocytic ability of the granulocytes and macrophages and depresses the cough reflex which normally would help remove mucus and bacteria.

WHAT REGULATES BLOOD FLOW THROUGH THE LUNGS?

In a physiological sense, the lungs can be thought of as lying between the right heart and the left heart. The lungs receive blood from the right ventricle and return it to the left atrium. The pulmonary circulation differs in some important respects from the systemic circulation. In the Chapter on the circulatory system, it was stated that the left ventricle pumps about 5 litres of blood/min. Of course, this means that if the heart is healthy, the right ventricle also pumps about 5 litres of blood/min. The myocardium of the right ventricle is considerably thinner than that of the left ventricle and generates much less force when it contracts. The resistance of the pulmonary vasculature is also much less. The pulmonary arteries possess less smooth muscle, are thinner and more distensible than the large arteries of the systemic circulation. While the "typical" arterial blood pressure in the systemic circulation is 120/80 mmHg, values in the pulmonary arteries are closer to 20/10 mmHg.

The pulmonary circulation has less resistance than the systemic circulation but equal blood flow. The arterioles of the pulmonary circulation have a sympathetic innervation, but sympathetic vasoconstrictor tone does not appear to play a significant role in setting resistance and regulating flow through the arterioles. Resistance can be changed by changes in the alveolar gas. An increase in CO_2 or a decrease in O_2 within the alveoli tends to increase resistance in the blood vessels supplying those alveoli. This serves as a mechanism where blood flow can be diverted from poorly ventilated alveoli.

Gravity plays an important part in determining what parts of the lungs are perfused with blood. If you are sitting or standing, more pressure will be required to overcome the force of gravity and perfuse the upper parts of the lungs with blood than is needed when you are lying down. Since the right ventricle generates much less pressure than the left, the upper portions of the lung will not be perfused as well as the lower portions.

If large areas of the lung are ventilated but not perfused, the patient will become hypoxaemic. Similarly, the patient may become hypoxaemic if large areas of the lung are perfused but not ventilated.

An area of the lung can be ventilated but not perfused following a pulmonary embolism. Emboli usually form in the veins of the lower limbs, travel to the right heart and often lodge in the pulmonary arteries of the lower lobes. The development of emboli is facilitated by trauma to, or infection of, the veins, or after prolonged inactivity. Pulmonary thromboemboli are not uncommon after surgery, particularly if the patient remains inactive.

Areas of the lung may be perfused but not ventilated if the airways are obstructed. Airways can be obstructed by smooth muscle contraction, tumours, mucus and inflammatory exudates among other things. If the lung tissue loses its normal elasticity and becomes stiff or inelastic, it will not be able to expand as well during inspiration; this will also reduce the amount of ventilation to the affected area.

It is not easy to differentiate between ventilation and perfusion disorders, and in most conditions there is an overlap between imbalances in ventilation and perfusion. For example, following a pulmonary embolism, the ability of alveolar cells to produce surfactant is reduced. This causes an increase in surface tension and collapse of the affected alveoli.

Pulmonary oedema may develop from a variety of causes including infection or damage to the pulmonary capillaries by toxic irritants. More common causes are mitral stenosis and failure of the left ventricle to pump sufficient blood into the systemic circulation. In both cases there is an increase in left atrial pressure which is reflected back through the pulmonary veins into the pulmonary capillaries. This upsets the normal balance of forces at the capillaries. More fluid leaves the capillaries than is reabsorbed into the capillaries or lymphatic channels, and this fluid accumulates in the interstitial space, causing a narrowing or closure of some of the smaller airways. If fluid continues to accumulate, it will enter the alveoli, which greatly reduces the ability of oxygen to diffuse into the bloodstream, so hypoxaemia results.

Treatment of pulmonary oedema is dependent upon the disorder that precipitated it. Usually the oxygen concentration of inspired air is increased. Fluids are restricted and the fluid intake and output are carefully recorded. Rotating tourniquets may be applied to the extremities to keep blood in the limbs and reduce the volume of blood in the heart and lungs. Drugs such as digitalis may be used to improve contractility of the heart and increase cardiac output. Diuretics may be used to mobilise fluid from the lungs.

Pulmonary oedema is not uncommon; it is a pathophysiological process worth understanding.

HOW IS THE RESPIRATORY SYSTEM EXAMINED?

This Section is intended to indicate a few of the whys and wherefores of the standard examination of a patient's respiratory system. For some reason most students have some idea of the significance of blood pressure and heart sounds, yet few students have any idea of the physiology or significance of breath sounds.

The examination begins with observation. The respiratory rate is counted and the noisiness and difficulty, if any, of breathing are noted. If the chest is injured or the airways are obstructed, the accessory muscles of respiration may be used; during inspiration the sternocleidomastoid, scalene and trapezius muscles may be seen to contract. One also notices any abnormal curvature of the spine which might interfere with the normal respiratory movements, and also any lack of symmetry in the chest and its movements. Skin colour is important in that it reflects blood flow through the skin and the amount of saturated haemoglobin in the blood. The pigmentation and texture of the skin may be changed in certain respiratory diseases.

Some questions are routinely asked before or during the examination. They should be asked in an open-ended manner. Even though the examiner may be well informed on the adverse effects of smoking, it is not appropriate to say; "You don't smoke, do you?" It is far better to ask; "How much do you smoke?" Other questions are asked concerning sputum, cough, haemoptysis, pain with breathing and dyspnoea (shortness of breath).

The patient's occupational history is very important as exposure to dusts or environmental toxins in the air can cause respiratory disease, particulary pulmonary fibrosis. The lungs become irritated, inflamed, scarred and fibrotic because of the irritants.

Persistent cough and/or sputum production are always abnormal, and the reasons for them must be found. Sputum can provide valuable clinical information. For example, in a bacterial pneumonia, the bacteria responsible for the pneumonia or respiratory infection may be identified in a stained sputum specimen and appropriate antibiotic treat-ment started on the basis of this identification. Haemoptysis, the coughing up of blood or blood-stained sputum, is reason enough for a thorough investigation to make sure there is no hidden serious disease or tumour responsible.

If you run 1500 metres you may well be short of breath and appropriately so. If you become short of breath trying to climb a single flight of stairs, shortness of breath is not appropriate to the amount of exercise involved. Dyspnoea can have many causes, not all of which are due to respiratory disease. For instance, many people become short of breath when they lie flat in bed but are comfortable and able to sleep when they are propped up with several pillows. This shortness of breath may be caused by heart disease. Sudden onset of dyspnoea in a healthy person might indicate a pneumothorax or a large pulmonary embolus, and recurrent spells of dyspnoea may be associated with asthma.

Percussion of the chest is used to determine the relative amounts of air or solid material in the lungs. The distal two phalanges of the middle finger are placed in the intercostal space parallel to the ribs. The tip of the middle finger of the other hand strikes the distal portion of the second phalanx, which is pressing on the chest. You know that if you tap on an empty box, the sound produced will be different from the dull sound produced if the box is full. In percussion of the lungs, the principle is the same. The examiner percusses from side to side to compare symmetrical areas of the chest. Dullness might indicate a pleural effusion, pulmonary oedema or a pneumonia. By percussion, one can also determine the level of the diaphragm and its ability to contract.

While the examiner auscultates (listens to) the chest with a stethoscope, the patient breathes through the mouth.

Ronchi are wheezing, almost musical sounds that may occur during inspiration or expiration. They are caused by rapid turbulent airflow through narrowed airways. Ronchi are usually more pronounced during expiration because there is then more compression of the smaller airways.

The sounds are frequently heard during an asthmatic attack when smooth muscle contraction narrows the bronchi and bronchioles.

Inspiratory crackles are also called rales, crepitations or moist sounds. If you rub your hair between your fingers near your ear you can approximate the sound of inspiratory crackles. To understand the physical basis for these sounds it will help to know why a balloon makes noise when it bursts — the air pressure within the balloon rapidly equalizes with the pressure outside it. In many diseases the smaller airways may become obstructed because of excessive secretion or by loss of retro-active forces around the airways, such as occurs with increased fibrous tissue in the lung or early pulmonary oedema when the interstial space is filled with fluid. Gas in the alveoli below the obstruction is absorbed into the bloodstream, therefore the air pressure below the obstruction is less than the pressure above. When the smaller airways expand during inspiration there is a series of minature crackling explosions when previously closed airways open suddenly and allow pressure upstream and downstream to equalize. The bigger the breath, the greater will be the number of openings of the previously closed alveoli. The timing of the inspiratory crackles is thought to depend on the nature of the disease.

Bronchial or tubular breath sounds have a blowing quality and are heard in inspiration and expiration. They are hard to describe but are somewhat similar to the sounds heard when the stethoscope is placed over the trachea. Bronchial or tubular breath sounds are heard when there is increased conduction of the sounds from the tubular airways. This can happen in pneumonia when the portions of the lung have become consolidated. The sounds are more easily transmitted from the airways and through the surrounding dense tissue, than when the alveoli are filled with air and the sound of air in the tubular airway is poorly transmitted.

A pleural friction rub is caused by the friction of the two inflamed pleural surfaces rubbing against one another. The sound is a crackling one but more localized than rales, and it occurs during both inspiration and expiration. Breath sounds may be diminished in pneumothorax, or if there is an acute obstruction of a large bronchus so that no air moves in or out of a lung segment.

This respiratory examination is somewhat superficial and a diagnosis can seldom be made on the basis of a single finding. One has to know the condition of the other physiological systems and know the full history of the patient. A chest X-ray is always an invaluable tool in any diagnosis of respiratory disease.

A FEW COMMENTS ON FIRST AID

As has been pointed out numerous times before, brain cells can live no more than a few minutes without oxygen. These cells may be deprived of oxygen by either a failure of the respiratory system to bring oxygen into the body, or a failure of the circulatory system to deliver oxygen.

If you come across an individual who is not breathing, first determine if his heart is beating. Try and feel for a pulse in the extremities. If there is no heart beat, press forcefully, firmly and rhythmically on the lower end of the sternum. The force should be applied at a rate of 1/sec for 10 seconds, and alternated with artificial ventilation after 10 seconds.

The recommended technique for artificial ventilation has changed within the last few years, and it is important that you understand the new technique. First, it is necessary to check the airway to ensure that the tongue, false teeth, vomit, a large piece of food or a foreign object is not blocking a part of the air passageway. Secondly, tilt the head backwards and pull the jaws forward to ensure that the airway is open as much as possible. Thirdly, pinch the nostrils of the victim closed, place your mouth over his or hers and blow forcefully into it — you will have sufficient oxygen in your expired breath. If your breath reaches the victim's lungs, the victim's chest will rise with your forced expiration.

11. The Urinary System

INTRODUCTION

The urinary system consists of:

(1) the two kidneys which form urine;

(2) two ureters which transport the urine to;

(3) the urinary bladder, where it is temporarily stored until it can be eliminated from the body by way of;

(4) the urethra.

The kidneys function to regulate the volume and composition of the body fluids. This is extremely important, for so much of the body is water, which is ever changing because it is almost always continually entering and leaving the body. A healthy individual is said to be in water balance; this means that the water taken in is approximately equal to the fluid output. Measuring fluid intake is a little more complicated than simply recording the volume drunk, as most solid foods have a very high water content and water is also formed in the body by the oxidation of foodstuffs. (Remember:

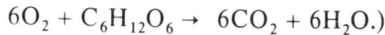

$$6O_2 + C_6H_{12}O_6 \rightarrow 6CO_2 + 6H_2O.)$$

An illustration of normal water balance is given by the following figures:

Intake		Output	
Drinking water	1200 ml	Urine	1400 ml
Water content of food	1000 ml	Loss through skin	600 ml
Water from oxidation	300 ml	Loss through respiration	300 ml
		Water in faeces	200 ml
	2500 ml		2500 ml

Of course, these figures can vary considerably and should be looked upon as a single example and not as average values. Although other systems help maintain the fluid balance of the body, the kidneys are the most important, for they handle the largest volume and can change in response to the changing needs of the body. The kidneys do more than simply adjust the fluid volume; they must rid the body of toxic substances, retain the plasma nutrients and help regulate the concentrations of the plasma ions — Na^+, K^+, Ca^{++}, Cl^-, HCO_3^- and H^+. One scholar has compared the kidney to an efficient homemaker, saving the good and getting rid of the bad. The kidney also has important metabolic functions. These include participation in the metabolism of vitamin D and production of the hormones, erythropoetin and renin.

WHAT IS THE ANATOMY OF THE KIDNEY?

Each kidney weighs about 140 grams, is bean-shaped and measures approximately 11 cm in length, 5 cm in width and is 3 cm thick. They are found on either side of the vertebral column behind the peritoneum on the posterior abdominal wall, are embedded in fat, which protects them, and extend from the 12th thoracic vertebra to the 3rd lumbar (see Figure 11.1). The left kidney is longer, thinner, and lies nearer, and a little higher to the midline than the right. The renal lymphatics blood vessels, nerves and the ureters enter and/or leave via a notch in the medial border of the kidney called the kidney hilum. Situated on top of each kidney like a fool's hat sit the adrenal (suprarenal) glands (see Figure 11.2). Each kidney is covered by a capsule of fibrous tissue.

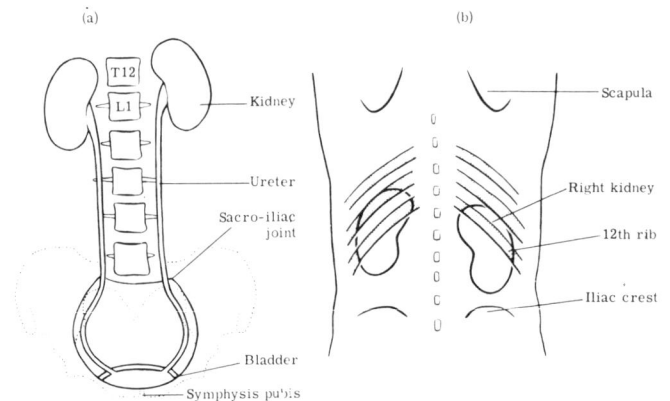

Figure 11.1 (a) Position of the urinary organs in relation to the vertebral column and the pelvis. (b) The position of the kidney as seen from behind

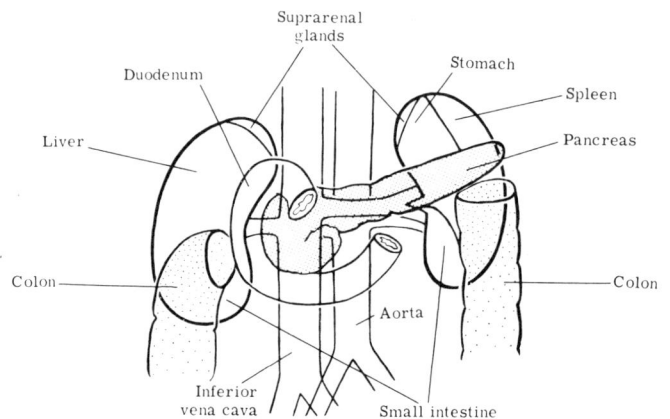

Figure 11.2 Organs related to the kidneys on the posterior abdominal wall.

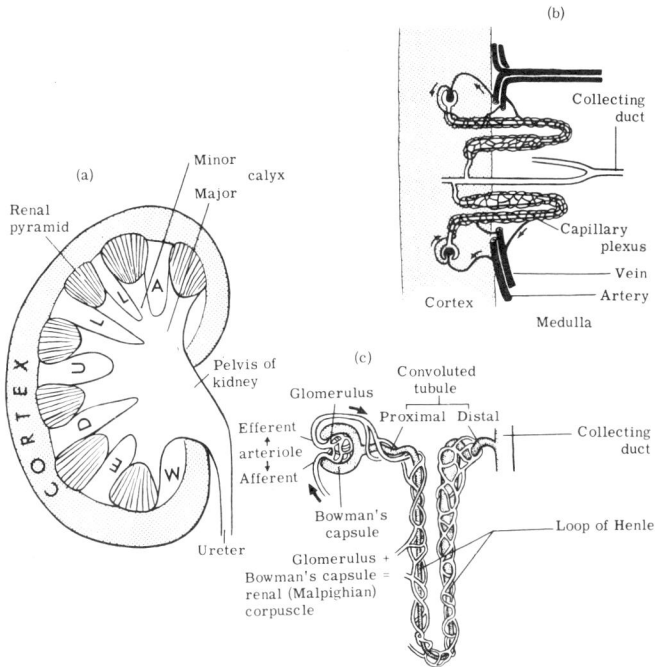

Figure 11.3 (a) Section through the kidney from the medial to the lateral border. (b) Relation of the nephron to the cortex and the medulla. (c) The structure of the nephron.

The outer solid area beneath the capsule is known as the cortex, while the inner area is known as the medulla and contains a series of projections called the pyramids, which converge towards the renal pelvis (see Figure 11.3a). The pyramids are formed from parts of the renal tubules, their blood vessels and the collecting ducts. These structures will be described later. Each pyramid is embraced by a cup-shaped tube called a minor renal calyx. Several of the minor renal calyces come together to form short tubes, the major renal calyces. These major calyces unite to form the renal pelvis which tapers to form the upper end of the ureter.

The gross structure of the kidney is meaningless unless you understand the fine structure of the kidney, for nowhere in the body is the close relationship between structure and function better illustrated. The structural and functional unit of the kidney is the nephron. Each kidney contains about one million nephrons and each nephron contains two parts: the glomerulus and a tubule.

To understand the glomerulus, it is necessary to have a knowledge of the circulation of blood through the kidney. Each kidney is supplied by either the right or left renal artery which arises from the aorta. As the renal artery approaches the hilum of the kidney, it divides and forms several smaller arteries. As these arteries enter the kidney and approach the cortex, they divide again and again forming still smaller arteries that branch out to supply the renal cortex. Within the cortex, they form many small arterioles called the afferent arterioles. These small afferent arterioles give rise to a delicately twisted and folded tuft of capillaries called the glomerulus. The capillaries of the glomerulus then form a single efferent arteriole. The efferent arteriole leaves the glomerulus and then forms a capillary plexus which entwines itself around parts of the renal tubule. The capillary plexus leaves the renal tubule to form a single venule which joins venules from other glomeruli to form small veins.

The efferent arterioles from some glomeruli do not surround the renal tubules but instead form straight capillary-like vessels which plunge into the pyramids and then return to the cortex. They accompany the loops of Henle and are sometimes called vasa rectae. In the cortex, the vasa rectae form small venules which join with other venules to form small veins.

The small veins in turn join to form larger veins. The veins generally accompany the arteries. The renal vein leaves the kidney and joins the inferior vena cava.

If you had to travel through the kidney via the circulatory system you could take the following route: renal artery → smaller arteries → afferent arteriole → glomerular capillaries → efferent arteriole → peritubular capillary plexus or vasa rectae → venule → small veins → renal vein → inferior vena cava.

Two things should be pointed out. First, the circulatory pathway, as described here, has been simplified to a certain extent; there are other possible routes. Second, you should understand that if all the blood that entered the renal artery returned in the renal vein, there would be no urine formation. To understand how urine is formed it is necessary to proceed with a more detailed anatomical description of the glomerulus and renal tubule which form the nephron.

The glomerulus is surrounded by a cup-shaped structure formed from epithelial cells. It has a membrane called either Bowman's capsule or the glomerular capsule (see Figure 11.3c). The glomerular capsule is the expanded, blind end of the proximal tubule. Since the glomerulus and the glomerular capsule have a close anatomical and physiological relationship, the two structures together form the renal (Malpighian) corpuscle.

The fine structure of the renal corpuscle deserves more consideration because of its great importance. There are three different cell types in the glomerulus. The glomerulus begins when the afferent arteriole gives rise to 4–6 capillary loops which, like capillaries everywhere, are formed from endothelial cells. These capillary loops are completely covered by an almost homogenous basement membrane that plays a significant role as a filtration barrier, working with the endothelium to prohibit large molecules from escaping from the circulation at the glomerulus. The basement membrane is in turn covered by epithelial cells forming the visceral layer of Bowman's capsule. In addition to the endothelial cells there are the mesangial cells, which give structural support to the glomerulus and also act as macrophages. Beyond the visceral layer of Bowman's capsule is the urinary space. Beyond this space is the parietal epithelial layer of Bowman's capsule, which begins the formation of the proximal convoluted tubule.

It has been estimated that if the glomerular capillaries were straightened out they would cover an area of about 1.5 m². This means that the two kidneys have a large surface area over which filtration can take place. Small molecules, like water, sodium and chloride ions, can pass through the glomerular endothelium, the basement membrane, the visceral epithelium and the urinary space to enter the proximal convoluted tubule. Blood cells and large molecules, such as the plasma proteins, cannot pass through the layers of the glomerulus and continue on into the efferent arteriole. The proximal convoluted tubule is made up of epithelium with small microvilli sticking into the lumen of the tubule. The proximal convoluted tubule twists and turns through the cortex, then turns and straightens out and heads towards the medulla as the descending limb of the loop of Henle (see Figure 11.3c). The descending limb of the loop of Henle makes a hairpin turn and heads back as the ascending limb of the loop of Henle. The length of the loop of Henle is quite variable; some loops project deep into the renal pyramids, although most loops are short and remain close to the cortex. The ascending limb expands to become the distal convoluted tubule. This tubule twists and turns a short distance before emptying into one of the straight collecting ducts. Several collecting ducts empty into a minor calyx.

At this point, it might be helpful to take another anatomical "journey" through the kidney. Again we begin in the renal artery, go to the smaller arteries, then to the afferent arteriole and finally to the glomerulus. This time we leave the glomerulus by crossing through the capillary endothelial cell, the basement membrane, the visceral epithelial cell and entering the urinary space.

The urinary space becomes the lumen of the proximal tubule. In the urinary space we are surrounded by the visceral epithelial cells of Bowman's capsule. These epithelial cells give way to the epithelial cells of the proximal convoluted tubule. From the lumen of the tubule we can see the many small, finger-like projections which these cells have that facilitate reabsorption. We twist and turn through the proximal tubule, descend and ascend in the loop of Henle and travel through the distal convoluted tubule. At this point we leave the nephron and enter the collecting duct which takes us down the medulla and empties into a minor calyx. Other minor calyces come together and we enter the pelvis of the kidney only to leave the kidney at its hilum and enter the ureter, which takes us to the urinary bladder, where we temporarily end the journey.

You should now have the anatomical basis needed to understand the formation of urine. This rather crude description should not conceal the exquisite structure of the nephrons and their compact arrangement within each kidney. It has been calculated that, if the million or so nephrons in each kidney were taken out and placed end to end, they could line the road running between London and Brighton, a distance of more than 110 kilometres. This long network of tubules enables the nephrons to function efficiently and to reabsorb most of the fluid that was filtered and crossed the glomerulus to enter the renal tubule.

One other structure should be noted: the juxta-glomerular apparatus (see Figure 11.4). Near the glomerulus of most nephrons, the afferent renal arteriole makes contact with the distal tubule of the nephron; this area of contact is referred to as the juxta-glomerular apparatus. The cells of the afferent renal arteriole are specialized in the area of the juxta-glomerular apparatus, and they contain and can release the hormone, renin.

The cells of the distal tubule which are in contact with the afferent arteriole are different from most other cells of the distal tubule and are known as the macula densa. The function of the macula densa is not known but these cells may participate in the release of renin from the cells in the afferent renal arteriole. The macula densa may be sensitive to the amount of sodium in the filtrate in the distal tubule.

Renin is a hormone which acts as an enzyme. (This will be discussed later in this Chapter and in the Chapter on the endocrine system.) Renin converts a plasma protein, angiotensinogen, to angiotensin I, which is converted to angiotensin II as it circulates through the lungs. Angiotensin II is a potent vasoconstrictor and also stimulates the release of aldosterone from the adrenal gland. (This will be discussed later, in the Chapter on the endocrine system.)

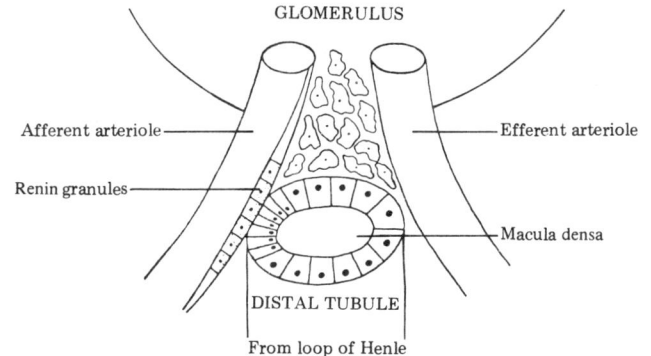

Figure 11.4 The juxta-glomerular apparatus.

An individual may live with just one kidney. If one kidney is removed, the remaining kidney will soon begin to grow and increase its functional efficiency. This is a phenomenon which has never been adequately explained.

WHAT IS URINE?

In 100 ml of urine, about 96 grams of this would be water, 2 grams would be urea. Urea is a nitrogen-containing molecule formed chiefly in the liver as a result of protein catabolism. The amount of urea formed in the liver will vary just as the amount of protein in the diet varies; however, in the healthy individual the amount of urea in the urine will be many times that found in the plasma. The remaining 2 grams urine solids contain other metabolites including creatinine, uric acid and the sodium, potassium and calcium salts of the phosphates, sulphates and chlorides. Sodium is usually less concentrated in the urine than in the plasma, while potassium has several times greater concentration in urine than in plasma. Hydrogen ions are also in the urine; urine tends to be slightly acid. The slight yellow colour of urine results from urochrome, a metabolite of haemoglobin. Since urine contains all these molecules, 100 ml of urine will be heavier than 100 ml of pure water. Specific gravity is defined as the ratio of weight of a substance to the weight of an equal volume of water. The normal specific gravity of urine ranges from 1.015 to 1.030; the greater the specific gravity, the more concentrated is the urine.

The specific gravity also correlates with the number of milliosmoles (mOsm) of solute per litre of urine. The greater the specific gravity of the urine, the greater the number of mOsm in 1 litre of urine. The number of mOsm in 1 litre of plasma is about 280. If a sample of urine has an osmolarity of 800 mOsm, you can see that the urine's specific gravity, as well as the osmolarity of the urine, would be greater than the plasma. The urine would be hypertonic relative to the plasma. If you are not clear on tonicity and osmotic pressure, go back and review them before proceding, as these concepts will become more important.

The molecules that are not normally found in urine are just as important as those which are found there. Blood cells, glucose and proteins are not usually found in the urine in more than trace amounts. If the glomerulus is injured, as it is in nephritis and glomerulonephritis, blood cells and proteins can cross the glomerulus and be lost in the urine.

HOW IS URINE FORMED?

Urine is formed by three basic processes: (A) filtration, (B) selective reabsorption and (C) secretion.

A. Filtration

Filtration at the glomerulus is much like filtration at the capillary. Pressure within the glomerulus is much greater than that in the capillary; the net filtration pressure is about 45 mmHg. Every minute, about 1 litre of blood enters the kidneys and, of this, from 100 to 140 ml of plasma will be filtered at the glomeruli and enter the proximal tubules. The filtrate will contain water, salts, nutrients, glucose, urea and other small molecules which can pass through the glomerular filter. Because of their size, blood cells and the larger proteins will be unable to fit through the glomerular pores and will, therefore, stay in the circulation, enter the efferent arteriole and continue to the renal vein. Disease and injury can destroy the ability of the glomerulus to act as a filter. The relationship between the glomerulus, disease and urine will be discussed later on in this Chapter.

B. Selective reabsorption

If 120 ml of plasma were filtered at the glomerulus every minute and there were no reabsorption, you would have the impossible task of eliminating 172.8 litres/day instead of 1400 ml/day. Since about 172.8 litres/day are filtered and about 1.4 litres/day may be excreted, 171.4 litres/day must be reabsorbed. But how is this brought about?

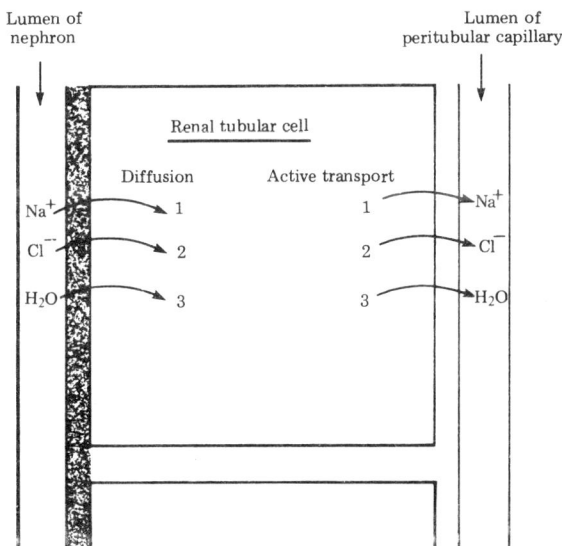

Figure 11.5 Outline of reabsorption in the proximal tubule.

Most reabsorption takes place in the proximal tubule (see Figure 11.5). Sodium ions diffuse into the proximal tubule cells but are rapidly pumped out into the peritubular capillary where they rejoin the blood. The negatively charged chloride ions will follow the positively charged sodium ions. Since these ions move from tubule to capillary and cannot move in the reverse direction, the membrane can be considered to be semi-permeable and the ions osmotically active. Water will now leave the tubule, because of the greater osmotic pressure in the tubular cells, and will follow the ions into the capillaries. In this manner, more than 80% of the filtered water and the ions are reabsorbed before the end of the proximal tubule. Reabsorption continues in the distal tubule and the collecting ducts; however, this is more variable than reabsorption in the proximal tubule because it is under the influence of at least two hormones:

(1) Aldosterone from the adrenal gland.

(2) Antidiuretic hormone (ADH) from the pituitary gland.

The loop of Henle participates by generating osmotic gradients to allow fluid to be reabsorbed from the collecting duct.

The generation of these osmotic gradients in the loop of Henle is significant because it permits the formation of a urine that is hypertonic (more concentrated than the plasma). This is accomplished because water can follow osmotic gradients and leave the collecting ducts, thereby concentrating the urine. The mechanism used to explain this is called the counter-current mechanism; you can understand the mechanism only if you understand osmosis and osmotic pressure (see Figure 11.6).

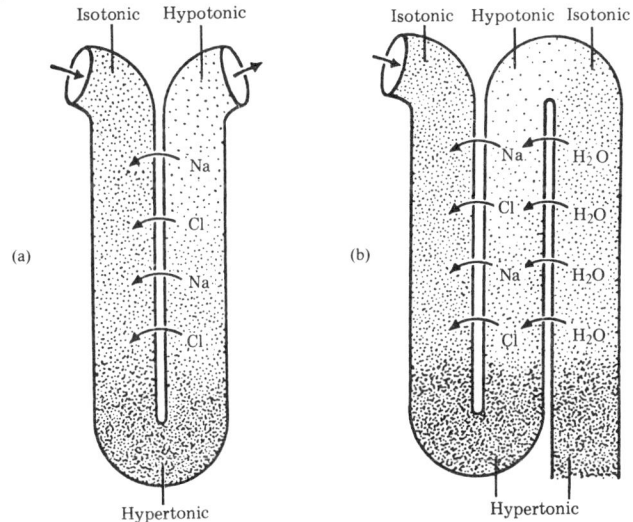

Figure 11.6 The counter-current system of the nephron. (a) The loop of Henle system. (b) The collecting duct system.

Assume that the plasma filtrate in the proximal tubule is isotonic to plasma and has an osmotic pressure of 300 mOsm/litre. This fluid descends in the loop of Henle and, in the ascending limb, sodium is actively pumped out, followed by chloride ions. Because of the special permeability characteristics of the cells in the ascending limb, water cannot follow the sodium and chloride ions. Now assume that the sodium and chloride ions diffuse through the surrounding fluid and the vasa recta and re-enter the descending limb of the loop of Henle. Since salt, but not water, is being added to the fluid in the descending limb, the osmotic pressure will increase. Assume that it increases to 400 mOsm/litre. This fluid, which is hypertonic to plasma, travels down the loop and again, in the ascending limb, more sodium is actively transported out of the ascending limb, diffuses through the surrounding fluid and vasa recta to enter the descending limb of the loop for a second time. Since water has again not followed the sodium and chloride, the osmotic gradient or pressure in the descending limb is increased. Assume that the addition of sodium and chloride to the fluid further down in the descending limb raises the osmotic pressure to 600 mOsm/litre. This hypertonic fluid circulates through the loop and, in the ascending limb, more sodium is pumped out with chloride, but no water. This causes the osmolarity of the fluid in the upper part of the ascending limb to go from 600 to 400 mOsm/litre. The salt diffuses through the lower medulla and enters the descending loop, further increasing the osmotic pressure of the tubular fluid. This process continues with sodium being pumped out, recycling through the fluid in the medulla and the vasa recta, and re-entering the descending limb, causing the fluid which surrounds the collecting duct to be hypertonic.

In the presence of antidiuretic hormone (ADH), the collecting duct can behave as a semi-permeable membrane and water can follow the osmotic gradients. Water leaves the hypotonic fluid in the collecting duct and moves to the hypertonic fluid which surrounds the tubule. This water will move into peritubular capillaries and capillaries surrounding the collecting duct, and be returned to the circulation. If flow through the capillaries is reduced, the reabsorption of water cannot continue. The fluid which remains in the collecting ducts is urine and it can, in the presence of ADH, become hypertonic. Emphasis should be put on the fact that the formation of a hypertonic urine is a means of conserving water.

The reabsorption of some substances is said to be threshold limited. This means that up to a certain point (threshold) all of a substance that is filtered will be reabsorbed. If the filtered load of the substance exceeds the renal threshold, that substance will appear in the urine. Glucose is an example of a threshold substance. Normally, no glucose is found in the urine although 100 mg of glucose, or more, may be filtered at the glomerulus every minute. This is because the normal filtered load of glucose is less than the renal threshold for glucose, and all glucose which is filtered will be reabsorbed by the nephron. In the disease, *diabetes mellitus*, plasma glucose levels rise to very high levels and the filtered load of glucose may exceed 200 mg/min. As the threshold for glucose has been exceeded, any glucose filtered past this point will appear in the urine.

If the plasma glucose is 100 mg/100 ml of plasma, and if 100 ml of plasma are filtered in 1 minute, then 100 mg of glucose is filtered in 1 minute, as:

100 mg glucose/100 ml plasma × 100 ml plasma/1 min = 100 mg glucose/1 min.

Since the kidneys are capable of reabsorbing 100 mg of glucose in 1 minute, there won't be any glucose in the urine.

If the plasma glucose is abnormally high, say 300 mg/100 ml, and 100 ml of plasma are filtered every minute, then 300 mg of glucose will be filtered in 1 minute, as:

300 mg glucose/100 ml plasma × 100 ml plasma/1 min = 300 mg glucose/1 min.

If the kidneys can reabsorb 200 mg of glucose in 1 minute and 300 mg of glucose are filtered in 1 minute, then about 100 mg of glucose will enter the urine every minute.

These calculations are not particularly difficult but it is worthwhile to go through them and understand them, as they help in getting at the concept of clearance (to be discussed later).

In Africa, long before *diabetes mellitus* was understood, a man was considered to be ill if ants came to his urine. The ants would not be drawn to the urine of a healthy man, for it would not contain sugar.

C. Secretion

This process involves the movement of molecules from capillary to tubule cell to lumen, even though the concentration in the tubule may be greater than that in the capillary. Hydrogen and potassium ions are commonly secreted into the tubules, so the kidneys play an important role in the regulation of hydrogen ion concentration (pH). These are complicated metabolic processes.

The secretion of the hydrogen and potassium ions is in some way co-ordinated with or coupled to the reabsorption of sodium. Thus, as the positive sodium ion is reabsorbed from the tubule, another positive ion, either potassium or hydrogen, is secreted into the tubule to take its place. The kidney also contains the enzyme, carbonic anhydrase, which produces carbonic acid (H_2CO_3). The carbonic acid breaks down to hydrogen ion, which can be secreted into the lumen of the kidney tubule, and bicarbonate ion, which can accompany the sodium ion into the peritubular capillaries.

The Table below shows a comparison of some substances in the plasma and in the urine of a "typical" adult. The differences between urine and plasma are, of course, caused by reabsorption and secretion processes that take place in the kidney.

Substance	Plasma (mEq/l)	Urine (mEq/l)	24-hour urine (grams)
Sodium	140	120	4.0
Potassium	4.5	50	3.0
Calcium	4.5	5	0.2
Chloride	105	180	9.5
Bicarbonate	25	15	1.5

Substance	Plasma (mg/%)	Urine (mg/%)	24-hour urine (grams)
Glucose	80	0	0
Urea	25	1600	24
Creatinine	1.5	100	1.5

There can be considerable variation in many of these values. In addition to the substances listed above, many drugs and toxic substances are removed from the circulation by the kidney. If the kidneys are diseased or damaged, the ability of the kidney to secrete can be reduced. This may make drug therapy hazardous, for the concentration of certain drugs can rise to harmful levels.

It is worth emphasizing again that whatever is retained by the kidney is returned to the blood, and whatever is excreted in the urine is eliminated from the blood. Thus, the composition of the blood is dependent upon what is retained and what is excreted by the kidneys. This relationship is illustrated in the case of kidney failure when the kidneys "shut down" and no longer function effectively. Urea, which normally is excreted in the urine, is retained and its concentration may rise to more than 30 times its normal plasma concentration.

The normal blood urea concentration is 15–35 mg/100 ml or 2.5–5.8 mmol/l. The blood urea is not quite the same as blood urea nitrogen or BUN. This determination is used in some laboratories, and the normal values are 8–17 mg/100 ml. The formula for converting BUN to urea is: Urea = BUN × 2.14.

Uraemia refers to the retention of urinary constituents in the blood, and to the toxic condition which they produce. It is often marked by nausea, vomiting, weakness, headache, mental confusion and sometimes even convulsions, coma and death. The signs and symptoms of uraemia are not all due to increased concentrations of urea in the blood. Other metabolites of protein are thought to be involved and for some of the effects there is no known explanation.

Uraemia is caused by the failure of the kidneys to excrete metabolic waste. Renal failure may be caused by conditions that lead to greatly reduced blood flow through the kidney. The kidney cells, like other cells of the body, may die or decrease in efficiency if they don't get adequate oxygen via the blood. Renal failure can follow after excessive blood loss through haemorrhage, reduced blood flow due to heart failure or because of hypertension. In the last-mentioned condition, the renal arterioles are pathologically narrowed, so flow is reduced. Some other causes of renal failure include mismatched blood transfusions and carbon tetrachloride and mercury poisoning. Diabetes and gout may also have devastating effects on the kidney.

Artificial kidney machines have been developed. They can reduce the amount of urea and wastes and help control the volume of fluid in the body when the kidneys are not able to function adequately. The process is known as dialysis or haemodialysis and requires the use of artificial, semipermeable membranes. Dialysis is really used on the principles of osmosis. Blood leaves the body, usually from an arterial cannula, and enters the machine where it is "cleaned" and returned to the circulation. Patients on dialysis are not cured of their renal disease, must be very careful with salt, fluid and protein intake, and have many other problems. The machines cannot synthesize erythropoietin, participate in the metabolism of vitamin D or do so many other things that living kidneys do. They are expensive and require constant care and maintenance, so their use has been quite limited. And yet their development has been an advance, considering the alternative for the people now dependent on them.

WHAT INFLUENCES URINE FORMATION?

A. Hormones. Hormones have a powerful effect on urine formation. Antidiuretic hormone (ADH) acts on the cells of the distal convoluted tubule and collecting duct. In the Section on reabsorption, the generation of osmotic gradients was discussed. It was pointed out that the collecting duct is surrounded by a hypertonic fluid. ADH acts on the cells of the distal convoluted tubule and collecting duct to increase their permeability to water. This action on the collecting duct is particularly important because more water than salt leaves the collecting duct, and a hypertonic urine results. If ADH secretion by the posterior pituitary gland is increased, the collecting duct cells will be more permeable to water, and more water will leave the collecting duct to return to the circulation.

An illustration of the importance of ADH is provided by patients who lack ADH and have the disease *diabetes insipidus.* Ancient physicians used the term, diabetes, for any disease in which there is a large urine flow. Insipidus means dull or tasteless. Patients with diabetes insipidus can each day pass as many as 20–30 litres of hypotonic urine, which is tasteless. Lest they die of dehydration, these patients are forced to drink many litres of fluid a day to replace the fluid they have lost. Some people have excessive urine flows because they drink excessive amounts of water. Their kidneys are intact, but these persons suffer from some psychological disorder.

How does the kidney change its output of urine in response to large differences in the fluid intake? There are cells in the hypothalamus of the brain which synthesize ADH and transport it to the posterior pituitary gland. These cells are sensitive to the osmotic pressure of the blood. Should you drink a large volume of water, the osmotic pressure of the blood will fall, as you are simply diluting the blood by adding water to it. This reduction in osmotic pressure is sensed by the hypothalamus and the output of ADH from the pituitary is reduced. With less ADH, less water is reabsorbed in the distal tubule and collecting duct. This leads to the formation of a less hypertonic, more dilute urine; the volume of the urine is increased. Conversely, if you do not drink water, the osmotic pressure of the blood will increase. This is sensed by the hypothalamus and it triggers the release of more ADH. The additional ADH causes more water to be reabsorbed, which tends to lower the osmotic pressure of the blood. Urine volume is reduced and it is more hypertonic.

The hypothalamus also receives information on the volume of blood in the circulatory system. Should the blood volume be reduced, ADH secretion will be increased. Thus, if a person haemorrhages, blood volume will be reduced and the increased ADH will cause more water to be reabsorbed. This will work to increase the blood volume. Stress can also increase ADH secretion. The kidney, responding to ADH, thus works to keep the blood volume and the osmotic pressure of the blood constant.

Aldosterone is synthesized and released by cells in the cortex of the adrenal gland. It acts upon the distal convoluted tubule to increase its reabsorption of sodium (and water) and simultaneously increases the secretion of potassium. The control of aldosterone secretion is not completely understood. More will be said about it in the Chapter on the endocrine system.

The role of renin and angiotensin II was mentioned earlier in this Chapter. Angiotensin II is a potent stimulator of aldosterone release, so the release of renin can lead to increased plasma volume because of the increased sodium and water reabsorption triggered by aldosterone (see Figure 11.7). The macula densa may be involved in stimulating renin release when sodium concentration in the distal tubule is low. Renin release is also stimulated when pressure in the afferent renal arteriole is reduced. There is some evidence that increased pressure in the afferent renal arteriole causes stretching of the cells in the juxta-glomerular apparatus, and this stretching inhibits the release of renin. Conversely, when pressure in the afferent renal arteriole falls, stretching of the cells is reduced and renin release increases. Since angiotensin II not only stimulates aldosterone release but also causes constriction of the arterioles, there is a link between the kidneys and arterial blood pressure. For example, if the renal artery is clamped so flow and pressure in the afferent renal arterioles are reduced, there will be a renin--angiotensin II–aldosterone-mediated rise in arterial blood pressure. If flow through the renal artery is blocked by the atherosclerotic plaque, renin release will be increased and hypertension may result. The role of the kidney and its relationship to essential hypertension is not known.

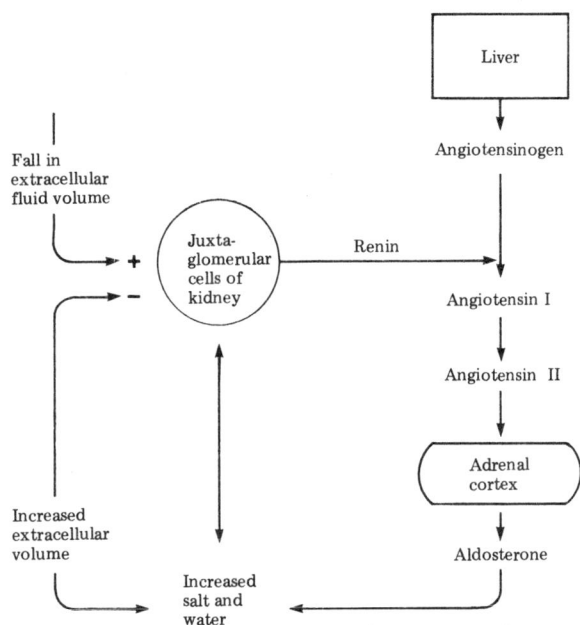

Figure 11.7   Outline of factors influencing renin release.

Other hormones, including prolactin and growth hormone, act on the kidney to retain water and salt.

B. Diuretics. Diuretics are chemical agents which lead to an increased urine output. Some diuretics act by reducing sodium reabsorption. If sodium remains within the tubule, water will have to remain also, for there will be less of an osmotic gradient to pull the water out. Other diuretics are molecules which can be filtered at the glomerulus, enter the tubule and yet cannot be reabsorbed, or are only partially reabsorbed. If the renal threshold for glucose is exceeded, as it is in diabetes mellitus, the glucose molecules which are not absorbed are osmotically active and will retain water within the tubule. These glucose molecules and their accompanying water molecules will be excreted in the urine. This explains the excessive urine production, polyuria, seen in severe diabetes.

Mannitol is an example of an osmotic diuretic; it is filtered at the glomerulus but is not reabsorbed in the tubule. There are also diuretics which work by antagonizing the action of aldosterone.

Alcohol produces a diuresis because it inhibits ADH release from the pituitary gland, and thus reduces water reabsorption from the distal tubule and collecting duct.

By increasing urine output, diuretics reduce blood volume and may thereby reduce blood pressure.

C. Blood flow. Filtration at the glomerulus is dependent on the blood pressure and blood flow to the kidney. Should the renal artery or the afferent arterioles be blocked or constricted, flow to the nephrons will be reduced and filtration and urine formation will go down.

The kidney possesses the ability to autoregulate the amount of blood which perfuses it. The kidney can compensate for changes in mean arterial pressure so that if arterial pressure is reduced, the arterial vessels of the kidney compensate for this and dilate, so flow is increased. The vessels can also constrict in response to increases in the mean arterial blood pressure, so flow through the kidney will not be increased. These factors work to keep renal blood flow and glomerular filtration rate relatively constant. There are circumstances, however, in which renal circulatory auto-regulation does not predominate, and blood flow through the kidneys is reduced.

Under resting conditions about one-fifth of the cardiac output or about one litre of blood/min goes to the kidneys. Since this is such a large volume, most changes in kidney flow will be reductions in flow rather than increases. The renal arterioles are well supplied with smooth muscle which has a rich sympathetic innervation. Sympathetic stimulation and adrenaline cause constriction of the renal arterioles, reduction in kidney blood flow and glomerular filtration. Renin output may also be increased as a result of this constriction. Physiological causes of reduced blood flow to the kidneys include exercise, pain and stress.

Clinically, there are two common causes of greatly reduced renal blood flow: loss of blood volume and heart failure. Loss of blood volume may occur with injury, surgery, diarrhoea and acute haemorrhage. Following loss of blood volume or failure of the heart to pump adequate amounts of blood, there may be an intense constriction of the renal arterioles and the reduction of renal blood flow. This can have at least two consequences. Firstly, the kidney may not be adequately perfused with blood, so the kidney cells die of anoxia. Secondly, the rate of glomerular filtration falls with the reduction of renal flow, and substances which are normally excreted can rise to toxic levels.

The renal arterioles may constrict following burns, blood loss or as the result of a traumatic injury. This constriction is brought about by sympathetic stimulation to the arterioles. This stimulation may be so intense that the renal arterioles become so narrow that adequate amounts of blood may not reach the kidney and renal cells may die. Again, urine formation is dependent upon perfusion with blood. One of the first signs of renal shut-down is a failure to eliminate urine.

HOW IS URINE ELIMINATED?

Urine travels via the collecting ducts to the ureter. Each ureter consists of an outer coat of fibrous tissue, a middle layer of smooth muscle and an inner layer of transitional epithelium, lying in loose connective tissue. Contraction of the smooth muscle squeezes the urine the 25–30 cm distance to the urinary bladder. The bladder is a pear-shaped structure lying in the pelvic cavity behind the symphysis pubis (see Figure 11.8). Its size and position will change depending on the amount it contains. The wall of the urinary bladder is similar in structure to the ureter, except that the muscle layer is thicker and the superior portion is covered by peritoneum. The two openings of the ureters into the bladder and the urethral orifice form a triangle which is called the trigone of the bladder (see Figure 11.1a). At the beginning of the urethra there is a sphincter of skeletal muscle which is normally contracted to prevent the urine from leaving.

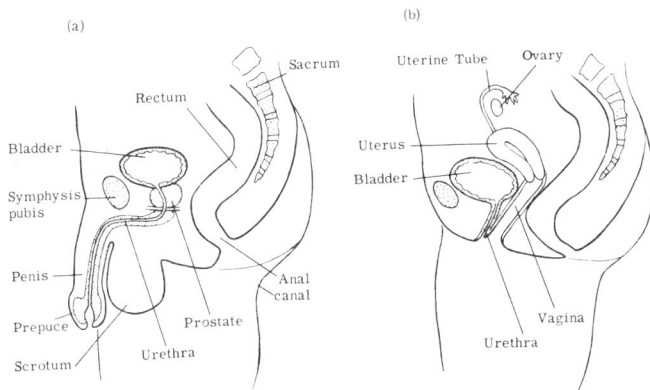

Figure 11.8 The pelvic cavity. (a) Sagittal section through the male pelvis. (b) Sagittal section through the female pelvis.

As more and more urine dribbles into the bladder, the bladder expands like a balloon. The stretch of the bladder wall stimulates receptors in it and initiates a reflex. Impulses leave the bladder via the nerves travel to the spinal cord and stimulate other neurones within the cord. These neurones, belonging to the parasympathetic division of the autonomic nervous system, will stimulate other neurones which send impulses back either to the musculature of the bladder causing it to contract, or to the motor neurones which normally stimulate the sphincter, and inhibit them, causing the sphincter to relax.

In the adult, impulses from higher conscious centres in the brain are necessary for the sphincter to be inhibited and open; in infants, the brain has only a minor influence so they will urinate whenever the bladder is full, regardless of social circumstances or parental convenience. About 300 ml will trigger the reflex in an adult bladder, though if it is inhibited, the bladder can stretch to hold nearly 2 litres.

The urethra is the single tube which extends from the bladder to the external orifice. The male and female urethra differ slightly in structure, for the male urethra functions in reproduction while the female urethra is used exclusively for urine transport (see Figure 11.8). Both contain an inner epithelial lining on top of loose connective tissue, a surrounding layer of smooth muscle and areolar connective tissue. The male urethra ends in the tip of the penis, while the female urethra reaches the exterior between the labia minor in front of the vagina.

Sensory nerves are also found in the urethra. Should some of the salts in the urine become insoluble and form little stones, they can block the tubes and cause an extreme amount of pain as the body tries to eliminate them. They are often called kidney stones.

Incontinence is the inability to control micturition. Diseases or injury of the spinal cord or nerves to and from the bladder and psychological factors may cause incontinence.

HOW IS KIDNEY FUNCTION AFFECTED BY DISEASE?

The kidney does highlight the exquisite relationship between structure and function. Disease may distort this relationship and thereby affect not only the kidney and its function but also other organ systems. Some understanding of these disease processes helps one's understanding of the normal kidney function and the relationship of the kidney to other systems.

Glomerulonephritis refers to disease in which the glomeruli of the kidney become inflamed. The response of the glomerular cells to inflammation is both variable and complex but usually involves the proliferation of the mesangial and endothelial cells, infiltration by white cells and disruption of the integrity of the basement membrane. As a result of these changes, the glomerulus can no longer act as an efficient filter and cannot prevent proteins and even blood cells from being lost in the urine. The reduction in the plasma proteins reduces the force favouring reabsorption in the tissue capillaries; this contributes to the oedema which develops and which is often detected by noticing puffy eyelids and a swollen face. Other complex factors cause increased salt and water reabsorption which also contributes to the oedema.

Many cases of glomerular nephritis have an immunological origin. Antibodies may be made to the glomerular basement membrane or, more commonly, antigen–antibody complexes may be caught in the glomeruli and initiate an inflammatory response. Glomerulonephritis may follow infections caused by certain strains of β-haemolytic streptococcus. The pathological process is thought to be similar to the development of rheumatic heart disease which follows β-haemolytic streptococcus infection.

The term pyelonephritis refers to an infectious process affecting both the renal tissue and the renal pelvis. Bacteria may gain access to the kidneys by following an ascending route — urethra, urinary bladder and ureters. Urinary catheters can be a source of infection. Infection often results if there is an obstruction in the urinary tract. Urine, like water, becomes contaminated if it is stagnant, and urine can be an excellent growth medium for some bacteria. The high osmotic pressure in the medulla prevents the white blood cells from responding effectively. The signs and symptoms of pylonephritis are variable and change with the severity of the disease. Fever and difficulty in urinating are not uncommon.

The kidney has important hormonal and metabolic functions and, if it is diseased, it may not be able to carry these out. Anaemia may result from the kidney's failure to produce erythropoietin, a hormone which stimulates red blood cell production by the bone marrow. The kidney plays an important part in calcium metabolism. It reabsorbs calcium, excretes phosphate and completes the metabolism of vitamin D. Osteomalacia is not an uncommon complication of certain renal diseases.

HOW IS KIDNEY FUNCTION TESTED?

Because of the importance of kidney function, clinical tests have been developed to evaluate it. Some tests are rather simple, others are more complex. Testing the urine for protein is really a check on the integrity of the glomerular membranes. Other tests investigate the ability of the kidney to form a dilute urine following ingestion of a water load and to form a concentrated urine following a period of water restriction. As the urine becomes more dilute, its specific gravity will fall and approach that of water, while a more concentrated urine will have a greater specific gravity. Injections of ADH (vasopressin) should increase water reabsorption by the kidney and lead to the formation of a concentrated urine with a high specific gravity.

The phenolsulphthalein (PSP) excretion test measures the ability of the kidney to secrete a dye, PSP. The patient receives an injection of PSP, urine samples are collected and the concentration of the dye in the samples is measured. Of course the secretory ability of the kidney may be normal, but because of poor perfusion of the kidney, the concentration of dye will be low.

Perhaps the most useful information about kidney function comes from the glomerular filtration rate (GFR). The GFR indicates how much plasma is filtered at the glomeruli in 1 minute. Information on the GFR comes from clearance studies. This concept is best illustrated by an example. In certain situations it is necessary to measure precisely the GFR. The latter may be learned by administering into the blood, at a constant rate, a compound known as inulin. Inulin is filtered at the glomerulus; there is no secretion or reabsorption of inulin in the renal tubules. This means that all the inulin filtered at the glomeruli will end up in the urine. Inasmuch as inulin is neither secreted nor reabsorbed, the input of inulin from the plasma into the tubules in 1 minute will equal the output of inulin in the urine in 1 minute. The inulin *output* is given by:

(ml of urine formed in 1 minute) × (concentration of inulin in 1 ml urine)

and the *input* of inulin is given by:

(ml of plasma filtered in 1 minute) × (concentration of inulin in 1 ml plasma)

Since, with inulin, input equals output, we can set an equation:

(ml plasma filtered/min) × (inulin concentration/ml plasma) = (ml urine formed/min) × (inulin concentration/ml urine)

We can find out three of the four variables in the equation: inulin concentration in urine, volume of urine, inulin concentration in plasma. By knowing three of the four variables, an equation can be set up giving us the fourth variable, the amount of plasma filtered at the glomeruli in 1 minute. Thus:

$$\text{amount of plasma filtered in 1 minute} = \frac{\begin{pmatrix}\text{ml of urine} \\ \text{formed in 1} \\ \text{minute}\end{pmatrix} \times \begin{pmatrix}\text{concentration} \\ \text{of inulin in} \\ \text{urine}\end{pmatrix}}{(\text{concentration of inulin in plasma})}$$

The following example with actual numbers might help. The plasma concentration of inulin is 1 mg/ml, the concentration of inulin in the urine is 120 mg/ml and the urine volume is 1 ml/min. By the equation:

$$\text{amount of plasma filtered in 1 min} = \frac{(120 \text{ mg/ml}) \times (1 \text{ ml/min})}{1 \text{ mg/ml}} = 120 \text{ ml/min.}$$

You might think that 120 ml is a lot of plasma to be filtered in 1 minute. It is an "average" value for a typical adult. At this rate, the entire circulating plasma volume is filtered and reasborbed twice within a single hour. Through selective reabsorption and secretion of this large volume, the kidney is able to protect the internal environment.

Students who are puzzled as to why inulin concentration in the urine is so much greater than in the plasma forget that the kidneys reabsorb water, not inulin, and that this leads to the increase in inulin concentration.

Since inulin is neither filtered nor reabsorbed, the amount of plasma filtered as determined by inulin will equal the GFR and this is often referred to as the inulin clearance. Other compounds have their own clearances too. The clearance of a compound may be defined as that amount of plasma containing the amount of that compound found in the urine in 1 minute.

The formula for clearance (Cl) is given as

$$Cl_x = \frac{U_x V_x}{P_x}$$

Cl_x refers to the clearance of compound x;
U_x is the urinary concentration of x;
V_x is the volume of urine formed in 1 minute;
P_x is the concentration of x in the plasma.

The development of this formula is the same as that used for inulin previously. The clearance of other compounds, of course, will not equal that of inulin if they are secreted or reabsorbed in the tubule. If the compound is secreted into the tubules, the clearance of that compound will be greater than that of inulin. If the compound is reabsorbed, its clearance will be smaller than that of inulin.

In clinical practice, inulin is seldom used to assess kidney function. The compound, creatinine, is used because it is released by muscle tissue into the plasma at a constant rate in a resting individual. Creatinine also behaves like inulin in that it is filtered at the glomerulus but not reabsorbed or secreted. An increase in the plasma concentration of creatinine indicates a failure of this compound to be excreted by the kidneys and might indicate kidney failure. Urea clearance is often also used.

You might be glad now to know that you don't need a computer and a chemistry laboratory to derive useful information from urine. Since the time of Hippocrates, men and women have been studying urine samples and gathered invaluable information from them. Today, a urinalysis is a relatively inexpensive but useful procedure that is almost routinely used as a screening test.

Haematuria refers to the presence of red blood cells in the urine. Less than 0.5 ml/l of blood in the urine may give the urine a hazy, ground glass appearance. More than 0.5 ml/l of blood will give the urine a reddish tinge. This can happen with many conditions including tumours of the urinary tract, infection or inflammation of the kidneys and in certain non-renal diseases, such as haemophilia. If there has been extensive breakdown of red blood cells in the circulation, haemoglobin and its metabolites may be lost in the urine and this can give the urine a dark, reddish brown colour similar to that of the cola drinks. Other abnormalities of haemoglobin metabolism can also colour the urine.

The presence or absence of glucose and ketone bodies in the urine can usually be tested by dipping a chemically treated paper in the urine and watching to see if it changes colour.

Protein in the urine can be tested for by either heating the urine and coagulating the protein, or adding acid to the urine and precipitating it.

The ability of the kidneys to concentrate urine (remove water) is indicated by the specific gravity test and is tested with a hydrometer. The first voided urine in the morning usually has a specific gravity greater than 1.018. In the absence of any glucose or protein, the urine with a specific gravity over 1.025 shows that the ability to concentrate is present.

The urine may be spun in a centrifuge and the sediment, if any, examined under the microscope. Red or white blood cells may be present, the latter often being associated with urinary tract infections. Bacteria or yeasts may be seen. Sometimes, casts are seen in the sediment. These are replicas of the renal tubular, collecting duct or lumens. Blood cells, proteins or even kidney cells which have entered the tubule, precipitate in the tubule and therefore are cylindrical in shape and resemble the lumen of the tubule in which they are formed. All casts are not always pathological but often they indicate renal disease and point to the kidney as the site of disease rather than to the other structures in the urinary system.

12. pH and Hydrogen Ion Regulation

INTRODUCTION

At the beginning of this book, the importance of homeostasis was pointed out. For life to continue, the concentration of glucose, salts and hydrogen ion within the blood must be kept within certain limits in spite of changing conditions. Hydrogen ion regulation is particularly necessary, for hydrogen ions are much more reactive than the other cellular and plasma positive ions, and small changes in hydrogen ion concentration can radically alter the structure of enzymes, reduce their efficiency and also affect other proteins and distort cellular structures. Should this happen to a significant extent, metabolism will be disrupted and life will cease.

WHAT IS pH?

The pH of a solution indicates the hydrogen ion concentration of that solution. Specifically, pH is defined as the negative logarithm (log) of the hydrogen ion concentration. In discussing pH and logs we are really discussing different ways of expressing numbers.

The words un, uno and moja are, respectively, the French, Spanish and Swahili words for the numeral, one. As all languages differ, there is a variety of words for the same numeral — and so it is with pH. Some examples might help illustrate how numbers may be expressed in different ways:

$$10 = 10^1 = 10$$
$$10 \times 10 = 10^2 = 100$$
$$10 \times 10 \times 10 = 10^3 = 1000$$
$$10 \times 10 \times 10 \times 10 = 10^4 = 10\,000$$
$$10 \times 10 \times 10 \times 10 \times 10 = 10^5 = 100\,000$$

$$1/10 = 1/10 = 10^{-1} = 0.1$$
$$1/10 \times 1/10 = 1/100 = 10^{-2} = 0.01$$
$$1/10 \times 1/10 \times 1/10 = 1/1000 = 10^{-3} = 0.001$$
$$1/10 \times 1/10 \times 1/10 \times 1/10 = 1/10\,000 = 10^{-4} = 0.0001$$
$$1/10 \times 1/10 \times 1/10 \times 1/10 \times 1/10 = 1/100\,000 = 10^{-5} = 0.00001$$

The shortest way of writing the numbers is to express them as a function of the base 10. For example $10^5 = 100\,000$. The number 5 is the power (exponent) of 10, the base. The exponent 5 says that the base 10 must be multiplied by itself 5 times to equal 100 000.

The logarithm of a number is the power (exponent) which 10 must have to equal that number. The logarithm of 100 is 2 because 10 with an exponent of 2 equals 100. The preceding statement is written in mathematical shorthand:

$$\log 100 = 2.$$

Again, $\log 0.01 = -2$ because 10 with an exponent of -2 equals 0.01. The logarithmic form of notation is useful in dealing with very large or small numbers. Thus:

$$\log 100\,000 = 5, \quad \text{because } 10^5 = 100\,000$$
$$\log 0.000\,000\,01 = -8, \quad \text{because } 10^{-8} = 0.000\,000\,01$$
$$\log 0.000\,000\,000\,001 = -12, \quad \text{because } 10^{-12} = 0.000\,000\,000\,001$$
$$\log 0.000\,01 = -5, \quad \text{because } 10^{-5} = 0.000\,01$$

Before proceeding further you should recall from your course work in mathematics the rule of signs which states that the product of two negative quantities is a positive quantity:

$$(-3) \times (-2) = 6$$
$$(-100) \times (-10) = 1000$$

You now have the essential material for understanding the definition of pH. Let us apply the definition to an example:

Assume you have 1 litre of solution and the hydrogen ion concentration of the solution is 0.000 01 Molar (0.000 01 mole/l). The definition states that the pH is the negative logarithm of the hydrogen ion concentration. First, it is necessary to express the H^+ concentration as a logarithm. The logarithm of $0.000\,01 = -5$. To get the pH we must take the negative of the logarithm and this is where the rule of signs is applied, for $-(-5) = 5$. You can now state that the pH of a solution with a hydrogen ion concentration of 0.000 01 mole/l is 5.

The following table lists the hydrogen ion concentration of various solutions and the corresponding pH.

Hydrogen ion conc. mole/l	Log. hydrogen ion concentration	pH
0.1	−1	1
0.01	−2	2
0.001	−3	3
0.0001	−4	4
0.000 01	−5	5
0.000 001	−6	6
0.000 000 1	−7	7
0.000 000 01	−8	8
0.000 000 001	−9	9
0.000 000 000 1	−10	10
0.000 000 000 01	−11	11
0.000 000 000 001	−12	12
0.000 000 000 000 1	−13	13
0.000 000 000 000 01	−14	14

This Table lists whole numbers, but not all logs or pH values are whole numbers. Another point that should be understood is that a little change in pH can mean a large change in hydrogen ion concentration. Therefore, a solution with a pH of 2 does not have twice as many hydrogen ions as a solution of pH 4, but has 100 times as many. A solution with pH 3 has $\frac{1}{10}$ the hydrogen ion concentration of a solution with pH 2.

The average (standard) pH of blood is 7.4. If the pH is 7.4, the hydrogen ion concentration is 0.000 000 04. The pH of arterial blood in a resting, healthy adult is almost always between 7.35 and 7.45; a pH less than 6.8 or more than 7.8 is seldom compatible with life. It may not be intuitively obvious to you unless you really know logarithms, but the difference in H^+ concentration as you go from pH 6.9 to pH 7 is not the same as the difference in H^+ concentration as you go from pH 7.7 to pH 7.8. If you wish, you can go to a mathematical text and calculate the H^+ concentration from the pH. The H^+ concentration is expressed in nanomoles per litre (nmol/l). One nanomole is 10^{-9} mole. If the pH is 7, there are 10^{-7} moles of H^+ (100 nmol/l).

pH	H^+ concentration nmol/l
6.90	126
7.00	100
7.10	79
7.20	63
7.30	50
7.40	40
7.50	32
7.60	25
7.70	20
7.80	16

It may not be necessary to memorize the above Table, but it is, however, necessary to understand that as pH decreases, H^+ concentration increases, and that the relationship between pH and H^+ is not a simple inverse relationship. If SI units are adopted, the usage of pH might be dropped in favour of expressing H^+ concentration in nanomoles. As it stands today, pH is more commonly used than nanomoles.

If you were to measure the pH of a solution of pure distilled water, you would find that the pH is 7. This means that in 1 litre of water there would be 0.000 0001 or 10^{-7} moles of H^+. But where do the H^+ in water come from? In 1 litre of water there will be millions upon millions of water molecules. At any one instant, however, a very few of these water molecules will dissociate into a hydrogen ion, H^+, and a hydroxyl ion, OH^-. The hydrogen ion and hydroxyl ion will come together again to form water, but while this is happening, another water molecule will dissociate, only to come together again.

The water molecule is said to be in equilibrium with the hydrogen and hydroxyl ions and can be written:

$$H_2O \rightleftharpoons H^+ + OH^-$$

The equation does not mean that the concentration of water and ions are equal, for there are many more undissociated water molecules than ions, but that for every water molecule which dissociates, a hydrogen ion and hydroxyl ion will associate into a water molecule. (Actually, some H^+ form a hydronium ion, H_3O^+, but as a practical matter we can consider all H^+ to be free or unbound.)

Water with a pH of 7 is said to be neutral. If the pH is below 7, the solution is called acidic; if the pH is greater than

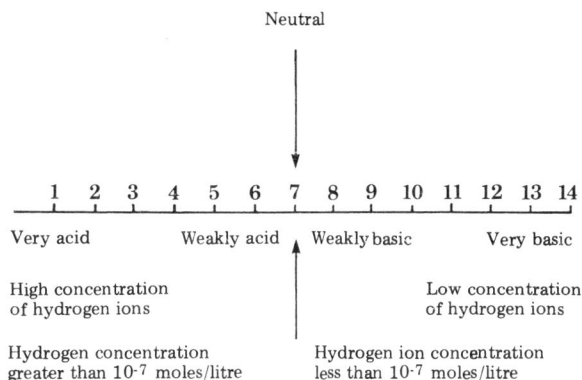

Figure 12.1 pH scale showing acidic and basic solutions.

7, the solution is called basic or alkaline (see Figure 12.1). Increasing the hydrogen ion concentration of a solution increases the acidity and lowers the pH. Reducing the hydrogen ion concentration reduces the acidity and raises the pH. Acidic and basic are adjectives and do not tell what an acid or a base is. A modern definition is: an acid is any compound which frees or gives up a hydrogen ion; a base is any compound which accepts a hydrogen ion. Acid molecules are hydrogen ion givers, while basic molecules are hydrogen ion acceptors. Although all acids are alike in that they give up a hydrogen ion, there are degrees of generosity among different acids — some give up their hydrogen ion reluctantly, whereas others readily give it up. Carbonic acid and hydrochloric acid are both acids because they give up hydrogen ions, but hydrochloric acid completely dissociates into H^+ and Cl^-, while only a few carbonic acid molecules give up hydrogen ions at any one time.

The hydrogen ion and the bicarbonate ion will recombine to form carbonic acid; hydrogen ion and the chloride ion will not.

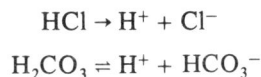

$$HCl \rightarrow H^+ + Cl^-$$

$$H_2CO_3 \rightleftharpoons H^+ + HCO_3^-$$

An acid which gives up most of its hydrogen ion is a strong acid; an acid retaining most of its protons is described as a weak acid. HCl is a strong acid and H_2CO_3 is a weak acid.

It is also necessary to know the definition of a buffer. A buffer is a chemical substance which helps resist changes in the pH of a solution. It can bind H^+ when the pH falls and releases H^+ when the pH rises. Proteins can act as buffers. Assume there are two solutions, A and B, which have the same pH (see Figure 12.2). Solution A has proteins, whereas solution B doesn't. The same number of hydrogen ions are added to both A and B but the fall in pH is greater in B than in A. This is because A has proteins which can act as a buffer.

The next example is more complex. Let us take a solution of lactic acid; lactic acid is a weak acid. If there are five molecules of lactic acid (LH) in solution, only one of these molecules may dissociate into the negatively charged lactate ion (L^-) and the H^+ at any one time. (These numbers are only used for illustration.) To this solution we add three molecules of the salt, sodium lactate, NaL (see Figure 12.3). Since sodium lactate is a salt, all of its molecules will

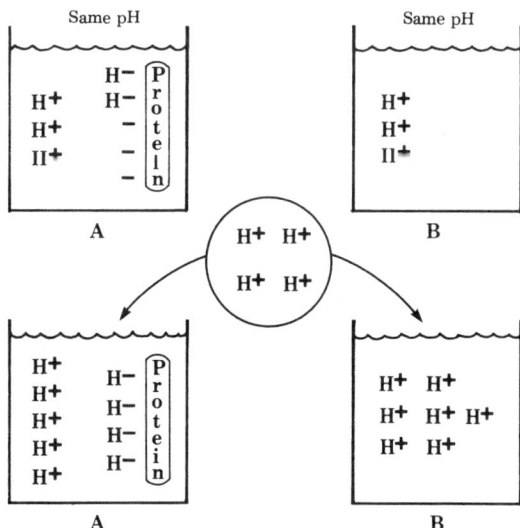

Figure 12.2 The action of a protein buffer.

stays within the range of 7.35–7.45. In a sense, healthy persons stay in hydrogen ion balance just as they stay in water balance. Hydrogen ions are constantly being produced as a result of metabolism and constantly being eliminated through the lungs and the kidneys. The rate of hydrogen ion formation is not constant. We take in different amounts of acids in our food and increase our acid production every time we exercise. Drugs, hormones and disease can influence our metabolism to produce more or less hydrogen ion. In a healthy person, increased H^+ production means increased buffering and increased elimination of H^+ so the individual can stay in hydrogen ion balance. As stated before, this balance is necessary, for hydrogen ions are more reactive than other positive ions, and H^+ can have significant effects on the charge and shape of proteins and therefore can powerfully influence enzyme activity.

Hydrogen ion concentration can influence the other plasma ions. For instance, if H^+ increases, some of the additional H^+ ions will displace K^+ ions from the intracellular proteins that bind K^+. This increased K^+ in the plasma is called hyperkalaemia and can have many serious consequences. One of the most serious effects of hyperkalaemia is on the excitability of the cardiac muscle and its conducting tissue. The heart may have arrhythmias or have reduced contractile force as a specific effect of hyperkalaemia.

The plasma proteins, such as albumin, normally bind some H^+. If the amount of H^+ is reduced, some of the free Ca^{++} ions in the plasma will bind to the negatively charged protein. This reduction in free Ca^{++} can affect cellular excitability and may lead to tetany. (Calcium and potassium are discussed in the Chapter on the endocrine system.) There are three control systems operating to keep H^+ within the normal limits:

dissociate into Na^+ and L^- ions; this will not change the pH, as it neither adds nor subtracts H^+.

Sodium lactate is, in fact, a buffer because it helps prevent pH changes. The solution (b) now contains four molecules of undissociated LH, $4L^-$, $3Na^+$ and one $H+$. To this we add three molecules of the strong acid HCl, which completely dissociates into $3H^+$ and $3Cl^-$ ions. If it were simply a matter of adding H^+, there would be a total of $4H^+$; however, the buffer helps resist this change in H^+ concentration by accepting the H^+. The lactate ions will accept some H^+ and form the weak lactic acid. The sodium lactate buffer would also help resist pH changes if H^+ were removed. Removing H^+ would increase the release of H^+ from LH.

HOW IS THE pH IN THE BODY REGULATED?

The pH of the arterial blood in a normal individual usually

a. The blood buffers. The plasma proteins and haemoglobin are important buffers, binding H^+ when pH decreases, and releasing H^+ when pH rises. (The proteins within cells also have a buffering capacity.) Another

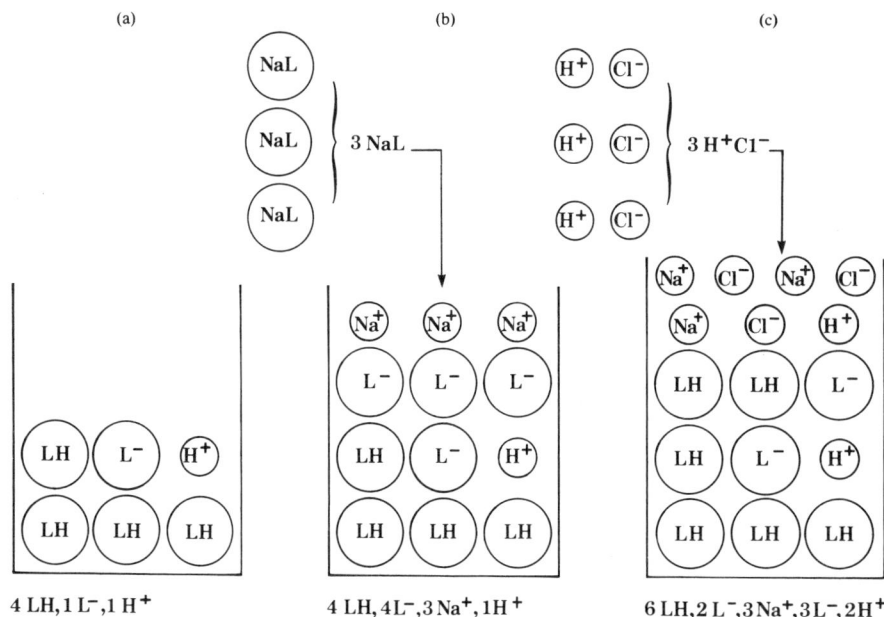

Figure 12.3 The action of sodium lactate as a buffer. Because solution b is buffered, the addition of $3H^+$ to a solution with $1H^+$ gives a total of $2H^+$ in solution c. The other $2H^+$ have combined with $2L^-$ to form the weak acid LH.

important buffer in the plasma is the bicarbonate ion which is part of the bicarbonate buffer system.

The addition of H^+ to HCO_3^- forms carbonic acid, H_2CO_3. This acid, like lactic acid, is a weak acid. It differs from other weak acids in one very important way. Carbonic acid, unlike other acids, can be broken down by the enzyme, carbonic anhydrase, to CO_2 and H_2O. The CO_2 can be excreted in the lungs. The concentration of the reactants determines the concentration of the products.

The normal value of HCO_3^- in arterial blood is 24–26 mEq/l. The concentration in venous blood is slightly higher because of the addition of CO_2 from the tissues. If acid or H^+ is added to the blood, the bicarbonate concentration will decrease, and more CO_2 and H_2O will be formed. If CO_2 is added to the blood, HCO_3^- will increase, while if CO_2 is taken away, HCO_3^- will decrease.

In a sense, the respiratory system adds CO_2 to the blood when ventilation is reduced, and it removes CO_2 from the blood when ventilation is increased.

b. The respiratory system. You remember from the Chapter on the respiratory system that the respiratory centre is responsive to both H^+ and CO_2. Increases in H^+ and CO_2 lead to increased activity in the respiratory neurones and increased removal of CO_2.

The respiratory controls are related to the bicarbonate buffer system of the blood. If there is an increased H^+ there will be increased respiratory activity and the reaction series will go in the direction of CO_2 and water formation. The CO_2 will be exhaled.

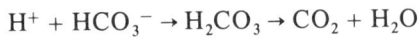

$$H^+ + HCO_3^- \rightarrow H_2CO_3 \rightarrow CO_2 + H_2O$$

increased respiratory system   increased removal
stimulation   in expired air

If there is a defect in the respiratory control system and CO_2 cannot be eliminated, it will accumulate. An increase in CO_2 will cause more H_2CO_3 formation and thus more H^+. The reaction will thus proceed toward increased acidity.

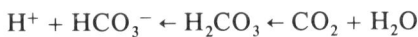

$$H^+ + HCO_3^- \leftarrow H_2CO_3 \leftarrow CO_2 + H_2O$$

respiratory system
not stimulated by
increased H^+ in
certain diseases

In arterial blood, the partial pressure of CO_2 is about 40 mmHg. In venous blood it is a little greater because CO_2 is added by the tissues. You can, within limits, control the amount of CO_2 in your blood and therefore adjust your own pH. If you hold your breath, your tissues will keep producing CO_2, but your lungs will not eliminate it. The longer you hold your breath, the more CO_2 will accumulate. This increased CO_2 will lead to an increase in HCO_3^- and H^+ and a decrease in pH.

If you choose to hyperventilate (take frequent deep breaths), you can influence the chemistry in a different direction. By increasing your ventilation, both the partial pressure of CO_2 and the amount of CO_2 in your blood will decrease. The decrease in CO_2 will lead to a decrease in H^+ and HCO_3^-, so pH will increase.

c. Renal control. The kidneys play some role in H^+ regulation. The kidneys are able to secrete H^+ and they either increase or decrease their secretion of HCO_3^-. Renal regulation is not as rapid as respiratory control however, but the kidneys are important in long range changes. The changes taking place during mountain climbing illustrate the functional changes that the kidney is capable of. The higher you climb the mountain, the more your respiratory rate increases. This is because at higher altitudes there is less oxygen and the chemoreceptors are stimulating the respiratory centre because of the lower partial pressure of O_2 in the blood. This oxygen hunger not only increases the ventilation rate but also reduces the H^+, HCO_3^- and CO_2 in the blood.

The kidneys respond to this alkalosis by reducing their H^+ secretion into the urine and increasing their secretion of HCO_3^- in the urine. By reducing the amount of plasma HCO_3^-, the kidneys permit the blood H^+ to increase faster, as there is less buffer to resist the change, so the blood becomes more acid.

If a patient has lung disease in which there is a defect or decrease in alveolar ventilation, the partial pressure of CO_2 will increase and the H^+ and the bicarbonate in the blood will also increase. The kidneys respond to these changes by increasing their secretion of H^+ and increasing retention of HCO_3^-. The additional HCO_3^- helps buffer the increased H^+. A rule to remember is that for every H^+ secreted by the kidney, one HCO_3^- is returned to the blood.

The kidneys can also produce ammonia, NH_3, which is able to act as a buffer and form the ammonium ion, NH_4^+. The reaction goes:

$$NH_3 + H^+ = NH_4^+$$

The ammonium ion will be excreted with a chloride ion. If there is some non-respiratory condition making the blood acid, there will be an increased production of NH_3 by the tubular cells. Hydrogen ions will be lost in the urine, in ammonium salts, and the urine will become more acid.

WHAT CAN CAUSE ABNORMAL pH CHANGES IN THE BODY?

There are four categories of disturbances in which the pH regulating systems of the body are upset. These four disturbances are metabolic acidosis, respiratory acidosis, respiratory alkalosis and metabolic alkalosis.

a. Metabolic acidosis. This condition is characterized by a decrease in HCO_3^-, pH and the amount of CO_2 in the blood. The condition may be caused by an excessive production of acid, such as takes place in diabetes mellitus when keto acids are formed. The loss of HCO_3^- from the intestines during diarrhoea, and the failure of the kidneys to excrete H^+, may also lead to metabolic acidosis. Treatment of metabolic acidosis is aimed at correcting the underlying disorder. In severe metabolic acidosis, sodium bicarbonate may be infused.

A person with metabolic acidosis may have an increased respiratory rate. This is because the increased hydrogen ion concentration stimulates the chemoreceptors and leads to greater respiratory activity. This helps reduce the acidosis by increasing the removal of hydrogen ion via carbonic acid and CO_2.

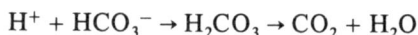

$$H^+ + HCO_3^- \rightarrow H_2CO_3 \rightarrow CO_2 + H_2O$$

If a person is in shock or circulatory failure and the tissues are not adequately perfused with blood, pH will decrease. This is because of the increased production of lactic acid by the tissues. (Lactic acid will be produced by anaerobic metabolism when O_2 levels are inadequate and tissues are hypoxic.) Often these people are so ill they are not able to compensate for the acidosis by increasing their breathing. This illustrates why it is often necessary to know arterial pH, CO_2 and O_2 levels, for the information they provide can be useful in monitoring a patient's respiratory and cardio-vascular status.

b. Respiratory acidosis. This condition is characterized by a primary increase in the amount of CO_2 in the blood, so the pH falls and the bicarbonate ion concentration increases. Respiratory acidosis may be caused by a condition in which the secretion of CO_2 by the lungs is hindered. CO_2 accumulates and this leads to an accumulation of $H_2CO_3^-$ and H^+:

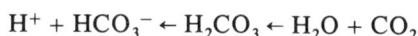

$$H^+ + HCO_3^- \leftarrow H_2CO_3 \leftarrow H_2O + CO_2$$

Respiratory acidosis may be caused by anything that depresses the activity of respiratory neurones in the brain; drugs and anaesthetics may do this. Another cause is weakness of the respiratory muscles or obstruction of the respiratory tract itself. In all forms of respiratory acidosis there is impaired alveolar ventilation. Treatment involves correcting the underlying disorder and may in some cases involve use of mechanical ventilators.

The kindneys try to compensate for the respiratory acidosis by increasing their secretion of hydrogen ion and returning more bicarbonate to the blood. This additional bicarbonate helps to buffer the increased hydrogen ion.

There are significant clinical differences between acute and chronic respiratory acidosis. Many patients with chronic obstructive lung disease, such as emphysema, are not able to compensate fully for the increased retention of CO_2. They may live in a state of continual, mild respiratory acidosis. The acidosis can suddenly become severe if a respiratory infection or pneumonia sets in.

c. Respiratory alkalosis. This condition is characterized by a primary decrease in the plasma CO_2, with a decrease in HCO_3^- and an increase in pH. In this disorder the ventilation exceeds the needs of the body and thus reduces the blood acidity:

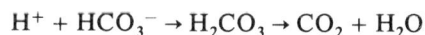

$$H^+ + HCO_3^- \rightarrow H_2CO_3 \rightarrow CO_2 + H_2O$$

Respiratory alkalosis may occur when there is hypoxia (revise the mountain climbing example) or fever. It may also occur during great fear as a result of some emotional disorder. A simple treatment is to have the affected individual breathe in and out of a paper bag. In so doing, he or she retains and inhales CO_2.

The kidneys respond to respiratory alkalosis but their response takes a matter of days before it can compensate for the alkalosis. The kidneys increase their excretion of HCO_3^- into the urine. This reduces the amount of bicarbonate in the blood and thereby reduces its buffering capacity which leads to a decrease in blood pH.

d. Metabolic alkalosis. This is a relatively rare condition in which there is a primary increase in HCO_3^- and an increase in pH. The condition may arise following prolonged vomiting and loss of gastric HCl, in certain endocrine disorders and after prolonged diuretic treatment. Patients who have gastric suction through nasogastric tubes can also develop a metabolic alkalosis. Again, treatment of the alkalosis requires treatment of the underlying disorder.

The increased pH of the blood means that there is a reduction in the H^+ and CO_2 which normally drives the respiratory system. The reduction in H^+ and CO_2 leads to a reduction in respiratory rate. The respiratory system thus compensates for the metabolic alkalosis by retaining more CO_2, which leads to a decrease in pH because:

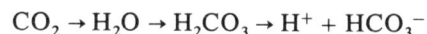

$$CO_2 \rightarrow H_2O \rightarrow H_2CO_3 \rightarrow H^+ + HCO_3^-$$

Of course, it is not always possible to classify an acidosis or alkalosis as purely metabolic or purely respiratory. Often these are components of both. You must have a knowledge of the initial problem and an understanding of how the body attempts to compensate for it before you look at the pH, HCO_3^- and CO_2 and diagnose a specific disorder. As an example, if a person takes an overdose of aspirin, a metabolic acidosis results because aspirin is an acid. The metabolic acidosis can lead to a profound respiratory alkalosis as the respiratory system attempts to compensate. From normal to acid to alkaline to normal again, with buffers, lungs and kidneys doing their part. Everything is connected.

13. The Digestive System

INTRODUCTION

We all eat, and yet the foods we eat are as many and diverse as the peoples of the earth. No doubt the pastoral Masai of East Africa think it strange that Europeans drink water that has been artificially coloured and sugared and which bubbles when poured from its bottle. The Masai prefer to drink slightly sour, charcoal-flavoured milk, sometimes mixing it with the blood of their cattle for added nutrition. The digestive tract, however, has no cultural or aesthetic preferences. West African foo-foo and French pastry are both broken down into individual glucose molecules by identical, carbohydrate-digesting enzymes and both share the same metabolic fate, if not the same consumer, culture and geography.

The digestive tract is essentially a long, hollow tube into which litres of acid and alkaline secretions, lubricating and emulsifying agents, and enzymes are secreted to ease and hasten the passage and breakdown of food into small, easily absorbed molecules. These secretions are produced by the salivary glands, the liver, pancreas and digestive tract itself. Movement is accomplished by contraction of muscles within the tract's walls. These contractions not only propel the food onwards but also mix and physically break down the larger food particles. The work of the digestive system is completed with the expulsion of faecal material which consists of water, a small amount of undigested food, bacteria and unabsorbed secretions. The whole process is controlled and co-ordinated by the nervous system and a series of related neural and hormonal reflexes.

WHAT IS THE ANATOMY OF THE DIGESTIVE SYSTEM?

The digestive tract includes the mouth, pharynx, oesophagus, stomach, small and large intestine. Secretions from the salivary glands, liver, pancreas and intestinal tract itself are emptied into the system.

A. The mouth

The lips surround the opening of the mouth. They consist mainly of muscle fibres and fibro-elastic tissue; their dark reddish colour results from the fact that the epithelium is relatively transparent and capillary blood shows through, so the lips, conjunctiva of the eyes and nail-beds are good spots to gauge oxygenation of the blood. The roof of the mouth is formed by the hard and the soft palates; the floor is made up mainly of the tongue and the walls are formed by the cheek muscles, the main one being the buccinator muscle (see Figure 13.1a). All the mouth is lined with a mucous

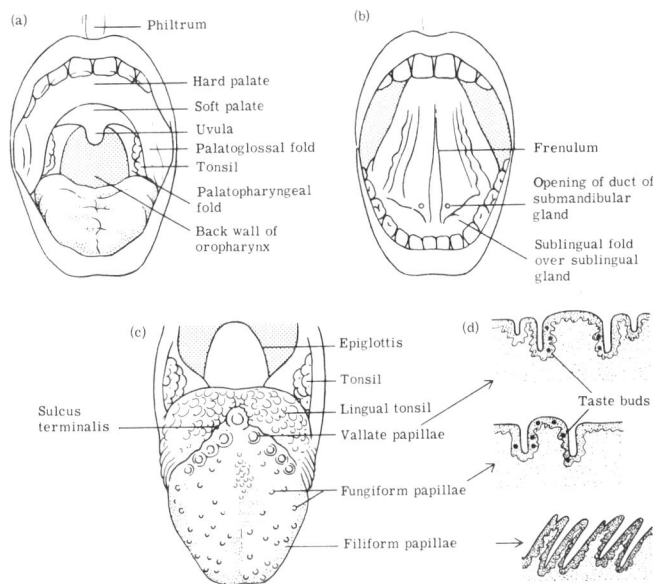

Figure 13.1 The mouth. (a) Inside the mouth. (b) The floor of the mouth after elevating the tongue. (c) The upper (dorsal) surface of the tongue pulled well forwards. (d) The papillae of the tongue.

membrane. If you look inside a friend's mouth you can easily see the uvula, a curved fold of mucous membrane which hangs from the middle of the soft palate. From each side of the uvula, two folds of mucous membrane pass downwards to the side of the mouth and form the posterior boundary of the mouth. Between the two folds is a mass of lymphoid tissue called the palatine (oral) tonsil (see Figure 10.5a). These tonsils are strategically placed to guard the entrance to the digestive and respiratory tracts so that antibodies against infecting agents can be produced. The tonsils are occasionally overrun with bacteria and viruses and become sources of infection themselves, necessitating their removal.

The tongue is mostly striated muscle wrapped in a special mucous membrane and attached at its back to the hyoid bone and towards the front to the mandible by the frenulum (see Figure 13.1b). The mucous membrane contains special projections known as papilla but more commonly called taste buds (see Figure 13.1c and d), which contain nerve endings that respond to the different tastes — sweet, salty, sour and bitter — and transmit taste information to the brain, via the glossopharyngeal (IX) or facial (VII) nerve. The striated muscle of the tongue is supplied by the hypoglossal (XII) nerve. Movements of the tongue are important in moving and mixing the food and in speech.

The position of the tongue in the mouth depends on the extrinsic muscles of the tongue and the muscles of the hyoid bone. The genioglossus muscle is fan-shaped, arises from the symphysis of the mandible and inserts into the front of the tongue and the hyoid bone. This muscle makes up the bulk of the posterior part of the tongue and its action is to depress the tongue. The mylohyoid muscle and the geniohyoid also run from the mandible to the hyoid bone. The mylohyoid muscles form a sling which supports the tongue, and can elevate the tongue, forcing it backward as occurs during swallowing. The geniohyoid muscle protrudes from the hyoid bone, thereby shortening the floor of the mouth. The styloglossus muscle arises from the styloid process of the temporal bone and inserts into the inferior aspect of the tongue. It draws the tongue backward. These extrinsic muscles of the tongue are innervated by fibres of the hypoglossal nerve (cranial nerve XII). The palatoglossus muscle arises from the soft palate and inserts into the side of the tongue. It is innervated by the accessory nerve (cranial nerve XI).

Many cells of the mucosa of the tongue are constantly being rubbed away by friction and must be replaced. It is not surprising that some diseases show their first signs in the tongue. This is particularly true of diseases caused by vitamin deficiency. The deficiencies hinder the process of cellular renewal and replacement.

Many glands secrete saliva into the mouth. The three largest pairs of salivary glands are the parotid, submandibular and sublingual glands (see Figure 13.2). The parotid glands are the largest and lie below the ear next to the ramus

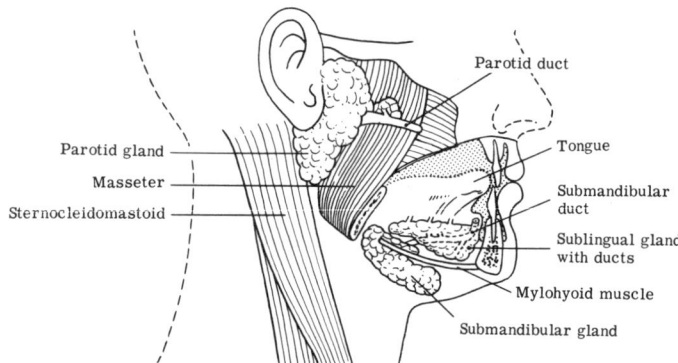

Figure 13.2   The salivary glands.

of the mandible. They have large ducts running through the cheeks and entering the mouth in the space between the cheeks and the second upper molars. In the disease, mumps, a virus infects the salivary glands (particularly the parotids), causing them to swell. The submandibular gland (sometimes called the submaxillary gland) lies on the inner surface of the mandible, near its angle. The sublingual glands lie behind that part of the lower jaw which makes up the chin. Like the submandibular glands, they empty their secretion into the floor of the mouth.

The 1–2 litres of secretion produced daily by the salivary glands is called the saliva. It is mostly water, but contains some salts, mucus and the enzyme, salivary amylase, which begins the digestion of starch. Saliva has many functions including:

(1) The moistening and lubrication of food so it can be easily swallowed and less damaging to the lining of the oesophagus.

(2) Prevention of tooth decay by washing the mouth of food which bacteria might feed upon.

(3) Increasing the taste of foods by dissolving them so they make contact with the taste receptors.

When an excessive amount of fluid has been lost, the glands stop secreting and the sensation of thirst arises.

These glands have both a parasympathetic and sympathetic innervation. Stimulation of the parasympathetic nerve supply to the salivary glands produces an abundant flow of watery saliva. The effects of sympathetic stimulation are more variable. Fibres of the facial nerve (cranial nerve VII) provide the parasympathetic innervation to the submaxillary and sublingual glands. The parasympathetic innervation of the parotid gland comes chiefly from the glossopharyngeal nerve fibres (cranial nerve IX). Sympathetic fibres to these glands originate in the spinal cord. Most leave the spinal cord in the thoracic region and ascend in the sympathetic chain ganglia and then synapse. Fibres from these ganglia ascend in the neck and ultimately reach the glands.

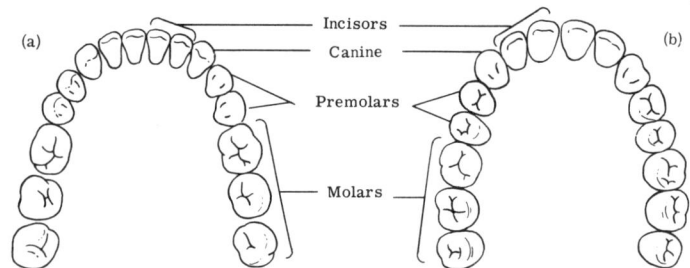

Figure 13.3   The teeth. (a) Upper jaw. (b) Lower jaw.

The adult mouth contains 32 teeth. There are 4 pairs of chisel-shaped incisors in the front of the mouth for holding food, 4 pointed canines, 8 premolar teeth (each with two cusps) and 12 molar teeth (each with four or five cusps) (see Figure 13.3). The premolar and molar teeth are for chewing and grinding food. The dental formula for one half of the jaw is:

Incisor	Canine	Premolar	Molar	
2	1	2	3	upper jaw
2	1	2	3	lower jaw

The molars are in the back of the mouth. The third molars are the last teeth to appear in the adult, so they are often referred to as wisdom teeth. Since they are such late arrivals there is often insufficient room for them so they cannot develop properly and must be removed.

Each tooth consists of:

(1) A crown visible above the gum.
(2) A root which binds the tooth into the bone of the jaw.
(3) A neck where crown and root meet (see Figure 13.4).

Most of the tooth is made of a calcified connective tissue called dentine. The visible part of the tooth is covered by an enamel reputed to be the hardest substance in the body. In the centre of each tooth is a space called the pulp cavity

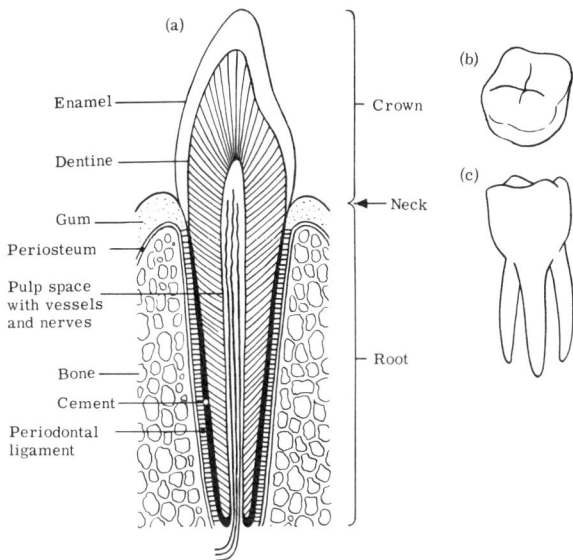

Figure 13.4 (a) Section through a typical tooth. (b) The upper surface of a crown molar (c) An upper molar with three roots.

containing nerves, blood vessels and specialized cells which make dentine for the life of the tooth.

Although the enamel is strong it can be decalcified and destroyed by the acids and enzymes produced by bacteria which have not been washed away by saliva or removed by brushing. This area of destruction is called a cavity or a dental carie. Cavities are neither harmful nor painful if restricted to the outer layer of enamel, but if the decay continues and reaches the dental pulp, infection, inflammation and oedema can result causing pain and the death of the pulp. Bacteria can also enter the blood stream and spread infection throughout the body if they reach the pulp.

An infant begins life toothless. From the 6th month to the 28th month, the primary (milk) teeth make their appearance. It is possible to determine the age of an infant by the number of milk teeth he or she has. The dental formula of milk teeth for one side of the jaw is:

Incisor	Canine	Molar	
2	1	2	upper jaw
2	1	2	lower jaw

There are 20 milk teeth. Begining with the 6th year and continuing sometimes as long as into the 21st year, the primary teeth are shed and replaced by permanent teeth.

B. The pharynx

The pharynx is a muscular cavity lined with mucous membrane. It can be divided into the oropharynx, nasopharynx, and laryngopharynx (see Figure 10.5a). The oropharynx is posterior to the mouth and is a common passage-way for both food and air. The nasopharynx and laryngopharynx were described in the Chapter on the respiratory system.

The muscular wall of the pharynx has two divisions: an inner longitudinal layer, which helps elevate the soft palate, and an outer circular layer, which constricts the pharynx. The inner longitudinal layer is formed from the stylopharyngeus and palatopharyngeus muscles. The arrangement of the superior, middle and inferior constrictors has been compared to that produced by stacking three flower pots, one within the other (see Figure 10.5b). All these muscles are important in swallowing. The stylopharyngeus and the palatopharyngeus both insert on the thyroid cartilage of the larynx. These muscles along with a muscle of the soft palate, the tensor palati, are important in raising the larynx during swallowing. The three constrictors and the palatopharyngeus are supplied by fibres from the vagus nerve (cranial nerve X). The stylopharyngeus is supplied by fibres from the glossopharyngeal nerve (cranial nerve IX).

C. The oesophagus

The oesophagus (gullet) connects the pharynx to the stomach and is found in the median plane of the body between the vertebral column and the trachea (see Figure 10.5a). The opening to the oesophagus is normally closed by the cricopharyngeal sphincter; in the act of swallowing, the muscle relaxes and the entrance is opened.

There are four layers found within the oesophagus which continue with modification throughout the rest of the tract. These four layers are: (1) the innermost mucosa, surrounded by (2) the submucosa, followed by (3) the muscular layers and (4) the outermost layer, called the serosa (see Figure 13.5).

(1) The innermost layer of the mucosa is epithelium. In the oesophagus and anus it is stratified epithelium, for it serves a protective function since very little absorption takes place. The epithelium from the stomach to the rectum is columnar epithelium and is better suited for absorption and secretion. Immediately behind the epithelium is some loose connective tissue which supports the epithelium and contains blood and lymph capillaries to transport the absorbed nutrients and

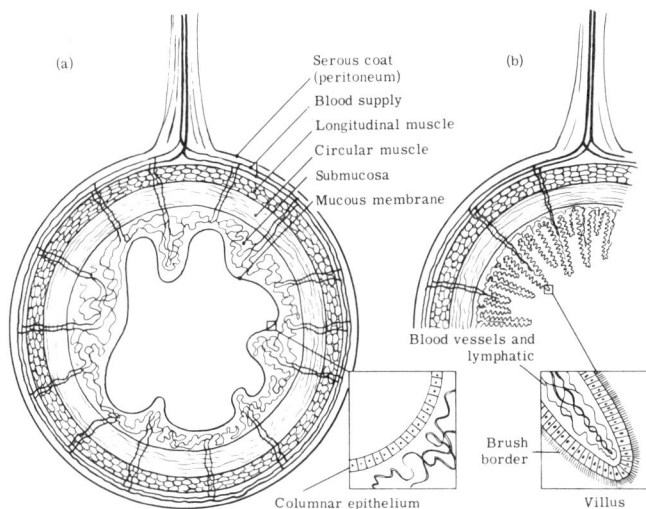

Figure 13.5 Cross-section showing the general histological construction of the gastro-intestinal tract. (a) Alimentary canal. (b) Small intestine.

food particles. In this tissue are found lymph nodules which help to prevent some of the micro-organisms which inhabit the nose and mouth from entering the oesophagus and to produce antibody against those that do. The oesophagus has relatively few lymph nodules, for the stratified epithelium is not very absorptive. The mucosa of the oesophagus has few secretory glands, but most of the other parts of the intestinal mucosa is richly supplied with glands. There is a small ring of muscle, the muscularis mucosa, which completes the submucosa.

(2) The submucosa connects the mucosa and the muscular layers. It is formed from loose connective tissue and contains many elastic fibres. Small plexuses of the blood vessels are housed in the submucosa and there are some ganglion cells and nerve fibres in the submucosa. The nerve plexus is called Meissner's plexus, and some of its fibres innervate the glands of the tract and the muscularis mucosa.

(3) There are two layers of muscle within the muscular layer. One layer is nearly circular while the other is more spiral and thus is at angles to the circular layer. In the pharynx, the upper third of the oesophagus and at the anus, the muscle is striated. Between these areas it is smooth and involuntary.

Between the circular and spiral layers of muscle throughout the tract are nerve plexuses which help regulate the tension and contraction. The muscle is supplied by both the sympathetic and the parasympathetic nerves. Most of the parasympathetic nerve supply comes from the vagus nerve. Fibres from the vagus synapse in the nerve plexuses between the two muscle layers. Fibres from the plexus then innervate the muscle. These fibres are very important for peristalsis.

(4) The outermost layer (serosa) is loose, connective tissue and supports the nerves, lymph and blood vessels which enter the tract. In much of the tract it is peritoneum.

The four layers are continuous throughout the tract and therefore will not be described for each portion of it. The circular smooth muscle fibres of the oesophagus are thickened at both ends of the oesophagus and they form sphincters. The upper oesophageal sphincter (cricopharyngeal sphincter) previously mentioned, separates the pharynx from the body of the oesophagus. The smooth muscle of this sphincter is tonically contracted so air doesn't enter the oesophagus with every breath. At the lower end of the oesophagus is the lower oesophageal sphincter. This sphincter is located at the level in which the lower oesophagus crosses through an opening in the diaphragm, leaves the thoracic cavity and enters the abdomen to open into the stomach. The lower oesophageal sphincter is tonically contracted so the food and acid fluids in the stomach can't travel backwards and irritate the oesophagus. Both the upper and lower oesophageal sphincters reflexly open during the act of swallowing.

D. The stomach

The oesophagus penetrates the diaphragm and opens into the cardia of the stomach. The size, shape and position of the stomach will depend on its contents. The area of the stomach near the junction with the oesophagus is called the cardiac region, and the pouch-like upper end of the stomach is the fundus. Beneath the fundus is the body of the stomach which

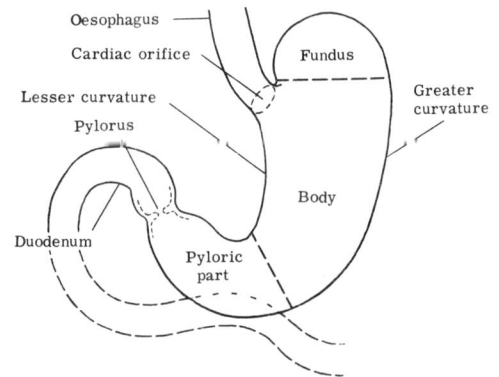

Figure 13.6 The stomach.

is its largest part (see Figure 13.6). The body gives rise to the pyloric part which ends at the pyloric sphincter (pylorus). The pyloric sphincter separates the stomach from the duodenum.

The mucosa and the submucosa of the stomach are arranged in deep longitudinal folds called rugae. The stomach has an additional layer of smooth muscle which runs obliquely. These three layers increase the force and variety of contractions that can take place in the stomach. Moreover, the stomach can stretch and temporarily store food. The muscular layers are covered by the serosa. The serosa contributes to the peritoneum (described in the Section on the peritoneum). The peritoneum above and below the stomach has a special name, the omentum (see Figure 13.7).

The lesser omentum is a double-layered membrane running from the liver to the lesser curvature of the stomach, and it supports the stomach and provides a route for the hepatic, coeliac and left gastric arteries that supply the liver and the stomach. As the lesser omentum reaches the lesser curvature, it separates. One layer covers the anterior surface of the stomach, the other the posterior surface. When the separate layers of the omentum cover the stomach they form the serosa.

At the greater curvature of the stomach the two layers of serosa, from the anterior and posterior surfaces, come together again and continue inferiorly as the greater omentum. The greater omentum covers the intestines, loops upward over the transverse colon and continues posteriorly as a part of the transverse mesocolon. The greater omentum can store considerable amounts of fat. Obese people do not have

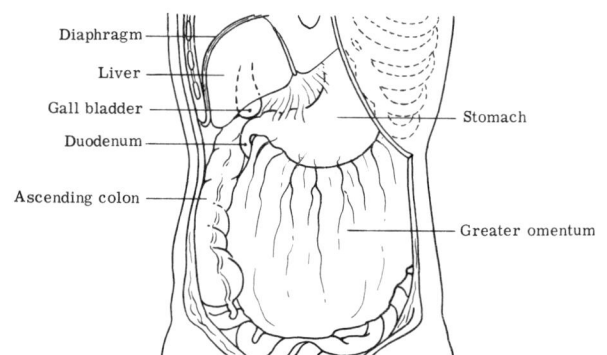

Figure 13.7 The abdominal cavity after removal of the anterior abdominal wall.

"fat stomachs", but their greater omentum stores large amounts of fat that contributes to the abdominal bulge.

The part of the stomach proximal to the pyloric sphincter in which the lumen of the stomach runs in a transverse direction is called the pyloric part (the antrum). The antrum is histologically distinct from the body and the fundus.

The mucosa of the body and the fundus is thick and folded, and contains many small openings. These openings are called gastric pits and are the openings into which the secretions of the gastric glands are discharged. The pits descend into the mucous membrane to reach the upper ends of the gastric glands (see Figure 13.8). These straight tubular glands extend almost to the muscularis mucosa. The junctional area between the gastric pit and the gastric glands is called the neck of the gastric gland and is the area where the cellular renewal and differentiation takes place. There are three types of cells in the gland: mucus-producing cells, parietal cells producing HCl and intrinsic factor, and chief cells producing pepsinogen, the precursor of the enzyme, pepsin.

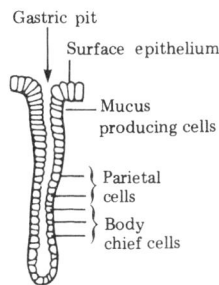

Figure 13.8 The fundic gland structure.

In the pyloric part (the antrum), the mucosa is thinner, but the gastric pits are deeper. The tubular glands are coiled and produce only mucus. Adjacent to the glands are "G" cells which produce the hormone, gastrin.

The gastric mucosa is covered by a 2–3 mm thick layer of mucus. The chief constituent of this jelly-like mucus is mucin. Mucin molecules are giant glycoprotein molecules which can stick to the mucosa and protect the lining of the stomach. Many cells of the surface epithelium of the stomach produce, store and release mucin granules. The mucin produced by the gastric glands and the glands in the antrum is soluble and is a constituent of the gastric secretions. Vagal stimulation can increase the secretion of mucus from these glands.

The mucus functions to prevent the pepsin and HCl from digesting and destroying the stomach. It is remarkably effective. Aspirin (acetylsalicylic acid) is a weak acid which is able to penetrate and disrupt this mucus barrier. If aspirin is taken in large quantities, HCl can penetrate the mucus, inflame and erode the mucosa and might cause bleeding from the stomach.

E. The small intestine

The small intestine is approximately 10 metres long. This great length ensures that the digested food particles and fluids will be digested and absorbed. The first and shortest part of the small intestine is the duodenum, which is closely attached to the head of the pancreas and curves around it, receiving a duct that empties secretions from both the pancreas and the liver (see Figures 13.6 and 13.15). The next 40% is called the jejunum and the remainder is the ileum.

The jejunum twists and turns throughout the abdominal cavity and is attached to the back wall by peritoneum called mesentery. The inner mucosa is arranged in folds and from these folds arise finger-like projections called villi, which greatly enlarge the surface area of the intestine and thus increase the chance that a molecule will come into contact with the mucosa and be absorbed into the capillaries contained within (see Figure 13.5b). The villi also contain specialized lymph capillaries called lacteals, important in fat absorption and transport. The columnar epithelial cells of the intestinal mucosa have microvilli, and these microvilli further increase the surface area for absorption.

Interspersed among these absorptive cells are goblet cells for mucus production, and Paneth cells for enzyme production. The crypts of Lieberkuhn are straight tubular glands which project, like deep crevices, into the muscular mucosa. In addition to producing mucus, enzymes and intestinal juices, the cells at the bottom of these crypts are mitotically active.

The cells at the tip of the villi are continuously being shed and are continuously being replaced by cells that have "migrated" from the base of the crypt. In the human, the migration time has been estimated to be about 3 days. Thus, the lining of the intestine is replaced every 3 days or so. Within the submucosa of the duodenum there are specialized mucus-producing glands called Brunner's glands.

The mucosa also contains many nodules of lymphoid tissue. In the distal portions of the small intestine, these small nodules together form large lymph nodes known as Peyer's Patches. The lymphoid tissue of the intestine is an important site in the development of those lymphocytes which become plasma cells and produce antibodies. It is strategically located for the body's defence, because micro-organisms which survive the journey to the intestine will be absorbed with other nutrients. The bacteria that cause typhoid fever, *Salmonella typhosa*, are particularly dangerous, for they are able to invade and over-run the lymph nodules and cause a severe inflammatory reaction, often severely injuring the tract.

Most nutrients are absorbed in the small intestine.

Hookworms can also inhabit the small intestine. The larval form of the hookworm enter the body through the skin or mouth and reach the small intestine, where they soon mature and reproduce. The adult hookworm is about 1 cm long and hooks on to the intestinal mucosa. Each hookworm can extract as much as 0.15 ml of blood each day and so, in many parts of Asia and certain tropical countries, hookworms are responsible for much of the anaemia found there.

F. The large intestine

The final 1.5 metres of the tract is the large intestine (colon) which functions to absorb water and store the faeces until they can be excreted. Although the large intestine is about 5 cm in diameter and therefore larger than the small intestine, it lacks villi and has less total surface area. It is also the home of many bacteria which play a small part in digestion and which produce vitamins and other metabolites. The ileum

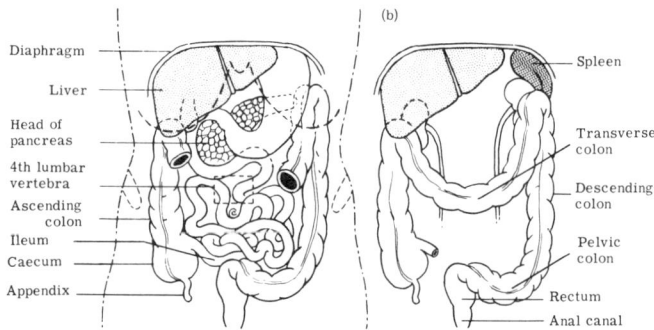

Figure 13.9 The abdominal organs.

is separated from the colon by the ileocecal valve after which comes a dilated pouch called the caecum to which the vermiform (worm-shaped) appendix is attached (see Figure 13.9).

The appendix is a short, closed tube which contains the same four layers as the rest of the digestive tract, except that the mucosa contains greater amounts of lymphatic tissue. It is similar to the tonsil in that the lymphoid tissue that it contains can enlarge in response to infection. If the opening of the appendix into the caecum is blocked, material from the intestine may be trapped within the lumen of the appendix. This can lead to the appendix becoming inflamed and infected, a condition known as appendicitis. Should the opening be obstructed and the pressure within the appendix be increased, the appendix can rupture and scatter infection throughout the intestine, a more serious and often fatal complication of appendicitis. Because of the response of the lymphoid tissue in the appendix to infection, obstruction of the lumen of the appendix, and appendicitis, are more common after viral gastro-intestinal infections. In the foetus, the appendix is considered an important site for lymphocyte production. In the adult, the appendix function is somewhat obscure.

The caecum is located in the right iliac region, resting on the iliopsoas muscle. The colon goes towards the diaphragm from here and is known as the ascending colon. Just beneath the liver, the colon turns at the right colic flexure and heads towards the spleen as the transverse colon. Below the spleen it turns right (caudad) as the splenic flexure and is then known as the descending colon. It soon makes another turn to the right, the sigmoid flexure, in the left iliac region and thereafter it is called the left pelvic colon. It then enters the pelvis where it becomes the rectum.

The mucosa of the large intestine contains goblet cells, absorptive cells and mucus-producing glands. The large intestine differs from the small intestine in that it lacks villi, and the crypts of Lieberkuhn are deeper, so the mucosa is thicker. The mucosal cells, like those throughout the tract, are continually being rubbed away by friction with passing food and faeces and are constantly being renewed. Occasionally, the control of this cellular renewal breaks down, the cells in the mucosa proliferate wildly and a cancer results. The mucosa of the large intestine is unique because the thin layer of muscle found in the mucosa disappears and there is thus no barrier between the submucosa and mucosa.

In the rectum and anal canal, the veins of the submucosa may bulge into the lumen of the tract; this condition is known

as haemorrhoids. The veins may tear and bleed during defaecation.

The muscular coat of the large intestine differs from that of the small intestine. Parts of the outer longitudinal muscle are arranged in three distinct bands called taeniae coli. Parts of the large intestine have puckerings or sacculations termed haustrae; they cause the large intestine to resemble a string of sausages. The taeniae coli may be responsible for the haustra. At the rectum, the taeniae coli fan out to completely surround the rectum.

The inner, circular smooth muscle layer of the colon also differs form that of the small intestine which precedes it. The muscle is arranged in thin bands which are separated by thin slits through which the blood vessels pass. The mucosa and submucosa may bulge outwards through these slits and form diverticula. If the diverticula are filled with mucus or intestinal debris and become inflamed, diverticulitis results.

The large intestine also differs from the small intestine in that parts of the large intestine contain appendices epiploicae. These are small finger-like masses of fat, enclosed in peritoneum, which project outward from the surface of the colon.

The left pelvic (sigmoid) colon gives rise to the rectum. This lies adjacent to the sacrum. The mucosa of the rectum is similar to that of the colon but the mucosa, submucosa and some smooth muscle form folds (valves) which project into the lumen of the rectum. Supposedly, they support the faecal mass as the rectum fills, but this is really speculation.

Peritoneum covers the front and sides of the upper part of the rectum. In the male, the peritoneum leaves the front of the rectum and attaches to the urinary bladder; the floor of this reflection is called the recto-vesical pouch. In the female, the recto-uterine pouch is formed by the reflection of peritoneum from the rectum to the back of the uterus.

The final few centimetres of the large intestine form the anal canal, whose opening is the anus. The anal canal passes through, and is supported by, the pelvic diaphragm. The most important supporting muscle of the diaphragm is the puborectalis portion of the levator ani. Below the levator ani is a large sphincter which has an internal and external component. The internal anal sphincter is formed from the smooth muscle of the anal canal. The external anal sphincter is a thick ring of striated muscle maintained in a state of tonic contraction. You can voluntarily increase the tone in the external sphincter, and during defaecation the tone of both sphincters is reduced.

The liver and the pancreas will be described now because of their contribution to digestion, although both organs have other functions independent of the digestive system.

G. The liver

The liver is the largest gland in the body. In an adult male, the average weight is 1.5 kg, and in women 1.3 kg. The liver is a dynamic organ, can shrink in size during starvation and can enlarge dramatically during certain diseases. Before going on with the anatomy of the liver you should first understand that this is a complex organ with a least five major interacting components:

(a) Hepatocytes are the basic cellular units of the liver and are metabolic marvels, carrying out a variety of biochemical functions such as glycogen storage, fat catabolism, protein synthesis and the production of bile.

(b) The circulatory system supplies the hepatocytes with oxygenated arterial blood from the hepatic artery and venous blood with nutrients from the intestines, and also with venous blood from the spleen and pancreas. The liver also has a supply of lymphatic vessels.

(c). The bile which the hepatocytes produce is secreted into the ducts of the biliary system which drain the bile out of the liver.

(d) The reticulo-endothelial system is well represented in the liver by Kupffer cells and other phagocytic cells, all of which defend and assist the liver in their various functions.

(e) A connective tissue network gives structure and support to the other elements of the liver.

Most of the liver is protected by the thoracic cage and lies beneath the dome-shaped diaphragm. The liver moves with the diaphragm during respiration. The liver is incompletely covered by peritoneum, and folds of peritoneum also form ligaments which support the liver (see Figure 13.10a). The falciform ligament attaches the liver to the diaphragm and the anterior abdominal wall. Posteriorly, the coronary ligaments extend from the superior surface of the right lobe of the liver to the diaphragm.

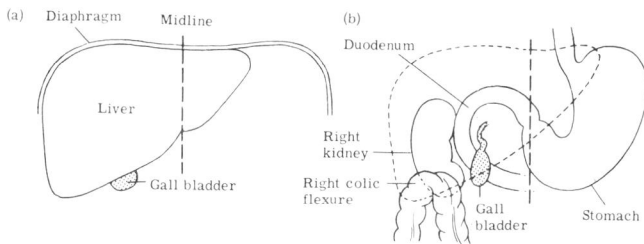

Figure 13.10 The liver. (a) Diagram to show the position. (b) Organs related to the visceral surface of the liver.

The liver has four lobes, only two of which are visible from the ventral view. The right lobe is the largest lobe and is separated from the left lobe by the falciform ligament; the right lobe may extend below the edge of the diaphragm. The two smallest lobes can be seen by viewing the liver from its inferior surface, for they are obscured by the large right lobe. These two lobes are the square-shaped quadrate lobe and the tail-shaped caudate lobe.

The position of the liver is described as lying beneath the right hypochondrium and epigastrium and also the left hypochondrium. Beneath the peritoneum the liver is covered by a connective tissue capsule called Glisson's capsule. This connective tissue also forms fine septa which project into the liver tissue. Connective tissue also accompanies the blood vessels, lymphatics and nerves into the liver, and this connective tissue branches extensively, forming the supporting network for the hepatocytes, the main functioning cells of the liver.

The anatomic unit of the liver is the lobule. The hexagonal lobules are formed by columns of hepatocytes radiating from a large intralobular (central) vein (see Figure 13.11a). The columns of hepatocytes are at least two cells wide but often

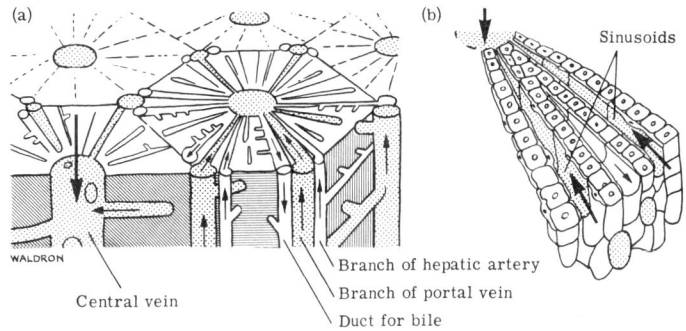

Figure 13.11 (a) Lobules of the liver with the circulation of the blood and the flow of bile. (b) The arrangement of liver cells in in relation to the flow of blood and bile.

only one cell thick. The width of the columns is not apparent in many microscopic sections, and the columns may appear to be only rows of single cells. Within the columns of hepatic cells are small bile channels called canaliculi.

The liver is a gland, and one of its many functions is to produce bile and secrete it into these bile channels.

The large spaces between the columns of hepatic cells are sinusoids (see Figure 13.11b). They are filled with blood, not bile. The liver has a double supply of blood, as the blood in the sinusoids which supplies the hepatocytes with oxygen and nutrients comes from two sources. Approximately 25% of the blood is oxygen-rich arterial blood, and about 75% is nutrient-rich venous blood from the intestines and also from the stomach, pancreas and spleen. The sinusoids drain into the intralobular veins.

The lining of the sinusoids is not the typical capillary endothelium. It is much more permeable and contains many specialized cells called Kupffer cells. These cells belong to the reticulo-endothelial system and are phagocytic. Besides defending the liver against bacteria, they phagocytose matter and are important in the body's recycling of iron from haemoglobin metabolites.

A small space separates the lining of the sinusoids from the hepatic cells; the space is called the space of Dissé. The sinusoids are very permeable but blood cells cannot leave the sinusoids. Plasma leaves the sinusoids by passing through large gaps between the lining cells, enters the space of Dissé and bathes the hepatocytes. Conversely, proteins and fats synthesized by the liver, or glucose that has been either synthesized or stored by the liver, can enter the circulation by leaving the hepatocytes, crossing the space of Dissé and sinusoid membrane and entering the circulation. Some fluid from the space of Dissé enters the small lymph capillaries, which form larger channels emptying into the cisterna chyli. Lymph enters the venous circulation after travelling through the cisterna chyli and thoracic duct (see Figure 9.2).

The microscopic structure of the liver makes no sense unless you understand the flow of blood and bile (see Figure 13.12). The liver receives blood from two sources:

(a) Oxygenated blood form the hepatic artery, and
(b) Venous blood from the hepatic portal vein.

The hepatic artery is a branch of the coeliac artery, and the coeliac artery is a branch of the abdominal aorta. The

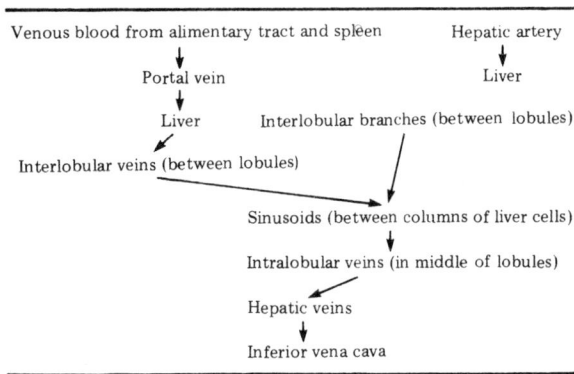

Venous blood from alimentary tract and spleen   Hepatic artery

Portal vein   Liver

Liver   Interlobular branches (between lobules)

Interlobular veins (between lobules)

Sinusoids (between columns of liver cells)

Intralobular veins (in middle of lobules)

Hepatic veins

Inferior vena cava

Figure 13.12   The blood flow to the liver.

hepatic artery breaks into many branches, which, in turn, divide into many still smaller branches, which supply the entire liver. Oxygenated arterial blood from these small interlobular branches of the hepatic artery enters into the hepatic sinusoids and, in doing so, supplies the hepatocytes with oxygen.

Venous blood from the abdominal wall, kidneys, adrenal glands and lower limbs does not enter the hepatic portal system. Venous blood from these structures enters the inferior vena cava and is returned to the right atrium of the heart.

The splenic vein which drains the spleen, pancreas and parts of the stomach, is joined by the inferior mesenteric vein which drains part of the large intestine (see Figure 8.17). The large hepatic portal vein is formed when the splenic vein joins the superior mesenteric vein; this vein drains the small intestines and part of the large intestine.

Smaller veins from the stomach also drain into the hepatic portal vein. The large hepatic portal vein breaks up into small veins, and within the liver these small veins break up into still smaller branches. These small branches of the hepatic portal vein run with branches of the hepatic artery, and they form still smaller interlobular branches which drain into the hepatic sinusoids. The hepatic sinusoids converge to form the interlobular (central) vein of the lobule. The central veins of the lobules come together to from fewer but larger veins. Ultimately, three large hepatic veins leave the liver, converge and empty into the inferior vena cava, which empties into the right atrium of the heart (see Figure 8.17).

The blood that enters the liver from the hepatic portal vein is low in oxygen but rich in absorbed foodstuffs from the intestines, hormones from the pancreas, stomach and small intestine, and haemoglobin breakdown products from the spleen. The fact that the liver is the only organ perfused with this rich concentration of nutrients, hormones and metabolites highlights its role as a centre of metabolic action.

To complete the description of the structure of the liver, and also to illustrate another metabolic function of the liver, the biliary system needs to be discussed. Between the rows of hepatocytes are small capillary-like channels that receive the bile produced by the surrounding hepatocytes. These small channels are sometimes called the bile canaliculi (see Figure 13.11b). Bile in the canaliculi flows towards small bile ducts located near the interlobular branches of the hepatic artery and vein in the periphery of the lobule. The small biliary ducts unite to form larger ducts. Ultimately, two large ducts,

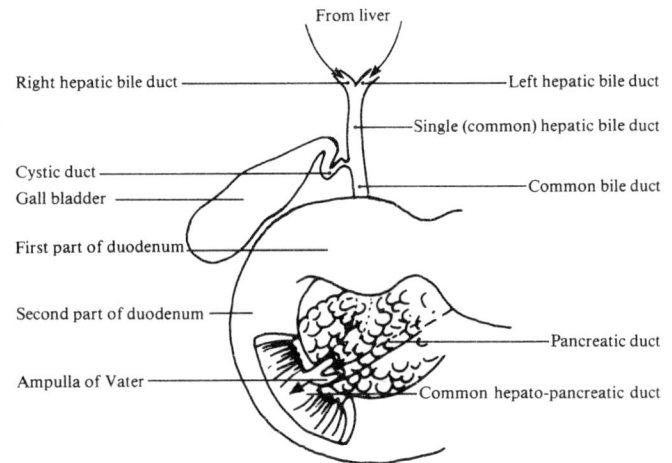

Figure 13.13   The extrahepatic bile duct system.

the left and right hepatic bile ducts, are formed and these two ducts form the single (common) hepatic bile duct (see Figure 13.13). The common hepatic bile duct leaves the liver and runs a short distance and is then joined by the cystic duct.

The cystic duct leads to the gall bladder (see Figure 13.13). The gall bladder is a small pear-shaped sac lying under the right lobe of the liver (see Figure 13.10). The typical gall bladder can hold an average of 30–50 ml of bile. The gall bladder is formed by three layers. The inner mucosal layer is not unlike the mucosa of the stomach, though it lacks glands and is much more absorptive. Water from the bile is absorbed into the gall bladder, and the bile becomes more concentrated. Over the mucosa is a smooth muscle layer which also contains fibro-elastic tissue. The outer coat of peritoneum binds the gall bladder to the liver.

Bile leaves the gall bladder the same way it entered, via the cystic duct. The cystic duct joins the hepatic duct to form the common bile duct. Bile travels down the common bile duct, which opens into the duodenum. The pancreatic duct often joins the bile duct and the two have a common opening into the duodenum. A thick muscular sphincter (the sphincter of Boyden) surrounds the bile duct before it joins the pancreatic duct. A second, much weaker sphincter surrounds the common hepato-pancreatic duct. This weaker sphincter is sometimes called the sphincter of Oddi.

Bile contains water, bile pigments, bile acids or salts, fatty acids, cholesterol, lecithin and mineral salts. In the liver canaliculi, bile is about 98% water but this is reduced to about 85% by the absorption of sodium chloride and water in the gall bladder.

You will remember that in the entire body, more than two million red blood cells are destroyed every second. Much of this takes place in the spleen. Haemoglobin is released from the red blood cells, and the reticulo-endothelial cells of the spleen metabolize the haemoglobin to bilirubin.

Bilirubin is basically a haemoglobin molecule from which the iron and globin have been removed, and the haeme exists in a linear rather than a circular arrangement. Bilirubin is not very soluble so it attaches to the plasma protein, albumin. The albumin–bilirubin complex travels to the hepatic sinusoids via the splenic vein and hepatic portal vein. The hepatocyte membrane removes the bilirubin from the albumin molecule. Within the hepatocytes the bilirubin reacts with uridine diphosphoglucose to form bilirubin diglucuronide (also known as conjugated bilirubin).

Bilirubin diglucuronide differs from bilirubin in that the former is much more soluble and can travel in the blood or bile without being bound to albumin. The hepatocytes secrete the conjugated bilirubin into the bile canaliculi. The molecule travels with the bile through the hepatic bile duct and cystic duct to the gall bladder, where it is temporarily stored. When the gall bladder contracts, the conjugated bilirubin travels back through the cystic duct to the common bile duct and, if the sphincters are open, will enter the duodenum.

Within the intestine, the very alkaline fluids cause some bilirubin to be reformed from conjugated bilirubin. Most bilirubin and conjugated bilirubin are excreted in the faeces. However, some bilirubin and bilirubin metabolites are reabsorbed into the hepatic portal circulation and recycled through the liver.

Bacteria in the colon can metabolize bilirubin to urobilinogen. Urobilinogen is very soluble and can be absorbed into the hepatic portal circulation. Urobilinogen may be reconverted to bilirubin by the liver, or, if present in sufficient quantities, excreted in the urine.

In the intestines bilirubin is also metabolized into sterco-bilinogen and mesobilfucsin. These compounds and their derivatives account for the brown colour of the faeces. If the flow of bile from the liver into the small intestine is obstructed, faeces will be light or clay-coloured and urobilinogen will be absent from the urine.

In contrast to the bile pigments, the bile acids play an important role in the digestive processes. The two primary bile acids are cholic and chenodeoxycholic acids formed in the liver from cholesterol. The bile acids may be further metabolized by intestinal bacteria, and these may be absorbed and recycled through the liver.

Bile salts function in digestion by acting as a detergent and breaking down large fat globules into much smaller particles. This increases the surface area of the fat and makes it easier for fat-digesting enzymes to come into contact with the fat and break down the triglycerides.

The formation and circulation of the bile pigments and salts are complicated processes, and they have to be studied thoroughly before they can be understood. Their importance is understood if we look at jaundice. Jaundice is not a disease but a syndrome. (A syndrome is a set of signs and/or symptoms which occur together.) Jaundice is defined as a syndrome characterized by excess bilirubin in the blood and deposition of bile pigment in the skin and mucus membranes, with the resultant yellow appearance of the patient. Since human skins come in a variety of colours, not all the patients will appear equally yellow. The sclera of the eye is a good indicator of jaundice, for the sclera is easily observed and has a high affinity for bile pigments. The normal level of bilirubin in the blood plasma is 0.8 mg/100 ml; patients will appear jaundiced when the bilirubin begins to exceed 2.5 mg/100 ml.

Jaundice has any one of numerous pathological causes. Red blood cells may be broken down in such large numbers that the capacity of the liver to metabolize and excrete bilirubin is exceeded. Breakdown of red cells may be normal, but the liver may be diseased. The hepatocytes may be diseased, and either unable to separate bilirubin from albumin or unable to conjugate it to uridine diphosphoglucose and secrete the conjugated bilirubin into the bile canaliculi.

Finally the common bile duct may be obstructed by gallstones or tumour. Gallstones are formed in the gall bladder from bile which has become insoluble, and may block the cystic duct, or they may reach the common bile duct and block it, so that bile flow backs up into the liver and circulation.

The function of the liver and its relationship to metabolism will be discussed in more detail in the following Chapters. Some of its functions are listed here in outline form:

(1) It stores glucose in the form of glycogen and is important in carbohydrate and fat metabolism.

(2) It synthesizes proteins, including the blood clotting factors and albumin.

(3) It is the chief producer of urea. This is an end-product of amino acid metabolism and is the chief molecular form in which nitrogen is eliminated from the body.

(4) The liver stores iron and certain vitamins.

(5) Because of its great metabolic activity, the liver is the great heat-producing organ of the body.

(6) As mentioned previously, the liver produces bile.

(7) The liver also produces a hormone. This is a protein called somatomedin, which seems to be necessary for the proper growth of the skeletal system.

Before going on, there is a topic that will relate the anatomy of the liver and its blood supply to material in the Chapter on the circulatory system. This is hepatic alcoholic cirrhosis. In the adult man, about 1500 ml of blood perfuse the liver in 1 minute. About 75% of this blood is supplied by the hepatic portal vein and 25% comes from the hepatic artery. Blood from both vessels perfuses the sinusoids and empties into the hepatic veins.

Chronic administration or consumption of large amounts of alcohol are harmful to the liver. The harm is increased by poor nutrition. The response of the liver to alcohol abuse is complex but can result in cirrhosis, which is defined as a disease in which there is progressive destruction of liver cells and their replacement by connective tissue and regenerating lobules. Excessive alcohol can cause the hepatocytes to become infiltrated with fat and to die; the resulting inflammation causes scarring, a replacement of diseased tissue with collagen. The liver enlarges, as some of the lobules do regenerate, but the normal "architecture" of the lobule is not preserved and blood cannot flow easily from sinusoid to intralobular vein. The lining of the sinusoids becomes thickened and resistance to blood flow through the hepatic portal system increases. Liver function decreases and there is a fall-off in metabolic efficiency as evidenced by reduced levels of albumin and blood clotting factors that are normally produced by the liver.

Because of the increased pressure within the liver and the great resistance to flow, some fluid may leave the veins and lymphatics and accumulate in the abdomen. The accumulation of fluid in the abdominal cavity is called ascites. Sometimes ascites can be present in such large amounts that the abdomen becomes grossly distended. The fluid pressure can compress other veins. The increased venous resistance leads to oedema in the lower limbs, particularly the ankles, and sometimes to haemorrhoids. A collateral venous circulation develops and blood is shunted away from the liver. Many other complications of alcoholic hepatic cirrhosis arise. About 10% of alcoholics develop cirrhosis, and alcoholism itself is becoming a disease of almost epidemic proportions in many parts of the world.

It should be emphasized that not all cirrhosis is caused by alcohol and that ascites may have other causes besides cirrhosis. Heart failure and parasites can also cause ascites.

H. The pancreas

This double gland lies in the hypogastric region with its head in the curvature of the duodenum and its tail touching the spleen (see Figure 13.9a). The adult pancreas averages about 20 cm in length and weighs about 85 grams.

Most of the pancreas is an exocrine gland. Secretions from the exocrine portions of the pancreas pass through the pancreatic duct to enter the duodenum (see Figure 13.13). The exocrine pancreas produces enzymes and an alkaline secretion. The alkaline secretion is watery and contains a high concentration of bicarbonate ion. The enzymes produced by the pancreas include trypsinogen and chymotrypsinogen which attack bonds between specific amino acids in protein, lipase and amylase. Lipase breaks down fats; amylase breaks down starch.

Scattered throughout the pancreas are clusters of cells called the Islets of Langerhans which make up the endocrine portion of the pancreas and do not empty their secretions into the duodenum via ducts. The islets produce three hormones, insulin and glucagon and somatostatin, which are secreted directly into capillaries that form the small veins which leave the pancreas and join the splenic vein, which goes on to the hepatic portal vein (see Figure 8.17). Insulin and glucagon and somatostatin have little effect on digestion but have a very great effect on metabolism and will be discussed later.

I. The peritoneum

The peritoneum is the largest serous membrane in the body. The peritoneum is not part of the digestive system but, since it covers the abdominal organs, it is best described here in this Section (see Figure 13.14). The peritoneum is a double membrane having two separate layers. The parietal peritoneum lines the abdominal wall, while the visceral layer covers the organs within the abdominal cavity.

The structure of peritoneum is rather complicated but can easily be understood if you begin with a membrane lining the abdomen. The space within the membranes is called the peritoneal cavity. Next, imagine that certain organs are pushed into the peritoneum from above, below and behind. If an organ is pushed far enough into this membrane it will be nearly surrounded by membrane. The membrane helps attach the liver to the interior surface of the diaphragm. The liver pushes into the membrane from above and is then covered with peritoneum on its dorsal and ventral surfaces. The urinary bladder which pushes in from below is thus covered only on its superior surface. The small intestine is pushed deeply into the peritoneum from the posterior wall so that it is both suspended and surrounded. The mesentery is the name

given to this double layer which encloses the ileum and jejunum and attaches them to the posterior wall. The kidneys, pancreas and spleen are pushed slightly into the peritoneal

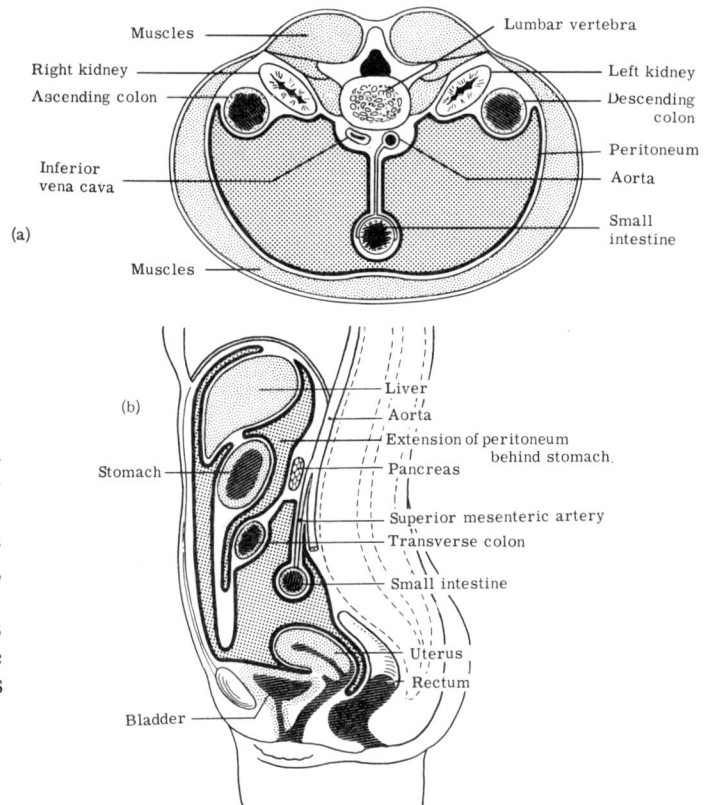

Figure 13.14 (a) The theoretical peritoneum and peritoneal cavity. (b) The actual peritoneum and peritoneal cavity in the female.

cavity so they are covered only on their anterior surfaces (see Figure 13.14).

The greater omentum hangs from the greater curvature of the stomach and covers the abdominal organs like an apron (see Figure 13.7). It is then reflected back to the posterior abdominal wall. The greater omentum stores a considerable amount of fat within its folds.

The peritoneum functions to support and protect the abdominal organs. The fluid secreted by the two layers reduces the friction as the two structures move over one another. The peritoneum stores fat and is richly supplied with lymph nodes to protect it against infection and to isolate an area of inflammation. This is important in appendicitis.

If the peritoneum becomes infected the condition is called peritonitis. In acute peritonitis, the abdomen will be very painful and the intestinal lumen may become blocked, hindering the passage of the many litres of fluid which normally pass through and are reabsorbed. Septic abortions are a frequent cause of peritonitis.

The male peritoneal cavity is a completely closed stucture. The uterine tubes open into the female peritoneal cavity (see Figure 13.14b). More will be said about this in the Chapter on the reproductive system.

HOW ARE FOODS DIGESTED AND ABSORBED?

Different foods are digested in different ways. The proteolytic enzymes which attack and break down the protein in meat will have no effect on the starch in potatoes. For learning purposes, it might be helpful to list the various steps in the digestion of carbohydrates, proteins and fats separately.

A. Carbohydrates

Most carbohydrate in the diet is in the form of starch, which consists of many glucose molecules linked together into single giant molecules. Such large molecules cannot be absorbed, so they must be broken down into individual monosaccharide units which can then enter the intestinal mucosa.

The process begins in the mouth with the secretion of salivary amylase from the salivary glands. This enzyme attacks the starch molecule and forms short strands of glucose molecules. There is relatively little digestion in the mouth, for the food stays there only a brief time before it is swallowed, but if you do chew a piece of potato and keep it in your mouth for a while you will note that it becomes sweeter as more and more of the starch becomes glucose.

The stomach acidity has some action in breaking down starch granules, but relatively little digestion occurs in the stomach. In the small intestine, pancreatic amylase is added and this breaks down the glucose chains into a disaccharide known as maltose. (In pancreatitis when the pancreas is inflamed, this amylase from the pancreas can be released into the bloodstream, and the amount of enzyme in the blood can be used to help diagnose and monitor the disease.) Maltose is split into two glucose units by the enzyme, maltase located on the border of the epithelial cells lining the intestine (see Figure 13.15).

Absorption of glucose into the mucosa is an active process, for glucose will enter the epithelial cells even if there is a greater concentration of glucose inside than outside. The other disaccharides, lactose and sucrose, are split into

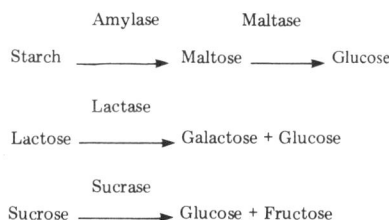

Amylase   Maltase

Starch ———————⟶ Maltose ————⟶ Glucose

Lactase

Lactose ———————⟶ Galactose + Glucose

Sucrase

Sucrose ———————⟶ Glucose + Fructose

Figure 13.15 Digestion of the main carbohydrates.

monosaccharides, galactose and glucose, and glucose and fructose, by the enzymes, lactase and sucrase, respectively. All the monosaccharides are absorbed into epithelial cells, then move into the capillaries of the villi and ultimately enter the liver via the hepatic portal vein.

Some individuals lack the enzyme, lactase, and cannot break down and absorb the milk sugar, lactose. The lactose molecule is thus osmotically active and retains water in the intestine; this leads to diarrhoea. Certain intestinal bacteria can ferment this lactose, and the bacterial growth and gas production will cause pain and cramps. This condition can be "cured" by removing lactose from the diet. Lactase deficiency is more common in infants of African and Asian ancestry, but should be suspected in all cases of infant diarrhoea. Many cases of lactase deficiency are not due to genetic causes. Sometimes lactase deficiency can develop as a result of infection or other injury to the intestinal mucosa.

Deficiencies of maltase and sucrase are less common but do occur.

B. Proteins

In order to be absorbed the proteins must be broken down into their individual amino acids. Not only can the individual amino acid be absorbed more easily, but if the protein were not broken down and were absorbed intact, the body would react to it just as it does to any other foreign protein or antigen and would synthesize antibodies against it. This rarely happens, but there are some individuals who become allergic to cow's milk, meat or egg proteins because of deficiencies in protein digestion and absorption.

The actual digestion of protein begins in the stomach, which secretes hydrochloric acid and the inactive enzyme, pepsinogen. The acid activates the enzyme and converts it to pepsin which splits the proteins into chains of amino acids. (Pepsin has to be stored as an inactive enzyme, otherwise it would digest the proteins in the cell which made it; this process of enzyme activation by pH is repeated for other digestive enzymes.) Most protein digestion is accomplished by enzymes from the pancreas, particularly carboxy-peptidase, which splits the protein chains down to even smaller groups of amino acids. These small chains of amino acids are called peptides: peptides can be di-peptides (2 amino acids), tri-peptides (3 amino acids), tetra-peptides (4 amino acids), etc. Other enzymes from the intestinal mucosa, also known as peptidase, make the final attack and leave nothing but separate amino acids. These are absorbed into the mucosa and travel to the liver via the hepatic portal system.

C. Fats

Fat digestion is unique in many ways. Most dietary fat is in the form of triglyceride. There is very little fat digestion before the small intestine because two things are needed: bile salts from the liver, and the enzyme, lipase, from the pancreas. These secretions enter the intestinal tract via the ampulla of Vater in the duodenum.

The bile salts do not digest the large globules of fat but act as a detergent and emulsify them. Emulsification means that the large globules are rearranged into small droplets. This change increases the total surface area of the fat particles so that pancreatic lipase can more easily come into contact with the triglyceride and split some of the fatty acids from the glycerol molecule.

The glycerol, fatty acids and incompletely digested triglycerides are absorbed into the mucosa of the intestine.

Here the fatty acids are rejoined to the glycerol molecules which agglomerate into small particles called chylomicrons. The chylomicrons do not travel to the liver via the hepatic portal system, instead they enter special lymph capillaries called lacteals. The lacteals empty into the larger lymph vessels which join the venous circulation at the thoracic duct. In this way chylomicrons enter the circulation and are distributed throughout the body. Some short-chained fatty acids are absorbed into the capillaries and go directly to the liver.

Normally all dietary fat is absorbed; the faecal fat is derived from rubbed-away cells and bacteria. Malabsorption of fat is called steatorrhoea and commonly results from either a deficiency of pancreatic lipase or of bile. Malabsorption of fat is more common in tropical and subtropical climates where the disease, tropical sprue, is common. This disease is characterized by poor absorption of fats and vitamins, and by atrophy of the intestinal mucosa.

D. Water, salts and vitamins

The salts and fluids which have been secreted into the digestive tract must be absorbed along with the water and salts ingested. In the jejunum, ileum and colon, sodium is actively transported from the intestinal mucosal cells into the blood. Chloride ions are thought to follow passively the positively charged sodium ions. Since sodium normally cannot diffuse back from the blood into the intestine, it can be considered an osmotically active molecule, and the mucosal cells a semi-permeable membrane. Water, a free-moving molecule, will move from the intestinal lumen to the blood. The active absorption of sodium followed by the passive absorption of water is similar to the absorption processes which take place in the nephron.

Of course, the movement of water from the lumen to blood can be reversed if a very hypertonic solution is rapidly introduced into the lumen of the intestine. This happens in children who have been eating sweets and drinking sweet beverages on an empty stomach. The glucose concentration is so great that it cannot be absorbed and thus there are more osmotically active molecules in the lumen than in the blood. Water will move from the blood into the lumen causing a decrease in blood volume and a swelling of the intestine, as well as nausea and vomiting. Similar effects can be induced by swallowing one or two tablespoons of ordinary table salt which is often used as an emetic, a substance which can induce vomiting.

The cholera-causing bacteria, *V. cholerae*, also reverse these absorptive processes. The bacteria produce a toxin which prevents absorption of sodium and, in fact, stimulates a secretion of sodium into the intestine; water follows. The toxin-induced intestinal hypersecretion is so great that serious diarrhoea results. This diarrhoea can be fatal. The bacteria do relatively little damage to the intestinal tract but the diarrhoea may be so massive that the patient becomes seriously dehydrated. It is therefore imperative that these patients be given fluids to replace the fluids that they have lost.

Fluid replacement is the first and most urgent step in treating cholera or any other diarrhoea. The formula for one of the all-purpose oral replacement solutions is given below to illustrate the nature of the fluid lost from the intestine:

	grams/litre
Sodium chloride	3.5
Potassium chloride	1.5
Sodium bicarbonate	2.5
Glucose	20.0

The above formula gives the following concentrations:

	millimoles/litre
Na^+	90
K^+	20
Cl^-	80
HCO_3^-	30
$C_6H_{12}O_6$	110

By drinking this solution, both infants and adults replace electrolytes and fluid lost from the tissues and circulating blood volume. Glucose is added to the mixture because it increases the absorption of the other ions. When glucose is not available, sucrose may be substituted.

Most calcium is absorbed in the duodenum. Vitamin D must be present if the calcium ion is to be absorbed. Iron is also absorbed in the duodenum. The rate of iron absorption depends on the body's needs. The epithelium of the duodenum can store iron and can increase its absorption of iron when its stores are depleted. Only a fraction of the iron in the diet is usually absorbed.

The fat-soluble vitamins (A, D, E and K) are, logically enough, absorbed with fat. Deficiencies in fat absorption can result in deficiencies in vitamins A, D, E and K.

Water-soluble vitamins are absorbed with water. The important exception is vitamin B_{12}. This is a large and highly charged molecule which needs a special protein to help "escort" it into the mucosal cells of the ileum. This protein is called intrinsic factor and is made by the parietal cells of the stomach's mucosa. Intrinsic factor combines with vitamin B_{12} and permits it to be absorbed in the ileum. If the parietal cells cannot produce intrinsic factor or if the stomach has been removed, vitamin B_{12} cannot be absorbed.

Vitamin B_{12} has many functions in the body and is required for the synthesis of blood cells. If there is vitamin B_{12} in the diet but no intrinsic factor present, an anaemia will develop. This is called pernicious anaemia and it must be treated by injecting vitamin B_{12}, as increasing the oral intake of vitamin B_{12} will be of little use. Many bacteria also require vitamin B_{12} for their metabolism. Should there be an overgrowth of these bacteria into the ileum, they will consume the vitamin B_{12} before it can be absorbed and the signs of vitamin B_{12} deficiency will develop.

HOW ARE DIGESTIVE PROCESSES CONTROL-LED AND CO-ORDINATED?

We have looked at digestive anatomy and the biochemical breakdown separately for the sake of clarity. It is necessary now to integrate the two and see how the physiological processes are co-ordinated.

The control of these processes is particularly important. Large volumes of fluid enter the digestive tract each day. These secretions must be released at the appropriate time, in the presence of the appropriate food. There are two solutions to this problem. One would be to have the stomach, pancreas, liver and intestine continuously secrete their products at maximal rates into the gastro-intestinal tract. A more efficient way would be to have the presence of particular foodstuffs trigger the release of the proper secretion and this is the way nature has chosen. Let us take another trip through the digestive tract in the company of a well-balanced meal.

a. The mouth. When food is put into the mouth, its touch, taste and the act of chewing stimulate receptors in the mouth which send this information to the brain. The brain in turn sends impulses via the sympathetic and parasympathetic nervous systems to the salivary glands, causing them to increase the volume of their secretions. These glands are always receiving some stimuli so there is always a low basal rate of flow. This flow decreases during sleep however, so those food particles which are lodged between the teeth after an evening meal will be less likely to be washed away. This accounts for the dentist's advice to brush your teeth after every meal, but particularly after the evening one.

After the food has been chewed and lubricated sufficiently so that it can be swallowed, it is pushed to the back of the mouth by the tongue.

b. Swallowing. There are three possible exits from the oropharynx that the food and fluid can take: the naso-pharynx, the larynx or the oesophagus (see Figure 10.6).

Entry into the nasopharynx is prevented by muscles which tense and raise the soft palate so that it presses against the posterior pharyngeal wall, preventing food from entering the nasopharynx.

Channelling food into the oesophagus rather than the larynx is more complicated. Food and fluid in the back of the mouth stimulate receptors. These receptors, located in the base of the tongue and near the tonsils, send impulses to the swallow centre of the medulla, which controls the reflex parts of the swallowing act. The swallow centre is near the respiratory centre and sends instructions to the respiratory centre so that respiration is inhibited; it also sends instructions to the muscles of the tongue, pharynx and larynx, mainly via the hypoglossal and glossopharyngeal nerves. The tongue presses against the hard palate. The larynx is drawn up under the base of the tongue and the lumen of the larynx is closed by the approximation of both the true and false vocal folds. The epiglottis partially covers the entrance to the larynx and fluids can cascade over it into the oesophagus. The action of the tongue pushes the food back and the superior constrictor muscle contracts, beginning the push down the pharynx into the oesophagus.

The circular ring of muscle guarding the entrance to the oesophagus relaxes immediately after the contraction of the pharyngeal constrictor muscles. Attention should be paid to the fact that if a patient is not fully alert or if the medulla is injured or the laryngeal muscles are paralyzed, the patient should not be fed orally or he or she may choke to death because of airway obstruction or may develop pneumonia because of the aspirated material.

c. The oesophagus. The chewed and lubricated mass of food is called the bolus. The bolus is propelled to the stomach by a series of contractions of the striated and smooth muscles within the oesophagus. These contractions, called peristalsis, are controlled by the swallowing and other medullary centres and actually have two components, an area of contraction preceded by an area of relaxation. Forceful peristaltic waves in the oesophagus depend to a large extent on the vagal nerve being intact.

In the stomach and intestines, vagal nerve stimulation increases motility; however, peristalsis can take place even if the vagal nerves are not intact. Peristaltic waves cannot occur if Auerbach's plexus, the nerve plexus between the circular and longitudinal smooth muscle layers, is damaged. Presumably, stretching of the gastro-intestinal mucosa stimulates receptors in the mucosa. The cell bodies of these receptors are in the submucosal plexus. They relay impulses from the submucosa to Auerbach's plexus, which in turn stimulates the smooth muscle to contract. This local reflex is a way of relating the muscular activity of digestive tract to its contents.

The last part of the oesophagus is the lower oesophageal sphincter. Although not a true sphincter in the strict anatomical sense, the muscle here is normally contracted, separating the stomach and oesophagus, and relaxing only when approached by the bolus and the peristaltic wave. In infants, the sphincter is poorly developed, which partially explains their greater frequency of vomiting. If the nerves within the gastro-oesophageal region are damaged, the sphincter will not open and a whole meal will become stuck in the oesophagus, entering the stomach only by drops; this condition is called achalasia.

Should the sphincter fail to close, however, hydro-chloric acid from the stomach could splash into the oesophagus and irritate the mucosa. This irritation is painful and is often called "heartburn" by lay people. It often begins as a burning sensation felt beneath the lower end of the sternum and it then spreads upwards to the chest. The medical name for "heartburn" is pyrosis. Pregnancy and herniation of the stomach through the diaphragm into the thoracic cavity can increase the incidence of heartburn.

Dysphagia means difficulty in swallowing; it is a symptom often associated with diseases of the oesophagus.

d. The stomach. The lumen of the empty stomach is a little bigger than that of the small intestine but this organ has a great capacity to stretch and contain a full meal. This stretching and change of shape indirectly leads to stimulation of the secretory units within the stomach and is called the local (gastric) phase of secretion.

However, even if food never reaches the stomach, gastric juices are secreted. This is brought about by the para-sympathetic stimulation from the vagus nerve. The sight, smell and taste of food initiate impulses within the brain which are relayed to the vagal nucleus in the medulla, and from this nucleus, they travel to the secretory units within the stomach via the vagus nerve. The volume of secretion can be influenced by the nature of the meal. Generally, the more appetizing the meal, the greater the volume of gastric secretions. This fact can be of importance in the planning and serving of meals to patients in hospital, for if the meal is not appetizing there will be less gastric juice and digestion will be made more difficult. Stimulation of secretions via the vagal nerves is called the cephalic phase of secretion. The local (gastric) phase of secretion is stimulated by food in the antrum or pyloric part. Food in the antrum stretches the antrum and brings about the release of the hormone, gastrin, from the G cells of the mucosa. This is released into the capillaries and enters the venous circulation. When gastrin reaches the fundus of the stomach, it stimulates the parietal cells to secrete HCl. This hormonal reflex ensures that the acid will be secreted in response to the presence of food in the stomach. Vagal stimulation can also increase gastrin secretion as can high levels of calcium in the blood or the presence of alkaline solutions within the stomach.

Cells within the pancreas can synthesize gastrin but their role in normal digestive physiology is not known. The control of acid secretion in the stomach is even more complicated. There is now evidence that two hormones produced in the mucosa of the duodenum — secretin and cholecystokinin — can inhibit the gastrin-stimulated release of HCl.

Gastric secretions have the following functions:

(1) The low pH (high acidity) kill many of the bacteria that enter with the food.
(2) The mucus protects the mucosa from the acidity.
(3) The acid denatures protein and converts pepsinogen to pepsin so that protein digestion begins.
(4) Intrinsic factor is secreted.

Not all gastric secretion is in response to food. There is a constant basic level of secretion which averages 50–75 ml/hour. This secretion contains water, mucin, Na^+, Cl^- and HCO_3^-; the concentration of HCl is less than that found in the gastric juice just before and after eating. The stimulus for this basal secretion is not known.

Often it is useful to measure the volume and acidity of the gastric juices. The juice is collected by passing a small, soft, plastic tube through the nose, nasopharynx, pharynx and oesophagus into the stomach. Suction is applied to the tube and the gastric secretions are collected for an hour or more. Secretion may be quite high when a duodenal ulcer is present, and secretion is low in pernicious anaemia and when there is a malignant ulcer in the stomach. A commercial preparation of the hormone, gastrin, may be given to increase HCl secretion.

The movements of the stomach are also important. The presence of food in the stomach generates peristaltic waves which mix the food and break it down into a thick mixture of smaller particles which is called chyme. The more the stomach is stretched by the chyme, the greater will be the strength of the contractions and the faster the chyme will pass through the pylorus into the duodenum. The word pylorus comes from the Greek work *pylouros*, meaning gatekeeper. The pylorus is like a gatekeeper and regulates the flow of chyme into the duodenum.

The stomach must store the food awhile and allow it to approach osmotic equilibrium with the blood. The actual control of gastric emptying is under both nervous and hormonal control. The rate at which the stomach musculature contracts is relatively constant; however, the force of these contractions varies considerably. Stretching of the stomach by its content increases the force of contraction as does vagal stimulation. A hormone produced by the intestinal mucosa, enterogastrone, inhibits the force of gastric contractions. This hormone is released in response to significant amounts of fat or acid in the duodenum.

It may take 4 hours for a normal meal to be completely evacuated from the stomach into the small intestine, although most of the meal is evacuated into the intestine within the first hour. A particularly acid meal or one with a high content of fat will reduce gastric motility and keep food within the stomach for a longer time.

People who attend official dinners where alcohol is served sometimes eat egg, take a teaspoonful of olive oil or a glass of milk before attending these functions so as to reduce gastric motility and reduce the absorption of alcohol by keeping it in the stomach where absorption is slower. This slows the rise of alcohol levels in the blood.

e. The small intestine. The secretions of the pancreas and liver are emptied in the middle of the duodenum through a common duct called the ampulla of Vater. There are no nerves going to the duodenum from the pancreas or liver, yet when chyme is placed in the duodenum, both the liver and pancreas release their secretions. The causal connection between these two events remained a problem until 1902, when two investigators, Bayliss and Starling, suggested that a hormone was responsible. At the time, this was a controversial idea and the investigators' data were not readily accepted. Today, we are familiar with the concept of hormone action and the list of hormones gets longer and longer.

We now know that two hormones from the duodenum, pancreozymin and secretin, stimulate the liver and pancreas. The presence of fat and protein fragments within the duodenum stimulates the duodenal mucosa to release the hormone, pancreozymin. This hormone is not released into the lumen of the intestine but is absorbed by the capillaries in the villi and travels in them to the superior mesenteric and the hepatic portal veins. Within the sinusoids, some of the hormone is absorbed and stimulates the liver cells to secrete bile and cause contraction of the gall bladder. Most of the hormone continues onward in the hepatic vein to the heart and the left ventricle, which distributes the hormone throughout all the arteries of the body. Some of the hormone gets to the pancreas via the pancreatic artery and causes the exocrine portion of the pancreas to release a secretion rich in digestive enzymes which enters the intestine by way of the pancreatic duct.

An acid solution in the duodenum causes the duodenal mucosa to release another hormone named secretin. This hormone takes the same route as pancreozymin and stimulates the exocrine portion of the pancreas to secrete a very watery alkaline solution which raises the pH and neutralizes the acid chyme in the duodenum. Secretin may have some role in stimulating the gall bladder to contract.

Vagal stimulation and pancreozymin seem to be the most important controls. Sometimes pancreozymin is called pancreozymin–cholecystokinin.

The acidic chyme in the duodenum can cause an ulcer or an erosion of the intestinal mucosa if there is an excessive secretion of acid or an insufficient secretion of mucus, which normally forms a protective layer about 1 mm thick. If the acid eats into the muscle and nerve, there will be a sensation of pain; if it reaches the blood vessels it can destroy them and lead to internal haemorrhaging, and if it continues to the serosa, the undigested foods can escape the tract into the abdomen causing serious infection. The initial part of the duodenum seems most susceptible to ulcer formation, though an ulcer may form anywhere in the tract. The stomach is well protected but aspirin and alcohol are especially irritating to it.

Duodenal ulcer is one of the most commonly encountered gastro-intestinal diseases. Approximately 1 in 10 adult males in Great Britain and the United States will suffer from this condition at some time in their lives. Understanding of the treatment of a duodenal ulcer depends upon an understanding of digestive physiology. Ulcer patients are urged to avoid alcohol, drinks containing caffeine (among them tea and coffee) and also to avoid pepper and ginger, as these substances directly stimulate the parietal cells to secrete HCl. Since distension of the antrum causes gastrin release, smaller, more frequent meals are indicated. In theory, a reduction in the stretch of the antrum also reduces gastrin release and HCl secretion. The frequent feeding benefits the patient in that the food acts as a buffer, raises the pH and reduces the concentration of free hydrogen ions.

The hypersecretion of HCl which occurs in most ulcer patients is due to the secretion of excess acid when the stomach is empty, rather than an increased secretion of acid in response to food in the stomach. Ulcer pain characteristically occurs 2–4 hours after eating when the stomach is empty, and the pain can be relieved by eating. There is no good evidence to show that bland or pureed diets are beneficial to the patient. Antacids also neutralize HCl, though they should not be taken immediately before or after eating, when the stomach is full of food, but an hour or more after eating, when they will be more effective. Anticholinergic drugs may be used. These block the acetylcholine which is released by the vagal nerves, preventing it from stimulating the parietal cells. New drugs are being developed which prevent gastrin from stimulating the parietal cells. These drugs seem to work by blocking the action of histamine, which is involved in parietal cell stimulation.

Stress, tension and anxiety can all increase HCl secretion. This is probably mediated via increased vagal stimulation, and this psychologically induced acid secretion can aggravate the ulcer. Simply telling the patient to relax and not worry does not usually work. Listening to the patient and making a serious attempt to be helpful may be more successful.

In a small fraction of all ulcer patients, medical therapy will fail, the ulcer will not heal and surgery will be necessary before the ulcer erodes into an artery and causes significant loss of blood. The surgeon may cut branches of the vagal nerves or remove part of the gastrin-producing antrum; both procedures reduce acid secretion. Surgery may be necessary for those rare patients whose ulcers are caused by gastrin-producing tumours of the pancreas.

Most digestion and absorption takes place in the jejunum and ileum. The intestine itself secretes about 2 litres of mucus and alkaline secretions each day while weak contractions of the smooth muscle propel the chyme along. Distension of the tract and parasympathetic stimulation increase contractions, while sympathetic stimulation reduces motility and thus slows the transit time through the small intestine. Neural stimulation is also important in contraction of the gall bladder and opening the sphincters of Oddi and Boyden, so allowing bile to enter the duodenum.

Parasympathetic stimulation tends to dominate most of the intestine. Peristaltic waves can occur without sympathetic or parasympathetic stimulation, as can segmentation contractions. Segmentation contractions are circular ring-like contractions that appear, then disappear at regular intervals along a section of the intestine. Tonus changes are local changes in the rate and degree of smooth muscle contraction. These changes are dependent on the relative strengths of sympathetic and parasympathetic stimulation.

The intestines are almost constantly active. Intestinal motility can be demonstrated by listening to the sounds produced while chyme and gastro-intestinal secretions are propelled through the tract. Just place a stethoscope over your abdomen and listen to the normal bowel sounds. If the intestines have been traumatized or handled during surgery, intestinal motility may be temporarily absent or reduced. This condition is called paralytic ileus. Infection or inflammation of the peritoneum can also cause paralytic ileus. Normal bowel sounds are absent with a paralytic ileus, and the character of the sounds changes if there is an intestinal obstruction. Often, food is withheld from post-surgical patients until bowel sounds are again present.

The smooth muscle of most of the intestine has β receptors. Stimulation of the β receptors causes relaxation of the intestinal smooth muscle. Thus, adrenaline (a β-receptor stimulator) reduces intestinal motility and tonus by causing the smooth muscle to relax. (The concept of α and β receptors is discussed more fully in the Chapter on the nervous system.)

f. The large intestine. Most nutrients and a great deal of fluid have been absorbed by the first half of the jejunum, so only 500 ml of chyme enters the colon. The colon is not particularly suited for absorptive work since it lacks convolutions and villi and therefore has a smaller absorptive surface area than the small intestine. Some active absorption of sodium does take place, followed by passive absorption of water. So, the colon has a storage function and also houses bacteria within its comfortably warm, moist and nutrient-containing environment. These bacteria synthesize vitamins, which is particularly important to individuals living on low vitamin diets. Within the colon these bacteria pose no direct hazard but, should they gain access to other parts of the body, serious infection could result. The most common colonic bacteria belong to the genus Bacteroides; these anaerobic bacteria make up more than 95% of the normal faecal flora. Since bacteria carry on metabolism, they produce gas (flatus) which has no redeeming biological value.

g. Defaecation. The time between the eating of a meal and its expulsion in the faeces is variable. Studies have shown that the transit time for a meal eaten by students in an English boarding school averaged 76 hours; 47 hours transit time for students in an African boarding school; 36 hours transit time for students in a rural African school. Transit time is defined as the time required for 80% of a meal to be eliminated in the stool (faeces).

The English diet was more sophisticated and higher in sugar, meat and fat, whereas the African diet contained more fibre. Fibre refers to an indigestible form of carbohydrate which is mostly cellulose. Cellulose is the chief constituent of plant cell walls and cannot be digested by humans because the glucose molecules making up the large cellulose molecule are linked together in such a way that the digestive enzymes cannot separate them. As these cellulose molecules cannot be absorbed, they are osmotically active molecules and retain water within the intestine. This is why people on high-fibre diets tend to pass large, soft, almost unformed stools. In general, the stool weight of African students was almost 2–4 times as great as that of English students. Fibre from wholegrain cereals, such as wheat, seems to stimulate intestinal motility more than fibre which is derived from fruit and vegetables. Bran from wheat is a much better source of fibre than lettuce and celery, although fruits and vegetables are of dietary importance; in fact, vegetarians in England have transit times and stool weights close to those of the African students.

You are probably wondering what the significance of transit time and stool weight is. In the past few years, there has been an increasing interest in the relationship between diet and disease. For instance, cancer of the colon is one fiftieth as common in many African countries as it is in parts of Europe and North America. If black Africans move to the United States and switch to a "typical" United States diet, their incidence of colon cancer increases. Scientists have speculated that cancer of the colon may be caused by certain metabolites in the faecal material, and that the longer the metabolites are in contact with the colon, the greater the chance of a malignant process in the colon being initiated. Other conditions, including constipation, haemorrhoids and diverticula in the colon, have been related to diet, fibre, transit time and faecal bulk. At the present time it cannot be said that adding fibre to the diet will definitely prevent or reduce cancer or certain other intestinal diseases, though there is evidence which suggests, but does not prove, that fibre may be beneficial.

Normally, there is little muscular activity within the large intestine but often after a meal there is a dramatic increase in which large portions of the colon contract in unison in quick forceful waves; these contractions are called a mass movement. The mass movement suddenly forces a large amount of faecal material into the rectum and causes its walls to be stretched. This stretching stimulates receptors within the wall which send impulses to the brain and trigger the desire to defaecate, and reflexly inhibit the internal and external anal sphincters which make up the final 3 cm of the rectum (see Figure 13.9). The external anal sphincter is striated muscle so the reflex inhibition can be overridden by impulses originating from conscious areas in the brain and the external sphincter will be closed until the individual chooses to defaecate.

Defaecation can be stressful, particularly for elderly persons who are constipated and who have to strain to pass their stool. It can be even more difficult when an individual is flat in bed and asked to defaecate into a bedpan. There is now a trend to let most patients defaecate sitting up out of bed.

Diarrhoea is the condition of frequent expulsion of highly fluid faecal material and is caused by excessive intestinal motility or by failure to absorb intestinal contents. Of course, the greater the frequency and force of contraction, the more rapid will be the progress of chyme through the tract and the less time there will be for the absorption of water, resulting in a more fluid stool. Contraction may be increased by parasympathetic stimulation (often caused by anxiety and tensions) or by intestinal irritants such as castor oil or certain bacteria and their toxins. In some countries, diarrhoeal diseases account for half the infant deaths, for the infant is less able to tolerate the loss of fluid and salts and the change in pH resulting from loss of bicarbonate ion, than can the adult. These infants cry, but they may be so dehydrated that they may not be able to form tears. Diarrhoea can often be a "social disease" for it may be caused by overcrowding, poor sanitation and contaminated food and water.

The opposite of diarrhoea is constipation, in which defaecation occurs at very prolonged intervals. This may result from a low bulk diet or sympathetic stimulation which will inhibit intestinal motility and thus greatly increase the transit time allowing more water to be reabsorbed and producing firmer stools. Constipation of itself is usually not debilitating. Occasionally, it is indicative of a more serious disorder.

Bowel movements, or the lack of them, are often a source of much humour. Unfortunately many people who are constipated are quite uncomfortable. The widespread sale of laxatives attests this. While many people do have bowel movement every day, others have one every other day or every third day. The chronic use of laxatives to increase the frequency of bowel movements is controversial. In a sense, it is a misplaced controversy, for it ignores the relationship of the diet to the frequency of bowel movement. If the diet lacks bulk or fibre provided by non-digestible cellulose, the intestinal muscle will not be stretched, peristalsis will be reduced and the transit time will be increased. A vivid example of this diet and transit time relationship was provided by the astronauts. During the early space flights, the disposal of human wastes was quite a problem. Part of the solution to the problem was obtained by feeding the astronauts very refined food with little fibre content. This caused constipation with 5 or 6 days between bowel actions.

Disorders of intestinal motility are more common than disorders of absorption. One of the most common disorders is the irritable bowel syndrome, also called the spastic bowel syndrome or functional diarrhoea and/or constipation. It may present an abdominal cramping, diarrhoea or constipation or a combination of these symptoms. The condition is due to disordered peristalsis related to abnormal sympathetic and parasympathetic stimulation. This nervous stimulation is brought about by anxiety, tension, physical or emotional stress, and it demonstrates the close relationship between the individual's environment and physiological processes.

A typical stool is two thirds water, the remainder being bacteria, cellulose, cellular debris and a very small amount of unabsorbed food and secretions. Since ancient times, stools have been examined for signs of disease. A particularly foul odour is often present in steatorrhoea and is due to unabsorbed fat. Thin strands of meat may be present if protein digestion is deficient. The stool can be cultured for pathogenic bacteria and examined microscopically for traces of parasites or ova. Mucus in the stool may suggest the irritable bowel syndrome or inflammatory disease of the bowel.

The colour of the stool is mainly dependent on the quantity of bile pigments from the liver reaching the small intestine. Blood may enter the stool as a result of a bleeding ulcer, inflammation of either the small or large intestine, ruptured haemorrhoids or a tumour. Tumours in the colon often ooze blood, which then mixes with the faecal material in the colon, so the faeces do not look bloody but appear their usual colour. There are tests for occult (hidden) blood in the stool. These tests are simple, inexpensive and invaluable, for the sooner a cancer is detected, the better the patient's chance of survival. In one such test, the guaiac test, a small amount of stool is spread on filter paper, reagents are added and, if haemoglobin is present, a blue-green colour will appear.

The stool should always be tested if a person has had a change in his or her pattern of bowel movements, as this may herald the appearance of a cancer. Large amounts of blood can colour the stool so it appears black and tarry. Iron, bismuth and certain berries can also cause a black-appearing stool.

h. Vomiting. Vomiting is the forceful expulsion of gastric, and occasionally intestinal, contents out of the mouth. In clinical situations, the word emesis is frequently used instead of the word vomiting, e.g. "Mr Jones had an emesis this morning".

The act of vomiting begins with an inspiration and is followed by a closure of the glottis. Next, the abdominal and thoracic muscles contract and cause the intra-abdominal and intra-thoracic pressure to increase. These pressure increases are transmitted to the stomach. When the gastro-oesophageal sphincter opens, the gastric (and sometimes the intestinal) contents will be forced out of the stomach and up the oesophagus. These actions are controlled by a special vomit centre within the medulla of the brain which sends impulses to the appropriate muscles in the proper sequence.

Vomiting is a reflex and the stimuli for its initiation can come from pain or irritation anywhere in the body, though the most common stimulus is irritation of the digestive tract itself. Acceleration of the head such as might be experienced on a rocking boat (nausea) or psychological factors such as fear or anxiety may also stimulate the reflex.

Vomiting can upset fluid balance and pH because of the loss of acid and ions from the stomach. Haematemesis is defined as the vomiting of blood and indicates gastrointestinal haemorrhage. Anyone vomiting blood should receive prompt medical attention. Blood that has been in contact with the gastric or intestinal juices will lose its typical red colour. It may become dark brown or black and resemble coffee grounds.

Vomiting can cause other complications. If the vomitus is not completely expelled from the mouth, some of it may get into the larynx, descend further in the respiratory tract and cause a pneumonia. This is called an aspiration pneumonia. Aspiration pneumonias are common in alcoholics who get sick in their stomach and whose gag-and-swallow reflexes are weak because of the depressant nature of alcohol on the nervous system. These pneumonias are occasionally seen in hospitalized and post-surgical patients whose nervous system is depressed by drugs or anaesthetics and who vomit when they are flat on their backs in bed.

Vomiting does, however, have its purpose. It is the useful way to expel unwanted material from the stomach. There are drugs that induce vomiting and may be used when people, particularly children, have taken unknown or too many pills. There are studies which show that in children vomiting is a more efficient way to remove material than suction by a gastric tube.

In ancient days, Roman citizens would often intentionally cause themselves to vomit by tickling the back of their throats with a feather after they had completed a meal. After vomiting they were fresh to begin eating a second meal. Alas, there are no citizens left of this once dynamic, prosperous and powerful empire to demonstrate for us. Perhaps there is a lesson here.

14. Metabolism and Nutrition

INTRODUCTION

The World Health Organization has chosen to define health as a "state of complete physical, mental and social well-being and not merely the absence of disease or infirmity". The wisdom of this definition becomes strikingly apparent when we consider nutritional disorders, under-nutrition and over-nutrition. Those suffering from them are not often found in hospital or considered sick in the conventional sense of the word.

Nutrition is the sum total of the processes by which the living organism receives and utilizes the materials necessary for growth, function and repair of the body tissues. The topic cannot be understood unless the essentials of metabolism are clearly in mind. So far we have been dealing with metabolism using statements like:

$$C_6H_{12}O_6 + 6O_2 \rightarrow 6CO_2 + 6H_2O$$

This is really an abbreviation and is like saying

John Kennedy; born 1916 — died 1963.

Although the statement is true, the life between and its significance are missing. Let us begin the study of metabolism with a consideration of energy.

WHAT IS ENERGY AND HOW IS IT MEASURED?

Matter occupies space and has weight; energy does neither. We can therefore never measure energy directly and must measure it indirectly by determining its effects on matter. This requires that energy be defined as the ability to do work, and the amount of energy is determined by measuring the work that has been done or can be done.

The most convenient unit of energy is the kilocalorie (kcal), which is that amount of energy which will raise the temperature of one kilogram of water $1\,°C$, from $14.5\,°C$ to $15.5\,°C$. Sometimes the kilocalorie is loosely referred to as simply the "calorie". A simple way to measure the energy contained within a substance would be to measure the number of calories produced by that substance when it is burned. An instrument known as a calorimeter has been specifically designed for this purpose (see Figure 14.1). The substance to be tested is placed in a chamber, surrounded by water, in the middle of the calorimeter. Oxygen is added and a spark introduced to ignite the substance. When the substance has burned, the temperature change of the water surrounding the casing is measured by a thermometer. You could find the number of kilocalories in a loaf of bread or a bunch of bananas by weighing a sample and

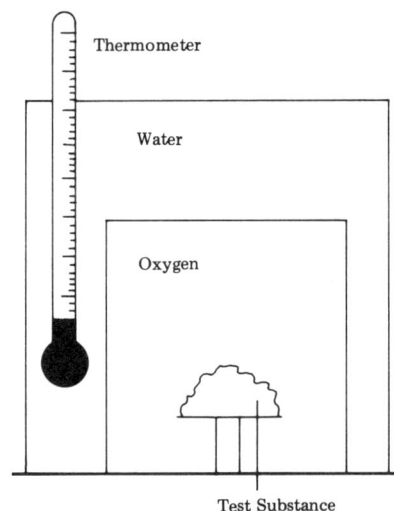

Figure 14.1 A calorimeter.

using this method. Since both bread and bananas are chiefly carbohydrate, they will be burned or oxidized to CO_2 and H_2O. This should not be too surprising to you when you consider that even the hardest and most expensive of diamonds could be converted to CO_2 in a calorimeter under appropriate conditions, for both bread and diamonds are carbon compounds and therefore burn.

Most fats, like carbohydrates, can be completely burned to CO_2 and H_2O in a calorimeter for they contain carbon, hydrogen and oxygen. Proteins cannot be completely oxidized to CO_2 and H_2O for they contain nitrogen and thus can only be partially oxidized. Fat, protein and carbohydrate each have a different calorific value. This means that if you determined the calorific value of 1 gram of fat or protein or carbohydrate they would each, when burned, yield a different number of calories. You probably remember from the Chapter on units, definitions, etc., that energy can also be expressed in units known as joules.

1 joule (J) = 0.239 kcal
1 calorie = 4.18 joules

There are 1000 kilojoules (kJ) in 1 megajoule (MJ). The energy contained in fat, protein or carbohydrate can be expressed in calories or joules. These values are listed below:

1 gram fat   = 9.3 kcal = 38.9 kJ
1 gram protein   = 5.3 kcal = 22.2 kJ
1 gram carbohydrate = 4.1 kcal = 17.1 kJ

Of course, we seldom eat pure fat or protein or carbohydrate, as most foods are a combination of these. Some calorific values of various foods are listed in Table 14.1.

Table 14.1 Some calorific values of various foods.

Food	Approximate values			
	kcal/100 g food	kJ/100 g food	g protein/ 100 g food	g fat/ 100 g food
Plantain	74	309	9	1
Yam	91	380	6	1
Irish potato	71	296	3	Insignificant
Maize	360	1505	9	4
Bread	250	1045	7	1
Rice	360	1505	7	Insignificant
Cow's milk	69	288	3	3
Eggs	146	610	11	11
Fish	32	134	8	1
Beef	155	648	16	10
Chicken	124	518	12	8
Peas	342	1430	27	3
Beans	342	1430	26	3
Groundnuts	389	1626	19	32
Soy bean flour	356	1488	40	25
Butter	716	2993	1	81
Ghee	902	3770	0	100
Dark green leafy vegetables	26	109	3	1
Light green vegetables	18	75	2	Insignificant
Banana	67	280	3	1
Orange	63	263	3	Insignificant
Pawpaw	25	102	1	Insignificant
Table sugar	418	1747	0	0
Beer (1 pint)	284	1187	1.7	0

A kilocalorie is a kilocalorie regardless of whether it comes from meat or potatoes; however, for reasons which will be seen later, good nutrition requires that kilocalories come from a variety of sources.

So far we have just considered the measurement of the calorific intake but have said nothing about calories within the body. The relationship between calorific intake and calories within the body is expressed by the formula:

$$\text{Calorific intake} = \frac{\text{calories used in}}{\text{biological work}} + \frac{\text{heat given off}}{\text{by body}} + \frac{\text{calories stored}}{\text{in body}} + \frac{\text{calories}}{\text{excreted}}$$

If we have a high calorific intake and do not use the calories in biological work, the body will store the calories. Calories may be used or saved but will never just disappear.

So-called light work is the type of work performed by those who are doctors, homemakers, teachers and office workers among others. The energy expenditure for men during 1 hour of work in these professions is 140 kcal (0.58 MJ); for women it is about 100 kcal (0.41 MJ). Of course, as the work increases, the energy expenditure must also increase. Men and women who engage in certain types of farm work, construction work, dancing or athletic activities will spend more calories than do less active workers. In 1 hour of these activites a man might spend 240 kcal (1.0 MJ) and a woman might spend 175 kcal (0.74 MJ).

Biological work within the body includes muscular contraction, sending neural impulses, absorption, secretion and synthesis of molecules. The body, of course, does not perform its work at 100% efficiency. Body heat results from the inefficiency of work processes. For example, if a food contained energy equal to 100 kcal, the body might form ATP which could do about 40 kcal worth of biological work; the other 60 kcal would be given off as body heat. It would be impossible to measure directly all the energy used in performing this biological work, so an alternative indirect method must be used.

We have seen that in the body, energy is obtained from the burning or oxidation of foodstuffs. We might gain some indication of how much energy was consumed if we knew how much oxygen was consumed and could use this knowledge to estimate the energy consumption. An analogy might help. If you had to, you could determine the distance you travelled in a car even if it had no distance indicator, or if you saw no signposts to tell you how many kilometres you have travelled. It could be done if you knew two things:

(1) the amount of petrol the car consumed and
(2) the number of kilometres the car goes per litre of petrol.

For example, if the car used 10 litres of petrol and the car gets 10 km/litre used, you could determine that the car went 100 km. It is the same with humans. If an individual consumed 15 litres of oxygen within 1 hour and it is known that each litre of oxygen consumed involves the expenditure of approximately 4.9 kcal, you could state that the individual is using about 73 kcal/hour, because:

15 litres/hour × 4.9 kcal = 73.3 kcal/hour.

The amount of energy a person is using can be determined. The clinical measurement of the individual's energy expenditure is known as the basal metabolite rate (BMR). Today, the BMR is seldom used in sophisticated clinical laboratories but it is still a useful teaching exercise. The term "basal" refers to the energy necessary to maintain the continuing activities of the body such as the heartbeat, the muscular work of respiration and kidney function. Since it does not include the energy spent when the individual engages in physical activity, such as walking or working, the individual must be completely at rest and not have eaten for 6–12 hours. The oxygen consumption of the resting individual is then measured for at least 10 minutes; this value is then converted into the oxygen consumption per hour. If 2.5 litres of O_2 were consumed in 10 minutes, then the O_2 consumption in 60 minutes would be 6 × 2.5 litres or 15 litres O_2 consumed per hour. This value is then multiplied by the calorific value of 1 litre of O_2 which is about 4.9 kcal/litre O_2. Thus:

15 litres O_2/hour × 4.9 kcal/litre O_2 = 73.5 kcal/hour.

In 1 day;

24 hours × 73.5 kcal/hour = 1764 kcal would be used.

The BMR can be expressed in any one of three ways:

(1) kcal/day.
(2) kcal/kg of body weight/day.
(3) kcal/m² of body surface area/day.

The third way is the most commonly used, for it gives the most uniform results. A tall and heavy man may have the same BMR as a tall and lean one; the tall and heavy individual will consume more oxygen than the lean one but he will also have a greater surface area.

Even the properly determined BMR is affected by many factors. Children have a higher BMR than adults, and men have a higher BMR than women. Starvation lowers the BMR whereas fever and living in a very cold environment raises it. Mental effort, studying and problem-solving do not affect it.

Clinically, a high metabolic rate usually indicates an excess of thyroid hormone, while a low BMR is an important diagnostic characteristic of too little thyroid hormone. This hormone is a general regulator of metabolic rate. It speeds up the metabolism in nearly all the cells of the body and this faster metabolic rate is reflected in the greater oxygen consumption. More will be said later about thyroid hormone.

WHAT HAPPENS TO CARBOHYDRATE, FAT AND PROTEIN AFTER THEY HAVE BEEN DIGESTED AND ABSORBED? HOW ARE THEY METABOLIZED?

A. Carbohydrate metabolism

After a meal there is a large increase in the sugar concentration in the hepatic portal vein, most of which is glucose. Some of the sugar leaves the liver sinusoids and enters the hepatic cells. Galactose and fructose are converted to glucose in the liver cells. Some glucose may be converted to glycogen. The remainder of the glucose passes on to the heart, which distributes glucose throughout the body so that it can be used by muscle cells, brain, viscera and the heart itself. Within most cells there are three paths that glucose can take:

(1) One possibility is that the glucose molecule may be converted to glycogen. This is accomplished by a series of four reactions, each enzymatically controlled. Since this is an anabolic process, ATP will be used to provide the energy to link the glucose molecules together to form glycogen. The liver, skeletal muscle and the kidneys store glycogen; the concentration of glycogen is greatest in the liver. After you have eaten a large evening meal, the glycogen concentration in your liver increases, but during the night some glycogen is broken down into glucose, which is released into the blood stream to nourish other tissues. If you have fasted for 48 hours or so, all the glycogen stores would be used up.

There is no qualitative difference between the glycogen found in liver and that which is found in muscle. Liver and muscle are different tissues, however, and have some different enzymes, so they will not metabolize glycogen and its breakdown products in an identical manner. Liver has an enzyme which permits glucose to be released into the blood stream, while muscle lacks this enzyme and thus cannot release glucose into the blood stream for the nourishment of other tissues.

There are diseases in which one or more of the glycogen- or glucose-metabolizing enzymes are deficient. In the most common of these diseases, the liver enzyme which permits glucose to be released into the blood is deficient. Infants with this disease can store glycogen in the liver but not break it down to glucose. As a result the liver becomes swollen with excessive glycogen and blood glucose levels can become quite low. More will be said about glycogen and

blood glucose in the Chapter on the endocrine system.

(2) A second path for glucose is its oxidation to CO_2 and H_2O with some of the energy released going into the synthesis of ATP. As pointed out earlier, this does not take place in a single giant step but in a series of enzymatically controlled reactions. There are really two phases to glucose breakdown: glycolysis and the citric acid cycle.

a. Glycolysis. The glycolytic reactions take place in the cytoplasm of the cell. Each glucose molecule produces a net yield of two molecules of ATP from ADP and two molecules of pyruvic acid; pyruvic acid consists of a 3-carbon molecule, so one glucose molecule will give two pyruvic acid molecules.

There are nine major reactions in the glycolytic series and all the reactions can take place without oxygen (anaerobically). If there is no oxygen or hypoxia, the pyruvic acid which has been formed will be converted to lactic acid, another 3-carbon molecule. During strenuous exercise there is often insufficient oxygen being delivered to the working muscles, so lactic acid is produced and some of it diffuses out of the muscle cells into the circulation.

b. The citric acid cycle. In the presence of oxygen, pyruvic acid is converted to an extremely important compound known as acetyl coenzyme A (see Figure 14.2). This molecule enters the citric acid cycle by combining with a

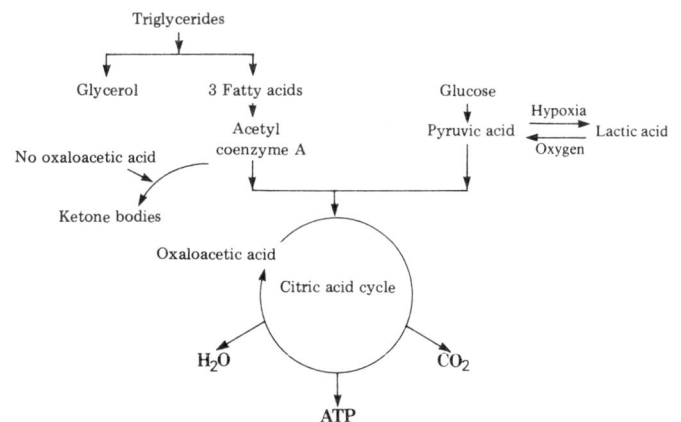

Figure 14.2 Outline of glucose metabolism.

molecule of oxaloacetic acid to form citric acid. The citric acid cycle, sometimes called the Krebs cycle, has nine major reactions in which 15 molecules of ATP, three molecules of H_2O and three molecules of CO_2 are formed for every pyruvic acid molecule that enters it. Oxaloacetic acid is regenerated at the end of the cycle, ready to combine with another pyruvic acid molecule to form citric acid and begin the cycle again. Since one molecule of glucose can form two molecules of pyruvic acid, these will produce 30 ATP, and $6CO_2$ and $6H_2O$ are formed as a result of the cycle. If there is inadequate oxygen only 2 ATPs will be formed from the glycolytic pathway, and lactic acid will be formed.

This fact helps explain the oxygen debt. If you have been exercising for a while and then suddenly and completely stop, you will continue to breathe heavily and consume large amounts of oxygen even though you are barely moving. The explanation for this behaviour is as follows:

(i) Because of the severity of the exercise, the oxygen requirements of skeletal muscles dramatically increase.

(ii) The circulatory system cannot completely meet these increased needs so insufficient oxygen is delivered to the skeletal muscles.

(iii) Glucose is metabolized anaerobically to lactic acid.

(iv) Lactic acid accumulates in the blood.

(v) When exercise stops, sufficient oxygen must be delivered to the muscles to meet their needs and to oxidize the lactic acid that has built up, waiting to go into the oxygen-requiring citric acid cycle.

(vi) Increased breathing continues until the lactic acid has been converted to pyruvic acid and completely oxidized in the citric acid cycle. Some lactic acid will be converted to glucose in the liver by means of a process known as gluconeogenesis. This process is described in sections to follow.

Thus the oxygen debt is the amount of oxygen required to convert lactic acid back to pyruvic acid and metabolize it.

(3) *Conversion to fat.* Intuitively you know that if you eat enormous amounts of carbohydrate you will get fat — from additional adipose tissue, just as surely as if you were on a high fat diet. Before glucose can become a fatty acid molecule, it has to go through the glycolytic pathway to acetyl coenzyme A. Two acetyl coenzyme A molecules then combine with each other to form a 4-carbon compound; another molecule of acetyl coenzyme A is added to the 4-carbon compound, forming a 6-carbon compound. Acetyl coenzyme A is added on again and again so that ultimately a long chain fatty acid with an even number of carbon atoms is formed. This synthesis requires ATP and can only occur if there is sufficient glucose within the cell to meet its needs. The fatty acids combine with glycerol to form a triglyceride. Triglycerides are stored in adipose cells found chiefly beneath the skin and in the abdominal cavity.

B. Fat metabolism

A major portion of the energy requirements of the body is supplied by fat. Though fats form a smaller percentage of most diets, they contain more calories per gram than carbohydrate does. Fats are a better energy storage form than carbohydrate. If you fast for 48 hours, nearly all the body's glycogen will have disappeared, yet there will be adequate fat stores to last for many days, the number depending on the size of the fat stores. There are two major metabolic pathways for fats:

(1) *Fat catabolism.* Liver, heart and skeletal muscle are the chief users of fatty acids and their breakdown products. The first step in fat catabolism involves the separation of the fatty acid molecule from glycerol (see Figure 14.2). Next, a complex molecule, coenzyme A, joins the fatty acid at one end and is enzymatically split off with the two end carbon atoms, forming acetyl coenzyme A, leaving the fatty acid two carbons shorter. If there is an oxaloacetic acid molecule available, acetyl coenzyme A will combine with it and enter the citric acid cycle and produce 12 molecules of ATP, $2CO_2$ and $2H_2O$. The shortened fatty acid recombines with coenzyme A, loses the two end carbons to form acetyl coenzyme A, which combines with oxaloacetic acid in the citric acid and the whole process is repeated again and again. Since most fatty acids have an even number of carbons, there are no "left overs" when the process is completed.

Successful fatty acid catabolism requires the presence of oxaloacetic acid and certain enzymes and their cofactors. If there is an enzyme deficiency or if there is an inadequate amount of oxaloacetic acid relative to the amount of acetyl coenzyme A, there is no way in which the excess acetyl coenzyme A can enter the citric acid cycle. In diabetes mellitus, both fat and glucose metabolism are disrupted. Fatty acids are broken down and more acetyl coenzyme A is formed than can enter the cycle. This causes large quantities of acetyl coenzyme A to build up. The acetyl coenzyme A molecules combine with one another and are metabolized to form ketone bodies (acetoacetic acid, β-hydroxybutyric acid and acetone) (see Figure 14.2). If the ketone bodies accumulate, the patient is said to be suffereng from ketosis, which is often detected by the strange fruity smell of the patient's breath.

The ability of the liver to metabolize fats can be seriously hampered. The accumulation of significant amounts of fat within the liver is a sign that the liver cells have been injured. Excessive amounts of alcohol are toxic to the liver and can cause fat accumulation among other things. The alcoholic's liver problems are frequently made worse because many alcoholics subsist on nutritionally poor diets. Fat may also accumulate in diabetes mellitus and as a result of exposure to certain drugs and anaesthetics. Carbon tetrachloride (CCl_4), a commonly used industrial solvent, also causes fat accumulation. This is thought to be the result of a direct action of CCl_4 on the membranes of the liver cell.

(2) *Fat synthesis and storage.* Dietary fat can be broken down or stored in adipose tissue. Fat may also be formed from carbohydrate (see above). This process is essentially the reverse of fatty acid breakdown, though synthesis requires much ATP.

Although fat synthesis can occur in the liver or adipose tissue, most fat is stored as triglyceride (three fatty acids plus glycerol) in the adipose tissue. Triglycerides from the circulating chylomicrons can also be catabolized or stored.

The release of fatty acids into the circulation from adipose tissue has been the subject of intense investigation. There is generally an inverse relationship between the fatty acids and the blood glucose. After a meal, when glucose concentration is normally highest, plasma fatty acids are low, whereas between meals, when blood glucose concentration is low, fatty acids are high. Hormones, including adrenaline from the adrenal medulla and growth hormone from the pituitary, are important in stimulating the release of fatty acids from adipose tissue, while insulin from the pancreas is necessary for the synthesis of triglyceride from circulating fatty acids. The regulation of fat metabolism will be covered more extensively in the Chapter on the endocrine system.

C. Protein metabolism

With 21 individual amino acids, each having its own metabolic pathways, protein metabolism can be quite complex. Fortunately, there are a few common features of protein metabolism so each amino acid does not need to be considered individually. These common features include:

(1) Manufacture of new protein. Cellular and plasma proteins must be continually synthesized for they are

continually being broken down. The liver is the site of most plasma protein synthesis. The amino acids which have been absorbed travel to the liver via the hepatic portal vein, and are linked together in the hepatocytes, under the control of the DNA–RNA code. Antibodies, which are plasma proteins belonging to the IgG class of immunoglobulins, are not synthesized by the liver — they are synthesized by the plasma cells. Most cells continually synthesize some proteins either for "export" as hormones or to replace enzymes and cellular structures which are continually being broken down and need replacing.

(2) Some amino acids may be converted to other amino acids. Essential amino acids, cannot be formed from non-essential ones, but non-essential amino acids can be formed from essential ones. It is for this reason that essential amino acids must be supplied in the diet.

(3) The amino acid may be broken down (catabolized) and energy obtained from its catabolism (see Figure 14.3). Before this can happen the nitrogen-containing group must be removed from the amino acid to leave a molecule containing only C, H and O. This process is called deamination, and the deaminated amino acid enters the citric acid cycle to give ATP, H_2O and CO_2.

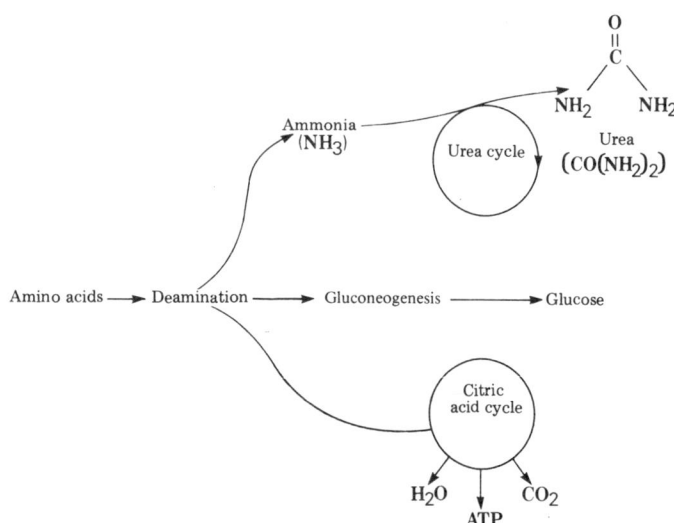

Figure 14.3 Outline of protein metabolism.

In the liver, some of the deaminated amino acids may be converted to glucose instead of going into the citric acid cycle. This formation of glucose is called gluconeogenesis. This long word is formed from three parts: *gluco* from glucose, *neo* meaning new and *genesis* meaning making. Gluconeogenesis refers to the making of new glucose from all sources other than glycogen; most amino acids are potentially gluconeogenic. Lactic acid, pyruvic acid and glycerol may also be converted to glucose within the liver.

Amino acids are not major sources of energy unless carbohydrate and fat stores have been completely exhausted. If an individual has been receiving insufficient calories, he will begin to metabolize protein. Ultimately the protein actin and myosin filaments of skeletal muscle are catabolized and the muscles begin to atrophy.

The nitrogen-containing group is removed from the amino

acid in the form of ammonia (NH_3) (see Figure 14.3). This compound is particularly toxic to brain tissue and is rapidly converted in the liver to urea ($CO(NH_2)_2$). Urea is very soluble in the blood and readily excreted by healthy kidneys. Within normal limits, urea is not harmful. The series of reactions by which ammonia is converted to urea is called the urea cycle and takes place in the liver. If the liver is seriously diseased, urea will not be synthesized from ammonia and the concentration of ammonia and other toxins in the blood will increase. This is why the intake of protein must be reduced in certain liver diseases. Certain bacteria which inhabit the colon can also form ammonia. These bacteria can be removed from the colon by certain drugs. Urea concentration in the blood will increase if there is excessive protein catabolism, if the individual is on a high protein diet or if the kidneys are working at reduced efficiency and cannot excrete urea.

Errors in protein metabolism do not upset the energy requirements of the body, yet they can have very serious consequences. An example of this is the disease phenyl-ketonuria (PKU), which is called an inborn error of metabolism because it results from a genetic deficiency. Some infants are born without the gene necessary to make the enzyme which converts the amino acid, phenylalanine, to tyrosine. Because of this deficiency, phenylalanine and its metabolites build up in the blood and can do serious damage to the brain, hindering its normal development and causing mental retardation. Since the cause of the disease is genetic it cannot be cured; however, the mental retardation may be prevented if the deficiency is detected early in life and the infant fed a diet which is low in phenylalanine. Some countries require a newborn infant's blood to be tested for high concentrations of phenylalanine so that the tragic effects of this disease may be prevented.

WHAT CONSTITUTES A GOOD DIET?

This question was asked by the early explorers who needed to keep their crews healthy on their long voyages in search of new lands and profitable trade routes. In one early experiment, the Japanese government sent out two ships with similar crews on voyages of the same length of time. The crew of the first ship ate their customary diet of polished rice and 100 of the crew came down with beriberi. The second ship reported only 16 cases of beriberi; these 16 men had preferred to eat only their polished rice and none of the meat and vegetables that had been provided to all the second crew.

A. Water

The first requirement for a good diet is an adequate amount of safe drinking water. Man may live for weeks without food, but only days without water.

B. Adequate calories

The emphasis here is on the word "adequate", for in industrialized societies the tendency is to consume excessive calories causing people to become overweight. Table 14.2 gives a list of average daily calorific (megajoule) require-

Table 14.2 Average daily calorific (megajoule) requirements.

	Calories (kcal)	Megajoules
Infant	weight in kg × 120	weight in kg × 0.5
Child of 1 year	1100	4.60
Child of 2 years	1300	5.43
Child of 5 years	1700	7.10
Child of 8 years	2000	8.36
Child of 11 years	2100	8.78
Boy 11–18	2500–3000	10.45–12.54
Girl 11–18	2250–2500	9.40–10.45
Adult male	2800	11.70
Adult female	2500	10.45
Nurses	3000	12.50
Men doing light work	3000	12.50
Men doing heavy work	4000	16.72
Pregnant woman (last months)	2800	11.70
Breast-feeding mother	3300	13·79

ments. The above Table provides a guideline for calorific (megajoule) intake. Infants and children who have a history of malnutrition will require more calories to provide energy for "catch-up" growth.

There are estimates that the calorific cost of a single pregnancy is 80 000 kcal (334 MJ). The energy needs are greater during the last trimester of pregnancy than during the 1st trimester.

An individual who does not have enough food suffers from starvation (marasmus). Marasmus is the scientific term applied to individuals suffering from inadequate calories and protein. A marasmic child is very thin with arms and legs that look like sticks. The skin will be wrinkled because there is no fat beneath it. A healthy adult may do without food (but not without water) for a considerable period of time. When the mayor of Cork, Ireland, was arrested in 1920, he fasted in jail for 73 days before dying of starvation. Thus, the biblical fast of 40 days is possible.

In societies where food is plentiful, obesity is a common problem. Obesity implies an excess of adipose tissue. The relationship between obesity and health is complex, but nevertheless it is clear that obesity is associated with an increased risk of many diseases, and aggravates others. High blood pressure is ten times more common in individuals who are overweight than in individuals who are not overweight. Cerebrovascular disease is likewise more common in obese people. Diabetes mellitus is made worse and pregnancy more complicated by obesity. In general, obese individuals do not live as long as those who are thin.

Obese persons take in too many calories and expend too few; the reason for this imbalance has not been ascertained. It is often said that obesity is caused by a metabolic disorder or some hormonal imbalance. There are cases in which an endocrine disturbance or neurological lesion can produce obesity. However, in most obese persons no endocrine or nervous disease which could cause the obesity can be found. Obesity can be the cause of certain endocrine disorders.

If obesity is a disease with an unknown cause, it is not surprising that the results of treatment for obesity are often so dismal. Many obese persons have great difficulty in reducing their calorific intake, and drug and surgical therapies may be more hazardous than obesity itself. Encouragement and psychological reinforcement are usually more effective than simply repeating orders or giving advice to reduce calorific intake and stop overeating.

Since obesity is difficult to treat, it is logical to think that the prevention of obesity is the best solution. Although not all obese individuals were obese as children, most obese children do grow up into obese adults.

C. Adequate carbohydrate, fat and protein

An adequate number of calories by itself is not sufficient for good nutrition. The calories must come from appropriate amounts of carbohydrate, fat and protein. In an "ideal" diet about 30% of the calories would come from fat; only one third of the fat calories should come from saturated fat. Carbohydrates would supply about 58% of the total calories. Most of the carbohydrate should be in the form of "complex carbohydrate" such as cereals and grains, with only 15% of the total calories in the form of sugar. Protein should supply the remaining 12% of the calories. In industrialized societies the typical diet contains more animal fat and sugar than is recommended. Diets adequate in calories but lacking in carbohydrate or fat are rare.

Protein deficiency is much more common and is usually, but not exclusively, found in tropical and subtropical countries. Kwashiorkor is the condition resulting from a diet which contains an adequate number of calories but an inadequate amount of protein. It is primarily a children's disease and those who suffer from it are often called "sugar babies" because of their high carbohydrate diet. Some symptoms of the disease include oedema (partially resulting from the fall in blood osmotic pressure due to reduced plasma proteins), loss and change in the pigmentation of hair, muscle wastage, anaemia and apathy.

Children with kwashiorkor may look fat and bloated if compared to marasmic children, because of the oedema which hides the weak muscles. A marasmic child will always be hungry, whilst a child suffering from kwashiorkor won't be because of the glucose and calories in the high carbohydrate diet. Although the child is quiet and not crying for food, he or she does have an urgent need for protein. Kwashiorkor is often associated with diarrhoea and infectious diseases.

People suffering from marasmus or kwashiorkor do not often die purely from either of these diseases. Instead they may die from infection or other illnesses. In a healthy person these infections or other diseases would be a relatively minor occurrence. In a malnourished person the ability to fight infection is reduced, and the person cannot compensate for the physiological imbalances induced by disease. The hungry of the world suffer terribly as a result of their malnutrition. The consequences of malnutrition include hindered growth, weakness, inability to do strenuous work and increased susceptibility to disease. Although the well-fed of the world do not feel the pain suffered by the malnourished, the well-fed do suffer a loss from the malnourished's reduced productivity and creativity, which cannot express itself. Kwashiorkor is as cruel a disease as cancer, and is even more frustrating than cancer because the "cure" for kwashiorkor is known.

Proteins are classified as either first class or second class proteins. First class proteins contain all the essential amino acids and are usually from animal sources — milk, meat, eggs and fish. Mother's milk is a first class protein particularly suited for growing children. Second class proteins do not contain all the essential amino acids, or contain them in very small amounts, and are usually of plant origin — wheat, rice, maize.

Since there is no storage form of protein, proteins should be provided in the daily diet so that cellular renewal and replacement of plasma proteins can continue. It is recommended that an adult should have 1 gram/day of protein for every kilogram of body weight; a woman weighing 58 kilos should have about 58 grams/day of protein. Infants and children need more protein in their diet because they are growing rapidly and building new protein; they should have 3 grams/day of protein for every kilogram of body weight. If most of the protein is supplied by milk, meat or other first class proteins, the protein requirement per kilogram body weight will be a little less than those mentioned.

D. Adequate minerals

The body requires sodium, potassium, chlorine, phosphorus, magnesium, some zinc and copper and other elements in very small amounts. Of all the elements there are only three in which deficiencies are commonly seen.

(1) *Iron* is necessary for cellular metabolism and haemoglobin synthesis. Beef and fish, green vegetables and pulses, such as peas and beans, are good iron sources. Although spinach has a high iron content, the body absorbs iron from spinach less efficiently than from other sources. Milk is a poor source of iron.

About 10% of dietary iron is absorbed, although there is considerable individual variation. Iron deficiency is often associated with blood loss. It is not uncommon in adolescent girls because of the additional iron requirements imposed by growth and menstruation; the requirements also increase in pregnancy. The body is able to store iron. If an individual develops an iron deficiency anaemia, it means that the person's diet has been deficient in iron for a considerable period of time, and the body's iron stores have been exhausted.

A healthy person is said to be in "iron balance". Every day a small amount of iron is lost when cells are shed from the skin and from the lining of the urinary and intestinal tracts. In an adult man this amounts to about 1 mg of iron every day; in a menstruating woman the loss would be greater.

A good diet contains 12–15 mg of iron per day, of which about 1 mg will be absorbed. This 1 mg will keep an adult man in iron balance, but it will not provide adequate iron for a menstruating woman. She may have to consume a diet containing approximately 25–28 mg of iron a day to absorb the 2.5–2.8 mg of iron which she may require every day. Many reasonable diets cannot supply this level of iron, so menstruating young and adult women may need some form of iron supplementation.

(2) *Calcium* requirements are greater in growing children than in adults because of bone formation. Calcium is also required for other body functions including blood clotting, strong healthy teeth and membrane stability. Milk is an excellent source of calcium. Pregnant women and nursing mothers also need additional calcium because of the drain on their calcium stores by the foetus.

Since calcium is present in all plant and animal tissue, diets usually contain sufficient calcium to meet the 500 mg recommended daily allowance. Some people may have adequate dietary calcium but they may not be able to absorb it because of a deficiency of vitamin D.

(3) *Iodine* deficiencies are seen in people who live some distance from the ocean, in high altitudes where the seas and oceans never reach or in the centre of large continents. Iodine is found in ocean water, in the land washed by the oceans in prehistoric times and in plants grown on that once covered soil. Iodine is necessary for the synthesis of thyroid hormone, the chief regulator of metabolic rate. Iodine is often provided in salt that has been iodized (it contains NaI in addition to $NaCl$).

(4) In addition to the three previous elements, there are other trace elements thought to be necessary for adequate nutrition. These elements include: chromium (Cr), cobalt (Co), copper (Cu), magnesium (Mg), molybdenum (Mb), selenium (Se) and zinc (Zn). Less is known about these elements, and dietary deficiencies of these elements are unusual. It is possible that these trace elements are more important than we presently realize.

In addition to the above elements, another element, fluorine (F), has been shown to reduce dental caries.

E. Adequate vitamins

Vitamins are compounds required by the body; they do not provide energy but are necessary for enzymes to function and synthetic processes to occur, though the precise functioning of all the vitamins has not yet been worked out. Since they cannot be synthesized by the body in adequate amounts, they must be supplied in the diet.

At the beginning of the twentieth century, when vitamins were beginning to be isolated, they were classified either as fat-soluble or water-soluble. With more modern analytical techniques and additional discoveries, the use of alphabet letters has been used to classify fat-soluble (vitamins A, D, E and K) or water-soluble (B-complex vitamins and vitamin C) vitamins.

Fat-soluble vitamins are most often found in dairy products and in the livers of fish. Human liver and, to a lesser extent, adipose tissue cells can store, within limits, the fat-soluble vitamins that have been absorbed. Steatorrhoea is a condition in which excessive fat is found in the stool because of some defect in fat absorption. Deficiencies of vitamins A, D, E and K may arise in steatorrhoea because these vitamins are soluble in fats and so are absorbed with them. If there is reduced fat absorption, a deficiency may arise, even though fats are included in the diet.

Water-soluble vitamins are found in cereals, fruits and vegetables and, in contrast to fat-soluble vitamins, must be taken more frequently as they may not be appreciably stored in the body.

Fat-soluble vitamins

(1) *Vitamin A (retinol).* Individuals who lack adequate vitamin A often have difficulty seeing in the dark. This is

because the rods (specialized light-receptive cells in the retina of the eye) are dependent on vitamin A for their function. Night-blindness is often the first sign of vitamin A deficiency. The vitamin is also necessary for the maintenance of skin mucous membranes and the epithelium of the eye. It is possible to go permanently blind as a result of vitamin A deficiency and the secondary disruption of the structure of the eye. In fact over 15 000 children become permanently blind every year because of vitamin A deficiency.

Vitamin A is found in fish and animal liver and in dairy products. The body can synthesize vitamin A from one of its precursors, β-carotene, which is a pigment found in many green, yellow or red plants and vegetables. Generally speaking, the more coloured the fruit, the greater is the β-carotene content. Thus, pink grapefruit is a better source for vitamin A than white grapefruit.

Excessive vitamin A can interfere with normal bone growth in children, cause skin eruptions, feeling of weakness, etc. Conditions caused by vitamin A excess are occasionally seen in children who have been given large amounts of cod liver oil or other high potency oils.

(2) *Vitamin D* (*cholecalciferol*). Sunlight acts upon the skin to produce vitamin D from its precursors: without sunlight, vitamin D cannot be synthesized in the body. The vitamin may be obtained directly in the diet from dairy products and fish liver oils. In many not-so-sunny countries, milk and margarine are artificially enriched with vitamin D since this is one of the most common deficiencies. These deficiencies are often found today in urban London with its concentration of immigrants from the West Indies, East Africa and Pakistan who have not increased their vitamin D intake even though their synthesis of the vitamin is reduced because of the relative sunlessness of the city.

The vitamin itself is specifically necessary for the absorption of calcium from the intestines and for the incorporation of calcium into bone. Children who suffer from vitamin D deficiency lack adequate calcium to form bone, and they are not able to mineralize the bone properly with what little calcium is available. The resulting condition is known as rickets. The bones of the lower extremities cannot bear the weight of the growing child and become bowed. Other deformities of the chest, spine and pelvis may develop. In adults, vitamin D deficiency will express itself in a different way. The adult form of rickets is osteomalacia, in which the bones lack adequate calcium, are weak and may even be a source of pain.

The adult daily requirement for vitamin D is 2.5 μg. Children less than 7 years old and women in the 2nd half of pregnancy may require 10 μg a day. Five ml (about a teaspoon) of cod liver oil will provide the 10 μg. This dose should not be exceeded.

In order for vitamin D to reach its full physiological potency, it must be converted to its most active form — 1,25-dihydroxy-vitamin D. The formation of 1,25-dihydroxy-vitamin D is carried out in the liver and kidneys and is regulated by parathyroid hormone (PTH) from the parathyroid gland. (This is discussed in the Chapter on the endocrine system.) Individuals with kidney disease may develop rickets because of the kidneys' inability to convert vitamin D into its most potent form. Vitamin D is like vitamin A in that excessive amounts may be harmful. Hypercalcaemia may be caused by large amounts of vitamin D. Old people often do not get adequate vitamin D.

(3) *Vitamin E* (*tocopherol*). There are several tocopherols which have a similar molecular structure and which function as vitamin E. Less is known about vitamin E deficiency in people than in rats, in which deficiency of vitamin E causes muscular weakness and sterility. This is not true in humans, though vitamin E has an unfounded reputation as a cure for fertility problems. In adult humans, vitamin E deficiency is not common, though it may cause anaemia.

There is some evidence to suggest that vitamin E is an antioxidant and can prevent the destructive, non-enzymatic oxidation by molecular oxygen of certain lipid components of cell membranes. The vitamin is given to premature infants who are receiving oxygen in higher than normal concentrations.

Vitamin E is distributed in seeds, leafy green vegetables and vegetable oils. The estimated daily requirement for vitamin E is 15 mg, although the real role of vitamin E is not presently understood.

(4) *Vitamin K* (*phylloquinone*). This vitamin is necessary for the liver to be able to synthesize prothrombin and other factors necessary for the clotting of blood. The daily requirement for vitamin K is about 30 μg. People who are vitamin K deficient will not form clots properly. The vitamin is found in green vegetables and in liver, and is also synthesized by intestinal bacteria.

Newborn infants are frequently deficient in vitamin K because the early diet lacks this vitamin and the infant does not yet have sufficient intestinal bacteria to produce enough vitamin K. This deficiency may be prevented by injecting the mother with vitamin K prior to delivery or injecting the infant immediately after birth.

There are times when it is medically necessary to reduce the likelihood of the formation of blood clots. Drugs which belong to the class known as coumarins reduce the ability of the blood to coagulate and form a clot. They are thought to work by interfering with the action of vitamin K.

A problem: On the basis of your understanding of the material in this and the preceding Chapter, can you explain why a patient with gallstones blocking the bile duct might be expected to develop a blood coagulation disorder characterized by an excessively long plasma prothrombin time? The answer is not difficult but does require you to integrate information.

Answer: The gallstones would block the flow of bile into the intestine. Bile is necessary to emulsify fat so that it can be broken down by lipase and absorbed. Without bile, fat could not be absorbed and steatorrhoea would result. Since vitamin K is a fat-soluble vitamin, it would not be absorbed and would be excreted in the faecal fat. The resulting vitamin K deficiency prevents the liver from synthesizing prothrombin and other factors which are necessary for clot formation.

Water-soluble vitamins

It used to be thought that there was only one B vitamin. Today, we know that there are many molecules in the B vitamin complex. Seven will be considered here.

(1) *Vitamin B_1* (*thiamine*). This vitamin plays a central role in carbohydrate metabolism; it functions as a coenzyme in the conversion of pyruvic acid to acetyl coenzyme A (see

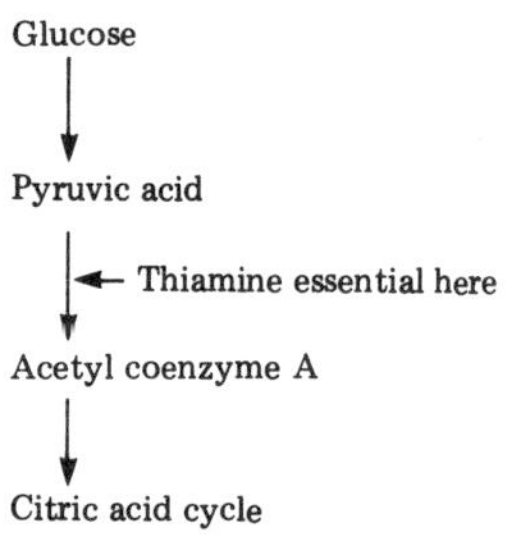

Glucose

↓

Pyruvic acid

↓ ← Thiamine essential here

Acetyl coenzyme A

↓

Citric acid cycle

Figure 14.4 The role of thiamine in metabolism.

Figure 14.4). Since the nervous system derives most of its energy from glucose metabolism, it is expected that the nervous system would be the first to show the effects of thiamine deficiency. Without thiamine, pyruvic and lactic acids will accumulate in the cell, and its normal metabolic pattern will be disrupted. Dry beriberi and thiamine deficiency were mentioned earlier. There is a "wet" form of beriberi in which the heart is affected, and which is associated with massive oedema.

There is a third important disorder due to thiamine deficiency called Wernicke's encephalopathy, which is due to acute thiamine deficiency and is most commonly seen in alcoholics. Wernicke's encephalopathy consists of visual disturbances, lack of proper co-ordination (ataxia) and lack of orientation. It is very often associated with Korsakow's psychosis, which is a thought disorder in which recent memory is markedly impaired and the patient makes up elaborate responses in answer to questions. Because Wernicke–Korsakow syndrome is caused by thiamine deficiency, one must be particularly careful not to cause the syndrome by giving intravenous glucose to hospitalized alcoholics or other thiamine-deficient individuals without first giving thiamine.

Thiamine is found in whole-grain cereals, organ meats, peas, beans and yeast. Thiamine is not found in many man-made or highly processed foods, and it is lacking in refined flour, rice and sugar. Large outbreaks of beriberi occurred soon after the introduction of steel rice mills which removed thiamine-containing husks. The recommended daily intake of thiamine is 115 mg. If a large proportion of a person's calorific intake is provided by alcohol, refined sugar and flour, thiamine should be increased.

(2) *Niacin (nicotinic acid)*. This vitamin functions as part of a coenzyme system which is important for glycolysis, fat synthesis and cellular respiration. A deficiency of niacin causes pellagra. This disease is remembered as the "3-D" disease because it is associated with diarrhoea, dermatitis and dementia. The severity of the three conditions depends on several factors, the chief one being the extent of the vitamin deficiency. Pellagra was epidemic in the countries of Mediterranean Europe and Africa during the 1800s. This epidemic was associated with the beginning of the cultivation of maize, and the subsequent reliance upon maize as a part of the staple diet. Maize is a poor source of both niacin and tryptophan.

The adult requirement is 15–20 mg a day. Meat, particularly liver, whole-grain cereals, peas and nuts are good sources of the vitamin. The amino acid, tryptophan, may be converted to niacin; the process is not, however, very efficient, because it takes 60 mg of tryptophan to produce 1 mg of niacin.

(3) *Riboflavin*. This vitamin also functions as a coenzyme in many oxidative reactions. Unlike thiamine and niacin deficiency, riboflavin deficiency is not associated with specific diseases such as beriberi and pellagra. Riboflavin deficiency is associated with dry, swollen, sore lips (cheilosis) and a swollen, painful tongue (glossitis). Riboflavin is found in leafy green vegetables, meat, fish and milk; it may be destroyed by heating or sunlight. Recommended daily intake is between 1.3 and 1.8 mg.

(4) *Vitamin B_6 (pyridoxine)*. This vitamin functions as a cofactor for several enzymes, many of which are involved in the synthesis and interconversion of amino acids. Deficiency of this vitamin is rare in humans, but the deficiency can produce irritability, convulsions and muscular twitching. Pyridoxine is found in many foods, including meat, whole-grain cereals, maize and many vegetables. The adult daily requirement is 2 mg.

Isoniazid, a drug used in the treatment of tuberculosis, often blocks the action of pyridoxine and similar molecules, so signs of pyridoxine deficiency may develop even though pyridoxine is included in the diet.

(5) *Folic acid (pteroylmonoglutamic acid)*. Folic acid is the parent molecule for a family of molecules called the "folates". The folates are essential for the synthesis of DNA, which precedes cell division in the process of mitosis.

The consequences of folic acid deficiency will appear in those systems where there is a rapid turnover of cells and new cells must be formed by mitosis. For example, diarrhoea may result from the failure of the epithelial lining of the intestines to adequately replace those cells which have been shed. An anaemia is also associated with folic acid deficiency. Since DNA synthesis is hindered more than haemoglobin synthesis, there will be fewer red cells, but each red cell will be larger and contain more haemoglobin than usual. Cells in which there is an unbalanced growth are called megaloblastic cells, and the anaemia which results from folic acid deficiency is a megaloblastic anaemia.

The word folic comes from the Latin word *folium* meaning leaf. Leafy green vegetables such as spinach, lettuce and asparagus are rich sources of folic acid. It is also found in organ meats and is synthesized by some intestinal bacteria. The daily adult requirement of folic acid is approximately 100 μg, and about double that for growing adolescents. In pregnancy, the requirement for folic acid may increase by more than five times. Pills containing iron and folic acid are commonly given to supplement the diet of pregnant women.

Within the body, folic acid is converted by enzymes to a metabolically active form. Rapidly dividing cancer cells, like healthy growing tissue, require this active form of folic acid to grow, form new DNA and divide. Without these folic acid derivatives, DNA synthesis and cell division are hindered. Drugs, which interfere with the enzymes that metabolize folic acid into its active form, have been developed and have been used in treating certain types of cancer.

(6) *Vitamin B_{12} (cyanocobalamin)*. This vitamin is required by all cells of the body, but those of the bone marrow, intestinal tract and nervous system have a special need for it. Cyanocobalamin participates in the metabolism of the folates and is necessary for DNA synthesis. It also plays a role in fat

metabolism and has several other functions, which in humans have not yet been completely clarified.

Disordered myelin formation is associated with cyanocobalamin deficiency. Myelin surrounds the neurone's axon and functions to speed impulse conduction. Disordered myelin synthesis secondary to cyanocobalamin deficiency may cause motor and sensory impairment and mental changes of varying significance and severity.

The anaemia of cyanocobalamin deficiency, like that of folate deficiency, is a megaloblastic anaemia because DNA synthesis is hindered more than RNA and protein synthesis. Many cases of cyanocobalamin deficiency are not due to a lack of the vitamin in the diet, but a failure of the vitamin to be absorbed.

Cyanocobalamin is a large and complex molecule, the structure of which was only determined recently. Because of cyanocobalamin's size and complexity, the vitamin needs assistance in being absorbed into the intestinal mucosa. The parietal cells of the stomach secrete intrinsic factor which is a glycoprotein (see Figure 14.5). Intrinsic factor binds to cyanocobalamin, helps the vitamin avoid destruction by gastric enzymes and permits the vitamin to be absorbed into the mucosa of the ileum. Without intrinsic factor there is no absorption of the vitamin.

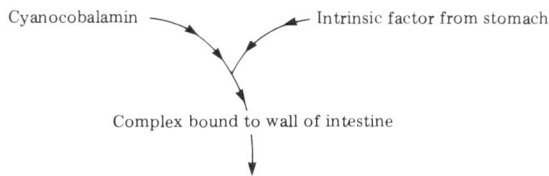

Figure 14.5 The absorption of vitamin B_{12} from the gut.

The megaloblastic anaemia which results from the failure of cyanocobalamin to be absorbed is often called pernicious anaemia. The word pernicious means deadly and pernicious anaemia often was fatal before the treatment for the disease was discovered. Pernicious anaemia will develop if the fundus of the stomach, which is the source of the intrinsic factor, is surgically removed. The disease may also develop spontaneously; it is thought that antibodies are made against intrinsic factor which prevent it from binding to cyanocobalamin. Pernicious anaemia may be treated by intramuscular injections of cyanocobalamin. The standard dose is 100 μg injected monthly.

The Schilling test is used to test the ability to absorb cyanocobalamin. Radioactive cyanocobalamin is given to the patient, who swallows it. If the patient can absorb the cyanocobalamin, some of the cyanocobalamin which has been absorbed will be excreted in the urine, and the urine can then be tested for the presence of radioactive cyano-cobalamin. Non-radioactive cyanocobalamin is also given to prevent the radioactive cyanocobalamin from being absorbed into the body tissues.

Plants do not need cyanocobalamin, so the vitamin is lacking in plants. Liver is the richest source of cyano-cobalamin, but it is also present in muscle meats, eggs, milk and fish. Vegetarianism is common among Hindus in India, and these individually may develop cyanocobalamin deficiency. They do not develop pernicious anaemia, however, because they can absorb cyanocobalamin if it is

included in the diet. The recommended daily intake is 2 μg for an adult and 3 μg for a pregnant woman.

In addition to the macrocytic anaemia seen in B_{12} deficiency, the tongue may be red and sore, and neurological manifestations indicative of peripheral nerve degeneration are seen.

(7) *Vitamin C (ascorbic acid)*. This vitamin is important in the synthesis of collagen, a structural protein in connective tissue. Vitamin C is found in fresh fruits especially citrus fruits (oranges, pineapples and grapefruit) and fresh veget-ables. It is found in mother's breast milk but not in boiled or pasteurized milk because high temperatures destroy the vitamin.

Vitamin C deficiencies are found today in individuals living in cold climates who cannot afford fresh fruits and vegetables and live on tinned foods. In past days, sailors on long voyages often developed scurvy, a vitamin C deficiency disease, in which the capillaries are extremely fragile, the individual bleeds from the gums, and wounds fail to heal properly. The British Navy recognized the relationship between the lack of fresh fruits and scurvy and required its ships to take limes for the crew.

The recommended daily intake of ascorbic acid is 30 mg, which is found in 50 ml of citrus fruit juice or half an orange. In a large controlled study in Canada involving hundreds of subjects, those who supplemented their diets with vitamin C missed significantly fewer days at school or work because of illness due to colds when compared with those subjects who were given placebos. Other studies have not duplicated these results. However, some recent experimental work suggests that vitamin C may work by increasing the efficiency of macrophages or blocking the action of histamine. Before vitamin C gains widespread medical usage, more research must be done to validate the efficacy of vitamin C and to investigate any possible harmful effects.

One often sees the term "minimal daily requirements" associated with specific quantities of vitamins. For example, the minimal daily requirement of niacin is approximately 18 mg/day. These values were arrived at by experimentally determining how much vitamin was necessary to prevent any symptom of vitamin deficiency. Originally, it was discovered that the individual needed a minimum amount of vitamin each month to prevent a vitamin deficiency. This monthly value was then divided by 30 to give the daily vitamin requirement. An individual need not worry if his diet is vitamin deficient for a few days. If he has been eating properly before the deprivation, there will be sufficient vitamin stored to last at least 2–3 weeks. Of course, if his previous meals have been deficient there will be much less vitamin stored.

In recent years more attention has been paid to roughage, the indigestible material in the diet such as fibres containing cellulose. Man's diet has changed during history, just as his clothing, shelter and way of living has changed. There is a tendency for industrialized society in modern times to reduce the amount of roughage in the diet. Grains and cereals are now highly refined, and sugar snacks have almost replaced fresh fruit, which contains fibre. A "balanced meal" of sausages, chips or french-fried potatoes and a glass of milk may contain adequate calories, vitamins and minerals but contains very little roughage. Some nutritionists believe that there is a daily roughage requirement and advocate adding bran to the diet. Bran is the cellulose-rich part of the wheat kernel which is removed when the wheat is turned into flour. In truth, the answer to what constitutes a good diet has not been completely answered.

CONCLUDING THOUGHTS

An infant's stomach is an extremely small structure and all too often it is filled with cheap, bulky food of poor nutritional quality. The infant may stop crying even though his or her urgent nutritional needs have not been met. This failure in nutrition can hinder growth, make him or her more susceptible to disease, can reduce his or her energies and affect a variety of other physical and intellectual functions. Some recent research indicates that even the development of the foetus in the mother's womb may be affected if the mother is malnourished.

Man with all the power of his technology cannot produce sufficient food to meet the special needs of today's children and adults. Tomorrow's technology will increase the production of food but this will not increase fast enough to meet the needs of a population which is increasing even faster. It is therefore necessary for techniques of responsible family planning to be adopted by nations and families alike so that a balance will exist between the amount of food available and those who need to be fed. Good nutrition is a requirement for all human life and not just a circumstance of the rich. All too often, nutritious foods are available but their great expense makes it impossible for the poor to purchase them. And finally, it is necessary for every health professional to use and spread his or her knowledge of nutritional requirements and find ways to help people to meet their need for the correct foods.

There is another side to the nutritional problem. The rich diets of the industrialized nations have been largely responsible for bigger and stronger individuals. Today the average American is more than an inch taller than his grandparents. It has been a mixed blessing however. There is increasing evidence that a diet high in animal fats contributes to atherosclerosis, an arterial disease which is the major cause of death in industrialized societies.

Eating and nutrition involve more than biochemistry and physiology. A meal eaten alone or in a hurry can be an almost mechanical act, yet the same meal shared with friends can be a rich, emotional experience. Beyond the strictly scientific and psychological perspective, there is another way of looking at eating and nutrition. This new view is necessitated by living in a world plagued by famine and food wastage, living with people crippled by starvation or obesity. In a broad sense, eating and nutrition can be seen within a framework of respect. Respect for the food-producing lands and waters, respect for one's own body and health and respect for the lives, needs and health of all with whom we share this earth.

15. The Endocrine System

INTRODUCTION

People travel. Some people have chopped their way through humid jungles and lush rain forests. Still others have trekked across the frozen wastes of the Arctic or climbed the highest mountains. Men and women have survived extreme changes in the *external* environment because of their ability to keep their *internal* environment constant.

Claude Bernard first used the term *milieu interieur* to refer to this internal environment, which consists primarily of the plasma and intercellular (interstitial) fluid that bathes and nourishes every cell of the body. The plasma and intercellular fluid make up the extracellular fluid. The volume of this extracellular fluid is large, more than one third of the total body water (12 litres). The constancy of this watery environment is not the cold of marble and death but is dynamic and results from the combined actions of the endocrine and nervous systems. The individual concentration of many of the molecules in the extracellular fluid may seem small and insignificant, yet changes in their concentration can mean the difference between life and death, sickness and health.

In this Chapter we shall consider part of the endocrine system, the glands and hormones which regulate the internal environment, control metabolism and permit normal growth and development. This does not cover all the endocrine systems; there are other glands and hormones that are important in digestion, reproduction and other systems which are being discussed separately. This Chapter considers the pancreas, the parathyroid, adrenal and thyroid glands and the pituitary gland and some of its hormones. The hormones are secreted directly into the blood and do not travel to their destination via ducts and for this reason the endocrine glands are sometimes called the ductless glands (see Figure 15.1). (To make sure you understand the important distinction between endocrine and exocrine glands you should revise the section on the pancreas in the Chapter on the digestive system.) The exocrine portion of the pancreas empties its secretions into the pancreatic duct through which they travel to the duodenum. The secretions of the endocrine portions of the pancreas are released into capillaries of the pancreas and travel to the pancreatic veins and finally reach the heart, which distributes them throughout the body. The secretions of exocrine glands are locally distributed, while endocrine gland secretions are universally distributed.

WHAT IS A HORMONE AND HOW DOES IT WORK?

A hormone may be defined as a chemical made by the specific cells of the body which travels in the blood to a specific site or

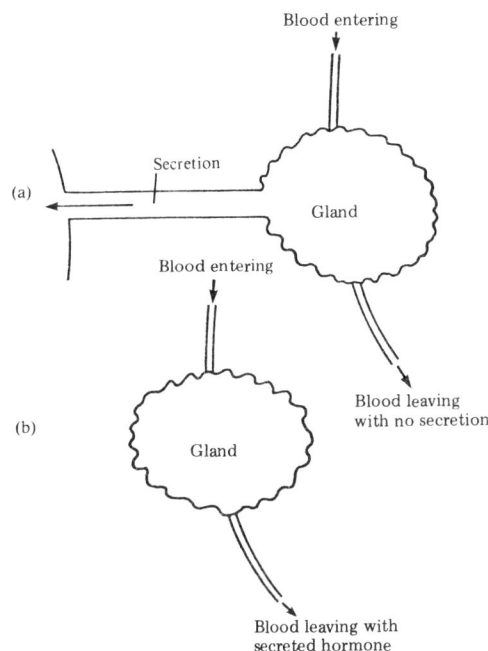

Figure 15.1 Glandular structure. (a) Exocrine gland. (b) Endocrine gland.

sites in the body where it regulates or initiates a chemical change; hormones themselves do not provide energy to the body. A hormone is a messenger. If the body were a single cell or made of many identical cells there would be no need for hormones, for all the cells would react the same way to a given stimulus. With a complex organism like man the work of different organs and tissues must be co-ordinated; messages must be sent back and forth. One problem that has puzzled endocrinologists for a long time is why a hormone which is distributed throughout the entire body will affect only certain cells. There is now good evidence, regarding protein hormones, which suggests that there are receptors on the cell surface which permit the hormone to recognize its target cell. A hormone would initiate its action by combining with its specific receptor on the cell membrane surface (see Figure 15.2). In contrast to the protein hormones, the receptors for the thyroid and adrenal cortical hormones are located within the cell. These hormones can easily cross through the cell membrane. If a cell lacks receptors for a hormone, this hormone cannot directly influence the cell.

Some theories on the mechanism of hormonal action include the following:

(1) *Hormones can affect membrane permeability and transport.* The cell membrane functions as a selectively permeable barrier, carefully regulating the kind and number of molecules it permits to enter the cell. Insulin, for example,

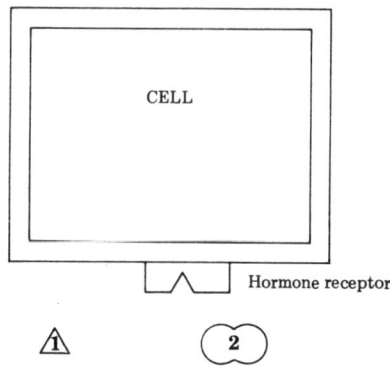

Figure 15.2 Hormone 1 will stimulate the cell because it can interact with the receptor, while hormone 2 will be unable to interact and will thus be ineffective in that particular cell.

can act directly on certain membranes, greatly increasing the amount of glucose which can enter.

(2) *Hormones can cause the synthesis of additional enzymes.* An increase in the amount of enzyme will lead to a change in the flow of molecules along different metabolic pathways. Some of the adrenal cortical hormones stimulate the synthesis of additional enzymes in the liver which deaminate amino acids. This means that the nitrogen-containing group is removed from the amino acid leaving only a carbon skeleton; this molecule can then either be metabolized via the citric acid cycle or converted to glucose via gluconeogenesis (see Figure 14.3). If there are more enzymes for deaminating amino acids, the probability of an amino acid in the liver being deaminated increases.

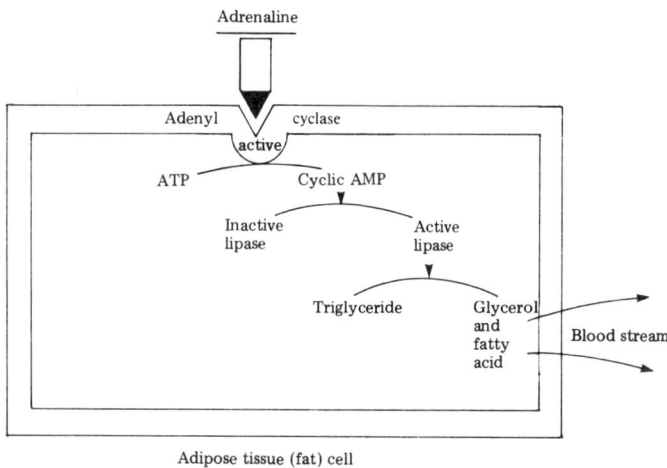

Figure 15.3 An example of the second messenger concept; the effect of adrenaline on adipose tissue.

The mechanism by which a hormone leads to an increase in enzyme synthesis is not fully known. In some cases there is evidence that the steroid hormones cross the cell membrane and bind to a specific receptor protein in the cytoplasm; this hormone–peptide complex then acts on the nucleus. Only those cells with the receptor protein will respond to the hormone. This hormone–receptor complex leads to DNA activation, messenger RNA synthesis and enzyme protein synthesis.

Hormones can also affect existing enzyme systems making them work more efficiently. This might be brought about by the hormone combining with the enzyme or by acting elsewhere in the cell and making cofactors or other molecules more available.

(3) *Hormones can stimulate or inhibit the formation of another compound which in turn affects enzymes.* This is something like a relay race in which the hormone's message is passed on in the cell to another compound, which in turn sends the message within the cell by changing the activity of enzymes.

The most famous "second messenger" is the intracellular compound, cyclic 3',5'-adenosine monophosphate, commonly called cyclic AMP. Cyclic AMP is formed from ATP by the action of the enzyme, adenyl cyclase. This enzyme system is located within the membrane of the target cell and is activated by hormones. The fact that adenyl cyclase is located in the membrane serves a functional purpose, for it means that the hormone does not need to cross the membrane to exert an effect within the cell. The one enzyme will affect many molecules inside the cell and this leads to an amplification of the hormone's effect.

The second messenger concept can be illustrated by the action of the hormone, adrenaline, on adipose tissue cells (see Figure 15.3). Adrenaline is released from the medulla of the adrenal gland, travels through the bloodstream to adipose tissue cells, where it activates the enzyme, adenyl cyclase. Adenyl cyclase converts ATP to cyclic AMP, which exerts its effects within the cell by activating the enzyme, lipase. This enzyme in turn breaks down the stored triglyceride into glycerol and fatty acids which are released into the blood.

Although this process seems long and complicated, it is far more rapid than those processes requiring the synthesis of new enzymes. The level of fatty acids in the plasma increases within minutes following the infusion of adrenaline. It should be pointed out that many other hormones can activate adenyl cyclase and that cyclic AMP can have many different intracellular effects. For example, the hormones, adrenaline and glucagon, can activate adenyl cyclase within liver cells, which converts ATP to cyclic AMP. The cyclic AMP then activates an enzyme sequence causing the breakdown of glycogen and an increase in blood glucose.

(4) *Hormones may act by some combination of the above mechanisms or by still unknown ways.* In your lifetime you will see many advances derived from a better understanding of hormones and enzymes.

A final point to remember is that once a hormone has been released into the blood it is soon metabolized by the liver and other tissues and/or excreted in the urine. So it is that the levels of hormones in the blood will fall unless they are replaced by newly synthesized hormones. For example, a molecule of the adrenal hormone, cortisol, will circulate an average of 30 minutes before it is metabolized. Should the liver or kidneys be damaged, the concentration of some hormones will increase.

HOW ARE BLOOD GLUCOSE AND FATTY ACIDS CONTROLLED?

The pancreas

One reason why glucose concentration in the blood must be

carefully controlled is because the brain is unable to store glycogen and so it gets most of its energy from the metabolism of glucose which comes from the blood. If glucose were suddenly removed from the blood, brain metabolism would stop and its cells would die; without glucose there would be no substrate to be oxidized. Because of its importance, blood glucose is frequently measured in the hospital. Even after hours of fasting, the blood glucose is in the range of 70–110 mg for every 100 ml of blood; this is equivalent to 3.89–6.11 mmol/l. In the day-to-day regulation of glucose and fatty acids, two hormones, glucagon and insulin, produced in the pancreas, are involved. Certain hormones, including the glucocorticoids, adrenaline and growth hormone, are also important.

The structure of the pancreas was described in the Chapter on the digestive system. The important point to remember now is that this gland has two divisions: an exocrine portion and an endocrine portion. The exocrine portion, which makes up a large part of the gland, sends its secretions directly into the duodenum via the pancreatic duct (see Figure 13.13). The endocrine portion of the pancreas is made up of many islands of cells called the Islets of Langerhans, which are scattered throughout the pancreas. The Islets of Langerhans have three different types of cells:

alpha (α) cells which secrete glucagon,

beta (β) cells which secrete insulin,

and a very few delta (δ) cells which secrete gastrin and somatostatin. (Somatostatin, also known as growth hormone-inhibiting hormone (GH-IH), is also found in the hypothalamus and other parts of the brain and body. Somatostatin may also reduce glucagon and insulin secretion in the nearby α and β cells.)

The islets also contain capillaries that receive the secretions from the α, β and δ cells. From these capillaries the hormones travel into the veins which drain the pancreas, ultimately to reach the hepatic portal vein, the sinusoids of the liver, the hepatic vein and, finally, the inferior vena cava (see Figure 8.17). After travelling through the right heart, the lungs and the left atrium, they are sent throughout the body by the left ventricle.

Glucagon and insulin are important metabolic regulators, whereas the roles of pancreatic gastrin and somatostatin are less clear. There are some tumours of the pancreas which produce gastrin. Patients having these will have ulcers because of the excessive gastrin-induced HCl secretion.

a. Glucagon. Assume you have had a large meal nearly 4 hours ago. The dietary carbohydrate has been stored as glycogen and the fatty acids as triglyceride. But now the blood glucose concentration is falling. This drop in blood glucose serves as a stimulus to the α cells of the pancreas to release glucagon into the blood. Glucagon has three major actions:

(1) It causes cyclic AMP formation in the liver, which in turn is responsible for activating the enzymes which break down glycogen into glucose — this glucose is released into the blood stream.

(2) In the liver it also stimulates gluconeogenesis to form glucose from amino acids.

(3) It causes cyclic AMP activation in adipose tissue. Triglycerides are spit into glycerol and fatty acids so plasma fatty acids will increase.

In summary, glucagon works to provide energy substrates to the tissues.

Glucagon has its uses in clinical situations. If a person is unconscious, due to hypoglycaemia or low blood glucose, glucagon can be injected to raise the blood sugar. Glucose also can be given intravenously. (An attack of hypoglycaemia may be caused by an overdosage of insulin.)

Other hormones, such as growth hormone, also increase plasma glucose and fatty acids. Their actions become more important as the fasting state is prolonged.

b. Insulin. Insulin is a protein hormone produced by the β cells of the pancreas. In contrast to glucagon, the stimulus for insulin release is a *high* blood glucose, so the plasma level of insulin will increase 10–15 times within 1–2 hours after a meal when glucose levels are highest. High levels of some amino acids also stimulate insulin release.

Insulin has very significant effects on fat, protein and glucose metabolism which include the following:

(1) Glucose cannot enter skeletal muscle cells by itself and needs the help of insulin to cross the cell membrane. This fact becomes particularly important when you remember that skeletal muscle makes up 40% of the body's weight and that glucose is a major source of energy for this tissue. Amino acid transport and protein synthesis in muscle are also increased by insulin.

(2) Insulin increases the formation of glycogen in the liver, and reduces the glucose output of the liver.

(3) Uptake of glucose and fatty acids by the liver and adipose tissue is increased, so triglyceride formation in fat cells is also increased.

(4) Insulin seems to inhibit gluconeogenesis and protein catabolism and, at the same time, leads to increased amino acid uptake and protein synthesis in the liver and muscle.

The actual mechanism by which insulin exerts these effects is not known. Studies in skeletal muscle have shown that one of the earliest actions of insulin is to cause an increased movement of potassium into the cell. This movement changes the membrane potential and precedes the increased transport of glucose and amino acids into the cell.

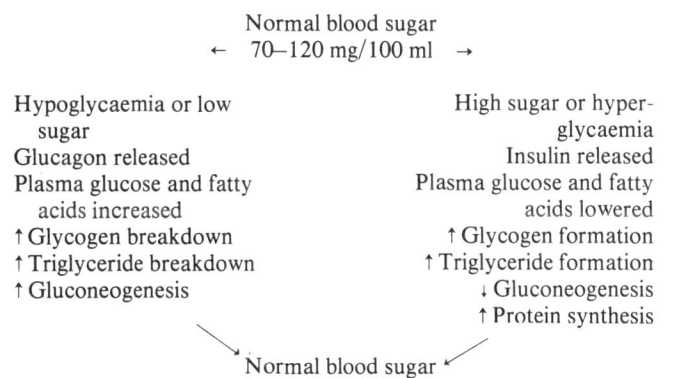

Normal blood sugar
← 70–120 mg/100 ml →

Hypoglycaemia or low sugar	High sugar or hyperglycaemia
Glucagon released	Insulin released
Plasma glucose and fatty acids increased	Plasma glucose and fatty acids lowered
↑ Glycogen breakdown	↑ Glycogen formation
↑ Triglyceride breakdown	↑ Triglyceride formation
↑ Gluconeogenesis	↓ Gluconeogenesis
	↑ Protein synthesis

Normal blood sugar

The glucose tolerance test is a test of the body's ability to regulate or stabilize glucose levels in the blood (see Figure 15.4). The patient drinks a solution containing either 50 or 100 grams of glucose. As the glucose is absorbed, the glucose concentration in the plasma increases. The high blood glucose levels stimulate the pancreas to release insulin and this will cause the blood glucose levels to fall as glucose starts

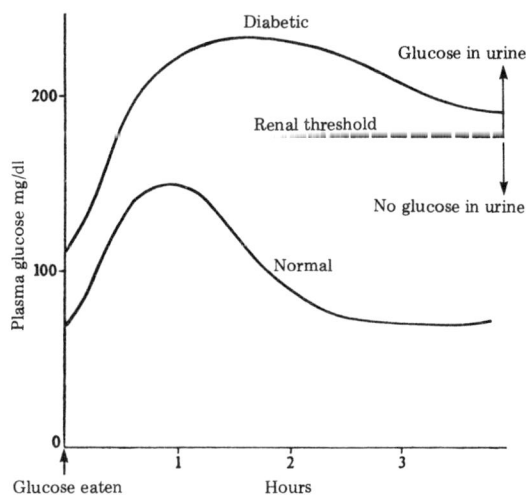

Figure 15.4 The glucose tolerance test.

to enter into muscle and adipose cells. Blood glucose is measured every half hour for 2 or 3 hours. In diabetes, the fasting blood glucose levels are often above 110 mg/dl and do not go below that level 3 hours after the ingestion of 100 grams of glucose. (Diabetes will be covered in more detail shortly.)

c. Growth hormone. This hormone is made by the anterior pituitary gland of the brain. It stimulates protein synthesis but in other respects its action is antagonistic to that of insulin. Growth hormone (GH) hinders the uptake of glucose by skeletal muscle which causes the amount of glucose in the blood to increase. The hormone also causes adipose tissue to break down triglyceride and release fatty acids. High blood glucose levels inhibit the release of GH, while low blood glucose levels stimulate the release of GH.

Muscle tissue can metabolize both fatty acids and glucose, but the brain can metabolize only glucose. It has been suggested that GH is a mechanism used by the brain to ensure adequate glucose for its own metabolism. The net effect of GH is to increase the metabolism of fatty acids by muscle and reduce the muscles' use of glucose, thus saving glucose for metabolism by the brain. GH also functions in growth; this is discussed in subsequent Sections.

Somatostatin (growth hormone-inhibiting hormone (GH-IH)), which is found in the hypothalamus of the brain, is able to inhibit growth hormone release from the anterior pituitary. The role of somatostatin and its full relationship to growth and glucose is not yet known.

d. Glucocorticoids. These hormones are released by the cortex of the adrenal gland during fasting or starvation because they help maintain blood glucose when glycogen levels are low or absent. They do this by stimulating protein catabolism in muscle and increasing amino acid uptake and gluconeogenesis in the liver. One reason why starving people are thin and weak is that the protein filaments of their muscles are broken down into amino acids which leave the muscle tissue and are converted to glucose in the liver.

e. Adrenaline. This hormone comes from the medulla of the adrenal gland and is a potent stimulator of fatty acid release and glycogen breakdown. Like the glucocorticoids, it is released in times of stress, but its effects are realized much more rapidly.

WHAT IS DIABETES?

This is one of the oldest known diseases and one of the most widespread with an estimated 200 million diabetics in the world today. In most industrialized societies, it is the commonest metabolic disorder and is still a poorly understood disease. Diabetes is a disease in which the levels of blood glucose are inappropriately high because of an abnormal secretion of, or response to, insulin. Some diabetic patients do not produce any insulin; some produce small amounts of insulin and some produce significant amounts of insulin, which, for an unknown reason, is less than is required or is less effective than would be expected. The primary defect causing this inadequate secretion of insulin is not yet known.

There are two clinical classifications of diabetes: juvenile-onset diabetes and adult-onset diabetes. As a general rule, juvenile-onset diabetes is much less common than adult-onset, is more severe, and its onset is sudden and usually occurs before 15 years of age.

Most cases of adult-onset diabetes are not diagnosed until after the patient is 40 years of age or older. It may not be as serious as juvenile-onset diabetes, as its development is more gradual and the patient's β cells are usually capable of producing some insulin. Certain individuals with adult-onset diabetes may have higher-than-normal levels of circulating insulin. Why these patients are "insulin resistant" is not known, although it is often associated with obesity, and the insulin resistance can be reduced if the individual manages to lose weight. Many adult-onset diabetics have normal levels of insulin between meals but their β cells cannot secrete the burst of insulin needed after the ingestion and absorption of a meal. Juvenile-onset diabetics almost always require insulin, as they produce very little or no insulin. It must be noted that there are patients with intermediate characteristics of both diseases and that the onset of either type of diabetes is not limited to people who are younger than 15 years of age or older than 40 years of age.

The symptoms and disorders resulting from this relative insulin deficiency will make sense only if you have understood the actions of insulin.

(1) *Diabetics will have high blood glucose levels.* Insulin is necessary for glucose to enter into many cells; if glucose is unable to enter the cells due to an insulin deficiency, blood glucose will increase. Since glucose can't enter cells, there will be less glycogen storage in cells. (It should be pointed out that most parts of the brain do not need insulin for glucose to cross the cell membranes. The brain will not be glucose-starved in diabetes. The one apparent exception to this is that portion of the brain which is important in appetite regulation and which appears to require insulin for glucose transport.)

Sometimes blood glucose can rise to such high levels that some of the glucose which is filtered in the kidneys will not be reabsorbed, resulting in the presence of glucose in the urine. One of the most common clinical procedures is to test urine for the presence of glucose, which may indicate diabetes. When glucose is not reabsorbed by the kidneys, it acts as an osmotically active molecule which retains water, so the volume of urine increases. The untreated diabetic will have to pass more urine (polyuria). Because of this increased loss of water, the untreated diabetic may constantly feel thirsty (polydipsia). The loss of glucose in the urine also represents a loss of calories. Because glucose cannot penetrate the appetite control centre in the brain, the diabetic may feel constantly hungry and eat excessively (polyphagia). It is also possible for the untreated diabetic to become seriously dehydrated due to considerable fluid losses in the urine. In addition, sodium and potassium ions are lost in the urine, and serious plasma electrolyte disturbances may result.

(2) *Insulin inhibits lipolysis (the breakdown of tri-glycerides into glycerol and fatty acids).* Without insulin, lipolysis and the concentration of fatty acids in the plasma will increase. These fatty acids can cross cell membranes and can be partially metabolized. They are broken down to acetyl coenzyme A but, because of the excessive fatty acid catabolism, more acetyl coenzyme A is formed than can enter the citric acid cycle. In the liver, these excess acetyl coenzyme A molecules will be converted to ketone bodies (see Figure 14.2). Some tissues can, and do, metabolize ketone bodies, particularly in times of starvation, but generally they are not a good source of energy and they contribute to the more acidic (low pH) blood which is found in a diabetic. Acetone is a ketone body and contributes to the abnormal, fruity-smelling breath of an advanced, untreated diabetic.

You should not infer from this that all diabetics have no fat stores. Many adult-onset diabetics are overweight before the disease is detected and some of them remain so as the disease develops. It has been suggested that these patients have sufficient insulin to convert glucose to fatty acids and to synthesize triglyceride, but insufficient insulin for other needs.

(3) *Insulin normally stimulates protein synthesis and inhibits gluconeogenesis.* Without insulin, protein synthesis will be reduced and more amino acids will undergo gluconeogenesis, increasing blood glucose levels but not helping the sugar-starved cells. In children, the lack of adequate insulin, and the subsequent hindered protein synthesis can cause stunted growth.

(4) *The long-term effects of diabetes.* Even if diabetes is treated and reasonably well controlled, the disease may express itself in a variety of ways. The mechanism by which an inappropriate hyperglycaemia might cause these effects is not known. (Some people think that the primary pathology of diabetes may involve more than a hormonal-metabolic imbalance.) The eyes, the kidneys and the peripheral nerves are most commonly affected, but significant pathology does not occur in all diabetics.

(a) *The eyes.* Diabetes is the major systemic illness causing blindness. The retina of the eye contains the rods and the cones, both of which are specialized light-responsive cells. With long-standing diabetes, parts of the retina might not be adequately perfused with blood, the capillaries of the retina may contain micro-aneurisms or may be unusually permeable. The net effect of these and other microvascular changes is partial, or even complete, blindness.

(b) *The kidneys.* Diabetes can manifest itself pathologically in the kidneys in two ways. Renal arteriosclerosis develops, the walls of the arterioles become thickened and the lumina become narrowed. Blood flow to the glomerulus is reduced and the glomerular basement membrane becomes thickened. These changes may give rise to protein in the urine (proteinuria) and hypertension. Urinary tract infections are more common in diabetics and renal failure is not unknown, particularly in adults with juvenile-onset diabetes.

(c) *The peripheral nerves.* Although the nerves going to the viscera may be affected in diabetes, the most common disorder is sensory impairment in the lower extremities. This is thought to be caused by deterioration of the myelin which surrounds the nerve fibres. As a practical matter, diabetics need to take good care of their feet. They should never go barefoot, should wash and inspect their feet daily. Great caution should be exercised when they trim their nails. Because of the sensory loss in the feet, diabetics may not know that their feet are injured or infected. Infection in the diabetic foot is often a serious problem, for it is often associated with reduced blood flow to the foot and diminished white blood cell efficiency in fighting the infection. Amputation of the foot is a common complication of an undetected or inadequately treated or persistent infection.

These complications do not occur in all or most diabetics, and if they do occur it is often after many years of a relatively healthy life. Most diabetics can learn to cope with their disease and lead happy, productive lives.

The treatment of diabetes has made many significant advances in the last 50 years but nevertheless many problems still remain. The diabetic is never cured but his or her condition may be prevented from deteriorating by careful daily treatment requiring much patience, perseverence, communication and co-operation on the part of both the patient and the health professional. Unfortunately, even with the best possible treatment, serious problems often arise. Treatment of the diabetic covers dietary control, insulin and oral hypoglycaemics:

(a) *Dietary control.* Everyone should try to balance their caloric intake against their energy expenditure. Diabetics must do this and, in addition, balance the carbohydrate content of their diet against the amount of functional circulating insulin. The latter is a delicate balance and is not always easily achieved. Diet therapy is not aimed at eliminating carbohydrate from the diet, only at keeping it within limits, along with the total number of calories. Intake of concentrated sucrose should be avoided and well-spaced meals of modest size are preferred. In some cases it is necessary to plan carefully the menus and actually measure and weigh the amount of food to be eaten.

(b) *Insulin.* In many cases of diabetes, insulin is required. As insulin is a protein it must be injected into the body, for it would be destroyed by the digestive enzymes if it were taken orally. Commercial insulin preparations come from the pancreas of sheep, hogs or cattle and are remarkably similar to human insulin. Crystalline insulin is the most rapidly acting insulin, while other insulin preparations are complexed with proteins and ions to reduce their solubility and thus slow their absorption into the blood. Care must be taken in the amount of insulin given, for if too much is injected most of the glucose will move into skeletal muscle and fat cells, plasma glucose levels fall, the brain will become glucose-starved and the patient may go into convulsions or die.

(c) *Oral hypoglycaemics.* These agents may at times have some use in the care of some adult-onset diabetics. Certain classes of oral hypoglycaemics, the sulphonylureas, are thought to work by stimulating the β cells to produce more insulin. The mechanism of action and the safety of some oral hypoglycaemics are controversial and cannot be stated with certainty.

Serious complications can arise when a diabetic, who requires insulin, does not receive it. The patient goes into keto-acidosis because of the excessive accumulation of ketone bodies and may even go into a coma, a state of unconsciousness from which the patient may not be roused even with powerful stimulation. Simply giving insulin to reduce blood glucose is inadequate therapy. There must be a correction of the acidosis of these patients, as they are usually very dehydrated and have disturbances in their plasma electrolytes because of the loss of sodium and potassium in their urine.

The troubles of the diabetic and the problems of treatment need to be viewed in an historical perspective. It was only a little more than 50 years ago that insulin was "discovered" and its role in diabetes was appreciated. The problems of the diabetic today are the problems of living with the disease. In the past, living with the disease was not an alternative. This is noted here to point out that advances in medical science and treatment do not always simplify or remove problems. Often one set of problems is exchanged for a different set.

HOW IS CALCIUM REGULATED?

Like glucose, calcium levels in the blood are carefully controlled and kept within a very narrow range. There is a hormone which can raise the blood level of calcium and another hormone which can lower it. Calcium control, like glucose control, is a dynamic, on-going process. In the plasma, calcium travels in two ways. About half the calcium in the plasma is bound to protein; the other half circulates independently as a free ion, not bound to anything. The total calcium in the blood is in the range 9–11 mg/dl (2.25–2.75 mmol/l) of plasma.

Calcium has many functions in the body. It is necessary for:

(1) The maintenance of the integrity of cell membranes, particularly nerve cell membranes, which become much more permeable in the absence of Ca^{++}.

(2) Muscular contraction and proper release of synaptic transmitters, such as acetylcholine, which transmits the order to contract from the nerve ending to the muscle.

(3) The maintenance of bone, which is a living tissue being constantly formed and broken down, with calcium being deposited and then released.

(4) The proper functioning of certain enzymes.

(5) The normal clotting of blood.

Should calcium ion levels become too low (hypocalcaemia) the neuromuscular system is affected first. Because the nerve cells lose much of their membrane stability, they become exceptionally excitable. Sometimes reflexes are triggered with very small stimuli and many muscles, particularly the extensors and those of the larynx, go into spasm and often maintain themselves in a contracted state. This condition is called tetany.

If blood calcium levels approach or exceed 15 mg/dl (3.74 mmol/l), impulse conduction in the heart is interfered with so that the heart rate is slowed or possibly even stopped. There are other conditions associated with hypercalcaemia that are mentioned later.

Calcium regulation also includes dietary consideration, for there must be adequate calcium in the diet to compensate for the small daily losses. Vitamin D must likewise be present in the diet for calcium to be absorbed. Excessive vitamin D can even cause hypercalcaemia. Large quantities of unabsorbed fat and the phosphate ion (PO_4^{--}) can lead to hypocalcaemia by impairing calcium absorption. Parathormone (a hormone produced by the parathyroid glands) also plays a role in calcium absorption.

The parathyroid glands

a. Anatomy of the parathyroid glands. These are four pea-sized glands located at each corner of the thyroid gland (which will be described later). It is not uncommon for some individuals to have three parathyroid glands or even five glands. These glands are very small, each with an average weight of 30 mg. In the past, surgeons removed them along with the thyroid, and many of their patients died because the plasma calcium levels fell so low. Although surgeons no longer remove the parathyroid glands, unless they are diseased, these glands are at risk during thyroid surgery because their delicate blood supply may be injured.

The chief cells of the parathyroid glands produce parathormone (PTH), and are small dark-staining cells arranged in clumps or irregular cords supported by reticular fibres.

b. Functions of parathormone (PTH). The stimulus for the release of PTH is a low level of Ca^{++} in the blood. The hormone leaves the veins draining the parathyroid gland and goes into the circulation. The hormone has three chief actions (see Figure 15.5).

(1) PTH stimulates the osteoclasts to attack the bone matrix and release calcium and phosphate ions.

(2) The kidney is stimulated to increase the reabsorption of the filtered calcium and to increase the excretion of phosphate; the combined effect of these actions is to increase plasma calcium.

(3) It increases the absorption of calcium from the intestine when vitamin D is present.

(4) It also causes a movement of calcium from the plasma into the cells — this effect is relatively small and does not lead to a reduction in plasma calcium.

Recent work has shown that magnesium is necessary for most of the actions of PTH.

c. Calcitonin (CT). This hormone is produced by the "C" (parafollicular) cells of the thyroid gland and also by the "C" cells of the thymus gland. It is sometimes called thyrocalcitonin (TCT) because of its origin in the thyroid gland. The principal action of CT is on bone. It seems to inhibit the action of osteoclasts and stimulate the conversion of

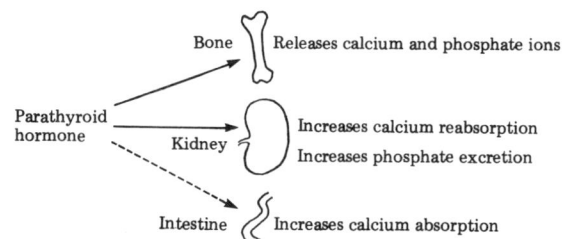

Figure 15.5   The actions of parathyroid hormone.

osteoclasts to osteoblasts. (Osteoblasts are the cells that build bone by depositing Ca^{++} on the protein matrix.) Because calcium is deposited in bone, the amount of calcium in the blood is reduced.

CT is now being used to treat certain bone disorders such as Paget's disease, in which the bones become weakened because of excessive bone resorption. The stimulus for CT release is elevated calcium. In humans, the complete control of CT has not been worked out. Hypercalcaemia may persist in spite of normal or high levels of CT, so there is still more to learn about the control and effectiveness of this hormone.

Both PTH and CT offer classic examples of negative feedback. The concept of negative feedback demonstrates that there is a specific relationship between the effect of a hormone and its rate of secretion into the blood. The effect of a hormone can regulate the amount of that hormone in the blood. Negative feedback is significant because it gives stability to systems that are not inherently stable. High levels of calcium inhibit PTH secretion. This inhibition leads to a reduction of plasma calcium. Low levels of calcium stimulate PTH which leads to an increase in calcium. High calcium ion levels stimulate CT release; as calcium ion levels fall, CT release is inhibited.

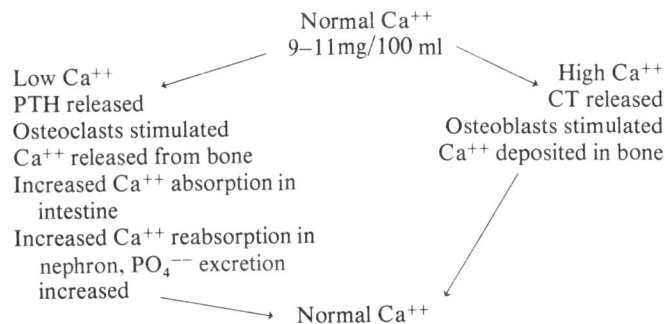

Normal Ca^{++}
9–11mg/100 ml

Low Ca^{++}
PTH released
Osteoclasts stimulated
Ca^{++} released from bone
Increased Ca^{++} absorption in intestine
Increased Ca^{++} reabsorption in nephron, PO_4^{--} excretion increased

High Ca^{++}
CT released
Osteoblasts stimulated
Ca^{++} deposited in bone

Normal Ca^{++}

Almost half of the calcium in the blood is bound to the protein, albumin, and is thus not free to act in physiological processes. The binding takes place because the positively charged calcium ions (Ca^{++}) are attracted to the negatively charged protein molecules. The amount of calcium binding is dependent on the pH of the blood. If the pH is low, the H^+ will bind to the protein and displace the calcium ions, so the free (unbound) calcium will increase. When the pH is high, more calcium will be bound to the protein and there will be less free calcium.

Sometimes the pH increase can cause the individual to go into tetany. Although the amount of calcium in the blood is within normal limits the unbound calcium is greatly reduced. Tetany resulting from excessive calcium binding is often seen in respiratory alkalosis. Women giving birth or frightened patients in the casualty ward take deep and frequent breaths, blow off CO_2 and thus raise their pH. If the patient breathes into a paper bag, he or she will retain more CO_2, decrease plasma pH, free more calcium and thus end the tetany.

There are other causes of tetany besides respiratory alkalosis. Should plasma calcium fall below 7 mg/100 ml plasma, tetany is likely to occur. Metabolic alkalosis, inadequate hormone secretion and poor absorption of calcium are among the conditions that may cause tetany.

You may remember from your work in basic chemistry the concept of the solubility product. This concept states that the product of the concentrations of the ions in equilibrium with a specific precipitate is a constant. Each slightly soluble electrolyte has its own constant product and this constant is called the solubility product. In biological systems, this can be applied to the equilibrium between Ca^{++}, PO_4^{--} and $CaPO_4$. It can be stated as follows:

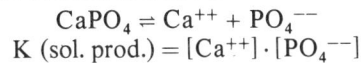

$$CaPO_4 \rightleftharpoons Ca^{++} + PO_4^{--}$$
$$K \text{ (sol. prod.)} = [Ca^{++}] \cdot [PO_4^{--}]$$

If you take a solution of plasma having no calcium or phosphate ions and start to add these ions to the solution, nothing will happen at first because the product of the concentration of these two ions will be less than the solubility product. All Ca^{++}, PO_4^{--} and $CaPO_4$ will be in solution. If you continue to add Ca^{++} and PO_4^{--}, there will come a point when the solution will become saturated and cannot hold any more $CaPO_4$ in solution. At this point, the product of the two ions will be equal to the solubility product. If any more ions are then added, insoluble $CaPO_4$ will precipitate out of the solution. The addition of more ions will cause the formation of still more precipitate. (It should be pointed out that the ions do not have to be added in equal amounts.) An insoluble precipitate may be formed if the solubility product is exceeded because of:

(1) High Ca^{++} and high PO_4^{--}
(2) Very high Ca^{++} and low PO_4^{--}
(3) Very high PO_4^{--} and low Ca^{++}.

Some non-malignant tumours of the parathyroid gland produce excessive PTH. The PTH raises the level of Ca^{++} and lowers the PO_4^{--} in the plasma and thus increases the likelihood of exceeding the solubility product and becoming the insoluble calcium salts. These insoluble salts are often first precipitated in the tubules of the kidney as small "kidney stones", which are extremely painful and can cause infection and injury within the kidney. The main source of the increased plasma calcium is the bones, which are more susceptible to fracture, because they contain less calcium. The high calcium also may lead to nausea and constipation. The likelihood of ulcer formation is also increased as HCl secretion is increased. For these reasons hyperparathyroidism has been summed up as "stones, bones, and abdominal groans."

HOW IS PLASMA SODIUM CONTROLLED?

Sodium is the most abundant ion in the plasma. Because sodium is so widespread in foods, the average individual receives many times the daily minimal sodium requirement. Sodium is lost in the urine, in small amounts in the faeces, in variable amounts in sweat or perspiration and, occasionally, in insignificant amounts in tears. Significant amounts of sodium can also be lost as a result of diarrhoea or osmotic diuretics. If the kidneys retain more water than sodium, plasma sodium concentration will be reduced. Excessive sodium loss results in too little plasma sodium (hyponatraemia). Hyponatraemia can cause muscle cramps — painful and persistent contractions. This often happens after strenuous exercise in a hot and humid environment when the individual loses both water and salt in perspiration. The drinking of water after exercise, without taking salt, only aggravates the situation by further diluting the plasma sodium concentration.

Since sodium is the most abundant plasma ion, it contributes the most to the total osmotic pressure of the plasma. If sodium levels are significantly reduced, the osmotic pressure of the blood will be similarly reduced. This means that water will move from the extracellular fluid into the tissues and the tissues will swell. The brain does not, however, tolerate swelling. Confusion and other behavioural changes can result from significant hyponatraemia.

Sodium ions are of great importance in the neuromuscular system, in the conduction of impulses across nerves and muscles; however, the real significance of the sodium ion is found in the relationship that exists between the sodium ion and the extracellular fluid volume. To review this relationship you will recall that sodium ion is the most abundant plasma ion and that every minute 120 ml of plasma are filtered in the glomeruli of the adult kidneys. When the sodium ions are actively reabsorbed from the lumen of the tubules into the capillaries, water molecules follow because of the greater osmotic pressure in the renal capillaries. The greater the amount of sodium ions that are reabsorbed, the greater the number of water molecules that will follow and be returned to the plasma; if few sodium ions are reabsorbed, less water will be retained and plasma volume will be decreased. Since the circulatory system cannot significantly change its size, the pressure in the system will increase with increased plasma volume and decrease with decreased plasma volume. The relationship between plasma volume and sodium is extremely important, because the plasma volume controls or influences the amount of sodium retained by the kidneys. The hormonal mechanisms by which this occurs are described in later Sections.

An individual's diet may include 4–10 grams of sodium chloride (NaCl) every day although 3 grams a day is adequate. Sodium is found in meat, milk and bread and in table salt, which is used as a preservative as well as seasoning for foods. Some individuals with heart or kidney disease may have to limit their total sodium intake to as little as 250–500 mg/day. The reason for this restriction is based on the relationship between sodium and blood volume. If these persons have a high salt intake and their kidneys aren't adequately perfused with blood or their kidneys can't excrete the excess sodium, salt and water will be retained, so their plasma volume expands. This can overload the heart and the circulatory system. Pulmonary oedema is a common complication of this fluid overload.

It is necessary to know that, since water is retained with sodium, the plasma concentration of sodium may not change. If you add salt and water in proportion to a solution containing salt and water, you can increase the volume of the solution without changing the concentration of the solution. Thus, a person may have an excessive blood volume and a normal sodium concentration.

An important hormone in conserving sodium is aldosterone. Aldosterone functions to reduce the loss of sodium in sweat and intestinal secretions; more important, it works at the kidney to increase sodium reabsorption by the distal tubule of the nephron. Within limits, increased aldosterone will lead to increased sodium reabsorption and increased plasma volume. Decreased aldosterone leads to reduced sodium reabsorption and decreased plasma volume.

The adrenal glands

a. Anatomy of the adrenal glands. The adrenal glands are flattened, cap-like structures which sit upon the superior pole of each kidney, roughly at the level of the 1st lumbar vertebra (see Figure 11.2). They are small structures (average size 2.5 cm in width, 4–6 cm in length and 3–6 cm in depth) and weigh about 5 grams in the adult. Although small, they consist of different types of cells and produce many hormones. The glandular tissue is surrounded by loose connective tissue and covered by a fibrous capsule attached to the gland by fibrous bands. The gland receives a rich blood supply from the aorta, phrenic and renal arteries and is also well supplied by sympathetic nerve fibres. The venous return is different for each adrenal: the right adrenal vein drains into the inferior vena cava while the left adrenal vein empties into the left renal vein. The gland is really a double gland, for it is formed from two separate tissues which unite early in development to form a single structure. The outer section of the gland is called the adrenal cortex, while the inner core is called the medulla (see Figure 15.6). The cortex and the medulla produce different hormones and are under different controls.

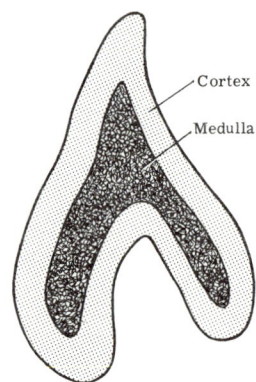

Figure 15.6   The adrenal gland.

b. Adrenal cortical hormones. The adrenal cortex produces over 40 hormones but only a few of them are present in significant concentrations and they can be grouped into either mineralocorticoids, glucocorticoids or sex steroids. All corticoids have steroid structures and are fat-soluble. These three classifications are not rigid, as there is a certain amount of overlap between classes; for example, glucocorticoids have some mineralocorticoid action.

Mineralocorticoids. The chief mineralocorticoid is aldosterone, a salt-retaining hormone. Aldosterone increases salt reabsorption in the intestine, reduces salt loss in the perspiration and, most importantly, increases sodium reabsorption in the distal tubule of the kidney nephron. In the absence of aldosterone, significant amounts of sodium are lost in the urine; with increased aldosterone more sodium is retained. The mechanism by which aldosterone acts is not understood, though it is known that for every sodium ion reabsorbed, a K^+ or H^+ is pumped into the tubule to be excreted in the urine. Therefore, as more Na^+ is reabsorbed, either more H^+ or K^+ will be secreted. Aldosterone thus retains sodium but promotes K^+ or H^+ secretion. The control of aldosterone secretion by the cortex has not been worked out but there seem to be three separate controls:

(1) *Potassium.* Increases in plasma K^+ levels will stimulate aldosterone release. This increased aldosterone secretion will cause greater renal sodium reabsorption and potassium secretion. As plasma K^+ levels fall, the stimulus for aldosterone secretion will fall proportionately. The normal serum level of potassium is 3.5–5.0 mmol/l.

This might be an appropriate time to consider briefly the role of potassium. More than 95% of the potassium in the body is found within the cells, thus the level of potassium that is measured in the plasma or serum can't give a true indication of the body's total potassium. Potassium is the most common ion within the cell; it is also the biggest contributor to the osmotic pressure within the cell and is, therefore, the primary determinant of intracellular volume. Certain enzymes require potassium, and potassium is necessary for protein synthesis and normal growth. The ratio between the intracellular and extracellular K^+ concentration is of critical importance in maintaining the excitability of cells, in particular all types of muscle cells.

Potassium is present in nearly all foods, so dietary deficiencies of potassium seldom occur. Hypokalaemia exists when there are abnormally low levels of potassium in the blood; hyperkalaemia results from abnormally high levels.

Vomiting, diarrhoea, some renal disease or use of certain diuretics can cause hypokalaemia, as can tumours which produce aldosterone. Muscular weakness and disturbances of impulse conduction within the heart are associated with hypokalaemia. The kidneys are able to excrete significant amounts of potassium without aldosterone, but reduced levels of aldosterone may be associated with hyperkalaemia.

Renal diseases in which the kidneys are not able to excrete potassium are a more common cause of hyperkalaemia. Acidosis, an increase in the hydrogen ion concentration, can cause hyperkalaemia; the increased intracellular hydrogen ion concentration causes a movement of potassium ions from the within cells out into the extracellular fluid. As most of the body's potassium is in the intracellular fluid within the cells, only a small proportion of this intracellular fluid potassium has to leave the cell to cause a large increase in the extracellular fluid potassium. This can occur rapidly and may be dangerous. Hyperkalaemia results in changes in neuromuscular excitability which can produce weakness or even paralysis. The effect of hyperkalaemia on the heart is most serious as it may cause the heart to stop beating or to have an arrythmia. Treatment of the hyperkalaemia involves the correction of the underlying disorder. Since insulin encourages a movement of potassium into the cells, glucose and insulin can be given to increase the movement of potassium from the extracellular fluid back into the cells.

Red blood cells, like other cells, have high concentrations of potassium. If a blood sample is drawn improperly, if the red cells haemolyze or if the sample sits too long, potassium from the red cells will escape into the plasma. This will cause a falsely elevated potassium determination.

(2) *The renin–angiotensin system.* The level of sodium in the plasma has a direct effect on the adrenal cortex and aldosterone release, and an indirect effect through the renin–angiotensin system.

Surrounding the walls of the afferent arterioles of the kidney are specialized cells, the juxta-glomerular cells, which secrete a hormone called renin (this hormone is also an enzyme). When renin is released from the cells, it reacts with a plasma protein secreted by the liver, angiotensinogen, to convert it to an active hormone called angiotensin I. Angiotensin II is formed from angiotensin I by an enzyme found chiefly in the lungs. Angiotensin II acts upon the adrenal cortex and causes it to secrete aldosterone (see Figure 15.7). Aldosterone in turn acts upon the kidney to increase salt and water reabsorption in the distal tubule and collecting ducts, leading to an increase in the extracellular fluid volume. Since stimulation of the renin–angiotensin system leads to an increase in the extracellular volume, it is not surprising that a fall in the extracellular fluid volume can stimulate the release of renin.

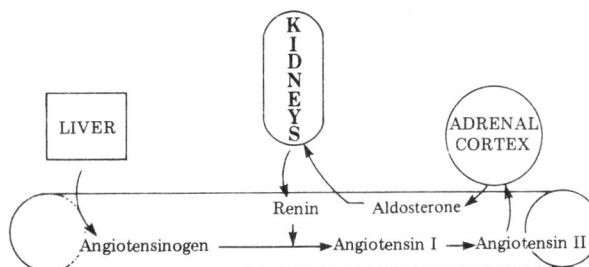

Figure 15.7 Outline of the renin–angiotensin aldosterone control system.

It is thought that the juxta-glomerular cells are able to monitor pressure within the renal arterioles. When the pressure is high these cells are put under increased tension and stretched, causing a reduction in renin secretion. Low pressure within the arterioles reduces the tension on the cells and leads to an increase in renin release. More renin ultimately leads to an increased plasma volume and increased blood pressure, which then reduces renin release.

Some recent work suggests that the juxta-glomerular cells can respond to changes in the Na^+ concentration within the renal tubule. Thus, if the Na^+ concentration is low, more renin is released, whereas if it is high, less renin is released. The net effect of these changes works to keep the sodium concentration within normal limits.

Angiotensin II is a hormone in its own right. It stimulates both aldosterone secretion and is a potent stimulator of arteriolar smooth muscle contraction. When angiotensin II stimulates the arteriolar smooth muscle to contract, resistance within the circulatory system is increased, resulting in an increase in arterial blood pressure. In addition, angiotensin II enhances the activity of the sympathetic nervous system, which increases cardiac output.

The renin–angiotensin system can be of clinical importance. It will be stimulated if the blood flow to the kidney is reduced. More salt will be retained, and both plasma volume and circulatory resistance will increase, so raising the blood pressure. If the heart is failing and/or blood pressure is already high, the renin response is inappropriate to the needs of the body. This is because it increases the stress upon the heart and may also increase oedema or its likelihood.

Figure 15.8 shows how renin might be involved in the regulation of blood pressure, and possibly in the production of hypertension.

increased cardiac output
↗
increased plasma volume
↗
increased salt and water reabsorption by kidney
↗
increased aldosterone
↗
increased renin → increased angiotensin II —
↘
increased arteriolar constriction
↘
increased resistance

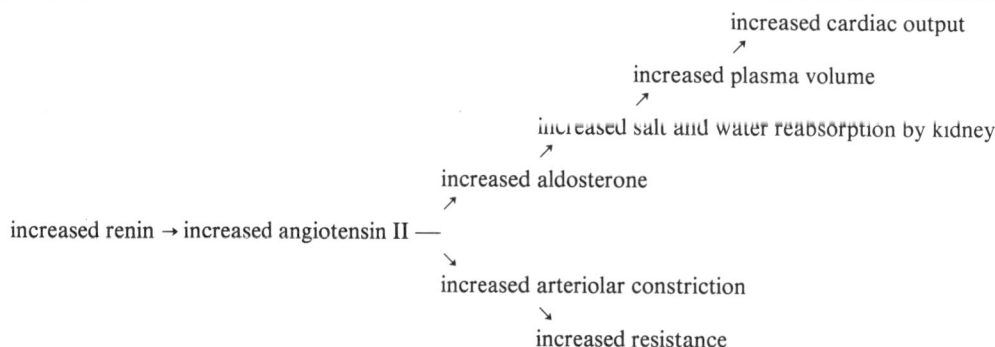

Figure 15.8   The role of renin in the regulation of blood pressure.

(3) *Adrenocorticotrophic hormone (ACTH)*. This hormone is produced by the anterior pituitary gland and plays a small part in the stimulation of aldosterone secretion, though it plays a more important part in glucocorticoid release.

It should be pointed out that other hormones are involved in sodium retention and secretion although less is known about them. Progesterone, glucagon and the prostaglandins all help to increase the excretion of sodium in the urine; prolactin retains it.

WHAT ARE THE ACTIONS OF THE GLUCOCORTICOIDS?

A. Metabolic effects

The adrenal cortex also produces glucocorticoids. In the human, the most important glucocorticoids are hydrocortisone (also called cortisol) and cortisone. In high concentrations these hormones have some sodium-retaining activity but, as their name suggests, they are more important in glucose regulation. Both hydrocortisone and cortisone can cause an increase in blood glucose and liver glycogen. This increase is mostly brought about by the breakdown of muscle tissue protein into amino acids, and the resultant increased uptake and conversion of these amino acids into glucose in the liver (gluconeogenesis). The inhibition of glucose uptake in muscle tissues raises blood glucose levels. The increased uptake of amino acids by the liver increases its synthesis of glycogen. This inhibition of glucose uptake and conversion of muscle protein into glucose can be very important during a fast or starvation when the normal glycogen reserves have been depleted.

The glucocorticoids also promote the mobilization of fatty acids from peripheral adipose tissue. The net effect of this and the other changes is to conserve the energy derived from glucose.

Many of the metabolic actions of the glucocorticoids have not yet been clearly demonstrated to occur in humans with the amounts of hormone that normally circulate. There is some acceptance, however, of the concept that glucocorticoids are necessary for the normal metabolic controls to be effective.

B. Effect on organ systems

Much of the information on glucocorticoids is derived from circumstances in which their concentration is either abnormally high or unusually low, and their actions in normal physiological concentrations are not yet clearly understood. They do, however, appear to be necessary for many organ systems to work normally and to respond to the usual physiological signals. All this is sometimes referred to as the "permissive action" of the glucocorticoids, which has a unique importance in two systems. In the cardiovascular system, the smooth muscle of the arterioles needs glucocorticoids to maintain tone. The actions of cortisol on the kidney are complex but it appears to be necessary when the individual has to excrete a water load. Psychiatric disturbances are common in both cortisol lack and cortisol excess, and the hormone also exerts a permissive action in erythropoiesis.

Perhaps the major permissive action on organ systems occurs during the body's response to stress. The human cannot withstand severe stress without glucocorticoids. The mechanism by which they do this is not yet known. Some evidence suggests that they prevent vascular collapse and induce the synthesis of additional enzymes which help in the metabolic response to stress.

C. Effects on inflammation and infection

Glucocorticoids and related steroids play a significant role in nearly all parts of the inflammatory response. In appropriate doses, they are frequently used to reduce inflammation and to treat diseases such as rheumatoid arthritis when the joints are inflamed. Glucocorticoids tend to inhibit the movement of white blood cells through capillaries by decreasing capillary permeability; they reduce phagocytic activity and stabilize the lysosomal membrane so that the powerful digestive enzymes within the lysosomes are less likely to be released and, depending upon the dose, the glucocorticoids can also cause atrophy of the lymphoid tissue and some depression of the immune response.

The use of glucocorticoids and similar steroids does have risks as well as benefits. By diminishing the ability of neutrophils to phagocytose and lymphocytes to produce antibodies and participate fully in the cell-mediated immune response, the body's defences are weakened, and the response to bacterial and viral infection is lessened. In addition, steroids can reduce the febrile response to infection so that fever, one of the physical signs of infection, does not always appear.

D. Adverse effects of large doses of glucocorticoids

Glucocorticoids are among the most commonly prescribed drugs, and their adverse effects often puts limitations on their use and usefulness. As mentioned above, infection and its control are often a problem. Muscle weakness and loss of muscle mass, secondary to protein catabolic action of the steroid, can occur. Bones can be weakened due to reduction in the protein matrix. Blood glucose levels may increase, so insulin requirements are increased. Fat may be distributed more centrally. Sodium and fluid retention can occur. The connective tissue of the skin is weakened, and the skin bruises more easily. Cataracts may develop. These adverse effects may not occur — generally they are dose-dependent.

WHAT CONTROLS THE SECRETION OF GLUCOCORTICOIDS?

The stimulus for glucocorticoid release (and to a small extent for other adrenal cortical hormones) is adrenocorticotrophic hormone (ACTH), which is released from the anterior pituitary gland. More will be said about the pituitary gland in the Chapter on the nervous system, but for now it can be said that the anterior pituitary provides many of the links between the nervous and endocrine systems.

The pituitary gland is about the size of a pea, weighs 600–700 mg and lies at the base of the brain in a protective cavity of the sphenoid bone called the sella turcica (see Figure 5.6). The pituitary gland is connected by a short stalk to an area of the brain known as the hypothalamus. Like the adrenal gland, the pituitary gland has a double embryological origin giving it two distinct parts, the anterior pituitary (adenohypophysis) and the posterior pituitary (neurohypophysis). Both the anterior and posterior pituitary communicate with the hypothalamus, though the means of communication are different in each case.

There is a small network of capillaries which begins in the hypothalamus, empties in the small veins that travel down the pituitary stalk and then forms another small capillary bed that empties into the anterior pituitary (see Figure 15.9). This capillary–vein–capillary network is called the hypothalamic–pituitary portal system and seems to be a one-way communication channel, as blood flows from the hypothalamus to the anterior pituitary. The hypothalamus itself has an endocrine function, for it makes a series of hormones called releasing hormones (releasing factors). These hormones are released into the capillaries and travel to the adenohypophysis, where they cause the release of specific anterior pituitary hormones.

One of the releasing hormones made by the hypothalamus is corticotrophin-releasing hormone or factor (CRF), which is a small polypeptide. CRF is released from the hypothalamus and travels via the hypothalamus–pituitary portal system to the anterior pituitary, where it causes the release of ACTH. This latter hormone enters the bloodstream via the veins draining the pituitary, and it ultimately travels to the adrenal cortex, where it rapidly causes cortisol and cortisone to be released. The control of CRF release from the hypothalamus is somewhat obscure, although it is known that CRF is released in response to information from higher centres in the brain. Stress, intense emotions and other factors can stimulate CRF release; CRF causes ACTH release, and ACTH release causes cortisol and cortisone release.

This shows the relationship existing between the hypothalamus, anterior pituitary and the adrenal cortex. Though it does not fully explain the control of adrenal secretion, this control can be considered in three sections: diurnal rhythm, negative feedback and stress.

(The posterior pituitary is not involved in the control of adrenal secretions. The posterior pituitary and its relationship to the hypothalamus is discussed in the Chapter on the nervous system.)

(a) Diurnal rhythm. The word diurnal refers to any event which happens every day. It has long been known that there is a daily rhythm or cycle for adrenal cortical secretions. Cortisol levels are known to be high in the early morning and low in the late evening. Refinements in techniques have made it possible to measure ACTH and cortisol levels more carefully. It appears that ATCH is not secreted continuously but in sporadic bursts. In a typical subject, these bursts peak between 4 and 8 a.m. Cortisol secretion by the adrenal cortex follows in response to the stimulus of ACTH. Presumably, ACTH is released in response to CRF, and CRF is released in response to events in the brain which take place during sleep. Plasma cortisol levels do not normally fall to zero because more cortisol is produced than can be immediately used.

(b) Negative feedback. If the adrenal glands are removed or cannot secrete cortisol, there is a dramatic increase in ACTH secretion. If cortisol is injected so that plasma cortisol levels are raised, ACTH secretion is depressed. This is because cortisol "feedback" inhibits CRF release from the hypothalamus. When there is very little plasma cortisol, the inhibiting action of cortisol on the hypothalamus is reduced, and CRF and ACTH secretion increases. This reciprocal relationship between ACTH and cortisol endeavours to keep cortisol levels within relatively constant limits, increasing cortisol when its levels are very low and reducing cortisol when its levels are high. This relationship does not appear to be the exclusive control, for it is overridden by the diurnal rhythm and in times of stress.

(c) Stress. Stress is a rather vague word. A stress can be the result of an intense emotional experience, pain, injury, surgery, extremes of temperature, loud noises, fear and anxiety. Recognizing the wide variance in the causes of stress, certain authorities choose to define stress as "any experience leading to a significant increase in adrenal cortical secretions". During stressful situations, the rate of adrenal

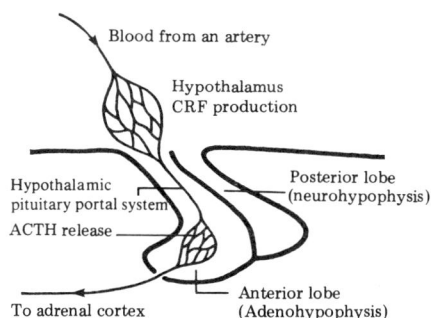

Blood from an artery

Hypothalamus CRF production

Hypothalamic pituitary portal system

ACTH release

To adrenal cortex

Posterior lobe (neurohypophysis)

Anterior lobe (Adenohypophysis)

Figure 15.9 The pituitary gland and its blood supply.

cortical secretions can increase by a factor of 10. It is thought that during stress, information from higher centres in the brain is relayed to the hypothalamus and causes CRF to be released. Stressful stimuli appear to be able to overcome the inhibiting action of cortisol on the hypothalamus because, in chronic stress, levels of both cortisol and ACTH are increased. The response to stress is rapid. In patients undergoing surgery, the adrenocortical secretions increase within minutes after the start of the operation if they have not already increased prior to surgery.

WHAT ARE THE FUNCTIONS OF THE ADRENAL SEX HORMONES?

The adrenal cortex also secretes the steroid hormones, androgens and oestrogens, called sex hormones because they are also made and secreted by the gonads or reproductive organs. The gonads secrete much higher levels of hormones than the adrenals. In both males and females, the adrenal androgens are released in greater amounts than the adrenal oestrogens. In the male, however, the amount is less than that produced by the testes. They are believed to be released by ACTH, though other factors may be involved. Some evidence indicates that they are responsible for the growth of hair in the axillary and pubic regions and the stimulation of oil secretion by the skin which sometimes cause acne, a skin disorder. Other work indicates that the adrenal sex steroids may exert some influence on the nervous system and behaviour. Women who have lost both their ovaries and their adrenal glands have a reduced libido (sex drive), while those who have lost their ovaries but retained their adrenals still have some libido.

WHAT HAPPENS IN ADRENAL CORTICAL INSUFFICIENCY?

Good insight into the function of the adrenal cortex can be gained by looking at the results of adrenal cortex deficiencies or excesses. Addison's disease is named after the Irish physician (working in England) who first described the clinical syndrome which arises following the destruction of the adrenal gland. Nearly 100% of the patients with Addison's disease will experience weight loss and weakness. This is due mainly to the loss of sodium and water in the urine because of the lack of aldosterone. Glucocorticoids, which have permissive action on skeletal muscle, are necessary for the tissue to maintain its normal capacity for work. Other common manifestations of Addison's disease are low blood pressure, loss of appetite, a darkening of the normal skin colour and a poor ability to tolerate stress. Addison's disease can be found in patients with tuberculosis who are not receiving treatment; the bacilli are able to infect and destroy the adrenal cortex. As the incidence of tuberculosis has declined, so too has the incidence of Addison's disease. The adrenal cortex may also be destroyed by other infectious processes, in rare autoimmune diseases and in atrophies following long-term administration of pharmacological doses of glucocorticoids — the cause of this being the inhibition of ACTH. Of course, glucocorticoid deficiency will occur if there is a defect in CRF or ACTH synthesis and release.

It is possible to distinguish between pituitary and adrenal disease. There are synthetic analogues of ACTH that will stimulate cortisol release. If there is no increase in plasma cortisol or its urinary metabolites following its injection, the defect can be assumed to be in the adrenal cortex. It is also possible to measure plasma ACTH.

WHAT HAPPENS WITH ADRENOCORTICAL EXCESS?

Cushing's syndrome is the disorder resulting from a chronic excess of glucocorticoids. Patients with this disorder are generally weak and more susceptible to infection. There is a breakdown of muscle protein and an increase in gluconeogenesis. The limbs may appear quite thin. Blood glucose is unusually high and occasionally so much glycogen is stored in the liver that it bulges outward. There is a redistribution of fat and more is deposited centrally. The face appears rounded (moonlike) because of an unusual deposition of fat in the cheeks; the abdomen appears quite obese and protrudes, and so much fat may be deposited in the back of the neck that the term "buffalo hump" is used to describe it.

There may be mineralocorticoid action which leads to salt retention and hypertension. High levels of adrenal androgens may also be secreted, and in the female this can cause them to have certain male characteristics such as a beard and a deep voice. Young boys will develop sexually earlier than is normal but there will be only minor effects in the adult male.

When a patient develops Cushingoid syndromes, it becomes necessary immediately to determine the reason why. It is possible that the cortex has developed a tumour which produces hormones independent of stimulation by ACTH. A more likely probability is that the defect is in the anterior pituitary, which produces excessive ACTH in spite of the high cortisol levels that would normally inhibit CRF and ACTH secretion. This high secretion of pituitary ACTH, which causes adrenal hypersecretion, is at times referred to as Cushing's disease. It is thought possible that the pathology is localized in the pituitary, not in the hypothalamus. This disease may be treated by microsurgery or irradiation of the pituitary. Occasionally tumours, not located in the pituitary, will produce ACTH; this is known as ectopic ACTH production.

The amount of aldosterone secreted in Cushing's disease is variable since ACTH is not the primary stimulus for aldosterone release. There is a tumour of the adrenal cortex which produces aldosterone and is independent of the normal hormonal controls. This condition is called Conn's syndrome after its discoverer. The excess aldosterone stimulates sodium and water retention by the kidney, which in turn leads to high blood pressure. Potassium excretion by the kidney is also increased, so plasma potassium is low (below 3.5 mmol/l), while urinary potassium is high. The changes in plasma electrolytes affect muscle tissue and reduce its strength.

WHAT ARE THE FUNCTIONS OF THE ADRENAL MEDULLA AND ITS HORMONES?

The adrenal medulla secretes chemicals which are classified as catecholamines rather than steroids. The two chief catecholamines produced by the medulla are called adrenaline (epinephrine) and noradrenaline (norepinephrine). Although adrenaline and noradrenaline have similar structures, there are some differences in their actions.

The adrenal medulla is really part of the sympathetic nervous system; medullary hormones reinforce and amplify the actions of the sympathetic nervous system. Sympathetic neurones within the thoracic region of the spinal cord travel to the adrenal medulla. Their endings release acetylcholine causing adrenaline and noradrenaline to be released. The neurones in the spinal cord have connections with the neurones in the hypothalamus.

In time of stress, the hypothalamic neurones are activated and send impulses, via the spinal cord and sympathetic nerves, to the adrenal medulla, which releases adrenaline and noradrenaline into the blood. Thus, in times of stress both the adrenal cortex and the adrenal medulla are activated, the cortex via ACTH and the medulla via direct neural stimulation.

Some of the many effects of sympathetic stimulation and catecholamine release from the adrenal medulla are:

(1) Glycogen breakdown in the liver leading to increased blood glucose.

(2) Increased triglyceride breakdown in adipose tissue leading to greater levels of fatty acids in the plasma.

(3) Increased contractility or efficiency of the heart leading to a greater stroke volume.

(4) A shifting of blood from the liver, skin, intestines, kidney, spleen, etc. to the skeletal muscles, this being brought about by contraction of arteriolar smooth muscle in the viscera and a relaxation of the arteriolar muscle in the skeletal muscles. In a stressful situation, it is difficult to separate the complex effects of adrenaline released from the adrenal medulla and noradrenaline released by the nerve endings. They do have some different effects, however. Adrenaline is a powerful constrictor of the arterioles in the skin and intestines, and, in low doses or amounts released by the medulla during stress, it is a dilator of arterioles in skeletal muscle. This effect is responsible for the reduced flow of blood into the viscera and increased flow of blood into skeletal muscle. In high doses, adrenaline can cause constriction of skeletal muscle arterioles. Noradrenaline constricts most arterioles regardless of the dose. Adrenaline has a direct stimulating action on the heart whereas noradrenaline does not.

(5) Adrenaline increases the relaxation of the smooth muscles in the bronchioles; this reduces the resistance to air flow so more air can enter the lungs with each breath.

(6) Dilation of the pupils to take in more light.

After catecholamine stimulation, the levels of cyclic AMP are increased in many cells and this leads to increased activity of many enzymes and helps explain how two hormones can have so many different actions. The response of α and β receptors to adrenaline and noradrenaline is also important. (These receptors and their actions are discussed in the Section on the sympathetic nervous system and in several other Chapters.) There is a rare disease in which the adrenal medulla cells form a tumour and produce excessive adrenaline and noradrenaline (pheochromocytoma). Patients with this disease have a very labile blood pressure which can suddenly become elevated; they are often troubled with heart palpitations. To be sure of the diagnosis of pheo-

chromocytoma, it is necessary to detect high concentrations of catecholamine breakdown products in the urine.

WHAT CONTROLS EXTRACELLULAR FLUID VOLUME AND PLASMA MOLARITY?

Aldosterone regulates sodium reabsorption and also indirectly the plasma volume. Glucocorticoids have a "permissive action" and are necessary for the excretion of a water load. If there is inadequate insulin, much of the filtered glucose will not be reabsorbed in the renal nephrons and so it will be lost in the urine, taking water with it.

Antidiuretic hormone (ADH) or vasopressin is the most important hormone in volume and molarity regulation. Some texts refer to ADH as a pituitary hormone but this is not entirely correct, for the hormone is made in the neurones of the hypothalamus and is released from their endings which terminate in the posterior pituitary. When these hypothalamic neurones are stimulated, their endings release ADH into the capillaries which drain the posterior pituitary. ADH then enters the circulation and travels to the kidneys, where it acts upon the distal convoluted tubule and collecting duct to increase their permeability to water. This cyclic AMP-mediated change increases the volume of water reabsorbed from the tubule into the capillaries; without ADH these cells have a limited permeability to water (see Figure 15.10). Increased secretion of ADH leads to increased water reabsorption and plasma volume and decreased urine volume.

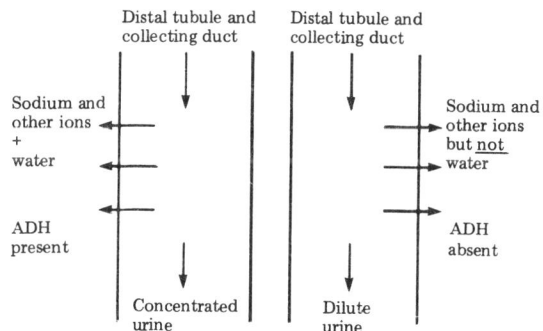

Figure 15.10 The action of antidiuretic hormone.

Injury to the hypothalamic neurones which produce ADH results in the disease, diabetes insipidus, in which the patient may pass as much as 15–30 litres/day of urine. The urine is tasteless, dilute and has a specific gravity less than 1.010. Without treatment the patient is forced to spend nearly all his or her time drinking water to prevent dehydration.

There are two important stimuli for ADH release: (1) a decrease in blood volume and (2) an increase in plasma osmolarity.

(1) Should the blood volume decrease, as it would in haemorrhage, more ADH is released, more water is reabsorbed and plasma volume is increased. If you were to drink a litre of isotonic salt water, you would increase your plasma volume without changing its osmotic pressure. This increase in blood volume inhibits ADH secretion, reduces water reabsorption and reduces plasma volume by increasing urine volume. The mechanism by which ADH regulates fluid volume has not been completely worked out. It is thought

that there are receptors within the left atrium of the heart responsible for this action; the more blood there is in the atrium, the greater the stretch of the receptors and the greater the inhibition of ADH release. If blood volume falls there will be less blood in the atrium, less stretch of the receptors and an increase in ADH release which will increase plasma volume and decrease urine volume.

(2) ADH secretion can be influenced if the osmotic pressure of the blood is changed whilst the blood volume remains constant. Clinical laboratory measurements of the osmotic pressure of serum give normal levels in the range of 285–295 mOsm/kg of serum water. Should blood salt or glucose concentrations be increased, more ADH will be released. As a result, more water will be retained diluting the sugar; so, as the blood is diluted by the increased water, the osmotic pressure of the blood will fall and be returned to normal. If you were to drink a litre or two of water, not only would you increase your plasma volume but you would also reduce the osmotic pressure of your blood. This change inhibits ADH release, which reduces renal water re-absorption and plasma volume, so that urine volume is increased. The receptors for this response are found within the hypothalamus of the brain.

Stress increases ADH release and alcohol inhibits its release. At times, the pituitary may release ADH when the osmotic pressure and plasma volume are within normal limits. Tumours may produce ADH. The net effect of this excess ADH will be an increase in water retention by the kidneys. The osmotic pressure will fall and the sodium ion concentration will be reduced because of the additional water. If the sodium concentration should fall below 125 mm/l, muscle cramps, nausea, vomiting, headache, confusion or even coma can result.

WHAT REGULATES METABOLIC RATE?

Many hormones regulate metabolism and the concentration of ions and substrates in the blood but here emphasis will be placed on the speed (rate) of chemical reactions rather than the reactions themselves. Just as glucose and calcium have optimal concentrations in the blood, there is an optimal rate for the metabolic processes of the body. The primary controls on metabolic rate are exerted by the hormones of the thyroid gland.

A. Anatomy of the thyroid gland

The thyroid gland is one of the largest of the endocrine glands. It consists of two lobes which are connected by a narrow band of tissue called the thyroid isthmus, and the gland is surrounded by a connective tissue capsule (see Figure 15.11a). The gland is closely attached to the trachea, and the lobes lie along the lower half of the thyroid cartilage (Adam's apple), while the isthmus is at the level of the 2nd or 3rd cartilaginous ring of the trachea.

The thyroid gland is well supplied with blood by the superior thyroid artery, which comes from the external carotids, and by the inferior thyroid artery from the sub-clavian. The gland is also supplied by sympathetic and para-sympathetic nerves; the laryngeal nerves pass in the lateral grooves between lateral lobes and the trachea. These nerves

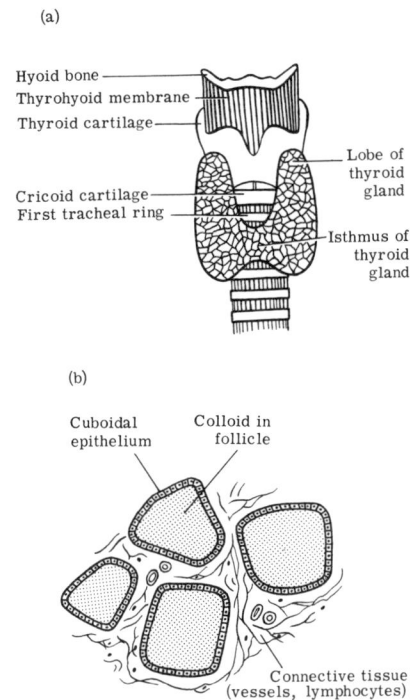

Figure 15.11   The thyroid gland. (a) Position. (b) Histology.

are occasionally injured during thyroid surgery, resulting in impaired swallowing and speech.

The microscopic structure of the thyroid gland is some-what unusual (see Figure 15.11b); it shows a circular arrangement of cuboidal epithelium surrounding a thick fluid containing protein and enzyme and called colloid (each droplet of colloid and the surrounding cells make a single thyroid follicle). Between the follicles are somewhat larger epithelial cells called parafollicular cells, which secrete thyrocalcitonin (TCT), which was discussed in connection with the control of calcium. The thyroid follicle cells actively absorb iodine in the form of iodide ions (I^-) from the blood and secrete it into the vesicle where the thyroid hormones are made and stored.

The thyroid gland is unique among the endocrine glands in that it stores much more hormone than any other gland. Thyroid hormone is made up of two molecules of the amino acid, tyrosine, and three or four atoms of iodine. Two atoms of iodine are added to each tyrosine molecule, and the two tyrosine molecules are joined together to form tetra-iodothyronine, which is also called thyroxine (T_4) or thyroid hormone (TH). If there are only three iodine molecules on the two tyrosine molecules, the hormone is called tri-iodothy-ronine (T_3).

Factors outside the thyroid gland may help to determine the amount of active thyroid hormone. Although most of the hormone secreted by the thyroid gland is T_4, some tissues can convert T_4 to T_3. Both T_4 and T_3 have the same effects, though T_3 is much more rapid in onset of its action. Some authorities consider T_4 to be a precursor (prehormone) of T_3, and believe T_3, not T_4, to be the important hormone. More recent work has shown that both T_4 and T_3 can be converted to an inactive form of tri-iodothyronine called reverse-T_3 (rT_3). This conversion makes possible an even greater degree of control over the amount of active hormone produced. At the present time, all that is known is that the conversion of T_4 and T_3 to rT_3 can take place, but the full significance is not yet appreciated.

Most T_4 and T_3 travels in the blood bound to plasma proteins. The protein which functions to transport most T_4 and T_3 is known as thyroid-binding globulin (TBG). Although most of the T_4 and some of the T_3 in the blood is bound to TBG, it is the free (unbound) hormone that is active.

B. Control of thyroid hormone secretion

TH is made within the thyroid follicle and stored there, being joined to a very large globulin protein molecule until it is released into the circulation. The stimulus for its release and for thyroid gland growth is a hormone from the anterior pituitary gland called thyroid-stimulating hormone (TSH). The general pattern of TH control is similar to that of the ACTH and glucocorticoids, though, of course, the individual hormones are different (see Figure 15.12).

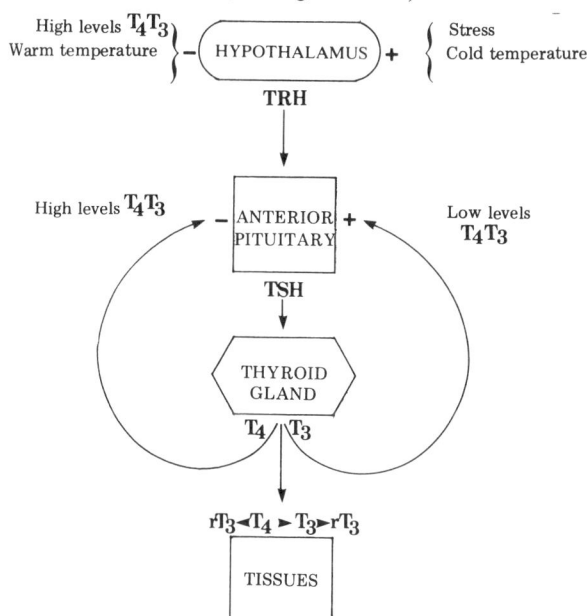

Figure 15.12 Control of thyroid hormone secretion.

Within the hypothalamus, there is another releasing hormone, thyroid-stimulating hormone-releasing hormone (TSH-RH), also known as thyrotropin-releasing hormone (TRH). TRH is a small peptide hormone consisting of three amino acids. TRH is released from the hypothalamus into the capillaries which drain into the anterior pituitary. An increase in TRH will cause an increase in release of TSH from the anterior pituitary, which will then stimulate the thyroid gland to synthesize and to release T_4 and T_3. (TRH can also increase the release of prolactin and other anterior pituitary hormones.) Some of the known stimuli for the release of TRH from the hypothalamus include stress, a cold environment and, to some extent, low levels of T_4 and T_3 in the blood. Day-to-day regulation of thyroid hormone levels depend upon a negative feedback relationship between T_4 and T_3 in the blood and TSH in the anterior pituitary. High blood levels of T_4 and/or T_3 will inhibit TSH release.

Should there be a deficiency of iodine in the diet, or some metabolic abnormality within the thyroid gland which prevents the production of T_4 and T_3, the negative feedback loop will be broken by the low levels of T_4 and T_3, and TSH will increase. This increased TSH will stimulate the growth of the thyroid gland in an attempt to compensate for the low T_4 and T_3 levels. As a result of the additional TSH stimulation, the thyroid gland may become quite enlarged. An enlarged thyroid gland is known as a goitre. The WHO estimates that there are 200 million people in the world who are goitrous. The most common cause of goitre is iodine deficiency in the diet which prevents hormones from being synthesized. Iodine deficiencies are more likely to be found in individuals who live in areas that are distant from or that were never covered by the iodine-rich seas and oceans. The centres of North America and Africa, Switzerland and the Himalayas are examples of places where goitre can be found because of lack of iodine. The lack can be prevented by adding iodine to the diet, usually in the salt, in the form of sodium iodide (NaI). There are certain compounds called goitrogens which can interfere with iodine absorption and metabolism by the thyroid gland so that TH cannot be synthesized. Vegetables belonging to the cabbage and turnip family contain small amounts of goitrogens. The amounts are so small however that they are usually insignificant but may become important if the individual is on a low iodine diet. Certain drugs also interfere with iodine metabolism. If TH cannot be synthesized there will be no inhibition of TSH, and TSH levels will increase and cause goitre. Goitre may also be caused by a tumour of the thyroid gland, metabolic abnormalities within the thyroid or autoimmune disease in which antibodies are made against thyroid tissue. A goitre may produce too much, enough or too little hormone.

The amount of TSH in the blood can be used as a clinical indicator of how much the thyroid gland is being driven to produce a given amount of thyroid hormone. As an example, a person with low-to-normal levels of T_4 and T_3 can have very high levels of TSH. This condition suggests that something is wrong with the gland, in that it has to be so highly stimulated to produce low-to-normal levels of T_4 and T_3. TSH levels may be so low that they are undetectable in certain hypothalamic and anterior pituitary diseases, or when T_4 and/or T_3 levels are very high. There are very rare tumours of the anterior pituitary gland in which excess TSH is produced and, consequently, excess T_4 and T_3 are released by the thyroid gland, which may become a goitre.

C. Action of thyroid hormone

The ultimate mechanism by which thyroid hormone works is not known, but it is necessary for normal growth and development and it affects nearly every tissue and organ in the body. The general effect of the hormone is to increase the rate of many metabolic reactions which leads to an increased oxygen consumption and greater heat production by most cells. Some of these changes are brought about by increased enzyme activity but the ultimate mechanism remains unknown.

There is a speeding up of both anabolic and catabolic reactions which can have different effects on different systems. For example, thyroid hormone tends to reduce the level of cholesterol in the blood. Although the rate of cholesterol synthesis is increased, the rate at which cholesterol is broken down is increased even more. Inasmuch as the thyroid gland affects so many systems and is poorly understood, it might be best to look at the signs and symptoms of an adult individual with too much thyroid hormone (hyperthyroid) and one with too little (hypothyroid).

Hypothyroid	*Hyperthyroid*
Cells:	
↓enzymes	↑enzymes
↓O$_2$ consumption	↑O$_2$ consumption
less turnover of fat and carbohydrate, impaired protein synthesis	more fat and carbohydrate turnover and protein breakdown
Digestive system:	
↓intestinal absorption	↑intestinal absorption
↓muscle activity	↑muscle activity
constipation	frequent bowel movements
↓appetite	↑appetite
Cardiovascular system:	
↓cardiac output	↑cardiac output
↓blood pressure	↑blood pressure
weak pulse	strong fast pulse
Muscle:	
weakness	weakness
low tension	tremor
Reproductive system:	
menstrual disorders	menstrual disorders
Whole body:	
greater susceptibility to infection	greater susceptibility to infection
↓BMR	↑BMR
Appearance:	
dry cool skin (↓blood flow)	warm moist skin (↑blood flow)
puffy oedema from protein in skin	prominence or bulging of eyes
↓weight	↑weight
Behaviour:	
slow reflexes	quick reflexes
mentally slow and sleepy	mentally quick, wakeful and often irritable
sensitive to cold	sensitive to heat
not very active	excessively active

This Table applies to an adult. Thyroid hormones are important for growth and development; these actions of the thyroid hormones will be discussed later on in this Chapter. It should be understood that the signs and symptoms of thyroid disease vary from patient to patient and that, at times, the disease may be quite difficult to detect. Of course, sometimes it is easy to detect, as the person may be in a coma due to an extreme thyroid hormone deficiency or be severely ill with a thyroid crisis due to the metabolic and cardiovascular disturbance produced by an excess of hormone.

WHAT CAUSES HYPOTHYROIDISM?

An individual may become hypothyroid for a number of reasons:

(1) Iodine deficiency is the most common cause in the world, though this cause is rare in societies where foods produced in different geographical regions are eaten frequently, and sodium iodide is almost always added to table salt. (The iodide is converted to iodine by the thyroid gland.)

(2) If there is a defect in the synthesis of either TSH or TRH, the thyroid gland will not be able to release hormones of its own.

(3) The thyroid gland itself may be at fault due to a metabolic defect such as an inability to take up iodide or convert it to iodine.

(4) The gland may be destroyed by autoimmune processes. These are not well understood but it appears that antibodies are made against the thyroid gland, thyroglobulin, and/or the cell-mediated immune response is directed against parts of the gland. This can lead to the destruction of the gland.

(5) Radioactive iodine is, at times, used in the treatment of hyperthyroidism and it is extremely difficult to give the optimal amounts. This drug reduces the size of the thyroid gland and also seems to prevent normal cells from replicating. Over a period of years many patients treated with radioactive iodine go from the hyperthyroid to the hypothyroid state.

Hypothyroidism may be treated by giving commercially produced T$_4$ or a preparation from dried animal thyroid glands.

WHAT CAUSES HYPERTHYROIDISM?

As you should expect to know by now, this condition can be caused in different ways:

(1) Disorders of the hypothalamus or pituitary which bring about uncontrolled excessive release of TSH can cause hyperthyroidism. (This is a rare occurrence and it is even more infrequent for the diseased pituitary to release excessive TSH.)

(2) A tumour of the thyroid gland could produce excessive T$_4$ and T$_3$. This hormone production would occur independently of TSH.

(3) The most common cause of hyperthyroidism is Grave's disease, characterized by a diffuse toxic goitre with excessive secretion of T$_4$ and T$_3$. Grave's disease is believed to be an autoimmune disease in which both T- and B-lymphocytes are involved. An IgG immunoglobulin is produced stimulating the thyroid to release hormone. This thyroid stimulator is known as long- (or late-) acting thyroid stimulator (LATS). The name is derived from the fact that LATS is slower than TSH in stimulating the gland but its action lasts for a longer time.

The eyes are commonly involved in Grave's disease;

mucopolysaccharide is deposited behind the orbit and it causes the eye, or eyes, to bulge forward — a condition known as exophthalmos. Some patients with Grave's disease experience a thyroid storm — a rare life-threatening event associated with a great excess of T_4 and/or T_3. There are problems not directly attributable to thyroid hormone but due to the fact that thyroid hormone potentiates the action of adrenaline and noradrenaline on tissues. This means that, although the amounts of catecholamines are within the normal range, their effects are much more potent. It is thought, for instance, that the rapid heart rate seen in these hyperthyroid patients requires drugs that block or reduce the effect of catecholamines. Drugs that block the β receptors of the heart are used, as the stress on the heart can be significant.

Treatment for hyperthyroidism must, of course, aim to reduce the amount of thyroid hormone in the blood. Surgery, radioactive iodine or drugs which inhibit hormone synthesis are used. Certainly, the diagnosis of either hypothyroidism or hyperthyroidism often requires laboratory confirmation. A common test is the protein-bound iodine (PBI), which measures the amount of iodine bound to the protein in the blood. This test assumes that most of the iodine in the blood is found in thyroid hormone. Better and more sophisticated tests measure the amount of either T_4 or T_3 through the use of isotopes and immuno-assay.

HOW DOES THYROID HORMONE AFFECT GROWTH?

The mechanism by which T_4 and T_3 affect growth is not known, but it is known that they are absolutely necessary for normal growth and development.

Hypothyroidism in infants and children can be due to maternal iodine deficiency, maternal dietary deficiency or a deficiency in the child's diet, or a defect in the gland itself. Unless this deficiency is detected early in infancy and treated with TH, the consequences are sad, serious and irreversible; the individual develops into a cretin. The cretin's nervous system fails to develop properly and he or she becomes permanently mentally retarded. Bones fail to grow properly so the cretin never reaches adult height and retains an infant-like face in spite of increasing age. Many of the other hypothyroid characteristics are also noted.

As mentioned earlier, TRH can also stimulate prolactin release from the anterior pituitary. TRH, like many of the other hypothalamic hormones, is also found in other parts of the brain and may have many actions that are not yet known.

WHAT REGULATES GROWTH?

The discussion of growth has been left until last because it involves many genetic, nutritional and hormonal factors. A wise man once said that growth is the best evidence of life. It can be said that normal growth and development is the best evidence of good health. To a certain extent one's growth potential is inherited from one's parents when the maternal and paternal chromosomes or genes of the egg and sperm unite to form the zygote. Pygmies are short and the Tutsi are tall primarily because of their genetic inheritance.

After conception, the growth of the foetus is dependent upon the mother for its nutrition. There is some evidence that poor maternal nutrition can impair foetal growth and later the full development and growth of the child. The dependence of the infant on the mother continues till after the period of breast feeding has been completed. The period between breast feeding and eating of adult foods is particularly critical for growth because it is during this time that kwashiorkor is most likely to develop from protein deficiency. If an infant or young child has been malnourished and then receives an adequate diet, some 'catch up' growth may be possible.

Besides the dietary and genetic aspects of growth, the endocrine system also plays an important role; thyroid hormone, insulin and the androgens and oestrogens contribute to normal growth. Also extremely important is growth hormone (GH). Growth hormone, sometimes called somatotropin, is a protein hormone made in the anterior pituitary. The hormone is found in the foetal pituitary and in both infant and adult blood, though there appears to be a greater concentration in infant blood.

WHAT ARE THE ACTIONS OF GROWTH HORMONE AND WHAT CONTROLS ITS RELEASE?

Growth hormone is an absolute requirement for normal growth. Like thyroid hormone, it has no specific target and affects nearly every organ, making them larger. If the epiphyses have not yet fused, GH will stimulate the bones to grow and the individual will become taller. He or she will not only be taller but bigger with larger muscle mass and bigger organs. Protein synthesis is also increased.

Excessive secretion of GH before closure of the epiphyses leads to gigantism. In spite of their big size, giants are usually not very healthy and often do not live as long as their smaller brothers and sisters because of an increased susceptibility to infection, diabetes and circulatory weakness.

If the epiphyses have closed and there is excessive GH secretion, then the individual will not grow taller but will develop a condition known as acromegaly which is characterized by enlarged viscera and increased deposition of connective tissue and cartilage, particularly in the joints and in the face and hands.

Insufficient secretion of GH leads to no known disease in the adult, but in infants and children normal growth will be hindered and dwarfism will result. These individuals have small but normal viscera and their intelligence is normal. This is in contrast to a cretin who not only is small and has deformed bones but also is mentally retarded. GH can stimulate growth in young individuals who are deficient in GH, but normal short people cannot be made taller by GH.

Certain recent work has shown that many of the actions of GH on cartilage and growing bone are brought about by an intermediate. It appears that GH stimulates the liver to release a hormone called somatomedin. This hormone works with GH and is able to stimulate the growth of cartilage and its conversion to bone. Recently a group of dwarfs has been found to have normal GH levels but no somatomedin. Thus, of the hormones mentioned in this Chapter, GH, somatomedin, insulin and thyroid hormone are among the hormones that promote skeletal growth.

In the adult, GH seems to increase the uptake of amino acids by most tissues and somehow antagonizes insulin so that glucose entry into muscle cells is hindered and plasma glucose is increased. Fatty acids also increase because of the action of GH on adipose tissue.

There is evidence that two hormones are made in the hypothalamus which influence GH secretion. They reach the anterior pituitary via the hypothalamic-pituitary capillary network. One hormone, growth hormone-releasing hormone (GH-RH) stimulates the release of GH. Growth hormone-inhibiting hormone (GH-IH), which is also known as growth hormone-inhibiting factor (GIF) or somatostatin, inhibits release of GH from the anterior pituitary. The manner in which GH-RH and somatostatin work is not known. Somatostatin is able to reduce GH secretion in people with acromegaly: it also has other effects outside the nervous system and is synthesized in the pancreas.

At the present time, it is not known what causes the hypothalamic hormones to be released. Some of the circumstances causing GH to be released are known. The levels of GH fluctuate during the day, and at night GH is secreted in outbursts. These outbursts of hormonal secretion are associated with the rapid eye movements that take place during dreaming. Metabolic factors likewise influence GH release. High blood glucose levels inhibit GH release, whereas low or falling blood levels tend to increase GH release.

The graph in Figure 15.13 contains information which might be helpful in reviewing certain hormones that influence GH release, and it shows how endocrinology can be applied to clinical problems. Children grow at different rates and some children grow more than others. Often parents are concerned that their child who is of short stature has an hormonal defect which might be responsible. Sometimes there is reason for concern and it is necessary to test the ability of the anterior pituitary to secrete GH. There are clinical laboratories that can measure the amount of GH in a sample of blood.

One way, but by no means the only way, to test the pituitary's reserve of GH is to inject glucagon. This causes the blood glucose to rise quickly. As glucose rises, insulin release will be stimulated, and insulin levels will increase. Insulin functions to lower glucose by increasing transport of glucose into muscle and fat cells. The insulin will thus begin to lower blood glucose levels. The falling glucose levels will then stimulate an increase in GH release. In a normal child, the GH level will more than double, while in a child with a hypothalamic or pituitary disorder it will remain low.

WHAT OTHER HORMONES ARE THERE?

There are other hormones in addition to the ones discussed here, as well as the ones mentioned in the Chapters on the digestive, reproductive and nervous systems. It is thought that the thymus gland, discussed in the Chapter on the lymphatic system, might secrete a hormone that stimulates lymphocytes and antibody production. The kidneys are thought to secrete erythropoietin, which acts upon the bone marrow to stimulate red blood cell production. A part of the nervous system, the pineal gland, is believed to secrete some hormones, though their importance and function in man are unknown.

A final class of hormones is the prostaglandins. The prostaglandins are a series of chemicals derived from fatty acids and found in blood, semen and within nearly every cell of the body. They can do a variety of things including lowering blood pressure, reducing salt and water reabsorption by the kidneys and acid secretion by the stomach. They are currently being investigated in the treatment of arthritis. Because of their very powerful action on uterine smooth muscle causing it to forcefully contract, they can be used to initiate labour, or the expulsion of the foetus. It has been suggested that aspirin reduces fever by inhibiting prostaglandin synthesis.

It should be restated that not all hormones are associated with the endocrine glands. As an example, some tumours found in the lung have been known to produce ADH, ACTH and parathyroid hormone.

Endocrinology is a rapidly changing field. We have only to consult a text-book that is 5 or 10 years old to learn the magnitude of the change. Biochemical techniques that permit reasonably accurate measurement of hormone levels have been responsible for much of this change. Not only are the measurements more accurate but also scientists are now measuring hormones whose existence was heretofore unknown. There are still more changes to come and more hormones to be discovered.

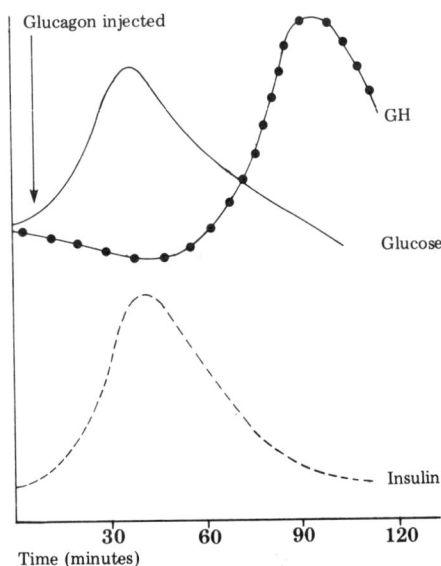

Figure 15.13 Changes in blood levels of glucose, insulin and growth hormone following injection of glucagon in a normal child.

16. The Reproductive System

INTRODUCTION

Bacteria reproduce quickly and simply by the process of cell division: one bacterium splits to form two bacteria. For humans the process is much more complex. Scientifically and medically the reproductive system is like any other, with its own structure, function and diseases.

Sexual acts and reproductive functions are like other processes of human life and involve glands, secretions, nerves, reflexes, muscular contractions, circulatory changes and so on. Because of the significance of human birth and the power, pleasure and beauty of the sexual act, more than biological processes are at stake; moral, physiological, social and even economic and political values are involved, though these cannot and will not be discussed here.

This Chapter will consider what is uniquely male and uniquely female. Previously we have talked about the differences between the sexes in quantitative terms, that is, differences in size — men in general having a larger vital capacity than women, women requiring more dietary iron than men, as examples. The differences between male and female are not just quantitative however, for there are qualitative differences, or differences in kind: women can become pregnant, men cannot. The differences between men and women are such that every cell in the body is marked either male or female. The basis of these differences is genetic. These differences are expressed in many ways including different susceptibilities to certain heart diseases. Men are more susceptible to heart attacks than are women, and women are more likely than men to have certain diseases of the thyroid gland. Weak minds have traditionally taken refuge in the idea that different implies inferior or inadequate. It does not. There is no evidence whatever that either sex is superior or inferior, more or less intelligent or competent, or biologically destined for either power or subservience.

WHAT IS THE ANATOMY OF THE FEMALE REPRODUCTIVE SYSTEM?

The female reproductive system is composed of external and internal reproductive organs, and the breasts (mammary glands) which are termed accessory reproductive structures.

A. The external reproductive organs

These organs are collectively called the vulva (see Figure 16.1). The external labia form the lateral border of the vulva. Each labium is a fold of skin which covers some fat and unites anteriorly to form the mons veneris, an elevation of fatty tissue which covers the symphysis pubis. At puberty,

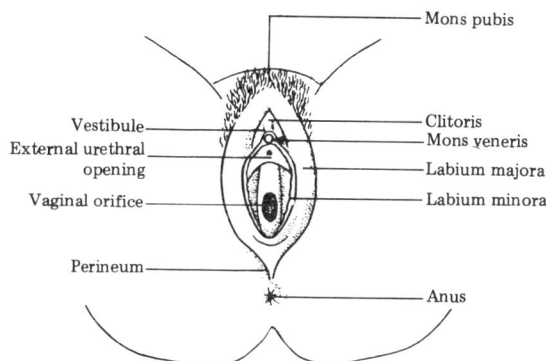

Figure 16.1 The external female reproductive organs.

the mons pubis becomes covered with hair. The labia pass backwards in a curve but do not actually unite. Within the labia majora are two thin folds of skin which cover some connective tissue and are called the labia minora; the labia minora enclose an almond-shaped area called the vestibule within which are the openings of the urethra, vagina and certain glands.

Anteriorly, the two labia minora meet to form a hood-like structure which partially surrounds and protects the clitoris. This is a small structure, about 2 cm long, located in the midline, anterior to the external opening of the vagina; it is attached to the symphysis by means of a suspensory ligament. Because of its rich nerve supply, the clitoris is a highly sensitive structure. The clitoris is an erectile tissue because it can be firm and rigid when filled with blood; developmentally it is similar to the penis in the male.

Posteriorly, the labia unite to form the fourchette, a small skin-fold which is often ruptured during the delivery of the first child.

Projecting from within the rim of the vestibule is a thin mucous membrane which incompletely covers the opening to the vagina and is called the hymen. The hymen is often ruptured during the first intercourse when the penis is thrust into the vagina causing a small amount of bleeding. It is a poor indicator of virginity, as it can be ruptured during certain non-sexual activities and in some women it is flexible and positioned so that it remains visible even after childbirth. Occasionally, it completely covers the vagina and it is necessary to puncture it surgically so the the flow of menstrual blood is not hindered.

The female urethra, which comes from the urinary bladder, exits between the clitoris and the vaginal opening (see Figure 16.2b). The area between the vagina and the anus is the perineum (perineal body). There are two Bartholin's (paravaginal) glands located between the labia minora and

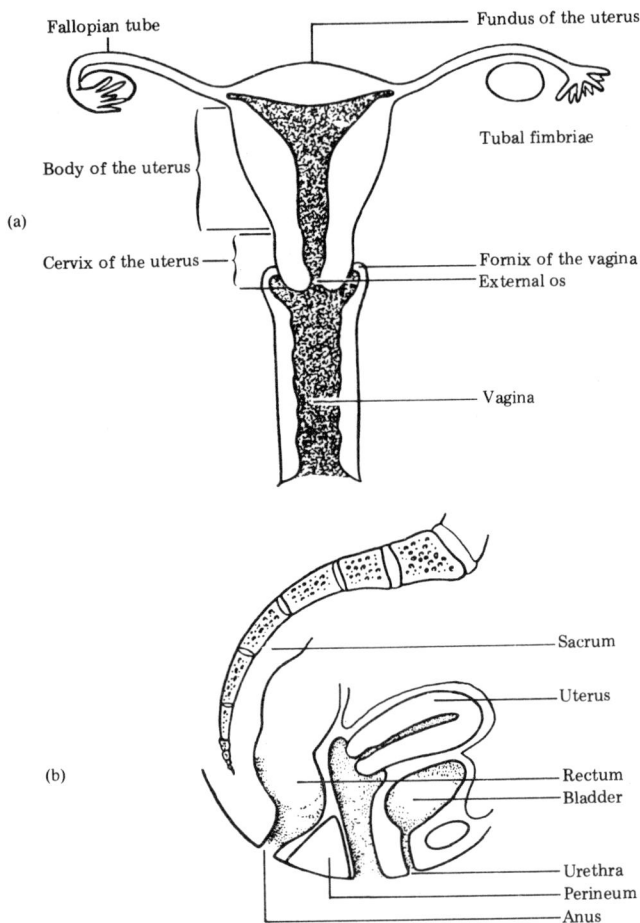

Figure 16.2   The internal female genitalia. (a) Posterior section. (b) Sagittal section.

the vaginal wall. The short ducts open into the lower vagina, one on either side. These are mucus-producing glands; as a result of certain infections, the ducts may become obstructed, abcessed and cystic.

B. The internal reproductive organs

These include the vagina, uterus (womb), two uterine tubes (oviducts) and two ovaries (see Figures 16.2).

a. The vagina. This tubular organ is about 8 cm long and connects the uterus with the external reproductive organs. The vagina lies between the urinary bladder and the rectum. Its walls are lined with mucous membrane of stratified epithelium. The middle layer of the vagina is the largest and consists of two layers of smooth muscle. The innermost muscular layer is formed from circular fibres, while the outer layer fibres are longitudinally arranged. The outermost layer of the vagina is connective tissue and contains nerves and blood vessels.

The mucous membrane lining the vagina is arranged in folds and its secretions are slightly acid. This acidity prevents some but by no means all micro-organisms from gaining access to the reproductive tract; many bacteria normally live within the warm and moist vagina, and their metabolites are responsible for the characteristic vaginal odour. This odour is

entirely normal and is not associated with any disease process. Vaginal deodorants work by killing the bacteria responsible for the odour, as well as some of the other bacteria which inhabit the vagina, and thus the deodorants upset the ecology of the reproductive tract. There is no physiological need for them and at times they may actually irritate the vagina itself. The small recess of the vagina which is above the entry of the uterus is called the fornix of the vagina.

The innermost lining of the vagina, like other membranes of the body, can become infected, inflamed and give rise to a copious discharge. Inflammation of the vagina (vaginitis) may be caused by bacteria, viruses or other micro-organisms such as *Candida albicans*, a yeast-like fungus, and *Trichomonas vaginalis*, a flagellated protozoan (more simply, a small single-cell organism that has a tail). Certain infections of the vagina are transmitted by sexual activity, others are not.

b. The uterus (womb). This is a hollow, pear-shaped organ lying in the pelvic cavity between the bladder and the rectum. The uterus has three parts: fundus, body and cervix. The fundus of the uterus is above the openings of the right and left uterine (Fallopian) tubes into the uterine cavity. The body is below the openings of the uterine tubes, but there are no significant histological differences between the body and the fundus. In the non-pregnant woman, the cervix is firm, about 3 cm wide and 2–3 cm long. About half the length of the cervix protrudes into the vagina. The attachment of the vagina around the periphery of the uterus divides into a vaginal and supra-vaginal portion. The external os is the opening into the vagina of the uterine canal and cavity. This opening is less than the size of a pencil. The cervix has a remarkable adaptability as, prior to delivery, the external os becomes dilated enough to permit the passage of the infant's head.

That part of the cervix which projects into the vagina is covered with stratified squamous epithelium, but beyond the external os there is a transition to a more glandular epithelium. Beneath the epithelium are circular, smooth muscle fibres which connect with the muscular myometrium of the body of the uterus above.

Cancer of the uterine cervix (cervical cancer) is the most common cancer of the female reproductive tract and is exceeded only by breast cancer in frequency of occurrence in women. Approximately 2% of all women will ultimately develop cervical cancer. There is an increased incidence of cervical cancer in women who become sexually active at an early age and who have many different sexual partners. Sexual activity does not cause cancer and there are women who are by no means promiscuous who may develop cervical cancer. There is no clear and certain explanation for these facts, but it is thought that a virus is responsible for initiating the malignant process. This virus may be transmitted by sexual activity and thus the young woman active with many different partners increases the statistical risk of making contact with the virus.

In 1928, Dr George N. Papanicolaou described a test in which cells were gently scraped from in and around the external os of the cervix. Microscopic examination of the stained cells may be more than 85% accurate in finding cancerous cells. This test has become popularly known as the

"Pap" test and is now widely used as a screening test for cervical cancer. The Pap test is a useful test, as early detection of cervical cancer increases the chances for successful treatment.

The entire uterus is about 8 cm long and 4 cm at its widest point. These measurements change dramatically during pregnancy. The fundus and body make up the largest part of the uterus. The uterine wall is composed of three distinct layers.

The innermost layer of the uterine wall, which lines the uterine cavity and canal, is the endometrium. The endometrium is a special mucous membrane which itself has two layers. The thick, superficial layer grows, bleeds and is shed periodically during reproductive life. Beneath the superficial layer is the basilar layer of the endometrium. This layer is more constant and regenerates the superficial functional layer after it has been shed. The fertilized ovum implants itself in the endometrium and it is here that its development first takes place.

The middle layer of the uterine wall is the myometrium and is the thickest of all the layers. The myometrium is made up of three layers of smooth muscle arranged circularly, obliquely and longitudinally. The myometrium of the fundus is thicker than that of the body. During pregnancy the uterus must increase its capacity hundreds of times, so the uterine muscle must be able to stretch and grow. The smooth muscle of the uterus should not contract till the foetus is mature and birth is imminent. Then the contractions must be strong enough to force the infant out of the uterus, down the vagina and into the outside world.

The outermost layer of the uterine wall is the perimetrium. This is really a covering which is draped over the uterus and functions to maintain the position of the uterus. The perimetrium covering the anterior surface of the uterus and the perimetrium covering the posterior surface of the uterus come together on both sides of the uterus to form a double layer called the broad ligament. Each broad ligament extends from the side of the uterus to the side wall of the pelvis. The broad ligaments are draped over and cover most of the uterine tubes. The broad ligaments, the floor of the pelvis and other ligaments maintain the position of the uterus. Pregnancy stretches these ligaments and during childbirth they are often stretched and torn. Since the uterus is no longer adequately supported, it descends towards the pelvic floor and puts pressure on the urinary bladder so micturition is interfered with and incontinence often results. This condition is known as prolapse of the uterus and can be repaired surgically.

Cancer of the uterine body and fundus is less common than cervical cancer. The uterine wall is, however, frequently the site of a non-cancerous tumour called by any one of several names — fibroids, leiomyomas, fibromyomas. These are non-malignant tumours composed of smooth muscle and connective tissue. The symptoms that fibroid tumours may produce depend on the tumours' size and location. They may cause pelvic pain, abnormal bleeding or failure of pregnancy to be completed.

Many hundreds of years ago, Arab traders were troubled by the problem of their camels becoming pregnant while the caravans were on long safaris. They solved this problem by placing an apricot stone in the camel's uterus. The exact mechanism by which the apricot stone prevents pregnancy is not known, but the same principle is involved in the use of the intra-uterine device (IUD) in pregnancy prevention in humans. The IUD is a plastic, curved or coiled loop inserted with a special device into the uterus. Expulsion of the IUD occurs in about 10% of the women who try to use it and pregnancy may take place if the expulsion is not detected. The IUD is usually a safe and effective contraceptive. Some women do experience irregular bleeding and cramping with use of the IUD; very rarely, the uterus may be torn or perforated by an IUD. Women who have given birth have more success with the use of an IUD than do women who have never been pregnant.

c. The uterine tubes (oviducts). These two tubes leave the uterus between the fundus and the body of the uterus. These tubes are narrow, about 10 cm long, travel away from the uterus and curve towards the ovary. The end of each tube is wide and open, something like the open end of a trumpet. Fimbriae, small finger-like projections, extend from this broad mouth and extend to near the ovary. These openings are important for two reasons. Since each is close to the ovary, which is the source of ova, it receives the ova and sends it on its journey down to uterine tubes where fertilization takes place in the uterus. Because the oviducts are open structures, they can receive ova and also serve as an entrance for micro-organisms into the pelvic and abdominal cavities from the uterine tubes; infection, for example, from an abortion performed under conditions that are not sterile, can spread to the uterine tubes and from there throughout the entire pelvic and abdominal cavities.

The tubes are lined with an inner layer of columnar epithelium. The columnar cells either produce a mucous secretion or are ciliated. The bacteria which cause the venereal disease, gonorrhoea, cannot penetrate the stratified epithelium of the vagina but they can infect the single epithelium layer lining the uterine tubes. The resulting infection can sometimes block passage of the sperm and ova, spread to the ovary and cause sterility.

The uterine tubes have a middle layer of smooth muscle and are covered by the broad ligament which is draped over them but does not cover the opening to them.

d. The ovaries. In a sense, all other parts of the reproductive system are accessory to the ovaries, for they are the source of the ova. They are also important endocrine glands, for they produce the important steroid hormones, oestrogen and progesterone. The two ovaries, right and left, are situated on either side of the uterus. Their positions vary, but usually they are attached to the posterior layer of the broad ligament by the ovarian ligament and lie below the uterine tubes which arch over each ovary (see Figure 16.2a). Each ovary is about the size of a large almond. The fine structure of the ovary depends on the age of the individual.

The mature ovary has an inner medulla of blood and lymph vessels, nerves and fibrous tissue, and an outer cortex with a connective tissue framework which contains the ovarian follicles.

A follicle is the egg (ovum) and its surrounding cells. The ovarian follicles are classified as:
(a) Primary follicles
(b) Graffian follicles
(c) Atretic follicles.
When an infant girl is born, each ovary contains hundreds

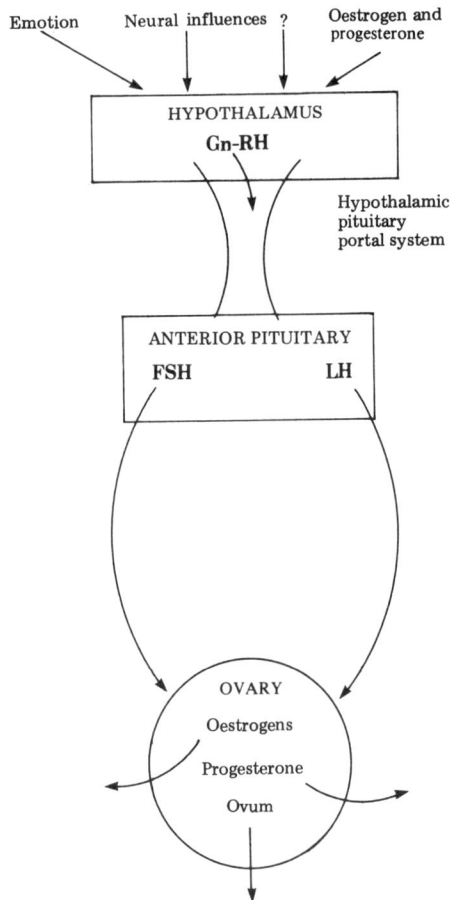

Figure 16.3 Outline of the hormonal control of the ovary.

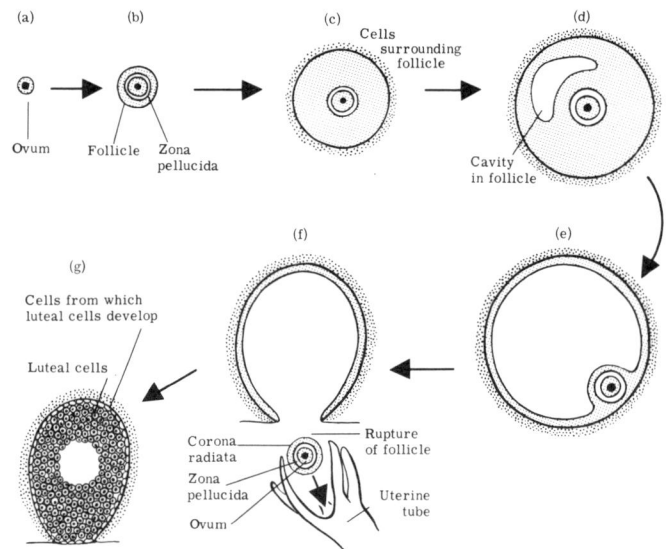

Figure 16.4 The ovarian cycle. (a) Ovum in the ovary. (b) (c) (d) The formation of the ovarian (Graafian) follicle. (e) The ripe follicle. (f) Rupture of the follicle, freeing the ovum. (g) The formation of the corpus luteum.

of thousands of follicles. A primary follicle is an ovum surrounded by a layer of epithelial cells. By the time of puberty, when reproductive life can begin, many of these follicles have already become atretic follicles; they are follicles that have degenerated and no longer contain a viable ovum. At puberty, it is possible for primary follicles to become Graafian follicles. These are mature follicles capable of releasing an ovum from the ovary.

The development of these primary follicles into Graafian follicles, which release an ovum, is complex and is chiefly under the influence of two hormones from the anterior pituitary gland (see Figure 16.3). The two hormones are follicle-stimulating hormone (FSH) and luteinizing hormone (LH). When a woman reaches the reproductive age, the monthly cycle in which FSH and LH are released from the anterior pituitary gland begins. This causes many primary follicles to grow and become Grafian follicles, and generally only one Graafian follicle releases an ovum (see Figure 16.4). As the primary follicle in response to FSH begins to grow, the zona pellucida (a thick membrane) covers the enlarging ovum.

The epithelial cells surrounding the ovum and zona pellucida increase in number and become known as the granulosa. The granulosa separates from the ovum and its zona pellucida forming a cavity which is called the antrum (see Figure 16.4d); the granulosa secretes a fluid into the antrum. (Many anatomists consider a primary follicle as having been converted into a Graafian follicle only after the

antrum has been formed.) The connective tissue surrounding the follicle becomes organized into a membrane known as the theca interna. The theca interna and the granulosa work together to produce the hormones known as oestrogens. FSH and oestrogens are powerful stimulators of follicular growth. The oestrogens are hormones produced in other parts of the ovary as well as in the theca interna and granulosa. (They are discussed in more detail later in this Chapter.)

Each month during the monthly cycle, many primary follicles respond to FSH and oestrogens and grow, but only a fraction of these become Graafian follicles. Each month, only one Graafian follicle fully matures and, under stimulation by FSH, LH and the oestrogens, ruptures and releases an ovum from the ovary and gives rise to the possibility of conception. During the reproductive life of the woman, only 300–400 of the primary follicles will come to full maturity in the process of ovulation. The follicles which do not mature and release an ovum will degenerate and become atretic follicles. The atretic follicles are ultimately replaced by connective tissue.

A special fate awaits the mature Graafian follicle that has released an ovum. Within the ruptured follicle, a temporary endocrine gland called the corpus luteum is formed from the cells of the granulosa and theca interna (see Figure 16.4g). The corpus luteum produces both oestrogen and progesterone. The life of the corpus luteum is brief, about 2 weeks. The gland begins to be formed after the ovum is released and is replaced by connective tissue in 2 weeks. This connective tissue forms a scar on the surface of the ovary and is called the corpus albicans.

To review in summary form: FSH stimulates primary follicles to grow and become Graafian follicles and produce oestrogens. FSH, LH and oestrogens cause one mature follicle to release an ovum each month. After the ovum is released, the corpus luteum is formed within the ruptured follicle. The corpus luteum produces progesterone for 2 weeks before being replaced by connective tissue. Further details about this monthly cycle will be presented later in this Chapter.

At this point, it is necessary to shift the focus from the ovary to the pituitary gland, which is part of the brain. FSH and LH highlight the close relationship between the nervous system and the reproductive system. In fact, a failure to ovulate may be due either to a disturbance of the nervous system or to a defect in the ovary.

Both FSH and LH are synthesized, stored and released from the anterior part of the pituitary gland. (The pituitary gland is sometimes called the hypophysis.) The release of these two hormones occur at different rates over the course of the monthly cycle. The release of FSH and LH from the anterior pituitary gland is partly controlled by a hormone made from the hypothalamus of the brain (see Figure 16.3). This hormone is called gonadotropin-releasing hormone (Gn-RH). It was once thought that there were two releasing hormones made in the hypothalamus, one for FSH and another for LH, but now there is thought to be only one hormone involved, and this may explain why Gn-RH is sometimes called luteinizing hormone-releasing factor (LH-RF). Gn-RH stimulates the release of FSH and LH and has been found to be made up of a chain of 10 amino acids. Commercial synthesis of this hormone is now possible and has been successfully used in the treatment of certain types of infertility.

Gn-RH travels from the hypothalamus in a short network of capillaries that begins in the hypothalamus and ends in the anterior pituitary and is called the hypothalamic–pituitary portal system.

The next question is; "What causes Gn-RH to be released from the hypothalamus and thereby help to stimulate FSH and LH release from the anterior pituitary gland?" The answer is that no one knows for sure. Several factors, including information from other parts of the nervous system and the levels of oestrogen and progesterone, are involved; they may act at either or both the hypothalmus and the anterior pituitary gland. (The hypothalamus and anterior pituitary gland will be covered in detail in the Chapter on the nervous system.)

Hormones from the pituitary influence the release of hormones from the ovary, and hormones from the ovary influence the release of hormones from the hypothalamus and the pituitary gland. The pituitary gland communicates with the ovary by means of hormones (FSH and LH) and the ovary communicates with the hypothalamus and the pituitary gland by means of hormones (oestrogens and progesterone).

C. The breasts (mammary glands)

The breasts are considered accessory reproductive organs as they are not essential for reproduction. They are described as hemispherical eminences extending from the 6th to the 11th ribs, and from the side of the sternum to the middle of the axillae. They are small before puberty, become very large during and immediately after pregnancy and atrophy during old age. The male has breasts but normally they remain undeveloped. The entire breast is located between the superficial and deep layers of the subcutaneous tissue of the skin.

Breast tissue contains adipose tissue, glands and their ducts, blood vessels and lymphatics, nerves and connective tissue. Fibrous bands of connective tissue run throughout the breast and come together to form fibrous bands known as the suspensory (Cooper's) ligaments. These ligaments attach to the deep layer of the subcutaneous fascia of the skin and they support the breasts. A brassiere (bra) supports the breasts artificially and thus can reduce the strain on these ligaments, so that they will remain firmer in old age and will not sag; there is no physiological advantage or disadvantage from wearing or not wearing a bra.

The glandular tissue of the breast forms 15–20 lobules arranged in a circular fashion around the nipple (see Fig. 16.5). Each lobule has a duct, and the ducts from each lobule join together so that they all drain into the nipple. The area around the nipple is called the areola and contains small glands which lubricate and protect the nipple during nursing. Adipose tissue both separates and completely surrounds the glandular lobules. The bulk of the breast tissue in a non-pregnant women consists of adipose tissue.

The growth of breast tissue is subject to many hormonal controls. Like other tissues of the body it has a requirement for small amounts of TH, GH, insulin and cortisol. Increasing these hormones will not increase breast development, but their absence can hinder it. Five other hormones are uniquely important for full breast development and milk production:

(1) Oestrogens and progesterone are produced by the ovaries at the time of puberty and trigger the growth of breast tissue which takes place then.

(2) A hormone made by the placenta called placental lactogen, together with oestrogen and progesterone stimulates maximal development during pregnancy.

(3) Prolactin, a hormone made in the anterior pituitary, is released during pregnancy and after birth (parturition), stimulates the glandular tissue to produce milk; it also has other actions. The release of prolactin from the anterior pituitary gland is under the control of a hormone from the hypothalamus which travels through the hypothalamic–hypophysial portal system to the pituitary gland. The

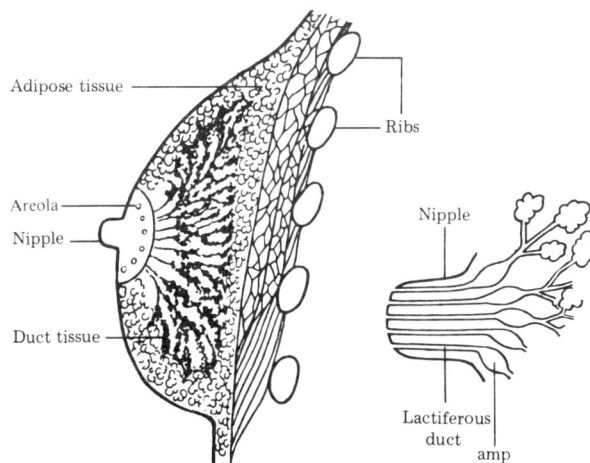

Figure 16.5 The female breast — longitudinal section.

hormone is called prolactin-inhibiting factor (PIF) and normally tends to inhibit the release of prolactin. Low levels of PIF tend to increase prolactin release.

(4) Oxytocin, a hormone released from the posterior pituitary gland, stimulates contractile cells around the gland to contract and force the milk into the ducts towards the nipple. The stimuli which act on oxytocin are complex but suckling and pressing upon the nipple seems to cause its release. This is a neuro-endocrine reflex. The infant's suckling and pressing upon the nipple stimulates receptors which send impulses to the hypothalamus of the brain and this causes the release of oxytocin from the posterior pituitary.

Oxytocin is also a powerful stimulator of uterine contraction and is thought to be involved in but not primarily responsible for the initiation of labour. Commercial preparations of the hormone are available and are used to facilitate uterine contractions during labour; they are also used after delivery to cause the uterus to contract, shrink in size and thus help reduce blood loss.

(5) Towards the end of pregnancy and for the first few days after parturition, the mother's breasts secrete a fluid known as colostrum; this milk-like fluid contains more protein and less fat than milk. Milk secretion begins about the third or fourth day after birth. In many of the developing countries, the introduction of artificial, powdered milk has sometimes led to an increase in the number of children suffering from kwashiorkor. Some mothers choose to feed their children with powdered milk in the foolish belief that it is superior to breast milk. Because of the great expense of the powdered milk, they often dilute it with too much water, so the solution contains lots of water but very little protein. A second factor is that the areola has certain glands whose excretion keep the breast remarkably safe and sterile, while improperly sterilized bottles used in artificial feeding may at times be a good source of infection which causes diarrhoea, gastro-enteritis and other ailments. Breast milk is always served at the proper temperature too, and with it the mother transmits antibodies to the infant which help to protect it. Artificial feedings are obviously necessary when the mother must work or cannot breast feed but the artificial milk fluid must contain adequate protein and be served in a sterile container. More recent work indicates that infants who have been breast fed are less likely to develop certain intestinal diseases and that breast-feeding facilitates "bonding", an important psychological step in the feeling of attachment between a mother and her child.

The breasts of infant girls often secrete a milk-like substance for the first day or two after birth. This is sometimes called "witches' milk", though there is nothing unnatural about it. The concentration of milk-producing and releasing hormones in the maternal blood is very high at birth. Some of these hormones pass through the placenta and stimulate the infant's breasts.

In the past, high doses of oestrogens, or a combination of oestrogen and testosterone (the male sex hormone), have been given to suppress milk production in those women who choose not to breast feed their infants. The wisdom of this treatment is currently being questioned.

No discussion of the breast would be complete without the mention of breast cancer, the most common cancer in women. In North America, 25% of cancers in women are

breast cancers; 1 in every 18 adult women will develop breast cancer sometime during her life. The statistics are essentially the same in European countries, but Japanese women have a low incidence of breast cancer. Breast cancer is not seen before puberty; from the age of 20 onward there is increasing incidence of breast cancer. A woman in her 60s has twice the chance of developing breast cancer than does a woman in her 30s. The cause of this cancer is not known.

If not treated, malignant cells from the tumour may enter the lymphatics and venous circulation and spread to the axillary lymph nodes, the vertebral bodies, the lungs, liver or brain. The most effective way to prevent the spread of cancer from the breast is to detect and remove the tumour before it has had a chance to spread. The sooner the tumour is detected, the better the chance for survival.

An examination of the breasts begins with observation of the breast while the patient is sitting. A tumour may cause dimpling or inflammation of the skin above it, or cause oedema or retraction of the nipple. The entire breast is carefully palpated with the tips of the fingers in a systematic manner. The axillary and supraclavular areas are palpated to detect any enlarged lymph nodes. The areolar area should be palpated and gently squeezed to see if any blood or abnormal secretions are discharged from the nipple. The patient then goes to a supine position and the entire breast is again carefully palpated twice — once with the patient's arm over her head and again with her arm by her side. (If the right breast is being examined, the patient should hold her right arm above her head — the left arm for the left breast.) Although the breast is a nodular structure, small masses may be detected; in fact, if a woman knows the proper methods of examination, she can usually more easily detect a small mass in her own breast than a physician can. It is recommended that a woman examine her breasts once a month and at the same time each month. Not all lumps and masses that are felt are malignant tumours. Cysts and non-malignant tumours can also be felt.

A biopsy of the suspicious mass is often needed to distinguish with certainty whether a malignant or non-malignant tumour is present. Men may also develop breast cancer, although it is about 1% as common in men as it is in women. Gynecomastia is the excessive development of the male mammary glands and may be caused by hormonal abnormalities.

WHAT ARE THE ACTIONS OF THE OESTROGENS AND PROGESTERONE?

A. The oestrogens

These hormones are a group of steroids with similar molecular structures. They are produced by the ovary, and, to a small extent, by the adrenal cortex. The most potent hormone is oestradiol-17β. It is produced by the ovary and is in equilibrium with oestrone. Oestrone is metabolized by the liver to oestriol.

The oestrogens have many important actions.

(1) The oestrogens are responsible for the development of the secondary female sex characteristics. Oestrogens do not cause "femaleness" but help the female structures develop properly. They stimulate breast development and have a

particular anabolic action on the female reproductive tract and cause it to grow and mature. They have some influence on the uniquely feminine hair and fat distribution.

(2) They have a very specific action on the endometrium of the uterus causing cells to grow and proliferate. The uterine glands increase in size and small uterine blood vessels also grow, pushing into the newly formed cell layers to nourish them.

(3) Oestrogens also stimulate the growth of the vaginal epithelium. This fact makes it possible to get a rough idea how much oestrogen is in circulation simply by staining vaginal epithelial cells.

(4) The oestrogens are produced by many cells in the ovary but particularly by the granulosa of the Graafian follicles and also by the corpus luteum. Oestrogens have local effects on the ovary itself, and they play an important role in stimulating follicular growth and ovulation. Oestrogens can reach their highest levels in the blood about a day before ovulation takes place. The peak level of oestrogen also precedes the peak levels of FSH and LH.

(5) Oestrogens have an effect on the nervous system. Oestrogens influence the release of Gn-RH from the hypothalamus, and this hormone stimulates the anterior pituitary gland to release FSH and LH. Oestrogens can also work at the anterior pituitary gland. Although one hormone, Gn-RH, influences the release of two hormones, FSH and LH, these two hormones are released at different rates from the anterior pituitary gland.

For a long time, it has been known that if the ovaries were taken out of an animal, and thus the source of most oestrogens was removed, the secretion of FSH and LH from the pituitary gland would be increased and maintained at high levels. If large amounts of oestrogens were then given to these animals, the secretion of FSH and LH would be reduced. From these and other experiments, it was concluded that there is a "negative feedback" relationship between FSH, LH and oestrogens; high levels of oestrogens inhibit the release of FSH and LH, whereas low levels of oestrogens stimulate their release. As a matter of fact, oestrogens may have a stimulating as well as inhibiting effect on FSH and LH release. This conclusion comes from more recent studies on women who have their pituitary gland and ovaries intact, as the majority of women do. These studies show that the highest levels of oestrogen come before ovulation when there is the greatest secretion of FSH and LH. It therefore appears that, at certain times, oestrogens may facilitate the release of FSH and LH from the pituitary. After ovulation, when the levels of oestrogens and progesterone are not at their highest levels but are still high, the release of FSH and LH from the pituitary is inhibited. Thus, oestrogens seem to have at different times in the menstrual cycle either a stimulating or an inhibiting influence on the pituitary gland.

B. Progesterone

Since the main source of progesterone is the corpus luteum, which is formed after ovulation, it cannot have the same role on sexual development as the oestrogens do.

(1) The hormone has a very specific action on the endometrium; it stimulates mucous secretions by the endometrial glands and glycogen storage by the cells. The immediate effects can be summarized by saying that it prepares the endometrium to receive and nourish the fertilized ovum. Progesterone is therefore necessary for the completion of pregnancy.

(2) Progesterone inhibits the contractility of uterine smooth muscle. You remember that the myometrium is smooth muscle and that smooth muscle can contract without neural stimulation. If during pregnancy the myometrium were to contract, the blastocyst (developing foetus) would not remain implanted and it would be expelled. If pregnancy occurs, progesterone concentrations usually remain very high till just before childbirth (parturition).

(3) Oestrogens and progesterone have an action on the nervous system and, in appropriate concentrations, can inhibit the release of FSH and LH from the pituitary gland.

For a long time, it has been known that pregnant animals do not ovulate. Pregnant animals produce oestrogens and progesterone throughout pregnancy, and appropriate concentrations of these hormones are thought to inhibit FSH and LH release by the anterior pituitary. These facts were used as the starting point in the search for an oral contraceptive. It was hoped that by finding the right chemical combination, it would be possible to "imitate pregnancy" and thus reduce the release of FSH and LH. If FSH and LH are not released, ovulation can't take place. Today, most of the oral contraceptive pills contain derivatives of oestrogens and progesterone. They prevent conception by preventing ovulation. This prevention is brought about by inhibiting the burst of FSH and LH secretion which precedes and triggers off ovulation.

Contraceptive pills have other effects, and their action is not limited to inhibiting FSH and LH release. In some women they lead to a "hypercoagulable" state of the blood, so that the likelihood of either thrombi or emboli being formed is increased. This risk is greater in women who have endocrine disorders or whose blood pressure is not within normal limits or who smoke cigarettes. In healthy women, the risk is not very great, and the risks are less than those incurred during pregnancy. This statement is not meant to discourage women either from having babies or from taking contraceptive pills, for the risks involved in either event are usually very small. Nothing in medicine — or life — is completely free of risk.

WHAT IS THE MENSTRUAL CYCLE AND HOW IS IT CONTROLLED?

Menstruation results when the ovum fails to be fertilized; it is the regular shedding of the superficial layer of the endometrium and its associated blood loss. This blood loss is often called the period.

The first menstruation is called the menarche and normally occurs sometime after the 9th year but before the 18th year, most frequently occurring during the 13th year. The cessation of menstruation, called the menopause, occurs between the 45th and 55th years but most commonly around the 50th year. Because of the reduced secretion of oestrogens, there is an atrophy of the reproductive organs that is associated with the menopause. It is important to note that the menopause is not necessarily associated with cessation of sexual activity. Sexual pleasure and problems often continue into and beyond middle-age for both men and women.

The amount of menstrual blood loss varies from 50 to 100 ml, the loss taking place during a period of approximately 5 days. The average length of the menstrual cycle, that is, the time between the beginning of one period and the beginning of the next, is 28 days. Emphasis here is placed on the word average. There is a fanciful story about a man who had one foot in a bucket of boiling water and the other frozen in a block of ice. When asked how his feet felt he replied: "On the average, quite well." The average temperature of his feet was a fairly comfortable 50 °C: (0 °C + 100 °C) ÷ 2 = 50 °C. This is simply pointed out to make the student wary of the word average. Many women do have cycles that last 28 days but there are healthy women with cycles ranging from 16 to 90 days; often there is a variation in the length of the cycle in the same woman. The individual's cycles are usually most variable near the beginning and near the end of reproductive life.

The menstrual cycle is not really so difficult to understand if you are familiar with the actions of FSH, LH, the oestrogens and progesterone. We shall call day number one of the menstrual cycle the 1st day that menstrual blood appears (see Figure 16.6).

a. Menstrual flow phase (the menses): approximately 5 days. Oestrogen and progesterone levels are low. The lining of the uterus, which is dependent on these hormones, is now being shed because the hormonal levels are too low to maintain it. The blood vessels which have pushed into the superficial layer are ruptured causing small haemorrhages

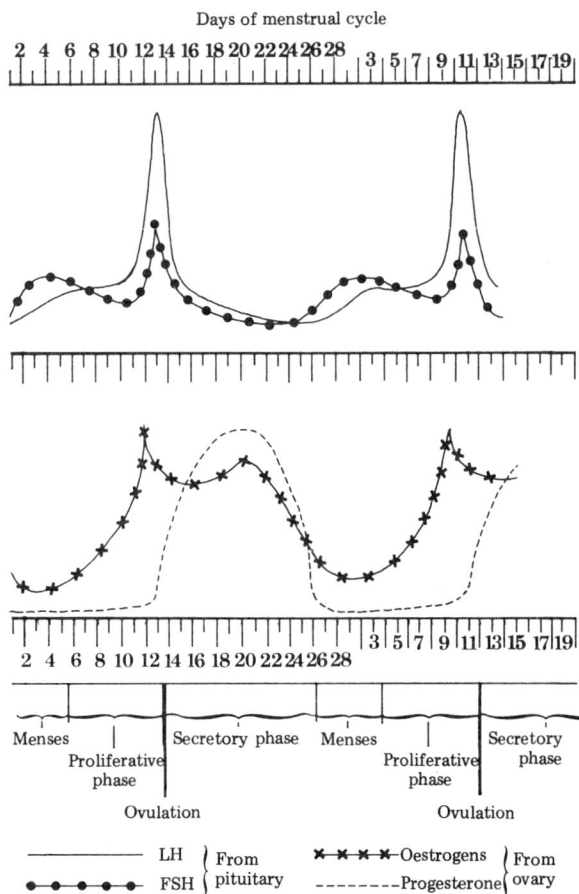

Figure 16.6 Hormone levels during the menstrual cycle.

and blood loss results. FSH levels are beginning to increase, and a group of primary follicles respond to this stimulation and begin to grow (see Figure 16.4b).

b. The endometrial proliferative phase: approximately 8 days. Some primary follicles become Graafian follicles, and oestrogen production increases. LH levels increase and oestrogen production increases even more. The oestrogens stimulate the cells, glands and blood vessels of the inner layer of the uterus to increase in size and number. At the end of the menstrual flow phase, the endometrial layer is about 1 mm thick, and at the end of the endometrial proliferative phase it is about 4 mm thick.

c. Ovulation: the 14th day. The oestrogens have prepared the Graafian follicles for the sudden burst of FSH and LH which will cause one follicle to release its ovum and begin its journey to and down the uterine tubes (see Figure 16.4f). Unfortunately, the reason why there is this dramatic increase in FSH and LH secretion at this particular time is not known. Of course, the effects of oestrogen and possibly progesterone on the hypothalamus are involved but the real reason for the burst of FSH and LH is not known. After ovulation, the corpus luteum is formed in the cavity remaining after the ovum's release.

d. The endometrial secretion phase: approximately 14 days. Graafian follicles are capable of secreting small amounts of progesterone in the corpus luteum. At one time, the corpus luteum was thought to be dependent on LH for its activity, but now this is not known with certainty. The corpus luteum has a life span of about 2 weeks before it is replaced with connective tissue. Oestrogen and progesterone combine to cause more growth in the endometrium, but the real change is a progesterone-induced change in the endometrium. This change stimulates glandular secretion and glycogen storage so that the endometrium is ready to receive and nourish the fertilised ovum. Progesterone production by the corpus luteum reaches its peak about 1 week after ovulation, then it declines.

The high levels of oestrogen and progesterone tend to reduce the secretion of FSH and LH, so the levels of FSH and LH start to fall. Oestrogen levels begin to decrease. In the latter phase of the endometrial secretion phase, progesterone levels fall as the corpus luteum deteriorates. Oestrogen levels fall as well. This reduction in oestrogen and progesterone levels causes a reduction in the thickness of the endometrium. This reduction in size compresses the blood vessels which have grown into the endometrium. Some parts of the endometrium become anoxic, the tissue dies and the small blood vessels supplying the endometrium go into spasm. Bleeding is incipient.

e. Menstrual flow phase: approximately 5 days. Two weeks after ovulation, oestrogen and progesterone levels are low, the shedding of the superficial endometrium and its associated blood loss begins. FSH starts to stimulate follicle growth. The cycle has begun again.

The main factor responsible for the shedding of the superficial endometrial layer is the decrease in progesterone levels. A pregnant woman does not menstruate because the corpus luteum continues to produce progesterone. Bleeding may be induced if a woman with a normal endometrium and normal oestrogen levels is given progesterone for several days. Soon after she stops taking the progesterone, the bleeding will begin, for without the progesterone the secretory endometrium can no longer be supported.

Bleeding in a woman who has reached menopause is a common problem. Inasmuch as the post-menopausal woman is no longer ovulating, the normal hormone mechanisms cannot account for the bleeding. This means an investigation is needed to determine the cause of the bleeding and be sure that a tumour is not responsible.

The description of the menstrual cycle given here is not complete. Some facts are not known, while others are not fully understood. The graph in Figure 16.6 is based on more recent work utilizing sophisticated techniques to measure the levels of circulating hormones. Even this graph is not completely accurate. The pituitary gland does not secrete its hormones at a constant rate but in bursts. The gland will secrete hormones, then stop awhile, then secrete again. This means that the level of the hormones in the blood will not be constant throughout the course of the day. The graph represents the average concentration of the hormones in the blood throughout the day.

WHEN CAN CONCEPTION TAKE PLACE?

The 100% honest answer to this question is that conception, the union of sperm and egg, can take place anytime there is sexual intercourse. Contraceptives properly used greatly reduce the chances of conception taking place and there are times during the menstrual cycle when conception is not very probable though not absolutely impossible. To answer this question further three things must be known:

(1) The length of time the sperm remains alive and capable of fertilization within the reproductive tract.

(2) The length of time the ovum remains capable of being fertilized.

(3) The time of ovulation.

Generally speaking, sperm remains viable about 24 hours, the ovum about 48 hours and ovulation takes place about 14 days after the first appearance of the menstrual blood. Again it should be emphasized that these are typical figures and not absolute ones, for life is variable and the ovary is not a clock-like structure which releases an ovum on the stroke of the 14th day. Even in a woman with a "regular cycle", ovulation may take place on the 12th, 13th, 15th or 16th day of the cycle. Assume that ovulation does take place on the 14th day. If sexual intercourse takes place on the 13th day, the day before ovulation, conception is possible because the sperm is capable of surviving till ovulation takes place. If intercourse takes place on the 15th or 16th day, conception is still possible, as the ovum which left the ovary on the 14th day can survive for 2 days. Thus a woman who ovulates on the 14th day may be fertile on the 13th, 14th, 15th and 16th days of the menstrual cycle. Since ovulation does not always take place on the 14th day, but can occur on the 11th, 12th, 13th, 15th, 16th and 17th day or frequently even other days, she may be fertile from the 10th through to the 19th day of the cycle. There is even evidence that menstruating women have become pregnant.

The division of the menstrual cycle into fertile and infertile (safe) periods forms the basis of the rhythm method of family planning, which is not highly reliable. The efficacy of the rhythm method can, however, be improved. The time of ovulation can often be approximated by accurately recording body temperature at the same time every day. Basal body temperature in the morning usually varies from 36.3 to 36.8 °C during the ovulatory phase of the cycle. The temperature increases by 0.3–0.5 °C at the time of ovulation, and continues at higher levels throughout the last half of the cycle, returning to the lower levels with the onset of the menses. This effect is believed to be caused by progesterone. Mucus from the cervix in the pre-ovulatory phase of the cycle forms a pattern resembling the leaves of a fern when it dries. Mucus in the post-ovulatory period does not form a ferning pattern but resembles raw egg-white. This postovulatory effect is also believed to be caused by progesterone.

Many animals including rabbits, giraffes and lions are reflex ovulators. This means that the sexual act reflexly triggers those hormonal changes which induce ovulation. Because ovulation closely follows intercourse, the likelihood of conception is increased. It has been suggested that there might be a reflex component in human reproduction, that under certain circumstances emotional intensity of the sexual act might trigger the release of hypothalamic releasing factors that lead to ovulation. This may help explain the high failure rate of the rhythm method and the high numbers of conceptions in young and relatively inexperienced women who do not use any contraceptives. On the other hand, severe emotional stress may inhibit the hormonal changes necessary for ovulation.

WHAT CHANGES TAKE PLACE DURING PREGNANCY?

Many changes take place as the mother must nourish, support and protect the life developing within her. When the fertilized egg implants itself in the endometrium, which has been made ready by the actions of oestrogen and progesterone, a specialized membrane called the placenta immediately begins to be formed. It functions to let gases, nutrients and certain substances dissolved in the mother's blood pass to the foetus and pass from the foetus to the mother.

The placenta also secretes hormones. Very soon after implantation it begins to secrete a hormone called human chorionic gonadotrophin (HCG). This hormone stimulates the corpus luteum to maintain production of oestrogen and progesterone so that the endometrium will not be shed; this explains why pregnant women do not menstruate. HCG can also be detected in the urine and its presence there serves as the basis for many of the pregnancy tests. Later on in pregnancy, the placenta itself produces oestrogen and progesterone till just before parturition. The placenta also secretes placental lactogen, a hormone which helps stimulate breast development. Relaxin is also synthesized by the placenta. This hormone weakens the ligaments of the pelvic joints and thus makes it easier for the infant to pass through the birth canal. It was discovered recently that the placenta secretes a hormone that stimulates the thyroid gland to secrete more thyroid hormone.

Two other hormones are important in pregnancy and parturition though they are produced by the pituitary gland instead of the placenta or ovaries. Oxytocin is released by the posterior pituitary gland and has a powerful action on uterine smooth muscle. It is released at parturition, stimulates uterine contractions and helps expel the infant into the outside world. In spite of much research, the precise reasons have not yet been determined as to why birth occurs when it does. Prolactin from the anterior pituitary is the final hormonal stimulus after the oestrogen and placental lactogen for converting the breasts into active milk-producing glands. Oxytocin stimulates the release of milk from the breasts; the stimulus for oxytocin release is the infant's suckling upon the nipple, so the release of milk is a neuro-endocrine reflex.

WHAT IS THE ANATOMY OF THE MALE REPRODUCTIVE SYSTEM?

The male reproductive system includes two gonads called the testes, which produce sperm, testosterone (the male sex hormone) and small but significant amounts of oestradiol and oestrone (the female hormones). In addition to the testes, the male reproductive tract includes a series of tubes that deliver sperm to the penis, which is an erectile organ. The tract also includes accessory glands whose secretions are necessary for sperm survival and transport (see Figure 16.7).

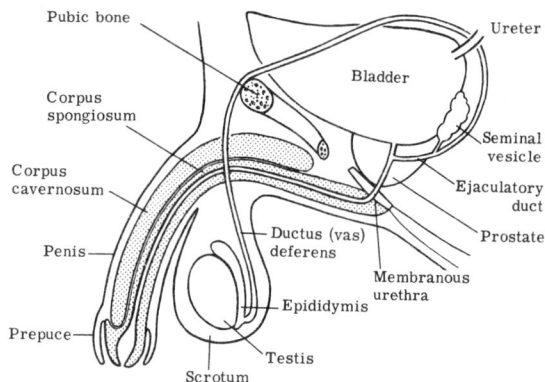

Figure 16.7   The male genital organs.

A. The testes, their coverings, and the vasa efferentia and epididymis

The two testes are contained in the scrotum, which is a pouch lying below the symphysis pubis, in front of the upper part of the thighs and behind the penis (see Figure 16.8). A layer of skin and the dartos tunic form the scrotum. The dartos tunic is tightly joined to the skin, and contains connective tissue and a thin layer of smooth muscle (the dartos muscle). This muscle contributes to the septum dividing the scrotum and separating the right testis from the left testis. Beneath the dartos muscle is a thin layer of connective tissue, the external spermatic fascia. This layer is continuous with the fascia covering the external oblique muscle of the abdomen. The cremasteric muscle and its fascia are found beneath the external supermatic fascia. This muscle arises as a continuation of the internal oblique muscle and its action is to draw the testes up toward the superficial inguinal ring.

Lying beneath the external spermatic fascia is the tunica vaginalis. This is a double-layered serous membrane containing a visceral layer and a parietal layer just as the peritoneum does. At one time during development, the tunica vaginalis was continuous with the peritoneum of the abdominal cavity. The peritoneum of the abdominal cavity sent a long, narrow, tube-like projection into the scrotum. The testes descended into the scrotum via the inguinal canal and became covered with the tunica vaginalis. Although the connection of the tunica vaginalis with the abdominal peritoneum becomes obliterated at birth or soon after, some peritoneum remains as a covering of the testis. This is the tunica vaginalis.

The next layer is the internal spermatic fascia (tunica albuginea). This is a dense fibrous membrane which projects into the testis forming septa. These septa divide the glandular structure of each testis into anything from 250 to 400 distinct lobules.

Finally, the innermost layer of the testis is the tunica vasculosa. This is formed by capillaries and small blood

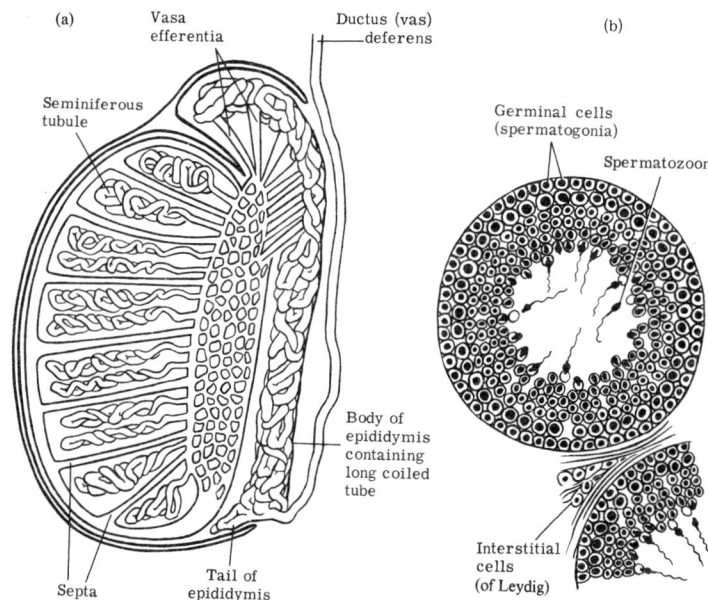

Figure 16.8   (a) The testis — vertical section. (b) Microscopic structure of seminiferous tubule.

vessels contained in a fine layer of connective tissue. The tunica vasculosa lines the tunica albuginea and accompanies it as it forms the septa which project into the testis. Each lobule of the testis is thus surrounded by a network of capillaries.

Each testis is an oval-shaped body; in the adult male it averages about 4–5 cm in length and 2.5–3.0 cm in width. The glandular structure of each testis is formed by numerous lobules that are contained within the septa. Each lobule contains from 1 to 3 tightly coiled twisted tubules, the seminiferous tubules. The testis feels like a solid structure because the many seminiferous tubules are so tightly packed within the lobules. If all seminiferous tubules in a single testis were completely unravelled, they would stretch for more than half a kilometre.

Attached to the basement membrane of the seminiferous tubule are the spermatogonia. These are the cells which ultimately give rise to the spermatozoa (sperm cells). The transition from spermatogonia to spermatozoa is complex and requires two intermediate cell stages: the spermatocyte and the spermatid. The significance of the cell changes and cell division that take place in this process are discussed in a subsequent Section. Within the seminiferous tubule the more mature spermatozoa are found closest to the lumen of the tubule, while the more immature cells are found closest to the basement membrane at the periphery of the tubule. In addition to the developing sperm cells, the seminiferous tubules contain supporting (Sertoli) cells. The spermatocytes are connected in some way to the Sertoli cells, and the spermatids remain attached to the Sertoli cells until they are released as spermatozoa. The Sertoli cells are thought to play an important role in sperm formation, and have been called "nurse cells" because of the help they give the developing sperm cells.

The connective tissue surrounding the seminiferous tubules contain clumps of cells, the interstitial (Leydig) cells. These cells are responsible for the production of testosterone and the small amounts of oestrogen which the testes produce. There are pores in the basement membrane that separate the cells of the seminiferous tubules from the interstitial cells. It is known that the Sertoli and Leydig cells co-operate together in the production of sperm. The formation and release of sperm into the lumen of the seminiferous tubule is a continuous one; it is estimated that it takes about 70 days for a spermatogonia to become a mature sperm. Different spermatozoa are maturing at different times in different parts of the tubules, but some are always being formed. The testes never release all their sperm at a single time. This is in striking contrast to the growth of the germinal cells in the ovary where a single critical event, ovulation, occurs approximately once a month.

The sperm leave the convoluted seminiferous tubules, pass through some short, relatively straight tubules and enter the efferent ducts (vasa efferentia). The vasa efferentia pass through the tunica albuginea and pass upward in a twisting fashion where they all empty into the epididymis, which is another set of coiled tubules.

Sperm complete their maturational processes within the epididymis and are stored at the distal part there for many days. If the spermatozoa are not ejaculated, they are thought to degenerate and be reabsorbed within the epididymis.

The crescent-shaped epididymis has a head, body and tail, all of which are draped upon the testis. The vasa efferentia empty into the head of the epididymis at the top of the testis, while the tail of the epididymis is located at the lower pole of the testis and empties into the vas deferens on the ductus deferens. The testes, vasa efferentia, epididymis and parts of the vasa deferentia are found within the scrotum.

B. The vasa deferentia, seminal vesicles, ejaculatory duct and prostate gland

The ductus deferens is continuous with the epididymis and can be considered to be the excretory duct of the testis (see Figure 16.9). It is lined with columnar epithelium, which is surrounded by a coat of smooth muscle and covered with

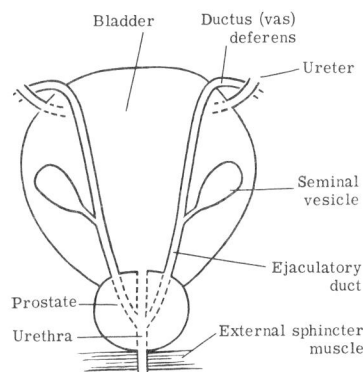

Figure 16.9 The ductus deferens, seminal vesicle and ejaculatory duct in relation to the posterior surface of the bladder.

fibrous tissue. The vasa deferentia become less twisted as they ascend upward along the border of the epididymis. Each ductus deferens continues as part of the spermatic cord that passes upward from the testis to leave the scrotum. The ductus deferens enters and then passes through the inguinal canal. At the internal inguinal ring, the ductus deferens separates itself from the spermatic cord. Each ductus then travels in the pelvis behind the urinary bladder and over the ureter towards the prostate gland (see Figure 16.7). A vasectomy is a surgical procedure in which each ductus deferens is cut and/or tied shut. It is usually an irreversible form of sterilization.

Before entering the prostate gland, each ductus deferens is joined by a duct from the seminal vesicle (see Figure 16.9). There are two seminal vesicles, each being about 7.5 cm long and pyramid in shape. The seminal vesicles do not store sperm but produce a secretion containing fructose and a thick proteinaceous material which serves many functions. This secretion travels in a duct to join the ductus deferens. The duct of the ductus deferens and the duct of the seminal vesicle unite to form a single duct, the ejaculatory duct, which then enters the prostate gland.

The prostate gland is about the size of a large chestnut and lies in the pelvic cavity behind the symphysis pubis, in front of the rectum (see Figure 16.7). This gland has an outer tough, fibrous capsule and an inner glandular substance composed of follicles. The secretions of the prostate gland include prostaglandins and the enzyme, acid phosphatase.

The two ejaculatory ducts join the single urethra whose

origin was in the urinary bladder. The male urethra thus transports sperm, secretions from the prostate, seminal vesicles and other glands as well as urine. This is in contrast to the female urethra, which carries only urine.

In elderly men, the prostate gland can hypertrophy, sometimes malignantly, so that the urethra is compressed. This interferes with the passage of urine out of the bladder and may cause difficulty in starting and stopping the urinary stream, difficulty in increased frequency and urgency, and nocturia. The male urethra enters the penis.

It was previously stated that the testes were formed in the abdominal cavity and descend through the pelvic cavity and inguinal canal into the scrotum. About 1 out of 25 full-term male infants have undescended testes at birth. Cryptorichidism is the name applied to the failure of one testis or both testes to descend into the scrotum. With bilateral cryptorichidism, spermatogenesis cannot take place because the higher temperature within the abdomen hinders spermatogenesis and the individual becomes infertile.

C. The penis

This organ is composed of special spongy erectile tissue which is arranged in three columns. There are two corpora cavernosa and a single corpus spongiosum through which the urethra passes (see Figure 16.10). The corpus spongiosum forms the enlarged ending of the penis called the glans penis and in its centre is the opening of the urethra (see Figure 16.7). The glans penis is covered with a fold of skin known as the foreskin (prepuce) (see Figure 16.7). Circumcision is the

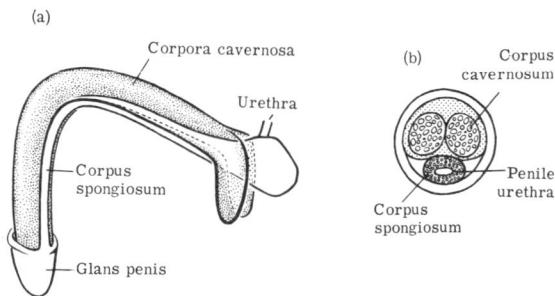

Figure 16.10 The penis. (a) Structure. (b) Transverse section.

surgical removal of the prepuce. Sometimes the prepuce covers the penis so tightly that micturition is interfered with; this condition is called phimosis and circumcision is necessary.

The two corpora cavernosa contain many small balloon-like cavities which are connected to the venous system. During sexual excitement the penile arterioles dilate and fill each corpus cavernosus with blood so that they expand; this expansion compresses some of the blood vessels which take blood away from the penis. Since more blood enters the penis than can leave it the penis fills with blood, becomes firm and erect.

WHAT ARE THE ACTIONS OF THE MALE SEX HORMONES AND WHAT CONTROLS SPERMATOGENESIS

The male sex hormones are collectively called androgens. These hormones, like the oestrogens and progesterone, have a steroid structure. Biologically, androgens are defined as hormones which stimulate the growth of the prostate gland and seminal vesicles.

The most important androgen is testosterone, and this hormone has many actions in addition to stimulating the growth of the prostate gland and seminal vesicles. Testosterone can also be metabolized within target tissues and it is the testosterone metabolite which is often the more potent influence within the cell. Testosterone is produced by the Leydig (interstitial) cells within the testes and, to a smaller extent, by the cortex of the adrenal gland.

A. Actions of testosterone and other androgens

(a) Testosterone is responsible for the male hair pattern. The increased beard growth which begins as boys approach or enter the teen years is correlated with increased levels of testosterone in the blood.

(b) Metabolically, testosterone stimulates many anabolic or biochemical building reactions; it promotes nitrogen retention and protein synthesis, and is responsible for the increased muscle mass found in the male.

(c) Androgens are also an important contributing factor to the skeletal growth-spurt that takes place at puberty. In males, puberty occurs at 9–16 years of age.

(d) Another change which takes place at puberty is the thickening of the male vocal cords that results in a deeper voice.

(e) The increase in testosterone secretion at puberty also stimulates the growth and maturation of the external genitalia and accessory sex organs such as the prostate gland.

(f) The androgens are also necessary for initiation and maintenance of sperm production in the testes.

(g) In addition, testosterone is thought to increase libido, a name applied to the sexual urge.

Other actions of testosterone on the nervous system are discussed in the next Section.

B. Control of male reproductive hormone secretion

Males, like females, have Gn-RH, FSH and LH. Gn-RH is made in the hypothalamus, and, after travelling through the hypothalamic–pituitary portal system, stimulates the release of FSH and LH from the anterior pituitary gland. The molecular structures of Gn-RH, FSH and LH are identical in males and females, but in males LH may be called interstitial cell-stimulating hormone because it acts upon the interstitial (Leydig) cells to synthesise and release testosterone. High levels of testosterone can inhibit the release of LH from the anterior pituitary gland. A simple negative feedback relationship between LH from the pituitary and testosterone from the Leydig cells does not seem to prevail in the day-to-day secretion of these hormones. LH is secreted in sporadic outbursts throughout the day. Within a few hours after the peak of secretion of LH, testosterone levels are at their peak, showing the rapid response of the Leydig cells to stimulation by LH.

Psycho-social factors are also able to influence testosterone secretion, and consequently, beard growth. In one experiment, a male subject noted an increase in beard growth in his anticipation of female company and a decline in beard growth during a period of isolation and sexual abstinence.

For most of their development, the maturing sperm cells are in close contact with the Sertoli cells, which nurse them in their growth and development to mature sperm. The Sertoli cells respond to FSH by providing the proper metabolic environment for spermatogenesis to begin and be maintained. Testosterone from the Leydig cells nearby is also necessary. The factors controlling FSH release are poorly understood. Although both FSH and LH can be released by Gn-RH, they are often not simultaneously released. There are several conditions in which FSH levels may be high and LH levels may be low or normal, or *vice versa*.

HOW DO SPERM FERTILIZE THE OVUM?

During sexual excitement, the labia majora, the labia minora and the clitoris become engorged with blood and enlarged. Glands within the vestibule secrete a mucous lubricating solution into the lower end of the vagina. After a period of time and appropriate stimulation the opening of the vagina becomes enlarged. Muscle tension increases in both man and woman. The enlarged penis is thrust into the vagina and the lumen of the vagina is reduced so that the vagina grips the penis. Movement of the penis in the vagina increases the pleasurable sensations of both partners because there is a greater stimulation of the sensory receptors in the tip of the penis, the vagina and the clitoris. If sexual excitement is sufficiently intense, the male's urinary bladder sphincter contracts, preventing urine from entering the urethra, the seminal vesicles, prostate and other glands increase their secretions, and the smooth muscles in the epididymis and vasa deferentia contract. This brings 2–5 ml of fluid (the ejaculate) into the urethra and from the urethra into the vagina. This process is termed ejaculation. Impulses from the autonomic nervous system are responsible for stimulating much of the smooth muscle contraction and glandular secretion. After ejaculation, the penis begins to return to its normal size. The ejaculate contains many millions of sperms and glandular secretions which nourish them and protect them against acidity in the vagina.

Associated with these intense muscular contractions and subsequent relaxation after ejaculation is an intense feeling of pleasure and psychological release. These phenomena are grouped together under the word orgasm. Although women do not ejaculate, they may also experience orgasm or orgasms during sexual activity — muscular contraction, pleasure, release and relaxation.

Sperm enter the uterine tubes from the vagina within 15 minutes after ejaculation, indicating that factors other than the sperm's motility are involved, though they are not understood. Although the number of sperm released in a typical ejaculation is greater than the population of the United States (200 million), relatively few ever reach the ovum and only one ever fertilizes it.

After the first sperm makes contact with the ovum and penetrates it, changes take place so that a second sperm cannot enter. The nucleus of the sperm and the nucleus of the ovum unite to form a single cell called the zygote, which develops by mitosis into the complete individual.

Fertilization usually takes place in the midpoint of the uterine tube and the developing embryo then travels down the tube to the uterus where it is implanted. Implantation of the embryo outside of the uterine cavity is referred to as an ectopic pregnancy. This can have very serious consequences such as maternal haemorrhage because other structures lack the strength to support the rapidly growing embryo.

Sexual performance and satisfaction are heavily influenced by psychological factors. Impotence is a condition in which the male is unable to achieve and maintain a firm and erect penis, so intercourse is impossible. This may be caused by disease or advancing age, but most commonly it is caused by psychological factors such as anxiety. One physician succinctly summarized the importance of psychological influences by saying that the brain is the most important sexual organ.

WHAT CAUSES INFERTILITY?

Infertility is the inability to produce children when they are desired and may result from either a male or female disorder. The male may suffer from some metabolic disease in which he is unable to produce sufficient normal sperm. A female's ovaries may fail to produce ova, or be unable to release them. Pituitary disorders may cause infertility in both sexes since the gonads are dependent on FSH and LH. Occasionally, the female may be "allergic" to certain sperm, perhaps even making antibodies against them, although this and other causes of infertility are not understood.

Infertility may be caused by venereal disease. Gonococcal bacteria may attack, infect and inflame the oviducts so that they become scarred and blocked. Infection can even spread to the ovaries, rendering them dysfunctional. This does not, however, happen in most cases of gonorrhoea.

WHAT ARE THE VENEREAL DISEASES?

The venereal diseases are somewhat inappropriately named after Venus, the Greek goddess of love. They are acquired during sexual activity with an infected person or are passed from an infected mother through the placenta to the foetus. There are many venereal diseases but the two most common are syphilis and gonorrhoea.

The first sign of syphilis may occur from 9 to 90 days after sexual contact with an infected individual when a chancre (painless hard sore) develops at the site where the bacteria, *Trepenema pallidum*, gained entry to the body. In men this is usually found in the glans penis and in women in the labia; many infected men and women do not develop a chancre though. In a few cases, this marks the end of the disease as the body's defences take over, but in most cases secondary syphilis develops.

The symptoms occur on an average from 10 to 12 weeks after sexual contact and include a mild skin rash and inflammation of the mucous membranes of the mouth and sexual organs, and the lymph nodes are swollen. Even if they are untreated, these symptoms may disappear and remain hidden or latent for a few months, or even from 2 to 10 years and occasionally even longer.

In late syphilis, small nodules (gumma) may be formed throughout the body including skin, liver, bone and nervous system. In addition, large blood vessels may be weakened and the smaller vessels inflamed and fibrosed. If not treated soon enough, neural tissue in the brain and spinal cord will be permanently destroyed, causing a variety of severe disorders, both physical and behavioural. Neurosyphilis occurs in about 10% of all untreated syphilitics.

If the disease is transmitted from the mother to the foetus, the disease is called congenital syphilis. Since the pregnant woman may show few outward signs of syphilis, many countries require that all pregnant women be tested for syphilis. If undetected, the chance of miscarriage is increased, the infant may die soon after birth or its development may be abnormal and it may have many deformities and mental deficiency, a truly sad situation.

It should be pointed out that syphilis does not require sexual intercourse to be transmitted. All that is required is for the causative bacteria to come into contact with a membrane and penetrate it. Thus kissing or homosexual acts might transmit the disease if one of the individuals is infected. The disease cannot be acquired from toilet seats and the like, for the bacteria do not survive outside the body.

Men who have acquired gonorrhoea often notice a white discharge from the urethra and have pain or difficulty urinating a few days after sexual contact with an infected individual. If the infection continues, the resulting inflammation may cause the urethra to be completely blocked so that it is necessary for it to be cleaned out with a catheter. Women may also detect gonorrhoea by a white irritating discharge from the vagina though most women do not have any outward symptoms of the disease and are thus often not aware that they are infected. If untreated, the uterine tubes may be blocked and scarred, and the ovaries affected. Gonorrhoea is a major cause of infertility in women.

An infected mother may pass the disease on to her child as the infant travels through the vagina. The infant's eyes are particularly susceptible to attack and blindness will result if untreated. Many countries require that all infants' eyes be treated with a silver nitrate solution or an antibiotic to prevent this. It is now rare for gonorrhoea to be found in infants who are born in hospitals, but it is much more common in children born outside them.

One of the ironies of the 1970s is surely that, in spite of increased knowledge of venereal diseases, a better spread of preventive knowledge and easier access to relatively cheap and effective treatment, the incidences of venereal disease have sky-rocketed. In one industrialized society, they are second only to the common cold as the most common infectious disease. Contracting a venereal disease is one matter, but contracting one and not having it treated immediately out of fear, embarrassment or shame is both foolish and dangerous.

WHY ARE SOME BORN BOYS AND SOME BORN GIRLS?

To answer this question we have to revise our knowledge of the human chromosomes. With one important exception, all human cells have 46 chromosomes arranged in 23 pairs. One pair of chromosomes is called the sex chromosomes; the larger of the two sex chromosomes is called the X chromosome and the smaller is called the Y chromosome. Genetic males have an X and a Y chromosome, while genetic females have two X chromosomes. Sperm and ova do not have 46 chromosomes but have 23 chromosomes and, thus, only one of each pair.

By a complex process called meiosis the cells which give rise to sperm and ova divide without chromosomal duplication; this reduces the number of chromosomes in each sperm and ova by one half so they each will have 23 chromosomes instead of 46 (see Figure 3.4). The paired sex chromosomes will also divide so that each sperm will have either an X or a Y chromosome, while each ovum will have a single X. The female parent cell has two X chromosomes which will enter two ova, each ovum having a single X chromosome. The male parent cell has both an X and a Y chromosome; when they divide, one sperm will have an X chromosome and the other a Y. Meiosis results in sperm which have either an X or a Y chromosome and ensures that a zygote will have 23, not 46 pairs of chromosomes.

If a sperm with an X chromosome fertilizes an ovum with another X, the zygote will have two Xs and will develop into a female. If a sperm with a Y chromosome fertilizes the X ovum the zygote will have an XY chromosomal pair, testes will develop and a male will result (see Figure 16.11). It is believed that the Y chromosomes contain the genes for enzymes which lead to the synthesis of testosterone.

Somatic cells contain the sex chromosomes, just as the reproductive cells carry the sex chromosomes and the other 22 pairs of chromosomes. This means that it is possible, with certain techniques, to determine or visualize the chromosomes within certain cells. Using these techniques, one can see if genetic sex is expressed appropriately in the chromosomes. A simple test for genetic sex requires scraping a few cells from the buccal mucous membrane and staining them. Cells from normal females have a "Barr body" in the nucleus. The Barr body is named after its discoverer and is thought to represent a condensation of all or a good part of the second X chromosome. Normal males would not have a Barr body, inasmuch as they only have one X chromosome.

There are certain types of syndrome associated with aberrations of the sex chromosomes. Persons with Turner's syndrome are females who lack true ovaries and certain secondary sex characteristics. These individuals have only one X chromosome and their sex chromosomal pattern is often referred to as XO. A Barr body is usually lacking in persons with Turner's syndrome. Males with Klinefelter's syndrome have an XXY chromosomal pattern and generally have a Barr body. These persons appear to be males though their testes are small, and sperm and testosterone production are grossly deficient, and they may have breast development; often Klinefelter's syndrome is not identified in boys till after they have reached puberty. There are other chromosomal abnormalities, although they occur less frequently.

Some newspapers and magazines have printed sensational accounts of sex-change operations. These operations usually involve plastic surgery and, in the male, castration. Since the basis of an individual's sex is genetic, surgeons cannot change a person's genetic sex any more than they can turn an eagle

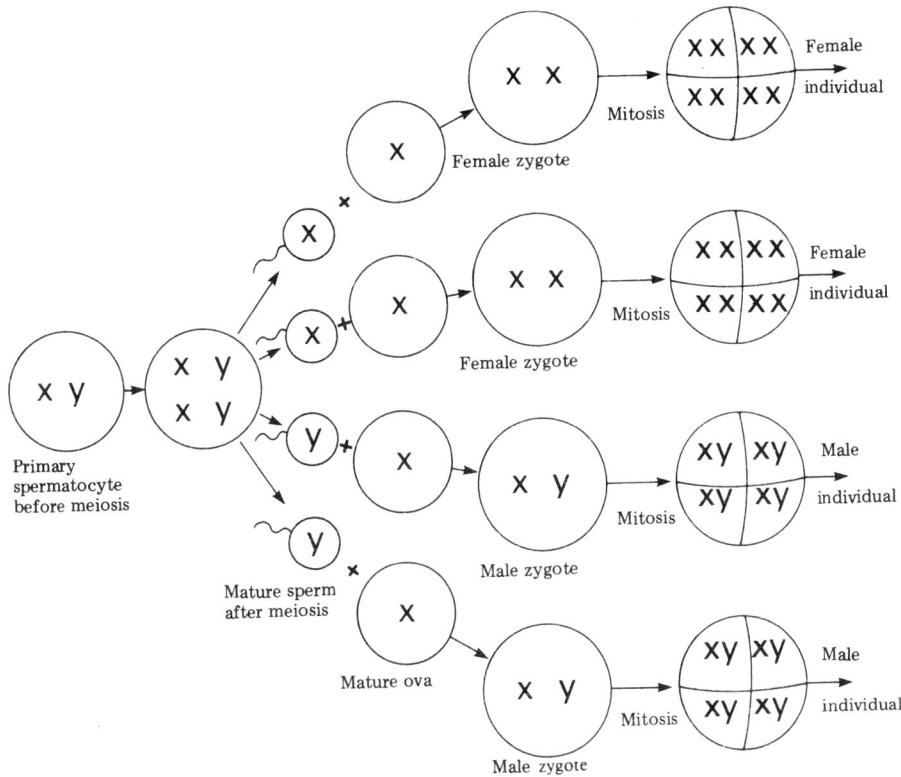

Figure 16.11   The development of the male and female zygotes.

into a fly. Surgery and appropriate hormones can, however, give the "appearance" of a different sex. These procedures may be useful for those individuals with genetic disorders and ambiguous sexual development, or those individuals who are strongly orientated towards a uniquely masculine or feminine way of life that is not compatible with their genetic male or female sex.

WHAT CAUSES TWINS?

Twins can be caused in two ways. Occasionally two ova are released from the ovary and both are fertilized. These are called fraternal twins. If a single ovum is released and a single zygote is formed but the dividing cells become split, each cell or cell group will form an individual. The resulting twins (or triplets) are called identical because they are alike in all physical aspects since they have the same genetic heritage, parent cell and identical chromosomes. About 1 out of every 3 pairs of twins is identical. Why this happens is still unknown. In West Africa, about 1 in 50 births results in twins, while in the United Kingdom about 1 birth in 95 results in twins. The increase in the number of multiple births in recent years is attributed to the use of the new fertility drugs.

CONCLUDING THOUGHTS

We often think that growth and development relates only to the development of the 3.5 kilo newborn into the 70 kilo adult. Actually, the most rapid rate of growth and development takes place in the first 2 months after conception. This is a particularly critical time, because this is when the organ systems are formed and when congenital malformations are most likely to occur. Unfortunately, many women don't know they are pregnant during these early critical weeks. The best way to ensure a healthy infant is to see to it that the woman is healthy before, during and after her pregnancy. Maternal nutrition is particularly important, with special emphasis placed on adequate dietary protein during the pregnancy and while breast feeding.

17. The Nervous System

INTRODUCTION

Past Chapters have indicated the function of the nervous system in relation to circulation, digestion, reproduction and the endocrine glands. The nervous system regulates these systems and is also influenced by these systems. For example, although the nervous system is important in regulating cardiac output and peripheral resistance, its ability to do so and to function in many other ways is dependent on the brain being perfused with adequate amounts of oxygenated blood by the cardiovascular system.

The nervous system sends instructions to muscles and glands and, in addition, is also the receiver, processor and storer of the information. The nervous system is likewise the centre of behaviour which includes conscious and unconscious thought processes. It is itself a paradox, seeming both incredibly simple and overwhelmingly complex.

The typical adult brain weighs about 1350 grams and more than 75% of this weight is water. The basic functional unit of the brain is the neurone, and the brain derives most of its energy from the metabolism of glucose to carbon dioxide and water. This simplicity gives way to complexity with the fact that the brain contains many more than a million million neurones.

The axons of some groups of neurones come together to form tracts (pathways) which channel information from one group of neurones to another, or to glands and muscles. Some of these pathways are large and fairly well defined and have great physiological significance.

Most students are interested in the relationship between the brain and behaviour. Behaviour encompasses all the things we think or do, consciously or otherwise, and it includes breathing, defaecating, dreaming, dancing, imagining, violent acts and acts of generosity and kindness among many others. In asking why we behave the way we do, you are asking how much the twig bends itself and how much the twig is bent by forces outside itself. That is asking how much behaviour is shaped by the anatomy, physiology and chemistry of the nervous system and how much it is shaped by the psychological, sociological and historical forces, and by conscious choice. The honest answer is that no one really knows. The reason for this is that research in this area is extremely difficult, and valid conclusions are hard to come by. Although you can compress someone's carotid arteries and cause the person to lose consciousness, you cannot conclude that the carotid arteries are the centre of consciousness; they supply a good portion of the brain with blood. You can study the actions of a single neurone but each neurone is surrounded by, and dependent upon, hundreds of other cells. A neurone can also be influenced by its synaptic connections with other neurones, which in turn are influenced by their surrounding cells and synaptic connection. Everything is connected to everything else.

There are also social, psychological and historical "synapses" or points of contact with one's human environment which influence our behaviour. Research into how psychological, familial or tribal and social values and forces influence behaviour is likewise complicated by the vast number of forces and their interconnections. One cannot breed humans to provide genetic identity, keep them all in cages to ensure a constant environment and then present them with a single experimental variable to see its effect. The needed experimental technique would destroy the validity of the experiment.

Although the ultimate reasons for many complex behaviours are not known, behaviour cannot be ignored. It may be important to note any difficulty that a patient has in getting up out of a chair, any abnormality in the patient's walk or an inability to perform "simple" acts like smiling, tying shoes or standing on one leg. Speech in all its aspects is likewise important — the ability to pronounce words as well as using them coherently and appropriately. Sometimes you may listen and be able to distinguish between a casual remark and the subtle cry for help. Ultimately, all your observations and judgements require some understanding of the anatomy and physiology of the nervous system.

This Chapter is admittedly, a difficult one. Much of what is not clear at first will be more clear when you have finished the Chapter and also the Chapters on the special senses. The pieces do all fit together and eventually make sense.

Finally, it is good to recall the statement of a prominent physician who said that he had never looked between the sheets and seen only a brain and spinal cord and not a person. It is impossible to isolate the nervous system from the other systems or from the human personality. All patients, but particularly those suffering from neural disorders, either physical or behavioural, need care, sensitivity, understanding and respect. Not all effective treatments come from the surgeon's knife, the psychiatrist's couch, or the pharmacist's pills.

WHAT IS THE BASIC UNIT OF THE NERVOUS SYSTEM?

The basic unit of the nervous system is the neurone. This is true despite the fact that most cells in the nervous system are not neurones but glial cells, which are cells that support nourish and influence the neurones. The glial cells are routinely classified as either astrocytes or oligodendrocytes. The shape of the astrocytes is variable but many of them have so many branches (processes) that they resemble bushy shrubs. Processes of the astrocytes extend from brain capillary to brain capillary or from brain capillary to neurone. Unlike neurones, the glial cells can undergo mitosis and can proliferate, even in an adult. This response is often noted after injury to the brain. As their name suggests, oligodendrocytes have few processes. These cells are often found lying in rows between the myelinated sheaths of axons and are thought to play a role in the formation and maintenance of myelin. Scattered within the brain and spinal cord are cells known as microglia. These are not derived from neural tissue but are thought to be derived from blood cells and to act as macrophages.

Neurones make functional contact with other neurones, muscles and glands at the synapse. A synapse is an anatomically specialized junction between two neurones (see Figure 3.13). The word synapse comes from a Greek word meaning to clasp. When people clasp or shake hands they come in contact with each other, but each hand remains separate and distinct. There is no continuity between the two hands. The same is true for neurones. The cell body and the dendrites of a single neurone have more than 10 000 synapses. The axon of a neurone may end in many branches with terminal buttons or specialized nerve endings. The terminal buttons may synapse with other neurones, muscle or glands. A chemical transmitter is released by the terminal buttons, diffuses across the synaptic space and affects the cell or cells on the other side of the synapse.

The reason why neurones are the basic functional unit of the nervous system is that neurones, and not glial cells, generate and transmit impulses. If you choose to move your toe, an impulse is generated in a brain cell and is transmitted down the neurone's axon to the end of the spinal cord where the terminal buttons of the first neurone synapse with the dendrites and cell body of the second neurone. The chemical transmitter released by the end button of the first neurone diffuses across the synapse to the second neurone, where it leads to the generation of a second impulse, which travels down the axon of the second neurone from the end of the spinal cord to the toe. The terminal buttons of the second neurone release acetylcholine, which diffuses across the myoneural junction to the skeletal muscle of the toe, which is stimulated to contract.

It appears that there are a number of chemical transmitters in the brain and spinal cord. In addition to acetylcholine and noradrenaline, the brain uses serotonin, histamine and dopamine as transmitters. There are also other transmitters which do not excite neurones; certain transmitters may inhibit the neurone and make it less excitable. The distribution and synthesis of these transmitters is extremely important. If you can pharmacologically alter synaptic transmission within the brain, you can change behaviour. It is believed that many of the tranquillizers and hallucinogenic drugs work by affecting synaptic transmission within the brain, though the mechanism and location of these actions are not well understood.

Before continuing it is necessary to introduce the concept of the resting membrane potential and the nerve impulse.

WHAT IS THE RESTING MEMBRANE POTENTIAL?

This is not intended to be a comprehensive discussion of a complex electro-physiological area but only to introduce some terms and touch upon a few concepts.

If you were to take a spoonful of salt and put it on one side of a plate and then put an equal amount of pepper on the opposite side of the plate, and then gently shake the plate, in time the salt and the pepper would be mixed and equally distributed over the surface of the plate. To separate the salt and the pepper and return them to their original position would require work, and work requires energy. In the Chapter on metabolism and nutrition, energy was expressed in calories. Energy may also be expressed in volts or millivolts: a millivolt (mV) is 1/1000th of a volt. But specifically what are volts? In physics, a volt is defined as a unit of measurement which is the force necessary to cause current (1 ampere of current) to flow against a resistance (1 ohm of resistance). The specifics of the definition might not be clear now but if you go on you will be able to make sense of it. You remember from the first Chapter that oppositely charged ions or particles attract one another, and like-charged ions or particles repel one another. To separate oppositely charged ions, e.g. K^+ and Cl^-, requires energy or work. Conversely, work can be done if oppositely charged ions come together, inasmuch as a force will be exerted over a distance. Volts or millivolts (mV) are units which express the *potential* of a separated electric charge (positive or negative ions, protons or electrons) to do work. Since voltage requires a separation of charge, voltage must be measured between two points.

With this as background, three facts can now be considered:

(1) Sodium, potassium and chloride ions can all cross back and forth across the nerve cell membrane.

(2) Although the ions can cross the membrane, they are not equally distributed on either side of the membrane. An approximation of the ionic difference is provided by the table below:

Ion	Intracellular concentration (mEq/l)	Extracellular concentration (mEq/l)
Na+	10	145
Cl-	5	120
K+	150	5

We have a separation of charges, e.g. the potassium ion is 50 times as concentrated inside the cell as outside the cell.

(3) It is not surprising therefore that a potential can be measured across the membrane between the inside of the cell and the outside of the cell. The potential that is measured across a typical nerve cell is about 70 mV. (By convention this is referred to as −70 mV since the inside of the cell is considered to be negative relative to the outside of the cell.) It might help to think of this potential as a measure of the amount of work necessary to maintain this separation of charges. The greater the magnitude of the membrane potential, the greater the separation of charge.

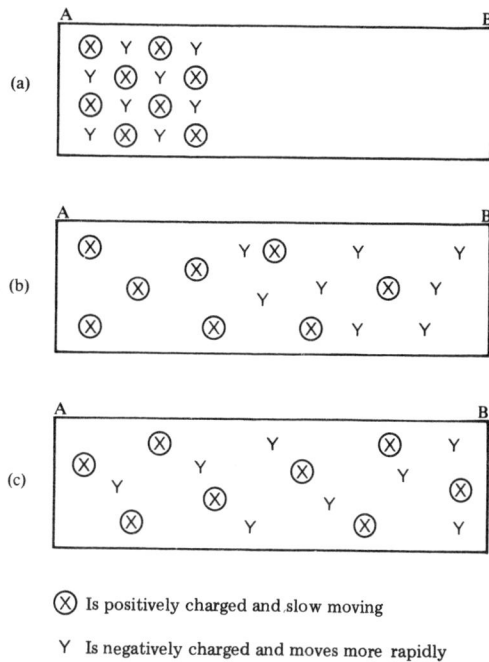

⊗ Is positively charged and slow moving

Y Is negatively charged and moves more rapidly

Figure 17.1 Differential potential. (a) At the start, there is no potential between A and B. (b) After a period of time, a small potential between A and B will develop because of the more rapid diffusion of the negatively charged ion. (c) Ultimately, the potential between A and B will disappear because the ions will equally distribute themselves, and there will be no separation of charge.

But how did this membrane or resting potential of -70 mV develop? Some insight into its development can be acquired by looking at diffusion potentials. Imagine that positively charged X ions and negatively charged Y ions are placed in one end of a tube filled with gelatin. Also assume that the negatively charged Y ions can diffuse through the gelatin at a much faster rate than the positively charged X ions (see Figure 17.1a). After a brief period of time, the rapidly moving Y ions will be more widely dispersed than the slower moving X ions (see Figure 17.1b). This will lead to a temporary separation of charge, and a small voltage will develop. The voltage will disappear in time as the ions distribute themselves equally throughout the gelatin (see Figure 17.1c).

In nerve cells, the resting potential is chiefly a potassium diffusion potential. Potassium's concentration is much greater inside the cell than outside. For sodium, the situation is the opposite, as its concentration is greatest outside the cell and it tends to diffuse into the cell. The resting potential is considered to be a potassium rather than a sodium potential because potassium can diffuse out of the cell much faster than sodium can diffuse in. This movement of positively charged potassium ions down their concentration gradient from inside the cell to the outside of the cell is chiefly responsible for the resting potential.

The accumulation of positively charged potassium ions outside the cell creates a positive charge. This positive charge tends to reduce the further diffusion of potassium outside the cell. This is because the like positive charges tend to repel one another. At equilibrium there will be a balance between equal opposing forces. The forces favouring diffusion will be opposed by the forces generated by the repellent effect

of like charges. At equilibrium the chemical force promoting the outward diffusion of K^+ down its diffusion gradient equals the electric forces of the positively charged potassium ions. This relative external positivity inhibits more K^+ from moving to the outside of the cell. In the resting nerve cell the membrane potential approaches but does not equal the K^+ equilibrium potential. When the cell is at rest, small amounts of Na^+ diffuse into the cell, and small amounts of K^+ diffuse out. This brings up the question of how the potassium diffusion potential is maintained over a period of time. The answer is that the ionic gradients are maintained by the Na^+–K^+ exchange pump (see Fig. 17.2). When a sodium ion diffuses into the cell, it is pumped back out into the extracellular fluid. This pumping out of a sodium ion is coupled to the pumping in of a potassium ion from the extracellular fluid into the nerve cell. Since one positive ion is exchanged for another, the sodium–potassium exchange pump is electrically neutral. The Na^+–K^+ exchange pump is located in the cell membrane and is thought to be a lipid–protein enzyme complex which requires ATP to do its work. Should the pump be poisoned, sodium would gradually leak into the cell, potassium would leak out of the cell and the membrane potential would disappear. The cell would not be excitable then.

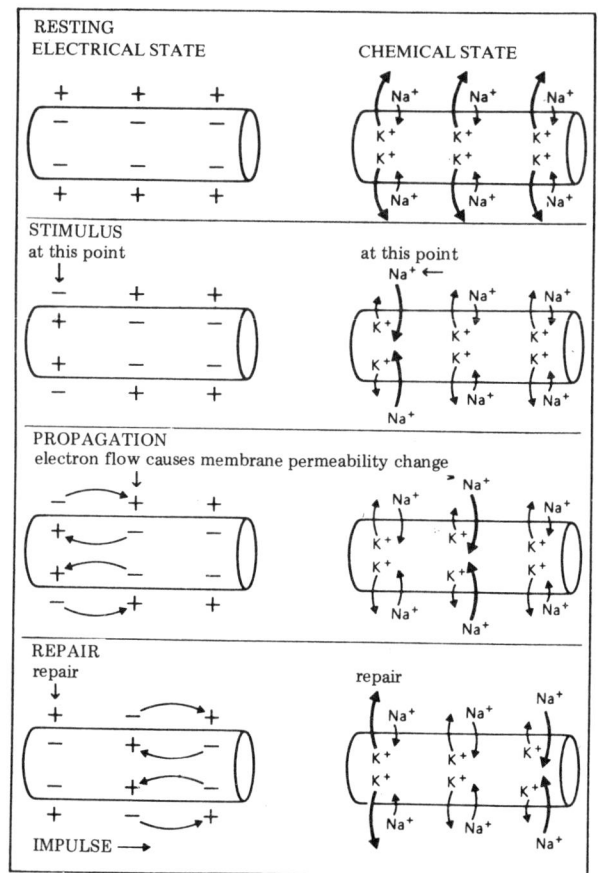

Figure 17.2 Electrical and ion changes in nerve conduction. The resting membrane potential depends on the Na^+–K^+ pump. The sodium ions that have diffused into the cell are pumped out; for every sodium ion pumped out, a potassium ion is pumped into the cell.

No mention has been made of the chloride ion. This ion is not thought to play an active role in the generation of the membrane potential but distributes itself passively as a result of its diffusion gradient and the potassium diffusion potential.

The above explanation is definitely an over-simplification. The resting membrane potential that is measured when electrodes are stuck into nerve cells approaches but does not equal the calculated potassium diffusion potential. The sodium–potassium exchange pump and other factors are involved. The resting potential of a nerve cell can be altered by chemical transmitters released at the synapse. If the transmitters are inhibitory in their action, the neurone will become less excitable and the membrane potential will be increased. The cell is then said to be hyperpolarized.

Chemical transmitters which increase the excitability of the cell tend to reduce the membrane potential by affecting the membrane's permeability to the surrounding ions. If the resting potential is reduced, the nerve cell tends to become depolarized. If the cell is sufficiently depolarized to a critical level, its threshold will be reached and an action potential (a neural impulse) will be generated.

WHAT IS A NEURAL IMPULSE?

Originally, the neural impulse was thought to be similar to the flow of electricity down wires. Generators derive energy from waterfalls, coal or petrol engines or even the atom itself to separate charge so that negatively charged electrons can flow down wires and do their work. An understanding of electricity is helpful in understanding the nervous system but it should be understood that impulses travelling in the nervous system and electricity are not identical. The biggest distinction between the impulse and electricity is that electricity results from the flow of electrons, whereas the neural impulse results from the flow of ions. An impulse may be defined as a brief, travelling, self-propagated, bio-electrical signal. The neural impulse is sometimes called an action potential; the terms are used synonymously. The definition of the neural impulse (action potential) requires some explanation.

The action potential can travel down an axon at speeds up to, or greater than, 100 m/s. This is faster than a train can travel but slower than a jet plane. An action potential can travel from the brain to the toe in less than 1/50th of a second. Impulse conduction is much faster in those nerves with myelin sheaths than those without these sheaths. There are gaps in the myelin sheaths surrounding the axons which are called nodes of Ranvier. Myelin is an effective insulator, so current cannot flow through it. The impulse is conducted from node to node and effectively jumps over the myelinated areas thus speeding the rate of conduction. Impulses are also conducted faster in larger neurones than in smaller ones. In certain diseases the myelin sheath is destroyed or it is not formed properly. Measuring the speed of impulse conduction may help in diagnosing these diseases.

The action potential does not last long; measurements have shown that the impulse lasts for less than 2/1000ths of a second. Because the impulse is so brief, the same neurone can send hundreds of impulses per second. The number of impulses that a neurone can conduct is limited by the absolute refractory period, e.g. if the impulse lasts for 1.5 ms, the nerve will not be able to conduct another impulse for at least 1 ms or so after the start of the impulse regardless of how strongly the neurone is stimulated. An important consequence of the absolute refractory period is that neural impulses in a single axon cannot summate (add up). Increasing the rate of stimulation can cause more neural impulses to be generated and to travel down the fibre but it cannot cause *bigger* neural impulses.

Describing the action potential as self-propagated is an indication that the energy for the transmission of the impulse comes from the nerve fibre over which it travels and not from the stimulus. An analogy is frequently drawn between the impulse and a spark travelling along a trail of gunpowder. Once the gunpowder has been ignited, the spark will travel down the gunpowder and will not need to be continuously reignited. The response of the gunpowder to ignition would be the same, no matter if it were ignited with one match, ten matches or a blow-torch. This analogy applies to the nervous system in that once the critical level of stimulation has been reached, the action potential will be the same even if the intensity of stimulation increases.

A stimulus that is too weak to cause a nerve impulse to be generated is called a sub-threshold stimulus. A stimulus which just causes a nerve impulse to be generated is a threshold stimulus, while one that is of greater intensity than a threshold stimulus is a supramaximal stimulus. There will be no difference in the action potential caused by a threshold stimulus and a supramaximal stimulus; this is to be expected from the all-or-nothing law.

One reason why this is often a confusing area is that much of the work involving action potentials has been done using single axons. Nerves, however, contain many different axons from different neurones. The record obtained by stimulating a nerve is complex and changes with the strength of the stimulus. This is because the different cells have different thresholds and different rates of conduction. A weak stimulus might stimulate only the large, fast-conducting fibres. A stronger stimulus would then stimulate all fibres.

Previous paragraphs have described some of the characteristics of the nerve impulse but have not described the impulse itself. Before doing so, it is necessary to revise certain facts concerning the resting state of the neurone. You will recall that the concentration of sodium ions outside the cell is many times that found inside the cell, while many more potassium ions are within the cell than are outside the cell. Sodium ions that cross the membrane and diffuse into the cell are quickly pumped out. For every sodium ion that is pumped out of the cell, a potassium ion is pumped into the cell. This pumping process requires energy and helps maintain a steady state in which concentration gradients are maintained. Thus, even though both sodium and potassium can penetrate the membrane, they do not achieve equal concentrations on both sides of the membrane. This steady state is interrupted by the action potential in which there is, first, an ever-increasing permeability to sodium ions, so that sodium ions can follow their concentration gradients and diffuse into the cell. This sudden movement of positively charged ions into the cell generates a small bio-electric current that can only be detected by very sensitive electrodes.

The next event is the outward movement of potassium ions from inside the cell. Since this creates a current flow which is opposite to the sodium-caused current, it will tend to reverse the direction of the action potential and return the potential towards the resting potential of -70 mV. As the potential approaches its resting value, the sodium–potassium exchange pump is reactivated. The excess sodium is pumped out of the cell and potassium is pumped back into the cell, and eventually the original resting conditions are restored.

The action potential is able to propagate itself. When the sodium ions rush in, they effectively reverse the polarity (charge separation) of the membrane. That is, the inside of the cell becomes positive relative to the outside of the membrane. This difference in potential between the depolarized membrane and that part of the membrane that has not been depolarized causes current to flow between the polarized and depolarized areas of the nerve. This current depolarizes both the area immediately adjacent to the area of membrane where sodium inflow is maximal and the adjacent membrane, so the action potential is conducted over the adjacent area of nerve fibre. The neural impulse cannot travel backwards over the area it has just crossed because the nerve fibre there is in an absolute refractory state.

WHAT INITIATES THE NEURAL IMPULSE?

The neural impulse (action potential) may be generated in two ways, either at the synapse or at a receptor nerve ending.

A. Synapses

It was previously stated that the cell body and the dendrites of a single neurone may have thousands of synapses. The neurone which contains the terminal buttons which release the chemical transmitter is referred to as the pre-synaptic neurone, whereas the neurone which receives the chemical transmitter is referred to as the post-synaptic neurone. An action potential travels down the axon of the pre-synaptic neurone to its end feet, where it causes the release of chemical transmitter. This chemical transmitter diffuses across the small synaptic space to the post-synaptic neurone, where it affects the membrane permeability of the post-synaptic neurone. Transmission of the action potential down the axon is bio-electric. Transmission across the synapse is chemical.

It is known that there is more than one chemical transmitter and that the effects of the different transmitters on the post-synaptic membrane may be either facilitory or inhibitory. When facilitory transmitter is released, the post-synaptic neurone becomes excited and is more likely to generate an impulse. If sufficient facilitory transmitter is released to excite the post-synaptic neurone to or above its threshold, an action potential will be initiated at the beginning of the axon and will proceed to travel down the axon. The release of additional transmitter may cause the initiation of more action potentials at the axon but will not affect the nature of the individual impulse. Not all transmitter is facilitory, however. The terminal buttons of some neurones release a transmitter which has an inhibitory effect on the post-synaptic neurone. The release of inhibitory transmitter makes it less likely for the post-synaptic neurone to initiate an action potential. Inasmuch as a neurone has thousands of synapses, it can receive thousands of inputs or signals from other neurones.

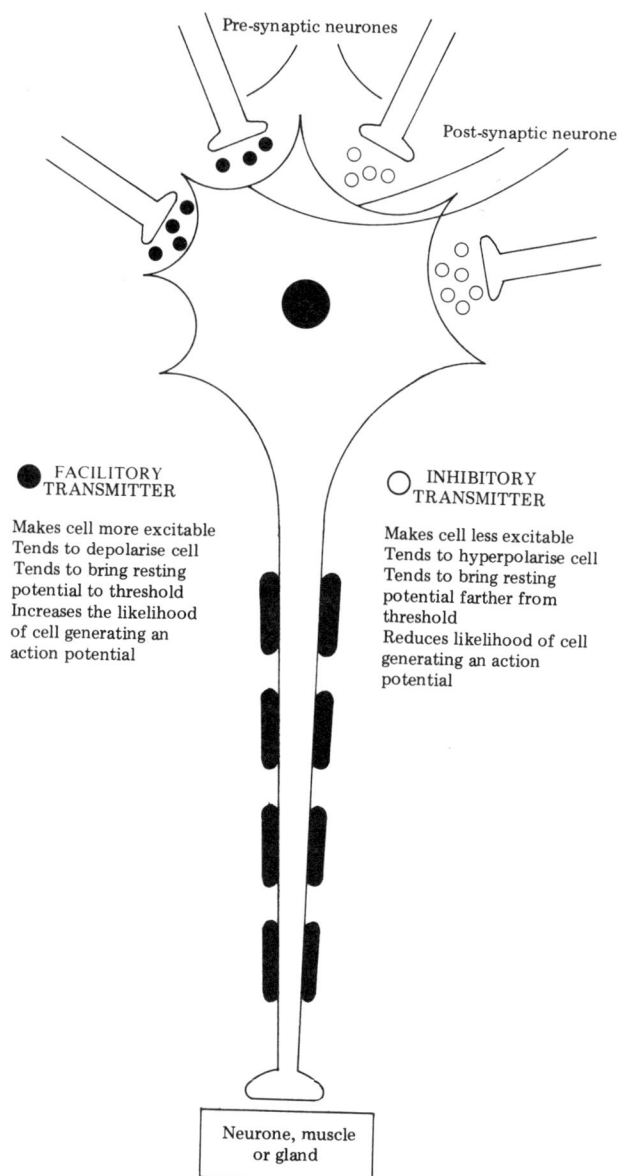

FACILITORY TRANSMITTER

Makes cell more excitable
Tends to depolarise cell
Tends to bring resting potential to threshold
Increases the likelihood of cell generating an action potential

INHIBITORY TRANSMITTER

Makes cell less excitable
Tends to hyperpolarise cell
Tends to bring resting potential farther from threshold
Reduces likelihood of cell generating an action potential

Figure 17.3 Facilitory and inhibitory transmission.

Some pre-synaptic neurones release facilitory transmitter while other pre-synaptic neurones release inhibitory transmitter (see Figure 17.3). The post-synaptic neurone thus receives stimuli in the form of facilitory and inhibitory chemical transmitter. The neurone has but one "decision" to make — it can either generate an action potential or not generate an action potential. The neurone's "decision" is based on the relative balance between facilitory and inhibitory influences. If enough facilitory transmitter is released to overcome the effect of the inhibitory transmitter and sufficiently excite the post-synaptic neurone, an action potential will be generated. The impulse will travel down the axon of the post-synaptic neurone to its end feet and cause the release of transmitter. The excitation or inhibition of a neurone can be looked at from another perspective. If electrodes are stuck within a neurone, the changes in the neurone's resting potential can be measured. These changes occur following release of transmitter from the nerve endings which synapse with the neurone.

The change in membrane potential is a function of the type of transmitter released by nerve endings.

If the transmitter is excitatory (facilitory), changes in the membrane permeability occur; ions flow across the membrane. Sodium ions diffuse into the cell. This movement of ions generates small currents which tend to depolarize the cell and reduce the membrane potential. If the membrane potential is reduced below a critical level, for example, from −70 to −55 mV, an action potential will be generated and conducted down the neurone's axon. The greater the amount of excitatory transmitter that is released, the greater the chance will be that the neurone's threshold will be reached and an action potential will be generated.

If the neurones release inhibitory transmitter, different changes take place in the membrane's permeability and potassium diffuses out of the cell. The ionic currents flowing across the membrane after the release of inhibitory transmitter are in a direction opposite to those following the release of excitatory transmitter. The resting potential increases in magnitude, that is, from −70 to −90 mV. The neurone then becomes less excitable, partly because its resting potential is removed even farther from the threshold level where an action potential is generated. This means that more excitatory transmitter will have to be released to generate an action potential when the resting potential is −80 mV than when it is −60 mV.

Although a neurone has but one decision to make, this decision is reached on the basis of information from many sources, that is, every synapse which releases transmitter which comes into contact with the neurone's membrane influences the neurone's decision by either increasing or decreasing the neurone's potential. The neurone is able to integrate this information and effectively add up all these excitatory and inhibitory currents, so an action potential will be generated only when the threshold is exceeded.

The neurone integrates information both spatially and temporally. Spatial summation refers to the fact that the synaptic end buttons of different nerve fibres synapse all over the cell body of a single neurone; the neurone is able to sum up the transmitter released by these end buttons, and possibly generate an action potential. Release of facilitory transmitter from a single end button or a few end buttons is not sufficient to stimulate the neurone. If many nerve endings simultaneously release facilitory transmitter, the neurone will integrate these excitatory influences. When the neurone is sufficiently stimulated, an action potential will be generated. If nerve endings release excitatory transmitter over a period of time, the transmitter will accumulate and its effects on membrane will be prolonged. The release of more transmitter will further depolarize the membrane, and in time an action potential will be generated. The ability of a neurone to integrate the effects of transmitter over a period of time is referred to as temporal summation. Thus, while a neurone may not respond to transmitter from a few neurones, it may respond if the same few neurones continuously release excitatory transmitter.

Because transmission at the synapse is chemical, an elaborate pharmacology of synapses and synaptic transmitters has evolved. Many pharmacological agents work by blocking the action of the transmitter on the post-synaptic membrane, facilitating or inhibiting the synthesis, releasing or destroying of the transmitter, or by imitating the action of the transmitter on the post-synaptic membrane.

It is worth stating again that synapses also impose an order upon the nervous system. This order results from the fact that transmission at the synapse is always only one way, from end feet to dendrites and cell body and never the reverse. Therefore, the pathway that the action potentials follow will be dependent upon the arrangement of the synapses. This means that the flow of information in the nervous system is directed by the anatomical arrangement of neurones and synapses.

B. Receptors

When a stimulus comes into contact with a receptor, the energy of that stimulus exerts an effect upon the receptor. If the stimulus is of sufficient strength, the receptor ending will respond by generating an action potential (see Figure 17.4). Receptors are specialized neurones and, therefore, the stimulus must be equal to or greater than the receptor's threshold for an action potential to be generated. The action potential generated by the receptor ending will travel to the brain or spinal cord. The end feet of the receptor will release chemical transmitter at its synapse in the brain or spinal cord.

The cell bodies of most receptors are located in a ganglion (see Figure 17.4). A ganglion is a collection of nerve cell bodies located outside of the brain or spinal cord. Ganglia

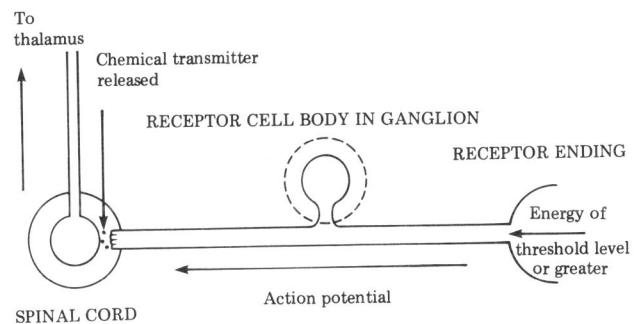

Figure 17.4 Diagram of the generation of action potential at receptor ending.

may contain receptor cell bodies or the cell bodies of neurones which relay signals to other neurones, glands or smooth muscle. For a sensation to be fully appreciated, the information from the receptor must reach a specific area in the brain.

The processing of sensory information illustrates two important points. The first refers to stimulus differentiation, that is, how do we tell something hot from something cold, or light from pressure. Part of the answer lies in the nature of the receptors themselves. Each receptor is especially sensitive to a particular form of energy. Shine the light of a torch into your ear and you will hear nothing, for the ear is sensitive to sound energy, not light. It might be helpful to think of receptors as transducers (energy translators), in that they translate specific forms of energy into action potentials. Thus the receptors translate energy from light, sound, touch, pressure and so forth into action potentials. The receptor's ability to translate is limited, in that each receptor is particularly sensitive to a specific form of energy. Even when it is possible to stimulate receptors pharmacologically, or by some other form of energy to which the receptor is not particularly sensitive, the receptor will generate action potentials which the brain will interpret as the energy form to which the receptor is most sensitive. Pressure upon the eye, for example, may stimulate the visual receptors in the eye, and the individual sees spots.

The action potentials generated by the receptor ending must reach a specific area in the brain where other neurones interpret the impulses as a specific sensation. How this perception takes place is not yet understood and is all the more remarkable, for there is no difference in the action potentials transmitting different types of sensory information to the brain. An individual can distinguish not only between different kinds of stimuli, but also between the intensities of a single stimulus. For example, if you hold a sliced onion at arm's length, then gradually bring it closer to your nose, the smell becomes stronger. The nature of the stimulus does not change, but its intensity increases. Bringing the onion closer does not necessarily stimulate additional or different receptors in the olfactory epithelium of the nose; the same receptors are stimulated but much more intensely, so more action potentials are generated and sent to the olfactory area of the brain. Thus, as the intensity of the stimulus increases, the frequency of impulses generated by the receptors increases. The brain interprets this increased frequency as a more intense sensation.

Often, if a receptor has been continuously stimulated, the receptor will adapt and send fewer signals. Perhaps you have walked into a room and noted an odour which seemed to have disappeared after a few minutes; this is an example of receptor adaptation. Generally, after a receptor has been stimulated for an interval of time, it generates fewer impulses and the stimulus appears to fade away or disappear; this phenomenon is called adaptation. Not all receptors adapt however, but some continuously report on certain conditions within the body. Those receptors which monitor blood glucose, temperature and body position, and also the baroreceptors, are examples of receptors that do not adapt. Pain receptors likewise do not adapt.

WHAT IS PAIN?

Pain is one of the most essential yet least understood physiological processes. It may be defined as a sensation of discomfort or agony resulting from the stimulation of certain nerve endings. It is pain that leads many people to seek medical attention. The significance of pain as a form of information is illustrated by the rare cases of children who are born without pain receptors. These unfortunate children will not feel pain and will not remove their hands away from fire even though the flesh is burning.

Pain receptors are widely distributed through the skin, are slow to adapt and will respond to many different forms of energy. The common denominator for these stimuli is that they are painful or injurious. If the stimulation of the pain receptors is at threshold level or above, action potentials will be generated and will travel down the pain fibre along the first sensory neurone, which synapses in the spinal cord. The second sensory neurone crosses to the opposite side of the

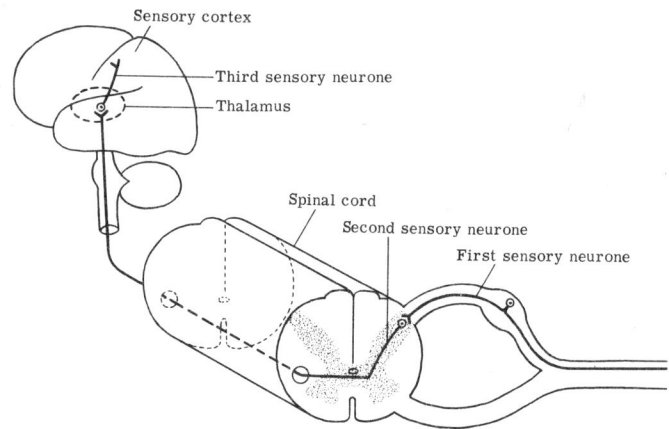

Figure 17.5 General arrangement of the sensory pathway in the central nervous system.

spinal cord and ascends to a part of the brain known as the thalamus, where it synapses. The group of fibres which transmits pain information are accompanied by fibres that carry temperature information. They ascend in the spinal cord to the thalamus on the lateral spinothalamic tract. A third sensory neurone in the thalamus relays the impulses to the cortex of the brain (see Figure 17.5). Both the thalamus and the cortex of the brain are important for the full perception of pain. In the hope that neurological anatomy will be more meaningful, this description of pain and its pathway is hereby presented before the anatomical description of the nervous system.

There are pain receptors within the viscera though they are less numerous than those in the skin, so that pain from the viscera is poorly localized or even incorrectly localized. Two examples illustrate this.

(1) If the coronary arteries are blocked and the heart is not getting sufficient oxygen, pain may be felt in the chest wall, the axilla or down the inside of the left arm.

(2) If the pleura covering the diaphragm is infected, the pain may be felt in the neck and the shoulder.

In both cases the pain is called referred pain because it is perceived as coming from a surface area of the body and not from the actual source. Referred pain is real pain and not just a figment of the patient's imagination.

Part of the explanation of referred pain rests upon the fact that the pain originating in a deep structure is referred to a surface structure which shared a common embryonic origin. Thus pain originating in the diaphragm may be referred to the neck because in its embryonic development the diaphragm was formed in the neck region and later migrated to its location in the abdomen. When the diaphragm moved from the neck to the abdomen it took its nerve supply with it. The suggestion has been made that both the deep and superficial pain fibres synapse on the same neurones within the spinal cord. These neurones relay the pain information to the thalamus and it is relayed to the cortex. Because pain from the skin is more common than pain originating in deep structures, the patient has "learned" to interpret these impulses as superficial pain rather than deep pain.

Pain originating in abdominal structures is common but is often difficult to localize and diagnose. It may be caused by the stretching of any of the hollow structures, or it may follow from obstruction or inflammation of them. Besides knowing the nature, location and severity of the pain, you must know when the pain comes, when the pain goes, what relieves the pain and what makes the pain worse. As an example, the pain caused by an ulcer may be relieved by eating. Conversely, the pain caused by a gallstone blocking the bile duct may be intensified by eating because the hormonal response to food in the duodenum induces contraction of the musculature in the obstructed duct.

Pain may be projected to structures which have been removed or severed from the body. For example, if a patient has had an arm amputated he may feel and behave as though the arm is still present. This is known as the phantom limb phenomenon. These phantom sensations are real to the patient and do not indicate any personality disorder on the patient's part, for most patients with amputations have these sensations at least once after surgery. There are many reports of patients with leg amputations who fall after rising from bed and attempting to walk as though the leg were still present. Some patients experience a strong sensation of pain, which they localize to the limb that has been amputated. There is no satisfactory explanation for this phenomenon of the phantom limb although it indicates that the pain is more than the report of pain receptors.

Learning and other psychological factors can influence an individual's perception of, and reaction to, pain.

WHAT IS THE ANATOMY OF THE NERVOUS SYSTEM?

Neuro-anatomy is a most complicated subject and is often taught as a separate course in many medical schools. It is neither necessary nor desirable to go into that much detail here.

The nervous system is a single unity, the branches of which extend through the body. For your learning purposes, it might be best to consider the nervous system to have three divisions: the central nervous system, the peripheral nervous system and the autonomic nervous system.

THE CENTRAL NERVOUS SYSTEM

This division consists of the brain and spinal cord. Both structures are covered by three membranes, which are collectively called the meninges and include the dura mater, the arachnoid membrane and the pia mater (see Figure 17.20). Again, for clarity, we can consider the brain to have three divisions, the forebrain, the midbrain and the hindbrain.

A. The forebrain

The major part of the forebrain is made up of two cerebral hemispheres, together forming the cerebrum, the single largest part of the brain which also covers the midbrain and part of the hindbrain. The outer part of the cerebral hemisphere is called the cerebral cortex. The cerebral cortex is a very convoluted (folded) structure; this arrangement increases the surface area of the cortex and permits more neurones to fit within the cortex. The outer layers of the cortex are often referred to as grey matter because of their dense concentration of nerve cells. In contrast, white matter contains no neurones but is composed of masses of myelinated axons; the fatty myelin has a white appearance.

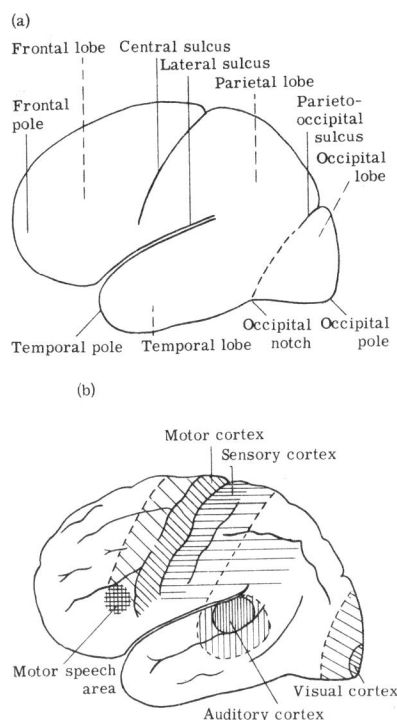

Figure 17.6 The cerebral hemisphere. (a) Subdivisions. (b) Functional areas of the lateral surface (wide-hatching indicates associative areas).

Although the right and left cerebral hemispheres are separated from one another by a tough fold of dura mater, they are connected below this fold by a band of fibres called the corpus callosum. Fibres from the right cerebral cortex pass downwards and across in the corpus callosum, then pass upwards to the left cortex. Fibres from the left pass in the same manner to the right. Each cerebral hemisphere has a frontal, parietal, temporal and occipital lobe which roughly corresponds to its position within the skull bones (see Figure 17.6a). There are three major landmarks in each hemisphere of particular importance:

(1) The central sulcus (groove), which separates and passes downward between the frontal and parietal lobes.

(2) The lateral sulcus, which separates the frontal and parietal lobes from the temporal lobe.

(3) The parieto-occipital sulcus, which separates the parietal and occipital lobes.

The convoluted surface of the brain appears grossly the same; the appearance hides the fact that different areas have very different functions. The cerebral cortex has been "mapped out" with certain areas assigned to particular functions. Unlike a map, however, the boundaries are often blurred; areas overlap and some areas' functions are still unknown, still unexplored.

The area posterior to the central sulcus in the parietal lobe is called the sensory cortex (see Figure 17.6b). The neurones here receive fibres from neurones in the sensory pathways, which carry touch and some proprioceptive information. The more sensitive an area is, the larger the sensory area in the cortex will be. For example, the face has a larger representation than the back; although the face is smaller than the back, the face has many more sensory endings.

Sensory information from the right half of the body travels via the spinal cord and thalamus to the sensory cortex of the parietal lobe of the left cerebral hemisphere where it is interpreted. The left half of the body is represented in the sensory cortex of the right cerebral cortex and *vice versa*.

Visual information from the eyes is relayed to the visual area in the occipital cortex. Below the lateral sulcus near the posterior end of the temporal lobe is the auditory cortex where most sound information is finally relayed (see Figure 17.6b).

The cortex is not just a receiver of sensory information. Some impulses which stimulate skeletal muscle to contract originate in an area of the frontal lobe anterior to the central sulcus. This area is called the motor cortex (see Figure 17.6b) and the neurones located there are called upper motor neurones. Most neurones leave the right motor cortex via the internal capsule and send their axons down on the right side of the brain stem, then they cross over to the left side before entering and descending in the spinal cord till they synapse with a motor neurone (see Figure 17.7). Some, however, descend on the same side of the spinal cord. The axons of the lower motor neurones leave the spinal cord and synapse with skeletal muscles. This pathway from the motor cortex to the motor neurone in the spinal cord is called the pyramidal tract. The representation of a body part in the motor cortex is proportional to the precision and complexity of movement it is capable of, thus the lips and tongue have a larger representation than the trunk, for they are capable of much finer movements and their muscles receive a rich supply of motor nerves.

The body is also represented on the motor cortex. This grotesque representation of the body is called the motor homunculus and is located in the frontal lobe, anterior to the central sulcus. The motor homunculus is similar but not identical to the sensory homunculus. The motor homunculus shows where in the body a response will occur if a particular area of the motor cortex is stimulated via an electrode (see Figure 17.8).

When you move the fingers on your right hand, impulses are generated in the cells of the left motor cortex. The impulses travel on fibres which leave the motor cortex *en*

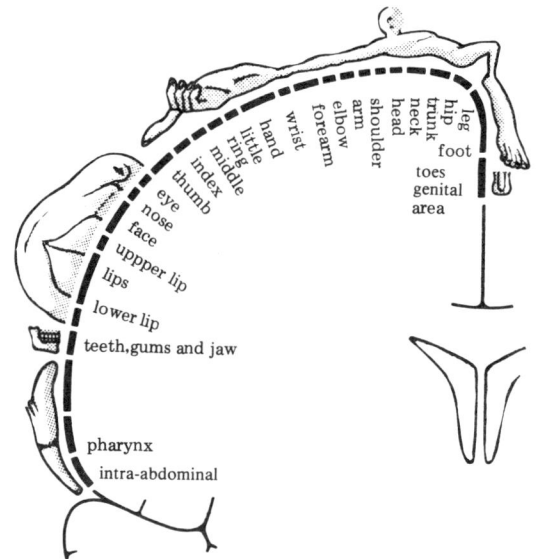

Figure 17.8 Diagrammatic arrangement of the motor cortex and the homunculus, showing the site and extent of sensory representation of different areas of the body.

masse in a fibre tract known as the internal capsule. These fibres descend in the brain on the left side till they reach the lowest part of the brain stem where most of them cross over to the right side and enter the spinal cord. Their crossover point is referred to as the pyramidal decussation. Most fibres from the right motor cortex cross over to the left side of the spinal cord. These fibres do not synapse but descend in the spinal cord in the lateral corticospinal tract till they come to the motor neurones whose axons innervate the muscles of the fingers. The descending fibres leave the corticospinal tract and synapse with these motor neurones. There are two sets of neurones in this direct or pyramidal pathway (see Figure 17.9). Those in the motor cortex are called the upper motor neurones, while those in the spinal cord are called lower motor neurones. Since the lower motor neurones innervate

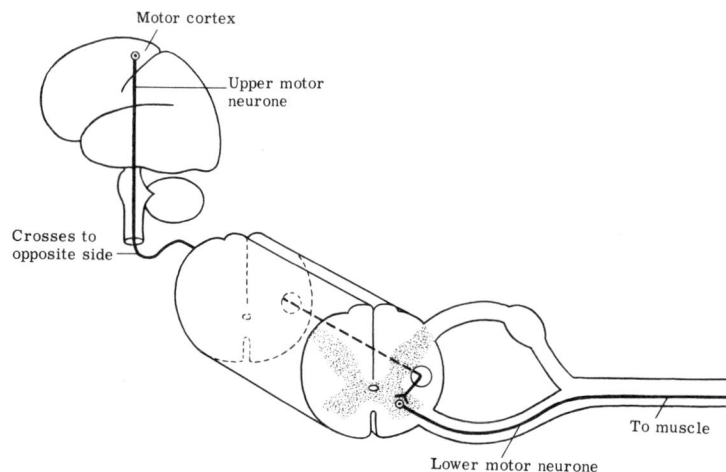

Figure 17.7   General arrangement of the direct motor pathway in the central nervous system (the pyramidal system).

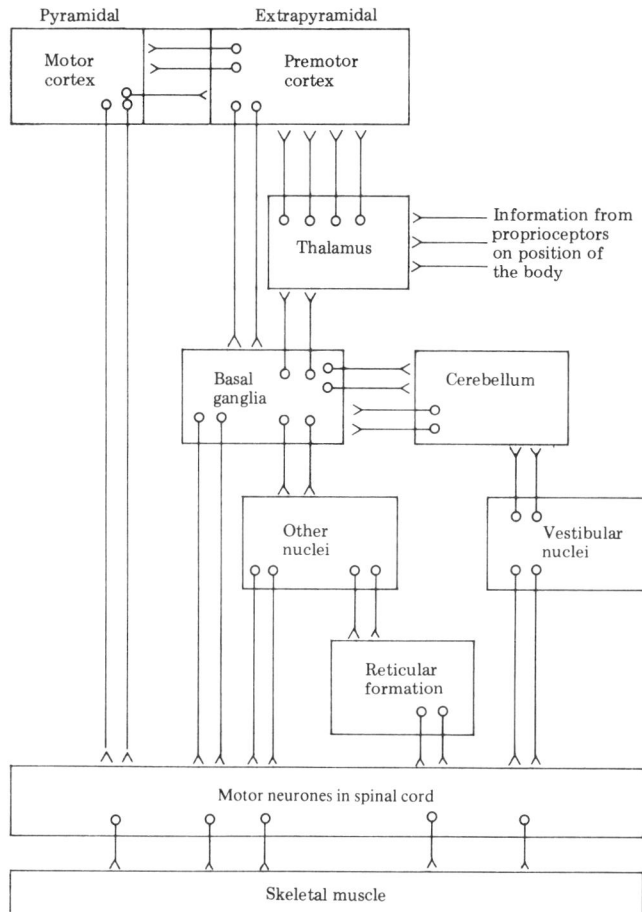

Figure 17.9 Outline of the pyramidal and extrapyramidal systems.

skeletal muscle, they are referred to as the final common pathway for neural impulses which stimulate movement. Many other fibres besides those from the motor cortex synapse on the lower motor neurones.

An insight into the organization of the motor cortex and the homunculus is provided by epilepsy. Epilepsy may be considered to be an uncontrolled outburst of neuronal activity within the brain which may result in convulsions, involuntary movements, strange sensory phenomenon, increased activity within the autonomic nervous system, loss of consciousness or, infrequently, psychological disturbances.

If an area of the motor cortex becomes hyperexcitable and generates an excessive number of impulses, the hyperexcitable state can spread along the homunculus. If the lesion is near the foot on the right motor homunculus, the seizure may begin with an uncontrolled twitching of the left foot or leg. These involuntary movements can continue to spread upward until the entire left half of the body is affected and may even spread to the other half of the body. (The primary lesion initiating the seizure need not be in the motor cortex; in fact, the temporal lobe is often the site of the primary lesion.) There are many conditions that may cause an area to be hyperexcitable. These include developmental defects, trauma to the head or conditions which interfere with the brain's blood and oxygen supply, or infections and metabolic

disorders. In an adult it is essential to rule out a tumour as the cause of the seizure.

At one time, a seizure was looked upon as an almost magical act by someone possessed by devils. Although this belief is not generally held today, the public is often frightened and upset by seeing a seizure, perhaps more so than the person having a seizure who may be in real need of assistance. Mozart, Cellini and Napoleon are amongst the famous people who were epileptics.

The area immediately anterior to the motor cortex is called the pre-motor cortex. Fibres from this area are involved in movement and its organization. Impulses from this area ultimately reach motor neurones but there are synapses in the nuclei of the cerebrum, the brainstem and the cerebellum. This indirect pathway is called the extrapyramidal tract. Most movements are not isolated gestures but involve balance, co-ordination, the shifting of weight and positioning of the body as a whole. For this to be possible, the lower motor neurones in the spinal cord which cause the movement must receive information from a variety of sources besides those in the motor cortex. This information cannot come from only the part of the body that is moving, but from the body as a whole. This requires a great deal of exchanging and comparing of information within the nervous system. The extrapyramidal system will necessarily be more complicated than the direct pyramidal system, for the instructions that the extrapyramidal system relays to the lower motor neurones are a function of the information it receives and processes.

The structures shown in Figure 17.9, which have not been explained, will be discussed in coming sections. The pyramidal and extrapyramidal do work together and their functions are neither as simple nor as separate as Figure 17.9 indicates.

Certain areas of the frontal lobes have little known motor or sensory function and are often referred to as "silent areas". The word "silent" needs explanation. To a deaf person the world may seem silent even though it may be filled with sound. So too with the so-called silent areas of the brain. Science does not yet have the experimental technique necessary to "hear" or to perceive the silent areas' function in humans. These areas are believed to be important in some of the higher functions such as reasoning, memory, learning, emotions and other complex behaviours. Fibres are sent from motor and sensory areas in the cortex, brain nuclei and other frontal areas, from the right to the left and the left to the right central hemispheres, so that most information is stored in both hemispheres. It is known that injuries or surgical lesions in certain of these areas may affect personality.

Finally, although the right and left cerebral hemispheres appear grossly similar, there are subtle anatomical differences and definite functional differences. It is said that as an individual grows, one hemisphere becomes dominant. This does not refer to the size of the hemisphere but to the fact that one hemisphere is superior to the other in performing certain actions. For example, most people write better with one hand than with the other. A person who is right-handed has his or her left cerebral hemisphere dominant; the right cerebral hemisphere may be dominant in left-handed people. More than 90% of people are right-handed. Almost all right-handed people and many left-handed people have left hemisphere dominance for speech.

If someone holds up a red tie and asks you, "What is this?", you have to go through a series of processes to respond properly. You must not only hear the question and see the object but you must also understand the question, identify and name the object, formulate your answer in a sentence and speak your answer with the muscles of the palate, lips and tongue. The diaphragm and vocal cords are also involved.

Many of the intellectual aspects of speech are localized in the adjacent areas of the parietal and temporal lobes (Wernicke's area) of the dominant hemisphere. Control of many of the motor aspects of speech appears to be located in the frontal lobe (Broca's area) near the pre-motor cortex of the dominant lobe.

Some investigators believe that different types of thought processes occur in different hemispheres. For instance, intuitive or creative processes may be localized in the right hemisphere, while logical, problem-solving processes may take place in the left hemisphere. Anyway, it is something to think about with either or both hemispheres.

Below the cerebral cortex, deep within the cerebral hemispheres, are important clusters or groups of neurones which receive, send and are surrounded by fibres to and from the cortex. The clusters of neurones also send fibres to other areas of the brain. Three of the most important of these groups of nuclei are the basal ganglia, the thalamus and the hypothalamus.

a. The basal ganglia

In spite of their name, the basal ganglia are really groups of nerve cells or nuclei located within the forebrain. The names of some of the structures that make up the basal ganglia include the putamen, the globus pallidus, the caudate nucleus and the amygaloid nuclear complex. The basal ganglia are an important part of the extrapyramidal system. The extra-pyramidal system is sometimes called an indirect motor pathway, for more neurones and synapses are involved here than in the two neurone pathways of the pyramidal system. It is a generally accepted over-simplification to assume that the pyramidal system is associated with the fine, precise aspects of movement, whereas the extrapyramidal system is associated with the less delicate aspects of movement. As an example of this, if you pick up a penny off the floor, the fine movements of your fingers would be chiefly controlled by the pyramidal system, while the bending over and associated postural adjustments would be influenced by the extra-pyramidal system.

The basal ganglia have many connections. Fibres from the motor and pre-motor cortex synapse in the basal ganglia. Some fibres leave the basal ganglia and synapse in the thalamus. Fibres from the thalamus project to both the motor and sensory cortex and to the basal ganglia as well. Thus a loop is established: motor and pre-motor cortex → basal ganglia ⇌ thalamus → motor and pre-motor cortex. It is this type of circuit that is thought to integrate fine movements with gross postural movements and to influence most motor activity. The basal ganglia also have important connections with nuclei in the midbrain. These nuclei are the red nucleus and the substantia nigra, and they send and receive fibres to and from the basal ganglia. The red nucleus also sends fibres

down the spinal cord which synapse the motor neurones. These connections between the basal ganglia, red nucleus and substantia nigra are thought to be important in the maintenance of muscle tone.

Disorders of the basal ganglia result in conditions characterized as either hyperkinetic or hypokinetic. Hyperkinetic disorders are associated with an abnormally increased motor activity. In hypokinetic disorders, motor activity is reduced.

Huntington's chorea is a very rare hyperkinetic disorder in which the pathological changes are most severe in certain of the basal ganglia. Movements are rapid, irregular, jerky and involuntary.

Parkinson's disease is much more common and is a hypokinetic disorder. These patients usually lack associated movements such as swinging of the arms when walking, or facial expressions when talking. Some muscular rigidity and an involuntary tremor (shaking) are also characteristic of the disease. This tremor commonly occurs in the fingers and thumb and is most severe when the limb is at rest. Sleep and purposeful movement of the limb reduce the tremor.

Major advances in the treatment of Parkinson's disease took place in the 1960s following research which showed that there was a deficiency of dopamine within certain nuclei of the basal ganglia. Dopamine is the immediate precursor of noradrenaline and both chemicals are significant in neuro-chemistry and brain function. Dopamine is released at many synapses within the brain. Giving dopamine does not remove the deficiency in Parkinson's disease, for dopamine cannot penetrate the nervous system to the deficient areas of the basal ganglia. The chemical precursor of dopamine is levodopa (L-dopa) and this can penetrate to the deficient areas. L-dopa presumably gets into the deficient cells, is converted by enzymes to dopamine and released into the synapses at the appropriate time. Treatment with L-dopa may lead to significant improvement in selected patients with Parkinson's disease.

L-dopa does not usually help patients with Huntington's chorea and, in fact, may induce irregular jerky movements. Some investigators look at these two conditions as being at opposite ends of a chemical spectrum of disease. They suggest that normal muscle tone and movement result from a balance of chemical forces in the nervous system. One force might be the dopaminergic force represented by those synapses that release dopamine. The other force might be the cholinergic force represented by those synapses which release acetylcholine. Drugs or disease may alter this chemical balance, and the balance may be tipped towards hypokinetic or hyperkinetic states. This last statement may be an over-simplification but there is no doubt that the thrust of research is aimed at understanding and modifying this synaptic biochemistry.

b. The thalamus

This area has been called the gateway to the cortex (see Figure 17.10). Axons carrying information from all the senses, except olfaction, synapse in the thalamus; neurones from the thalamus then go to the sensory areas of the cortex. They radiate to the cortex via the internal capsule. The thalamus is a large and complicated structure with at least 40

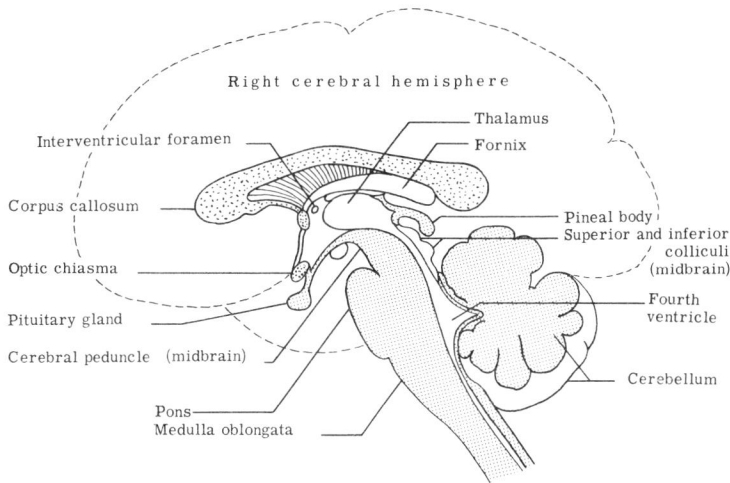

Figure 17.10   The brain — sagittal section.

major nuclei located within it. It is not merely a relay station however, because it is able to integrate sensory information and even modify it. The thalamus also sends and receives fibres from the cerebral cortex, particularly the "silent areas" (see Figure 17.11b). It has been said that many sensations are not simply sensory phenomena. This implies that many sensations have an "affective" component. A sensation can be very pleasant, very disagreeable or even painful, so sensation normally cannot be separated from an emotional reaction. No doubt this thalamus → cortex → thalamus circuit is involved. If the thalamus is injured there may be a loss of some sensory perception. In some types of thalamic injury however, the patient may appear to over-react to stimuli that are not particularly painful. Stimuli that are usually not painful may become so distorted in these individuals that great pain results.

The thalamus is also important in movement. If you are going on a long journey, you had better know precisely where

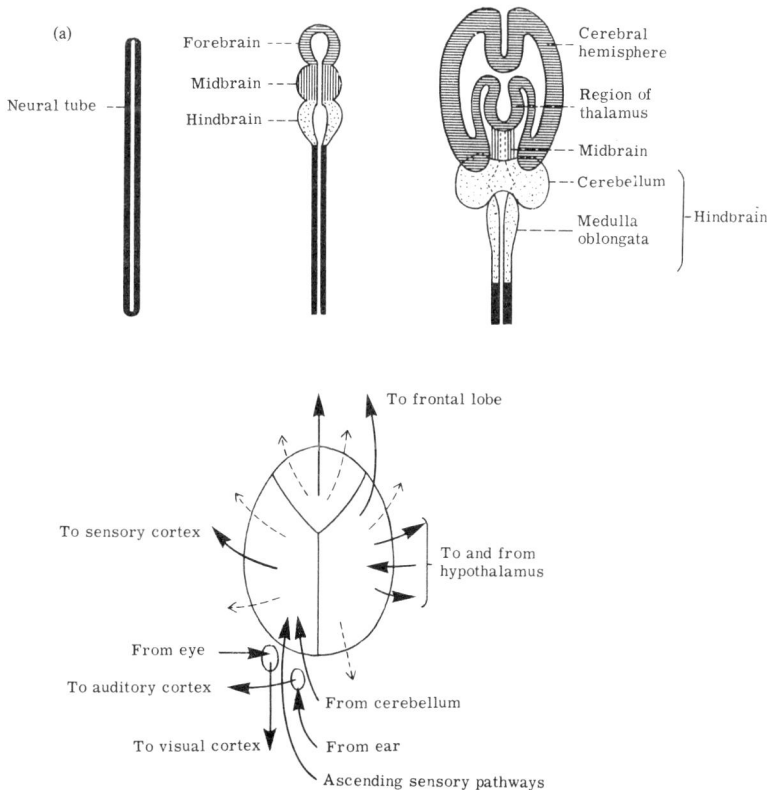

Figure 17.11   (a) Development of the brain. (b) Connections of the thalamus (dotted arrows indicate that the whole thalamus has connections with the whole cerebral cortex).

you are leaving from before you start to travel. The thalamus informs the motor and pre-motor cortex on the position of the body's parts, and the cortex can then appropriately modify the actions it initiates. Proprioceptive information reaches the thalamus from two nuclei in the medulla, the nucleus cuneatus and the nucleus gracilis. These nuclei receive information from proprioceptors in the joints and muscle spindles, as well as touch and pressure information from receptors in the skin. The thalamus also receives information on movement from the basal ganglia, the red nucleus and the cerebellum.

The thalamus also receives fibres from the reticular formation. There is some evidence that signals from the reticular formation which are relayed to the frontal lobes by the thalamus are important in maintaining the level of alertness.

c. The hypothalamus

This group of neurones which lies below the thalamus has been mentioned previously in connection with the endocrine and the reproductive system. Hormones called releasing factors are synthesized in the anterior cells of the hypothalamus and are released into a short network of capillary vessels which transport them to the anterior pituitary gland, where they affect the release of hormones. The releasing factors are summarized in the Table below.

Recent research suggests that many of these releasing hormones made in the hypothalamus may also be found in other parts of the brain and may have other actions in the nervous system and other parts of the body. For example, GHIF (somatostatin) may reduce glucagon secretion in the pancreas. (Material on this is best revised in the appropriate preceding Chapters.)

The pituitary gland used to be called the master gland of the body. The hypothalamus is now called the master gland of the body because the hormones (releasing factors) made in the hypothalamus do control the secretion of the hormones from the anterior pituitary. In addition, the two hormones which are released from the posterior pituitary are actually

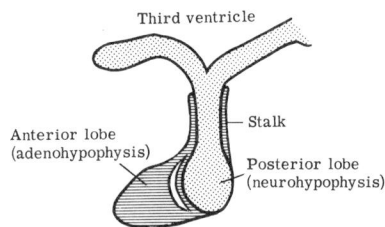

Figure 17.12   The pituitary gland.

synthesized in the hypothalamus. The hypothalamus receives fibres from many places in the brain including the thalamus and frontal lobes of the cortex. These inputs are essential in stimulating the release of the hormones from the hypothalamus. Everything is so connected.

One connection that has been recently investigated is the relationship between sleep and the release of hormones from the hypothalamus and the pituitary. Many of these hormones are released in sudden, dramatic outbursts while the individual sleeps. Sleep is a complex state, has many dynamic components and is much more than a reduction in the level of consciousness. It is interesting to note that you can store surplus calories in fat but that nature has not provided a way of storing sleep.

The posterior pituitary is really an outgrowth or down-pocketing of the hypothalamus (see Figure 17.12). Two sets of neurones begin in the hypothalamus and pass, by way of a connecting stalk, to the posterior pituitary where they end (the neurohypophysis). One group of neurones synthesizes antidiuretic hormone (ADH); another produces oxytocin. These hormones travel down the cytoplasm to the nerve endings in the posterior pituitary. From here they are released into capillaries which drain into the general venous circulation. Hormones from both the anterior and posterior pituitary travel in these capillaries to the veins, are sent to the heart and distributed throughout the body.

Hypothalamic hormones or releasing agents:	FSHRF—LHRF		ACTHRF	TSHRF	GHRF	GHIF	PIF
Anterior pituitary hormones:	FSH*	LH*	ACTH*	TSH*	GH*	GH†	Prolactin†
Target organs:	gonads		adrenal cortex	thyroid gland	many organs		breasts

* increased secretion.
† decreased secretion.

FSHRF	=	follicle stimulating hormone releasing factor	
LHRF	=	luteinizing hormone releasing factor	In humans these two releasing hormones are probably the same hormone or a single molecule; may be called gonadotropin releasing hormone
ACTHRF	=	adrenocorticotropic hormone releasing factor	
TSHRF	=	thyroid stimulating hormone releasing factor	
GHRF	=	growth hormone releasing factor	Growth hormone is sometimes called somatotropin
GHIF	=	growth hormone inhibiting factor	GHIF is often called somatostatin and seems to have other metabolic actions besides decreasing growth hormone secretion
PIF	=	prolactin inhibiting factor	

If the osmotic pressure of the blood perfusing the hypothalamus is increased, the posterior lobe neurones are stimulated to release ADH, which increases the amount of water reabsorbed by the kidneys, so the osmotic pressure is reduced. Oxytocin stimulates uterine contractions in childbirth and contraction of the myo-epithelial cells of the breasts, causing milk release. Suckling on the breast stimulates the hypothalamus and causes oxytocin release.

The hypothalamus has many functions besides producing hormones and hormonal releasing factors. Depending on where they are, lesions in the hypothalamus may cause obesity or induce the individual to reduce his or her food intake. Cells within the hypothalamus appear to be sensitive to levels of glucose in the blood. It has been suggested that when glucose levels are normal, or above normal, a satiety signal is generated. When blood sugar falls below a certain level, these signals are no longer sent and a conscious feeling of hunger results.

The hypothalamus also functions in temperature regulation, for it contains thermoreceptors or cells sensitive to the temperature of the blood which supplies them. Temperature receptors from the skin also send information to the hypothalamus. Body temperature is not rigidly fixed at 37 °C (98.6 °F) but varies in healthy individuals, peaking in the early evening and falling to its lowest levels in the early morning. Emotions, exercise and disease can raise body temperature; 110 °F (43.3 °C) is the highest temperature that is compatible with human life, though temperatures above 106 °F (41 °C) are seldom seen.

The body's responses to environmental temperature changes are mediated by the hypothalamus which sends fibres to the vasomotor centre. This centre sends impulses through the sympathetic nervous system, which regulates the diameter of the arterioles. Information on temperature reaches the thalamus indirectly from temperature receptors in the skin via the thalamus and also from the temperature of the blood which perfuses the hypothalamus. Cold stimulates the vasoconstriction of blood vessels in the skin (reducing heat loss), stimulates shivering (which increases heat production) and perhaps even increases the output of thyroid hormone (which accelerates metabolic rate). Heat stimulates vasodilation of blood vessels in the skin (increasing heat loss), stimulates sweating and perhaps reduces thyroid hormone and adrenaline release. Heat energy is not directly lost in sweat, but in the energy required to evaporate it. People are generally more uncomfortable on hot, humid days when the air is saturated with water vapour, so sweat runs off rather than evaporates. Temperature regulation is also discussed in more detail in the Chapter on the skin.

Hypothalamic neurones are also activated in fear, rage and anger. Fibres from the frontal lobes go to the hypothalamus, synapse, and the hypothalamic neurones leave the hypothalamus to synapse with neurones which function in the sympathetic nervous system. Much of the sympathetic nervous system's response to stress is mediated via the cerebral cortex and the hypothalamus.

Before proceding to the midbrain, mention should be made of the pineal gland. This small cone-shaped gland is located above the posterior portion of the thalamus (see Figure 17.10). The hormones produced by the pineal gland in the human are not yet known.

B. The midbrain

This is the smallest section of the brain and is between the cerebrum above and the pons below (see Figure 17.11). The upper surface of the midbrain is marked by two elevations caused by nuclear masses. These are the superior colliculi and the inferior colliculi. The midbrain also contains neurones which receive information from the ear and the eye. The oculomotor (III) and trochlear (IV) nerves begin with neurones located in the midbrain.

There are connections between the afferent sensory fibres from the eye and the efferent motor neurones of the oculomotor nerve which go to the iris sphincter. If you shine a light in the eye of a friend, you will notice that the pupils of both eyes constrict and reduce the amount of light which enters the eye. This is a reflex in which sensory information from the retina of the eye is sent to the midbrain, which then sends instructions to contract via the oculomotor nerve to the iris and ciliary muscle. Because of the crossover of fibres from the eye in the midbrain, both pupils will constrict, even if the light enters only one eye. If the midbrain is injured, the reflex will be slowed or abolished, and so the reflex serves as an important clinical test. (The eye and its innervation are discussed in more detail in the Chapter on the eye and the ear.)

Two important nuclei in the midbrain are the substantia nigra and the red nucleus. The substantia nigra receives fibres from, and sends fibres to, the basal ganglia. The substantia nigra is considered to be part of the extrapyramidal system and is also thought to be involved in the pathogenesis of Parkinson's disease.

The cells of the red nucleus contain a small amount of reddish pigment and hence the name. The red nucleus receives fibres from two main sources. Some fibres from the motor and pre-motor cortex synapse there, as do fibres from the cerebellum. Fibres leave the red nucleus to synapse in the cerebellum or descend and synapse at various levels in the spinal cord. These fibres have either an excitatory or inhibitory influence on lower motor neurones. The red nucleus is considered to be part of the reticular system which will be discussed in subsequent Sections.

In addition to the nuclei mentioned, large tracts of fibres pass through the midbrain. These fibres include descending fibres from the motor and pre-motor cortex, and ascending fibres carrying sensory information to the thalamus.

C. The hindbrain

The hindbrain has three components: the cerebellum, the pons and the medulla oblongata.

a. The cerebellum

The cerebellum is smaller than the cerebrum and similar, in that its outer surface is convoluted and contains neurones. It is separated from the cerebrum by a hard fold of dura mater called the tentorium cerebelli (see Figure 17.10).

In some animal experiments, the cerebellum has been surgically removed. The animals were in no pain, were able to move voluntarily and had reflexes, though both movements and reflexes were abnormal and the animals could not walk properly. When these animals were thrown into deep water they appeared happier and swam almost normally. In deep water, the animal is supported on all sides, so the force of gravity is eliminated. This evidence suggests that the cerebellum also functions to help regulate muscular movement with respect to the force of gravity and to help position the body with respect to the ground. This information originates within the labyrinthine system of the inner ear and is relayed to the cerebellum via the vestibular nuclei. (More will be said about the ear in the next Chapter.)

Removal of the cerebellum in humans leads to a reduction in muscle tone. Most patients with cerebellar diseases however show few symptoms when they are at rest. Often, when they initiate a voluntary action, a tremor begins; this is in contrast to Parkinsonian patients who have a resting tremor, but the tremor is reduced when a purposeful motion begins. A frequent symptom of most cerebellar disorders is a movement which is inappropriate for the action intended.

The cerebellum has two hemispheres, somewhat oval in shape. Fibres to and from the cerebellar cortex go via three separate bundles known as the cerebellar peduncles. Nerve fibres from nuclei in the cerebellum proceed anteriorly via the superior cerebellar peduncles. Many of these fibres synapse in either the red nucleus or the thalamus. It is through these connections that the cerebellum can influence or modify a movement.

Much proprioceptive information reaches the cerebellum via the inferior cerebellar peduncle (see Figure 17.13). Fibres from the tendon and muscle stretch receptors enter the spinal cord and synapse on neurones there. Fibres from these neurones ascend in the spinal cord in the spino-cerebellar tracts, and most of these fibres reach the cerebellum and synapse there via the inferior cerebellar peduncle (see Figure 17.13). Additional information on the position of the body with respect to the ground is also sent to the cerebellum from the vestibular system. The sense receptors for this information are located in the vestibular portion of the inner ear. Finally, the cerebellum also receives information from, and sends information to, the visual system. This is essential in the co-ordination of eye movements with body movements.

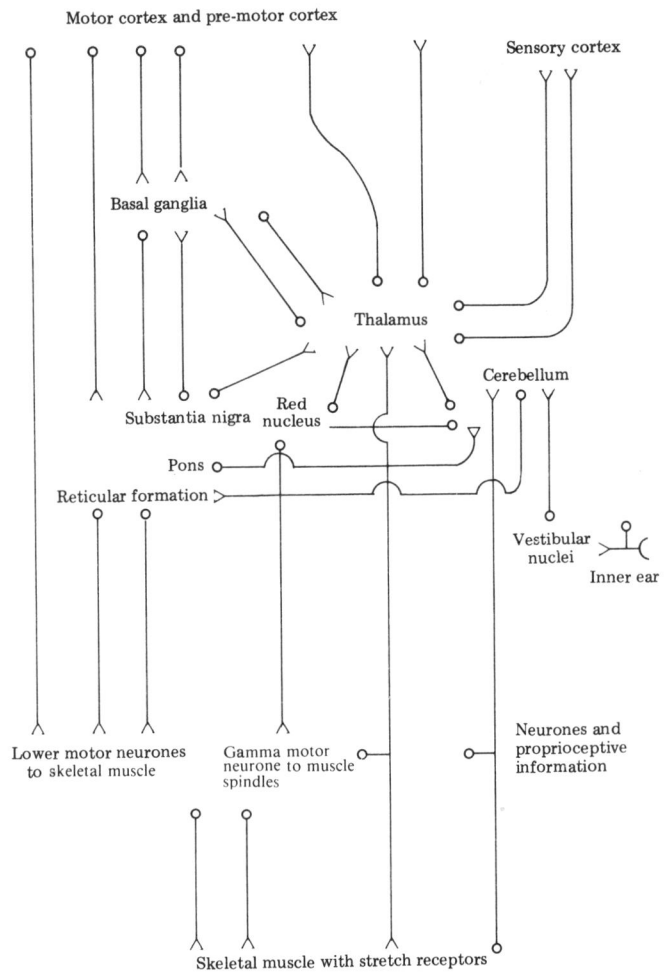

Figure 17.14 Diagram of some of the connections between motor neurones, the cortex and the cerebellum.

Although the cerebellum receives sensory information, there is no conscious sensory perception within the cerebellum.

Fibres from the motor and pre-motor cortex synapse in the pons (see Figure 17.14). Neurones in the pons send their axons to the cerebellar cortex via the middle cerebellar peduncles. Fibres also leave the cerebellum and synapse in the pons by way of the middle cerebellar peduncle.

One way to organize this information might be to construct a pathway chart utilizing in sequence the connection of the various structures mentioned. You could, as an example, construct a pathway chart connecting indirectly the motor cortex with the motor cortex by means of the cerebellum. Suppose, for example, you move your right hand. A possible pathway might be: left motor cortex → decussation at pyramid → motor neurones in spinal cord on right side → contraction muscles of right hand → increased discharge of tendon and muscle spindle receptors → neurones of the spino-cerebellar tract (unconscious proprioception pathway) → right inferior cerebellar peduncle → cerebellum and intra-cerebellar connections → superior cerebellar peduncle → cross to red nucleus on left → thalamus → left motor cortex.

Memorizing the cerebellar pathways is of little value unless you understand their functional significance. When a move-

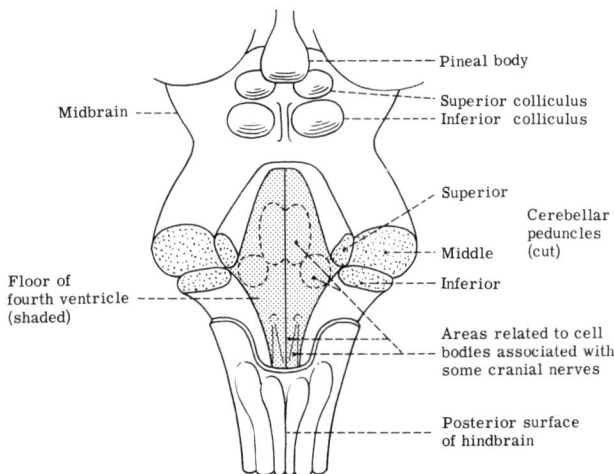

Figure 17.13 Posterior surface of the hindbrain and midbrain after removal of the cerebellum.

ment is initiated, signals from the motor and pre-motor cortex reach the pons and are relayed from the pons to the cerebellum. As the movement takes place, information from the proprioceptors reaches the cerebellum and informs it of the progress of the movement (see Figure 17.14). In a sense, the cerebellum receives information on an intended movement and information on the progress of the movement. It can compare these two sets of information and send corrective instructions to the motor neurones, indirectly, via its connections with the thalamus, red nucleus and the vestibular system. These corrections reduce errors in the force, range and speed of the movement.

b. The pons

The pons is located between the midbrain and the medulla, and is below and slightly anterior to the cerebellum (see Figure 17.10). In Latin pons means bridge; the pons is a bridge between the two cerebellar hemispheres. Neurones from the left cerebellar hemisphere cross to the right, and *vice versa*, via the middle cerebellar peduncles with which the pons is continuous (see Figure 17.13). The pons contains the nuclei of cranial nerves V, VI, VII and VIII. These nuclei receive fibres from the cortex. The pons also contains a diffuse scattering of neurones which belong to the reticular formation. One distinguished neurologist has called the reticular formation a "synaptic swamp". This is in reference to the extensive, diffuse nature of the reticular formation and its many synaptic connections with other parts of the brain. Fibres from the motor and pre-motor cortex synapse there, as do fibres from the cerebellum. Neurones from the reticular formation send their axons down the spinal cord in the reticulo-spinal tract. Because of the diffuse nature of the reticular system and its many interconnections, it is difficult to assign a single specific function to them. Reticular spinal neurones synapse on both the large motor neurones and on the small γ motor neurones which influence the sensitivity of the muscle spindles. Different fibres of the reticular system may have either an inhibitory or facilitory influence on the neurones in the spinal cord.

Fibres of the pyramidal system also pass directly through the pons, as do ascending fibres carrying sensory information to the thalamus.

c. The medulla oblongata

This structure is below the pons and above and continuous with the spinal cord below (see Figure 17.10). Although the structure is only a few centimetres thick, it is extremely important. On the dorsal surface of the medulla are two elevations called the pyramids. These represent the place where 80–90% of the fibres from the motor cortex in the pyramidal system cross over before descending in the spinal cord to synapse with lower motor neurones. Fibres of the extrapyramidal system pass deep within the medulla. Scattered within the medulla are groups of neurones which belong to the reticular formation (reticular system).

(1) Some neurones in the reticular formation in the medulla, like the reticular neurones in the pons, descend in the spinal cord. These neurones receive information from the motor and pre-motor cortex, the cerebellum and other parts of the reticular formation; they are important in the maintenance of muscle tone and they participate in the postural changes associated with movement.

(2) Neurones in the reticular formation also have a rich sensory input. Information from sense receptors in the skin and also from the visual and auditory system is sent to the reticular system. Fibres from the reticular system synapse in the thalamus and fibres from the thalamus go to the cortex. There are many complex interactions between the reticular formation, the thalamus and the cortex. While you were reading the last few sentences, you probably were not conscious of the temperature of your feet, the pressure caused by wearing a belt or the sound of a clock nearby, though this temperature, pressure and sound information was being reported to the nervous system. Only a small fraction of the sensory information received by the brain ever reaches the level of conscious attention. Presumably, the reticular formation and thalamus filter out a great deal of this information, so it never reaches the cortex. These interactions must be quite complex for certain subtle discriminations to be made. You might, for instance, be able to sleep through loud traffic noises, but awake instantly at the soft sound of strange footsteps near your bed. There is some electro-physiological evidence indicating that when a sleeping person is awakened, the sensory information from an alarm clock, for example, triggers the reticular system, which then arouses or alerts the cerebral cortex and thereby returns the individual to consciousness.

Other information relating the reticular formation to sleep and altered levels of consciousness comes from individuals with lesions or tumours within the reticular system, who behave as though they are asleep, that is, not fully conscious. Certain general anaesthetics are thought to work by reducing the activity of the reticular system. The relationship between the reticular system and sleep is a subject of great research interest. The more that is learned about sleep, the more complex the phenomenon seems. Sleep is more than a reduced level of consciousness though, for there are many active physiological processes which occur only during sleep.

(3) The medulla contains large nuclei known as the nucleus cuneatus and the nucleus gracilis. Fibres from these nuclei cross to the opposite side of the medulla and proceed to the thalamus where they synapse. They also have connections with the reticular formation. The input to the nucleus cuneatus and nucleus gracilis comes from proprioceptors in the joints and muscles, as well as receptors in the skin which are sensitive to light pressure. Fibres from these receptors enter the spinal cord and ascend in the same side they enter until they reach the medulla, where they synapse in the nucleus cuneatus or nucleus gracilis. This is in contrast to fibres from pain and temperature receptors, which enter the spinal cord and synapse (see Figure 17.15). Fibres from the secondary neurones cross the spinal cord and ascend till they synapse in the thalamus. All sensory information from the right half of the body ultimately reaches the sensory cortex in the left half of the brain, and conversely, information from the left half of the body reaches the sensory cortex in the right half of the brain.

(4) The neurones of the respiratory centre are also located in the medulla. The neurones here are stimulated by decreases in blood pH or increased plasma carbon dioxide. They are

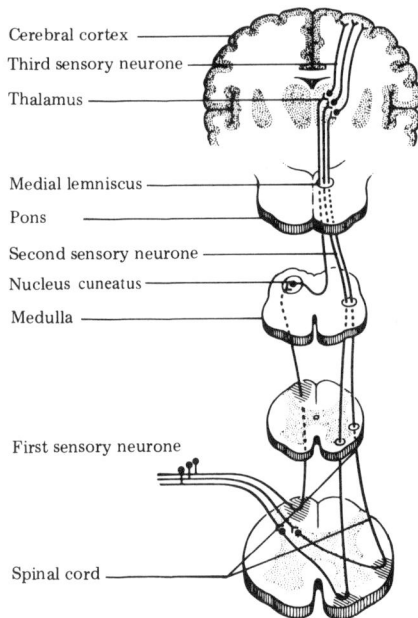

Figure 17.15   The central pathway for proprioception.

influenced by information on blood pH and the partial pressure of carbon dioxide and oxygen sent from the chemoreceptors via the glossopharyngeal (IX) and vagus (X) nerves or by information from the cerebral cortex. Information concerning the pH of the cerebrospinal fluid is also sent to the respiratory neurones from chemoreceptors located on the surface of the medulla. Neurones from the respiratory centre travel down the spinal cord to the cervical or thoracic levels, where they synapse with motor neurones which leave the spinal cord and innervate the respiratory muscles via the phrenic or inter-costal nerves. The respiratory neurones are cyclically active, discharging regularly at brief intervals. A suggested explanation for this is that the neurones are arranged in a loop or loops, so that some activity is maintained. A certain amount of sensory input does appear necessary for continuous cyclic activity.

(5) The vasomotor centre is located in the medulla. The neurones of the vasomotor centre are tonically active, but their activity may be increased with increases in plasma carbon dioxide or changed by information on the pressure perfusing the carotid sinus and by changes in the composition of the blood detected by the carotid and aortic bodies. This information is relayed via the glossopharyngeal (IX) cranial nerve. Information from the cerebral cortex and from the hypothalamus is also sent here. The vasomotor centre responds by changing its rate of discharge. Impulses travel down the spinal cord to the thoracic or lumbar levels, where they synapse with the first neurone of the sympathetic nervous system. These neurones go to a ganglion and synapse with a second neurone which travels to the smooth muscle of the arterioles. An increase in the number of impulses from the vasomotor centre will lead to contraction of the smooth muscle and increased resistance and blood pressure. The vasomotor centre works in conjunction with the cardiac centre, so changes in vasoconstrictor tone are co-ordinated with appropriate changes in heart rate.

(6) The centres which regulate the reflex acts of swallow-

ing, vomiting, sneezing and coughing are also located in the medulla. The presence of food or fluid stimulates receptors in the back of the mouth and this information is relayed to the swallow centre via the glossopharyngeal (IX) nerve. This sends instructions to a large number of muscles and co-ordinates this complicated act. Irritation of the gastro-oesophageal intestinal tract stimulates the vomit centre. Irritation within the nasal passage will stimulate a sneeze, while irritation further down triggers a cough.

D. The spinal cord

This structure is almost cylindrical in shape, about the thickness of your little finger, and, in a typical adult male, is approximately 45 cm long. Thirty-one pairs of nerves known as the spinal nerves leave the spinal cord. The spinal cord is continuous with the medulla oblongata, passes through the foramen magnum in the occipital bone of the skull (see Figure 5.6) and runs within the neural canal of the vertebral column to the level of the 1st lumbar vertebra, so the spinal cord is shorter than the vertebral canal. The spinal nerves from the lower spinal cord pass downward and exit between the lumbar vertebra or through the foramina of the sacrum. This downward and flowing arrangement gives the lower spinal nerves the appearance of a horse's tail so it is named from the Latin, the cauda equina (see Figure 17.16). The spinal cord is incompletely divided into right and left halves by a posterior median fissure and the deep anterior median fissure.

A cross-section of the spinal cord shows a sharp distinction between the white matter and the "H"-shaped grey matter. The white matter of the cord is arranged in three columns: anterior, posterior and lateral columns (see Figure 17.17). These columns contain fibres in very organized tracts (pathways); fibres going to the same place travel together (see Figure 17.18). For example, all the fibres in the pyramidal tract travel in a narrow tract in the lateral column before leaving the tract to synapse with motor neurones in the anterior horn of the grey matter. Some of the descending tracts are the rubro-spinal fibres (from the red nucleus), the reticulo-spinal and vestibulo-spinal tracts.

Before the spinal nerves enter the spinal cord, each spinal nerve divides. The posterior division contains the cell bodies of the sense receptors; fibres from the cells form rootlets which enter the posterior half of the spinal cord. Fibres from pain and temperature receptors synapse and secondary neurones cross to the opposite side of the spinal cord and ascend to the thalamus in the lateral spino-thalamic tract. Fibres from the proprioceptors ascend and synapse in the cerebellum via the spino-cerebellar tract (see Figure 17.15). Other information from the proprioceptors ascends in the fibre tracts in the dorsal (posterior) part of the spinal cord to synapse in the nucleus cuneatus or nucleus gracilis. These fibre tracts, which ascend to the nucleus cuneatus and nucleus gracilis, are referred to as the fasciculus cuneatus and the fasciculus gracilis, and they carry information concerning conscious proprioception. These, and other ascending pathways, also carry information concerning touch.

Fibres from sense receptors may also synapse with interneurones. Interneurones may synapse with motor neurones or ascend or descend within the spinal cord to

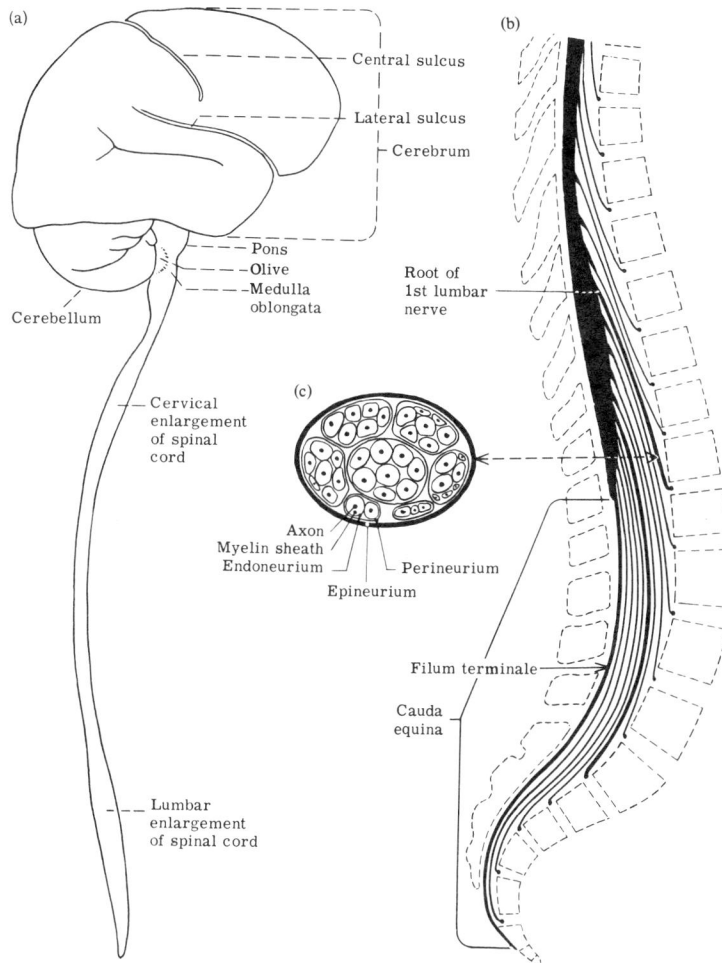

Figure 17.16   (a) The spinal nerves and the enlargements of the spinal cord.(b) Longitudinal section. (c) Transverse section.

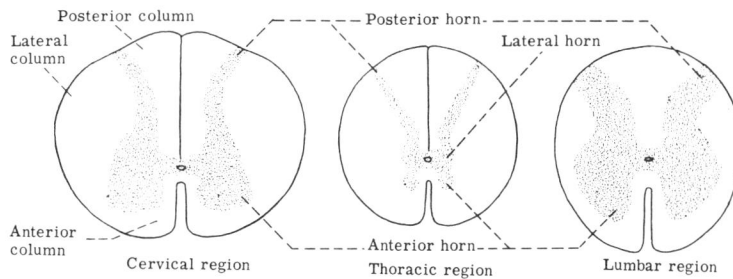

Figure 17.17   The spinal cord — transverse sections.

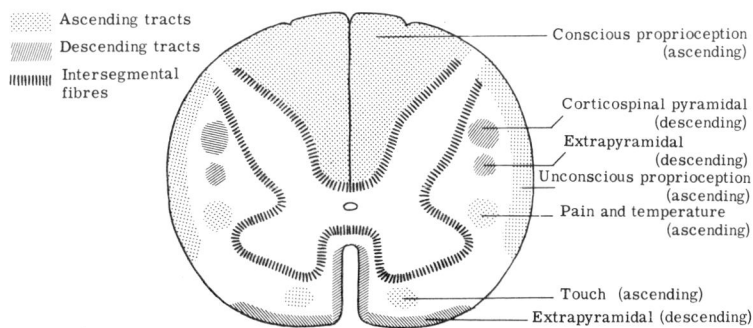

Figure 17.18   The spinal cord — transverse section, showing the position of the main tracts of nerve fibres.

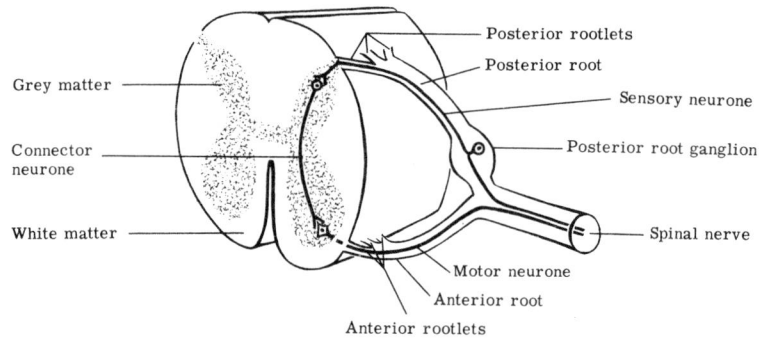

Figure 17.19 The formation of a spinal nerve.

synapse with other neurones; these are important in co-ordinating activities within the spinal cord itself. Motor neurones leave the spinal cord to form the anterior roots. The posterior roots thus carry sensory information and the anterior roots carry instructions to glands and muscles (see Figure 17.19). The anterior and posterior roots unite, so the spinal nerves can be considered mixed nerves.

E. The membranes of the brain and spinal cord and the cerebrospinal fluid

There are three membranes which cover the entire brain and spinal cord and are collectively called the meninges (see Figure 17.20).

The innermost membrane is the pia mater (tender mother). As the name suggests, it is a delicate structure composed of collagen and elastin fibres, squamous epithelium and blood vessels, which are distributed over the surface of the brain. The pia mater closely follows the surface of the brain, dipping and rising, covering all its irregularities.

The middle membrane is the arachnoid (cobweb) mater, which lines the dura mater but is attached to pia mater by a cobwebby connective tissue network of collagen and elastin fibres. Between the pia mater and arachnoid mater circulates the cerebrospinal fluid (CSF) in the subarachnoid space.

The dura mater (hard mother) is the outermost layer and is made up of dense connective tissue. It forms the falx cerebri (which separates the right and left cerebral hemispheres), the tentorium cerebelli (which separates the cerebrum from the cerebellum) and the falx cerebelli (which separates the two cerebellar hemispheres). In the vertebral canal, the dura mater is separated from the periosteum, while it is fused to it in the cranium. The dura mater extends below the spinal cord and merges with the periosteum of the coccyx.

The brain is not a solid structure. Embryologically, the brain is derived from a simple neural tube which folds back onto itself. The adult nervous system retains signs of this hollow beginning. Deep within each cerebral hemisphere is a cavity called the lateral ventricle (see Figure 17.21). The right and left cerebral hemispheres are connected by the inter-ventricular foramina to a centrally placed cavity, the third ventricle. The posterior part of the third ventricle narrows to form a duct which expands below the cerebellum to form the fourth ventricle. Continuous with the fourth ventricle is a narrow central canal which extends down the centre of the spinal cord. The fourth ventricle contains openings through which the CSF can leave the interior of the brain and circulate in the subarachnoid space over the surface of the brain and spinal cord.

The brain literally floats in this fluid, which protects it

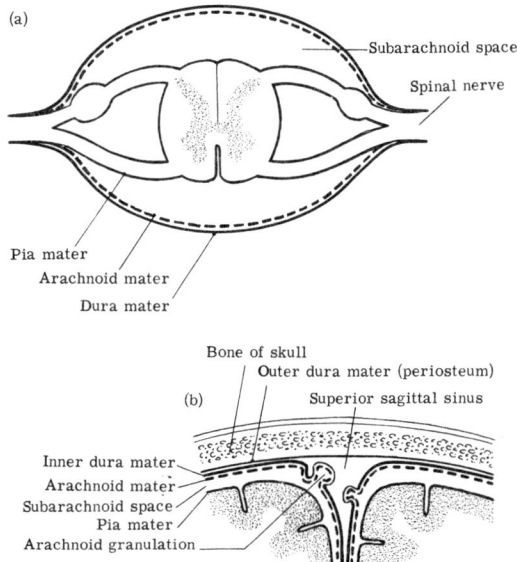

Figure 17.20 (a) Transverse section through the spinal cord and meninges. (b) Coronal section through the skull, cerebral hemispheres and meninges.

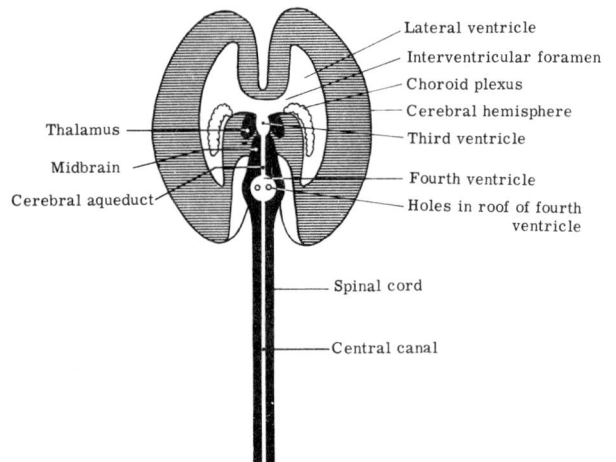

Figure 17.21 Ventricles of the brain.

against drying and mechanical trauma, acting like a watery shock absorber. There are about 130 ml of fluid in the adult — enough to fill a teacup. The fluid is similar but by no means identical to a plasma filtrate. The pH of the CSF is carefully regulated; a slight decrease in pH stimulates receptors on the surface of the medulla, which in turn stimulate the respiratory neurones to increase the respiratory rate. The CSF is secreted by the choroid plexuses, small tufts of capillaries which are found in each of the four ventricles. The volume of CSF formed in a day should be equal to the volume reabsorbed. Reabsorption is accomplished by hollow button-like villi which project from the arachnoid membrane into the venous sinuses and return CSF to the venous system.

Examination of the CSF may provide essential clinical information so that a "spinal tap" is not an uncommon procedure. Generally, the patient lies on his side in a position of extreme flexion, with his head flexed and his knees drawn upward. An extremely aseptic technique is followed to prevent infection, and a local anaesthetic should be administered to reduce pain and lessen the chance of sudden movement. A hollow needle is inserted in the midline of the body between the 4th and 5th lumbar vertebrae. This area is below the level of the spinal cord. (In identifying the intervertebral space it is helpful to draw an imaginary line connecting the top of one iliac crest to another.) Careful palpation is necessary to reveal the depression between the spines of the vertebrae. When the needle penetrates the dura, the resistance will be reduced and there will be a slight give. Fluid should be removed slowly. The needle may be connected to a manometer so that the pressure of the CSF may be measured. Normally, the pressure falls within the range of 50–180 mm of water. CSF should not be removed if the pressure is abnormally high. Usually a total of 5–10 ml is collected in three separate test tubes for different determinations.

The fluid should be clear, colourless and odourless. A cell count and differential should be performed. In normal CSF there are no red cells or granulocytes and less than five lymphocytes/mm^3. Red cells may be present if the spinal tap is traumatic or if there had been a previous haemorrhage into the subarachnoid space, as can happen with a ruptured aneurysm. The presence of polymorphonuclear leucocytes is always abnormal and suggests an infection or inflammation of the brain or meninges. Bacterial toxins may directly injure brain tissue, and pus formation may block the circulation of CSF and lead to an increase in CSF pressure. More than five lymphocytes may be seen in viral infection or infection with other conditions including tuberculosis or syphilis. Fluid should be smeared, stained and cultured for micro-organisms. The normal amount of protein in the CSF is 15–45 mg/100 ml. The amount of protein may be normal or increased in certain diseases of the nervous system. In multiple sclerosis, the total protein may be normal but the amount of IgG may be increased.

Glucose is usually present in the fluid at about 50–80% of the glucose concentration in the blood. If there is an infection in the brain or its coverings, the glucose is often decreased in the acute phases. There are several other measurements and tests that may be made on the CSF and which provide useful information.

THE PERIPHERAL NERVOUS SYSTEM

This division of the nervous system is concerned with bringing information to the brain and spinal cord, and relaying instructions to the glands and muscles. The peripheral nervous system has two divisions: the 12 pairs of cranial nerves and the 31 pairs of spinal nerves.

A. The 12 pairs of cranial nerves

Each pair of nerves is numbered in the order in which they leave the brain, moving from anterior to posterior (see Table 17.1). (There is a mnemonic for remembering the first letter of the proper names of each cranial nerve's order. On Old Olympus's Towering Tops a Frenchman Viewed Grapes, Vines and Hops.)

I. *The olfactory nerves* convey smell information to the brain. Within the nasal mucosa are different receptors which are sensitive to odour. In theory, there are different receptors which respond to molecules only of a certain shape. Thus the molecules responsible for the smell of coffee have a shape different from those which smell like peppermint; different-shaped molecules stimulate different olfactory receptors or a different combination of them. Fibres from these cell bodies pass through the cribriform plate of the ethmoid bone and synapse with neurones in the olfactory bulb (see Figure 17.22). Cells in the olfactory bulb pass posteriorly in the

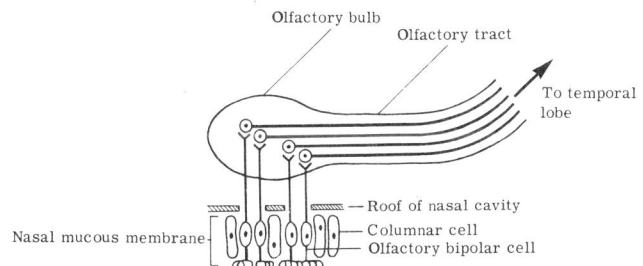

Figure 17.22 The olfactory nerve.

olfactory tract. Most of them go to the medial part of the temporal lobe where the impulses are interpreted as smell. Olfactory information is the exception, in that it reaches the cortex without passing through the thalamus. Occasionally in head injuries, the olfactory bulbs are injured and the individual loses his or her sense of smell, a condition known as anosmia. In testing smell, the individual should be asked to identify odours from samples, e.g. coffee or peppermint. One nostril is closed and the other nostril is tested. Infection can sometimes follow the olfactory pathway and infect the meninges, or, rarely, the brain tissue itself. If the frontal bone is fractured and the dura and arachnoid membranes torn, CSF may leak out of the nose. This is called cerebrospinal rhinorrhoea.

II. *The optic nerve* fibres carry visual information from the ganglion cells of the retina of the eye and pass backward through the optic foramina of the sphenoid bone. Fibres from the lateral portions of the right and left halves of the retina

Table 17.1   The cranial nerves centre.

No.	Name	Origin	Type	Enters or leaves skull through	Functions
I	olfactory	mucous membrane of nasal cavity	sensory	roof of nose	smell
II	optic	retina of eyeball	sensory	optic canal (foramen)	vision
III	oculomotor	midbrain	motor and parasympathetic	superior orbital fissure	motor to four muscles moving eyeball; motor to ciliary and sphincter pupillae muscles
IV	trochlear	midbrain	motor	superior orbital fissure	motor to superior oblique muscle of eyeball
V	trigeminal	pons			main sensory nerve to skin and mucous membrane of head (face, scalp, nasal cavity, mouth, palate); motor to muscles of mastication
	a. ophthalmic		sensory	superior orbital fissure	
	b. maxillary		sensory	base of skull	
	c. mandibular		mixed	base of skull	
VI	abducent	pons	motor	superior orbital fissure	motor to lateral rectus muscle of eyeball
VII	facial	pons	motor, taste and parasympathetic	temporal bone	motor to muscles of facial expression; taste from front of tongue; motor to salivary glands
VIII	vestibular-cochlear (auditory)	pons	sensory	temporal bone	
	a. vestibular				a. balance, position of head
	b. cochlear				b. hearing
IX	glossopharyngeal	medulla	sensory and parasympathetic	jugular foramen	sensory including taste from back of tongue and pharynx; motor to parotid salivary gland
X	vagus	medulla	parasympathetic	jugular foramen	motor to muscle of heart, lungs, alimentary tract; motor to glands of alimentary tract
XI	accessory	medulla	motor	jugular foramen	motor to laryngeal, pharyngeal and palatal muscles; motor to sternocleido-mastoid and trapezius muscles
XII	hypoglossal	medulla	motor	occipital bone	motor to muscles of tongue

pass directly back to the right and left divisions of the thalamus and optic cortex. Fibres from the medial half of the retina cross at the optic chiasma. Fibres from the medial half (nasal side) of the right retina cross to the left side, and those from the medial half (nasal side) of the left retina cross to the right (see Figure 17.23). After crossing, the fibres go to the thalamus, midbrain and the occipital lobe of the cortex. The crossover of fibres at the optic chiasma is clinically significant, for if the lesion is before the chiasma, the visual field in one eye will be abolished; posterior to the chiasma, half of the visual field of both eyes will be affected. Fibres from the retina go to the midbrain and are important in the pupillary light reflex. (This reflex and the optic pathways are discussed in greater detail in the Chapter on the eye and the ear.)

III, IV and VI. *The oculomotor, trochlear and abducent nerves* work together in the control of the eye.

The oculomotor nerve begins with neurones in the midbrain. It innervates the superior, inferior and medial recti and the inferior oblique muscles, which are all responsible for the movement of the eye. The oculomotor nerve also supplies the ciliary muscles, which alter the shape and thickness of the lens and are important in focusing the eye, as well as the muscles of the iris which produce constriction of the pupil and thus regulate the amount of light entering the eye. The upper eyelid is also innervated by the oculomotor nerve. When the oculomotor nerve is injured, the upper eyelid may droop (called ptosis), the pupil may dilate and the eye may deviate laterally.

Some of the fibres of the oculomotor nerve belong to the parasympathetic nervous system. These fibres leave the nucleus in the midbrain and synapse in the ciliary ganglion, which lies toward the back of the orbit. Fibres from the ganglion then travel a short distance to the muscles which constrict the pupil and the ciliary muscles of the eyeball.

Fibres of the trochlear nerve arise behind the oculomotor nucleus and supply the superior oblique muscles of the eye.

The abducent nerve supplies the lateral rectus muscles of the eye. Injury to these nerves prevents the eye from being turned outward, so they deviate medially.

All three pairs of nerves pass anteriorly into the orbit of the eye through the superior orbital fissure. The motor nuclei of these three nerves are connected to one another and to the vestibular system by a fibre tract in the brain known as the

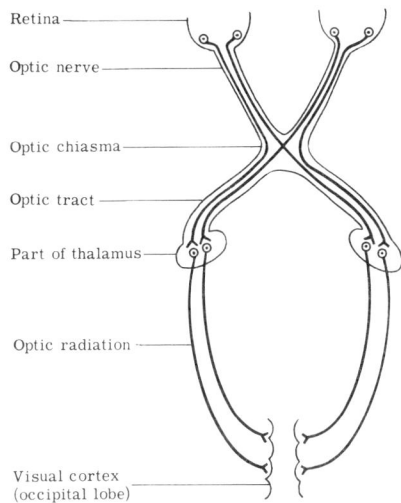

Figure 17.23   The optic nerve, tracts and radiations.

medial longitudinal fasciculus. A simple way to see if these nerves are intact is to have the patient follow the examiner's finger as he or she makes an "H", moving the finger up and down, across, then up and down again. (The muscles of the eye are discussed in the following Chapter.)

V. *The trigeminal nerve* is a predominantly sensory nerve which also contains some motor fibres. A short distance from the brain, the nerve splits into three branches.

The ophthalmic branch is entirely sensory and supplies the eyelid, the eyeball, the forehead and anterior aspect of the scalp (see Figure 17.24); it enters the orbit through the superior orbital fissure.

The maxillary branch supplies the cheeks, upper gums and teeth and lower side of the scalp (see Figure 17.24). It leaves the skull through its base, passes anteriorly along the margin of the orbit and enters the face just below the lower margin of the orbit.

The motor division of the mandibular branch supplies the muscles of mastication such as the masseter. The sensory portion supplies the floor of the mouth, the anterior two-thirds of the tongue (this does not include the sense of taste), the lower jaw and lateral part of the scalp (see Figure 17.24); it also leaves through the base of the skull.

Damage to this nerve causes sensory loss from the face and abolishes the corneal reflex — blinking with both eyes when the cornea is touched. The motor component is tested by feeling the contraction of the masseter muscles when he or she bites his or her teeth. Damage to the motor division of the mandibular branch can cause great difficulty in chewing food.

VII.   *The facial nerve* is predominantly a motor nerve with a small sensory component carrying taste information from the tongue. It leaves between the pons and the medulla, passes backwards and downwards, emerging from the skull in the temporal bone. The nerve splits into many branches which supply the salivary glands, the lacrimal glands (which secrete tears) and the muscles of facial expression. Injury to the motor portion of the facial nerve paralyses the facial muscles on the side of the lesion. Sensory injury interferes with the sensation of taste along the anterior surface of the tongue.

The motor portion of the nerve is tested by asking the patient to wrinkle up his or her forehead, to close the eyes, to close lips as tightly as possible, as the facial nerve innervates the frontalis, orbicularis oculi and orbicularis oris muscles (see Figure 7.2).

Those fibres of the facial nerve which innervate glands belong to the parasympathetic nervous system. Some fibres of the nerve synapse in the spheno-palatine ganglion before going on to innervate the lacrimal gland. Those fibres which innervate the submaxillary and sublingual salivary glands synapse in the submaxillary ganglion.

VIII.   *The vestibular-cochlear nerve* is so called to indicate its two distinct functions — hearing and balance. Some authorities call it the auditory nerve. The nerve is formed from two branches, the first of which carries sound information from the cochlea of the ear to the cochlear nucleus in the pons (see Figure 17.25a). From here the information is relayed to the thalamus and auditory cortex.

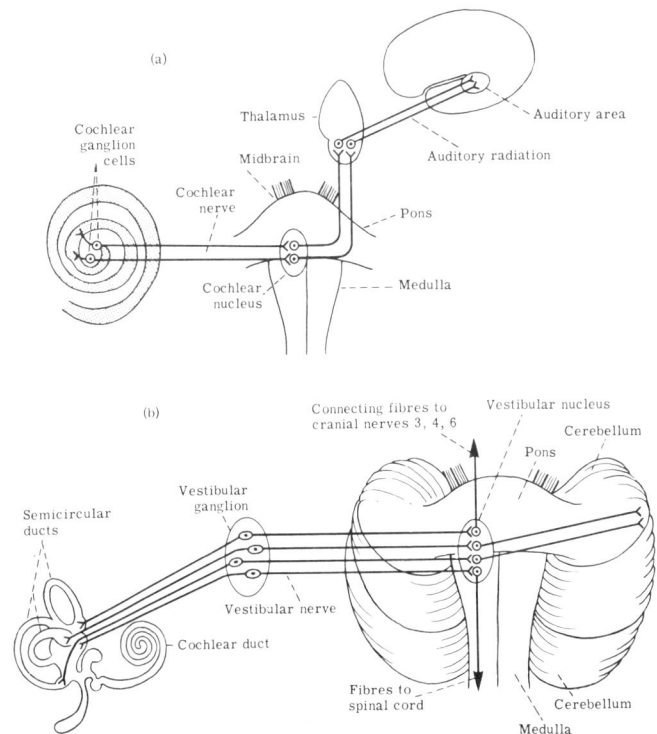

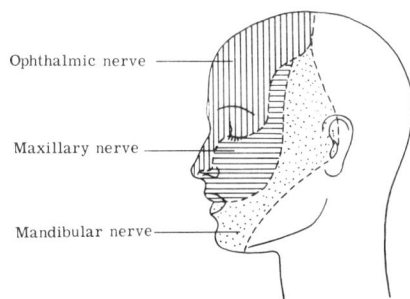

Figure 17.24   Distribution of the branches of the trigeminal nerve to the skin of the scalp and face.

Figure 17.25   (a) The cochlear nerve and its connections to the brain. (b) The vestibular nerve and its connections to the brain.

The semicircular ducts (canals) send information important in maintaining balance from the canals to the vestibular ganglion (see Figure 17.25b). Neurones from this ganglion enter the brain in company with the cochlear branch at the lower border of the pons. They synapse in the pons with neurones which make connections with the cerebellum, motor neurones in the spinal cord, or other nuclei of cranial nerves III, IV and VI. Some proceed directly to the cerebellum. (The vestibular-cochlear nerve and its connections are discussed in the following Chapter.)

IX. *The glossopharyngeal nerve* is predominantly a sensory nerve. It conducts taste, touch, pain and temperature information from the posterior third of the tongue, the soft palate and upper part of the pharynx. Information on the amount of stretch in the carotid sinus is also conducted to the brain via the glossopharyngeal nerve and its branch, the carotid sinus nerve. The parasympathetic portion of the glossopharyngeal nerve supplies the parotid glands after synapsing in the optic ganglion. The nerve leaves the brain at the medulla and passes through the jugular foramen of the skull.

X. *The vagus nerve* is predominantly a motor nerve. In Latin *vagus* means wanderer and is an appropriate name for this nerve because it wanders through the neck, thorax and abdomen. It passes through the jugular foramen of the skull and travels downward through the neck, accompanied by the carotid artery and jugular vein, and sends branches to the muscles of the pharynx and larynx. It enters the thorax and sends branches to the lungs and heart, continuing into the abdomen via the oesophageal opening in the diaphragm. In the abdomen it supplies the glands and smooth muscle of the alimentary tract as far as the transverse colon. It also supplies the pancreas, liver and spleen. There are also sensory fibres in the nerve from the larynx, heart, lungs and gastro-intestinal tract.

The vagus is an important part of the parasympathetic nervous system. The parasympathetic ganglia of the vagus are distributed in the thoracic and abdominal viscera. Fibres leave from the ganglia and travel a short distance before synapsing in the appropriate structure. Parasympathetic activity tends to slow the heart rate, stimulate intestinal peristalsis and increase gastric, hepatic, pancreatic and other glandular activity. (The parasympathetic nervous system is explained more fully in the next Section.)

XI. *The accessory nerve* is a motor nerve whose fibres arise from fibres in both the spinal cord and the medulla. The spinal fibres pass upward through the foramen magnum then loop downwards through the jugular foramen and innervate the trapezius and sternocleidomastoid muscles (see Figure 17.26). Injury to this branch causes inability to turn the head or shrug the shoulders. The cranial fibres join the vagus and soon leave it to provide the bulk of the supply to the pharyngeal and laryngeal muscles and some of the soft palate muscles.

XII. *The hypoglossal nerve* supplies the muscles of the tongue. It begins in the medulla and exits through the hypoglossal canal in the occipital bone. The hypoglossal nerve can be tested by asking the patient to stick out his or her tongue so that it protrudes in the midline.

The ability to speak properly involves the hypoglossal nerve; however, speech is a very complicated phenomenon

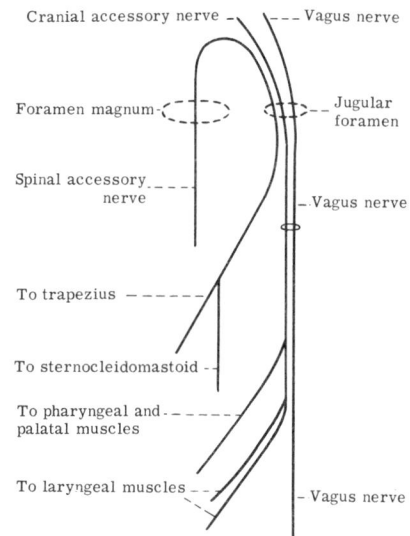

Figure 17.26 Connections between the accessory and vagus nerves.

and much more than the tongue musculature and its innervation must be intact.

B. The 31 pairs of spinal nerves

Unlike the cranial nerves, these nerves do not have individual names but are numbered according to the level of the spinal cord from which they emerge. There are seven cervical vertebrae but eight cervical nerves, as the 1st cervical nerve emerges between the occipital bone and the atlas, and the 8th cervical nerve emerges below the 7th cervical vertebra. There are 12 thoracic, 5 lumbar, 5 sacral and 1 coccygeal nerves in pairs. As indicated, the posterior roots are sensory and the anterior roots are motor. Both unite a short distance from the cord to form the complete spinal nerve. The meninges cover the roots till they unite. After the union of the roots, each spinal nerve splits into a smaller posterior primary ramus and a larger anterior ramus. In some areas, there are also branches to the sympathetic chain ganglia. The posterior rami pass backwards, branch out and supply the skin and muscle on the dorsal surface of the whole trunk. The anterior rami unite and supply the ventral and lateral aspects of the whole trunk and the upper and lower limbs. In the cervical, lumbar and sacral regions, the anterior primary rami unite on each side of the vertebral column to form plexuses. There are five large plexuses formed consisting of motor and sensory fibres which divide and join again to form the mixed nerves which distribute themselves throughout the body.

a. The cervical plexus lies beneath the jugular vein and opposite the first four cervical vertebrae and is formed from the anterior rami of the first four cervical nerves. Its superficial branches supply the skin of the neck, part of the ear and scalp. The deeper branches supply the muscles of the neck and contribute to the supply of the sternocleidomastoid and trapezius.

The most important branch is the phrenic nerve, which passes downward through the thoracic cavity to the diaphragm. The phrenic nerve is formed from branches of cervical nerves III, IV and V. Originally, the diaphragm develops in the neck and is pushed downward by the force of the developing heart and lungs bringing its nerve supply with it. This is important in the relationship of referred pain. One mnemonic with which to remember the nerves forming the phrenic nerve is: C three, four and five keep the diaphragm alive.

b. The last four cervical nerves and the first three thoracic nerves make up the *brachial plexus* situated above and behind the subclavian vessels and partly in the axilla. The nerves unite to form trunks which branch and unite to form cords, which branch and unite to form the various nerves. Branches of the brachial plexus supply the skin and muscles of the upper limb and some of the chest muscles (see Figure 17.27). Its chief branches are: the axillary, radial, median and ulnar nerves:

(1) The axillary (circumflex) nerve winds around the surgical neck of the humerus and supplies the deltoid muscle, which is the chief muscle responsible for lifting the upper limb sideways. When the shoulder is dislocated, this nerve is frequently injured and this motion is not possible.

(2) The radial nerve is the largest branch of the plexus and passes behind the middle of the humerus to supply the triceps, continuing to pass downward and supply the extensor muscles of the forearm; it also supplies the skin of the limb

and the hand, the thumb and first two fingers. Because of overlap with other nerves, injury to the radial nerve causes only a small sensory loss, which is greatest on the dorsal lateral (radial) surface of the hand. The radial nerve is most frequently injured after it has passed the humerus, so the patient is unable to bend back his hand at the wrist or straighten bent fingers, the condition being known as "drop wrist".

(3) The median nerve passes down the middle of the arm in the company of the brachial artery, supplies some muscles of the forearm and those which flex the hand and fingers and supplies the skin of the thumb and first two fingers. Injury to this nerve most frequently occurs above the wrist and results in the inability to oppose the thumb and first two fingers, and in loss of sensation from them. The thenar muscles may atrophy and become partially paralysed, and sensory disturbances in the first three fingers may arise if the median nerve is compressed in the carpal tunnel at the wrist. This is called the carpal tunnel syndrome.

(4) The ulnar nerve passes through the upper arm medial to the median nerve, then curves posteriorly behind the epicondyle of the lower end of the humerus where it is in close contact with the bone and quite superficial. Any forceful blow in this area produces pain and a tingling sensation in the little and third fingers which indicates its sensory distribution. Past the elbow, the nerve passes forward and runs down the medial side of the front of the forearm, continuing to the hand where it supplies many muscles of the hand, including the third and fourth fingers. Injury to the ulnar nerve causes inability to flex the proximal or distal phalanges of the third and fourth fingers and weakens flexion of the hand at the wrist. Because of their close anatomic relationship the median and ulnar nerves are often injured together.

c. The lumbar plexus is formed from the first three nerves and part of the fourth anterior ramus of the lumbar nerves and is located in front of the transverse processes of the lumbar vertebra.

The largest nerve of this plexus is the femoral nerve which passes under the inguinal ligament with the femoral artery and vein to enter the femoral triangle in the front of the thigh (see Figure 17.28a). It supplies the skin of the thigh and anterior and medial aspects of the leg and also the muscles which extend the leg and cause flexion of the hip — the quadriceps and the psoas.

The smaller branch is the obturator nerve, which leaves the pelvis through the obturator foramen of the innominate bone and gives branches to the adductor muscles on the medial surface of the thigh (see Figure 17.28a).

d. The sacral plexus is formed by the first three sacral nerves and by parts of the fourth and fifth lumbar nerves, and lies low in the posterior wall of the pelvic cavity. It forms the sciatic nerve which is the longest nerve in the body (see Figure 17.28b and c). The sciatic nerve leaves the pelvis via the greater sciatic foramen. It sends a branch to the gluteal muscles before descending down the back of the thigh, supplying muscles there — the biceps femoris and adductor magnus. Before reaching the lower third of the femur, it divides into the tibial and common peroneal nerve. The tibial continues to descend posteriorly, sending branches to the gastrocnemius before innervating the sole of the foot and the toes. The common peroneal descends in the lateral aspect of

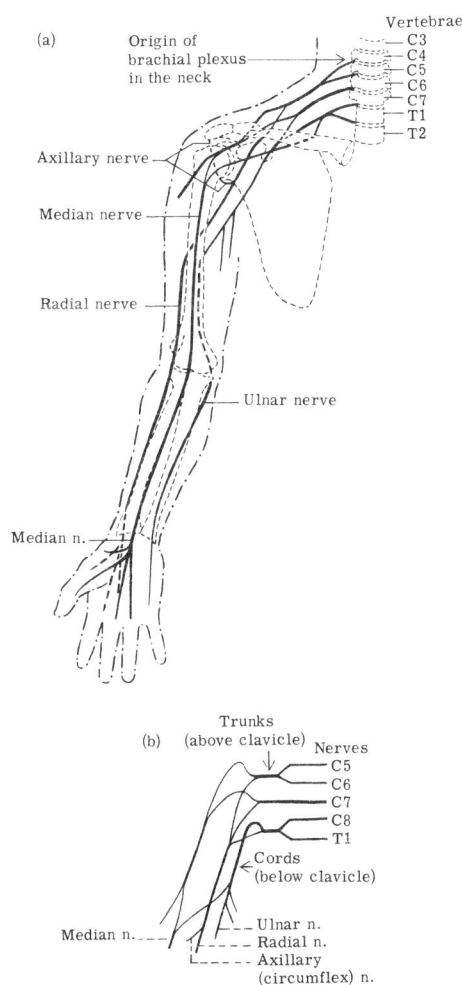

Figure 17.27 The brachial plexus nerves. (a) The distribution in the upper limb. (b) Formation of the brachial plexus.

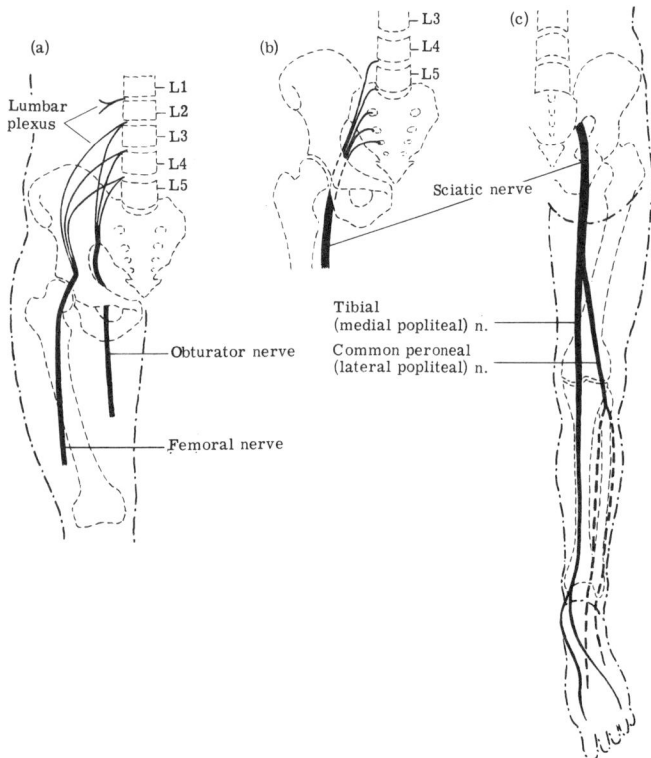

Figure 17.28 (a) The main branches of the lumbar plexus. (b) Formation of the sciatic nerve. (c) Distribution of the sciatic nerve in the lower limb.

the popliteal fossa, then curves anteriorly over the tibia and supplies the extensors and dorsum of the foot and toes. Because the nerve is quite superficial as it passes over the tibia, it is frequently injured and a "dropped foot" results. This injury means that the affected individual has to lift his foot higher than normal when walking, lest he scrape the toe on the ground.

e. The coccygeal plexus. This is the smallest of the plexi, being formed from the fifth sacral and coccygeal nerves, and supplies the muscles of the pelvic floor.

There is no thoracic plexus but there are 12 pairs of thoracic nerves. Each nerve passes to the intercostal space, then between the ribs to supply the intercostal muscles. They are known as the intercostal nerves and are important in respiration.

THE AUTONOMIC NERVOUS SYSTEM

This division supplies the heart, smooth muscles of the viscera and blood vessels, and secretory cells. The autonomic nervous system is not generally under the control of the will: we cannot will to have a greater volume of blood flow through the liver or kidneys or choose to stimulate intestinal secretions. The system functions as a regulator of visceral function, increasing and decreasing secretions and smooth muscle contractions so other systems can work more efficiently and can respond to the immediate needs of the body. Like the endocrine system to which it is related, the system helps maintain the constancy of the internal environment. Dilatation of the pupils when an individual enters a dark room, enhanced gastric secretion during a meal and

more forceful heartbeats during stressful situations are some examples of its work. Although an individual is not conscious of its function, it is extremely significant.

The basic unit of the autonomic nervous system contains two neurones. The first neurone is in the brain or spinal cord which synapses with a second neurone or neurones in a ganglion located between the brain and spinal cord, and the structure. There are two divisions: the sympathetic and parasympathetic (see Figure 17.29). Usually they are said to oppose one another, but this statement needs amplification. While the two systems usually have different effects on an organ they do work together. If you want to stop your car, you take your foot off the accelerator and then apply it to the brake; to start again you release the brake and step on the accelerator. You never step on both the brake and the accelerator at the same time. Similarly, when heart rate increases, there is a reduction in the inhibitory (heart-slowing) effects of the parasympathetic vagus nerve and an increase in sympathetic activity, which accelerates heart rate. The two divisions thus give a fine degree of control over a structure. It should be noted that the heart will continue to beat and the intestine will show peristalsis even if they have been

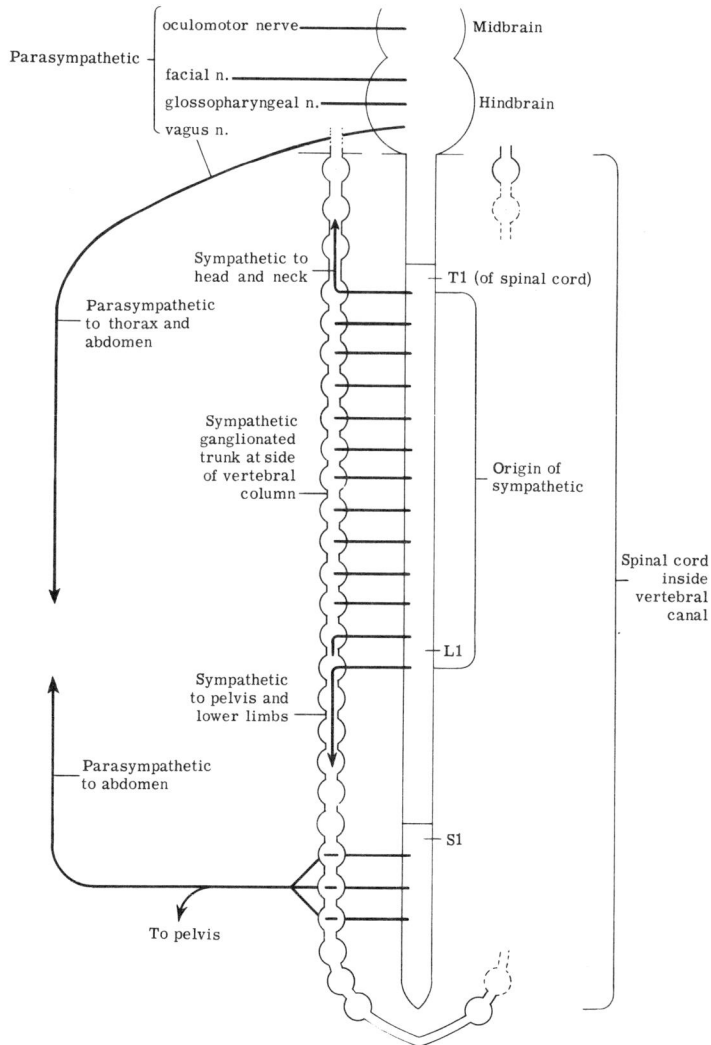

Figure 17.29 The formation and distribution of the sympathetic and parasympathetic nerves.

"disconnected" from the autonomic nervous system. This is in contrast to skeletal muscle, which will not contract if it has been severed from its neural innervation.

A. The parasympathetic division

Sometimes this division is called the cranio-sacral division because its first neurones are located in the nuclei of cranial nerves III, VII, IX and X and in the sacral division of the spinal cord whose fibres leave in the first four sacral nerves. The first neurones of the parasympathetic division have long axons which travel close to the structure they will innervate before synapsing with a second neurone in a ganglion. The second neurone has a short postganglionic fibre which innervates the structure. Both the preganglionic and post-ganglionic nerve endings release acetylcholine. Generally, the cranial division is concerned with conserving and protecting resources — constricting the pupil, increasing absorption. The sacral division is concerned with emptying the bladder, colon and rectum, and is involved in sexual function.

B. The sympathetic division

The first neurone of the sympathetic division is located in the thoracic and lumbar regions of the spinal cord. It is some-times referred to as the thoraco-lumbar division. Most fibres from these neurones travel a short distance before synapsing in one of the two sympathetic chain ganglia which lie on both sides of the spinal cord; some pass further to synapse in either the coeliac, superior or inferior mesenteric ganglia (see Figure 17.30). The postganglionic fibre then proceeds to the structure it innervates. Because the preganglionic neurone synapses so close to the spinal cord, the postganglionic fibres are longer than those of the parasympathetic system, and the postganglionic neurones more distant from the structures they innervate. This arrangement means that the distribution of postganglionic fibres is generally more diffuse than those of the parasympathetic system, whose ganglia are close to the structure they innervate. The preganglionic fibre releases acetylcholine, and the postganglionic fibre, in most cases,

releases noradrenaline. The preganglionic neurones in the spinal cord continually receive information and instructions from local and higher centres such as the vasomotor centre. Many sympathetic neurones are tonically active, con-tinuously sending impulses to the heart and arteriolar smooth muscle. Changes in their activity are important in the regulation of blood pressure and flow of blood through the viscera and skin. Regulation of flow through the skin is of course important in temperature regulation. Other fibres reach the bronchiolar smooth muscle, the intestine, bladder and sex organs.

Not only does the sympathetic division contribute to normal maintenance of vital functions, but also the sym-pathetic activity dramatically increases in times of fear, stress, pain etc. This response mobilizes additional resources and increases the level of functional efficiency so that the individual is more prepared to "take flight or fight". Since blood glucose levels are raised, and the brain metabolizes only glucose, a better description may be that the sympa-thetic nervous system prepares the individual to "take flight, fight or negotiate".

Table 17.2 The differences between sympathetic and para-sympathetic activity.

The sympathetic causes

The dilator pupillae to contract so that the pupil becomes bigger,
The blood vessels to constrict except the blood vessels of the heart and striated muscle which dilate,
The sweat glands to secrete,
The hairs to stand on end,
The smooth muscle of the bronchial tree to relax,
The heart rate to increase,
The longitudinal muscle of the alimentary tract to relax and the circular muscle to contract,
The glycogen of the liver to be mobilized,
The adrenal medulla to secrete adrenaline,
The urinary bladder to relax and its sphincter to contract.

The parasympathetic causes

The ciliary muscle to contract with the result that the lens becomes more biconvex,
The sphincter pupillae to contract so that the pupil becomes smaller,
The lacrimal and salivary glands to secrete,
The smooth muscle of the bronchial tree to contract,
The heart rate to decrease,
The longtitudinal muscle of the alimentary tract to contract and the circular muscle to relax,
The glands of the alimentary tract to secrete,
The urinary bladder to contract and its sphincter to relax.

Table 17.2 lists the differences between sympathetic and parasympathetic activity. One exception to the autonomic system in general, and the sympathetic division in particular, is the innervation of the adrenal medulla. Fibres pass directly from the thoracic region of the spinal cord to the adrenal medulla. These fibres release acetylcholine, which stimulates the medullary cells to release adrenaline and noradrenaline. The amount of adrenaline released is greatly increased in times of stress.

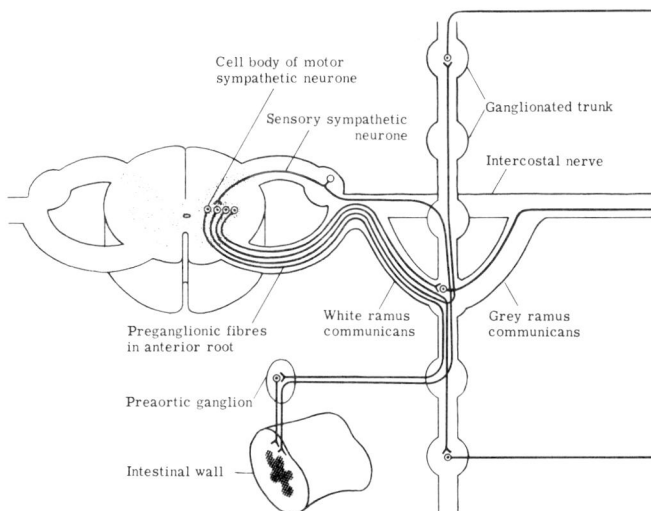

Figure 17.30 Different ways in which the sympathetic nerves synapse in sympathetic ganglia.

The example of stress also illustrates that the autonomic nervous system is "connected" to the rest of the nervous system. Although the basic unit of the autonomic nervous system consists of two neurones, the first of these neurones, the preganglionic neurone, is located in the brain or spinal cord and therefore receives inputs from many other places in the nervous system.

The hypothalamus, in particular, serves as an integrating centre for the autonomic nervous system. The hypothalamus receives information from a variety of sources including the thalamus and the cerebral cortex. Many fibres leave the hypothalamus and synapse on the preganglionic neurones of both sympathetic and parasympathetic neurones. Fibres from the hypothalamus also go to the vasomotor centre in the medulla, and fibres from the vasomotor centre to the preganglionic neurones. There are also reflexes involving the autonomic nervous system. (These will be discussed in a later Section.)

Many clinically useful drugs work at synapses within the autonomic nervous system. By blocking or facilitating transmission at these synapses, a wide range of physiological processes can be regulated. The following clinical examples help to illustrate the use of these drugs and the functioning of the autonomic nervous system:

The mucous glands of the tracheo-bronchial tree and some of the salivary glands of the mouth have a parasympathetic innervation; parasympathetic stimulation increases the release of secretions from the glands.

Parasympathetic stimulation also slows the heart rate. Prior to going to surgery many patients are given atropine or one of its derivatives as a pre-anaesthetic medication. In the doses employed, atropine blocks the acetylcholine receptor sited on the effector organ. This means that acetylcholine, released by the end feet of the post-synaptic neurones, diffuses across the synapse but is unable to stimulate the organ because of the receptor site blockade caused by atropine. This blocks the effects of the parasympathetic system, reduces glandular secretion and removes the inhibitory parasympathetic influences on the heart. These effects are useful, for they lessen the patient's need to swallow, stop excessive mucus from accumulating in the lungs and prevent any reflex slowing of the heart mediated by the parasympathetic nervous system.

Atropine has many other clinical uses and is commonly used to dilate the pupil of the eye. It works chiefly by blocking the action of acetylcholine on glands, the heart and smooth muscle; it has no effect on skeletal muscle.

Curare, which was first discussed in the Chapter on the muscular system, blocks the action of acetylcholine on skeletal muscle and causes paralysis. It does not block the action of acetylcholine on glands, the heart and smooth muscle.

The receptor for acetylcholine on skeletal muscle differs from the acetylcholine receptor on glands, the heart and smooth muscle. Though both types of receptors respond to acetylcholine, one receptor will not be significantly affected by those drugs which block the other receptor. In a sense, acetylcholine is like a master pass key that fits many different locks — it has many different effects.

The next example concerns the sympathetic nervous system. Asthma is characterized by recurrent periods of difficult, wheezing-type breathing caused in part by contraction of the bronchiolar smooth muscle which increases the resistance to air flow. Parasympathetic stimulation tends to cause narrowing of the bronchioles by increasing smooth muscle contraction, while sympathetic stimulation has the opposite effects. In an acute attack, adrenaline or isoprenaline (isoproterenol) may be given. These compounds mimic the effects of sympathetic stimulation and cause a relaxation of the bronchial and bronchiolar smooth muscle which widens the airways and makes breathing easier.

Drugs which imitate the action of the sympathetic nervous system are called sympathomimetic; those which inhibit its action are sympatholytic. This response to adrenaline or isoprenaline is because smooth muscle may contain one or two types of receptors, called alpha (α) receptors and beta (β) receptors. The events that follow stimulation of α and β receptors are listed in the Table below:

α Receptor stimulation	β Receptor stimulation
(1) Vasoconstriction. α Receptors are plentiful in the arterioles which supply the skin, stomach and intestines and kidney. They are found to a lesser extent in the arterioles supplying skeletal muscle and the pulmonary circulation.	(1) Vasodilation. β Receptors are plentiful in the arterioles in skeletal muscle and those blood vessels which supply the heart.
(2) Pupillodilation. α Receptors are found in the smooth radial muscle of the iris of the eye. When this muscle contracts, the pupils dilate.	(2) Bronchial and bronchiolar smooth muscle relaxation. β Receptors are plentiful in the smooth muscle of the respiratory tract.
(3) Contraction of uterus.	(3) Relaxation of the uterus. These effects on the uterus are modified by certain hormones.
(4) The sphincters of the intestinal tract generally have α receptors that cause contraction of the sphincter when stimulated.	(4) β Receptors predominate in the intestinal muscle (excluding the sphincters). When these receptors are stimulated, intestinal tone and motility decreases.
(5) Triglyceride breakdown leading to increased free fatty acids in the blood. Adipose cells are thought to have α receptors.	(5) Glycogen breakdown leading to increased blood glucose. β Receptors are thought to be located in the liver.
(6) Sweating in the palms of the hands. The sweat glands in the palms have α receptors.	(6) Increased heart rate. The sino-atrial node has β receptors.
	(7) Increased contractility of the heart. Both atria and ventricles have β receptors.

Drugs which stimulate the receptors are called agonists; those which prevent them from being stimulated are called blockers. Adrenaline is both an α and β agonist, whereas noradrenaline is chiefly an α agonist with very little or no β activity. Isoprenaline is a pure β agonist. Phenoxybenzamine blocks α receptors, while propranolol can block β receptors. For a drug to have an effect it must interact with the appropriate receptor. If there are no receptors or if the receptors are blocked, it can't have any effects. Thus phenoxybenzamine would have no direct effect on the heart because the heart has no α receptors. Both adrenaline and isoprenaline could stimulate the heart to increased contractility, as both can interact with the β receptors of the heart. If propranolol is first given so the β receptors are blocked, the subsequent addition of either adrenaline or isoprenaline will have no effect, as the β receptor is blocked and the agonist cannot make contact with its receptor. If a structure has both α and β receptors and phenoxybenzamine is given, subsequent addition of adrenaline will cause it to act as a β agonist, because the α receptors are blocked and only the β receptors are free. Adrenaline can reduce blood flow through the skin, kidney and intestines by stimulating their α receptors while simultaneously increasing heart rate and blood flow through skeletal muscle by stimulating their β receptors.

The possibilities are endless and at times can be confusing. They do show, however, the potential for intervention that drugs do have. By looking at the Table, you can see how many of the changes that take place when you are stressed can be related to α and β receptors.

For the sake of completeness, it should be noted that not all β receptors are alike. They can be subdivided into those which excite (E) and those which inhibit (I). The β receptors of the heart which can cause increased force of contraction, and in the liver which stimulate glycogen breakdown, are known as the β_E or β_1 receptors. The rest of the β receptors are generally inhibitory when stimulated and are referred to as β_I or β_2 receptors.

WHAT IS THE CIRCULATION THROUGH THE BRAIN AND WHAT CONTROLS IT?

A. Anatomy

Before going on, it might be good, in case you have forgotten what and where the carotids are, to go back to the Chapter on the circulatory system and re-read the Section on blood supply to the brain. To cover here in great detail the entire circulation of the brain would be impractical; however, certain points should be emphasized (see Figure 8.14).

At the base of the brain is a group of arteries forming a circle and giving off branches to supply much of the brain. This arterial circle is named the Circle of Willis after the seventeenth-century anatomist, Sir Thomas Willis, and within the approximate centre of this circle are found the pituitary gland and the optic chiasma. As each internal carotid artery approaches the base of the brain it gives off three arteries which contribute to the formation of the circle. These are:

(a) The anterior cerebral artery.
(b) The middle cerebral artery.
(c) The posterior communicating artery.
The two anterior cerebral arteries are connected by the short

anterior communicating artery. Vertebral arteries unite to form the single basilar artery. As the single basilar artery approaches the pituitary gland, it gives off paired branches which include the anterior inferior cerebellar artery and the superior cerebellar artery.

The basilar artery splits into the right and left posterior cerebral artery. Each posterior cerebral artery connects with the posterior communicating artery.

Let's try to convince ourselves that a circle has just been described. You travel up the basilar artery until it ends, and you turn right into posterior cerebral artery. Travel a short distance, then make a left turn to enter the posterior communicating artery. You travel in this artery a short distance and see where it arises from the internal carotid, which also gives off the large middle cerebral artery and the anterior cerebral artery. You leave the posterior communicating artery and enter the anterior communicating artery via the middle cerebral artery. You travel in the anterior cerebral artery to the very short anterior communicating artery, which takes you to the opposite half of the brain and the anterior cerebral artery.

You proceed posteriorly to the posterior communicating artery via the internal carotid. The posterior communicating artery joins the posterior cerebral artery, which takes you back to the basilar artery, where you started.

Blood cells don't usually follow this circular route; if they all did, none would reach the brain. However, the Circle of Willis is an anatomical mechanism that helps insure adequate blood flow to all parts of the brain. For example, suppose one internal carotid is partially occluded (blocked). Blood can enter the anterior and middle cerebral arteries and the posterior communicating artery through the anterior communicating and basilar artery if pressure and flow is adequate. (You should check Figure 17.31 to get a picture of what artery supplies which part of the brain.)

The middle cerebral artery is the largest of the branches of the internal carotid, and it runs within the lateral (Sylvian) fissure and supplies much of the lateral surface of each

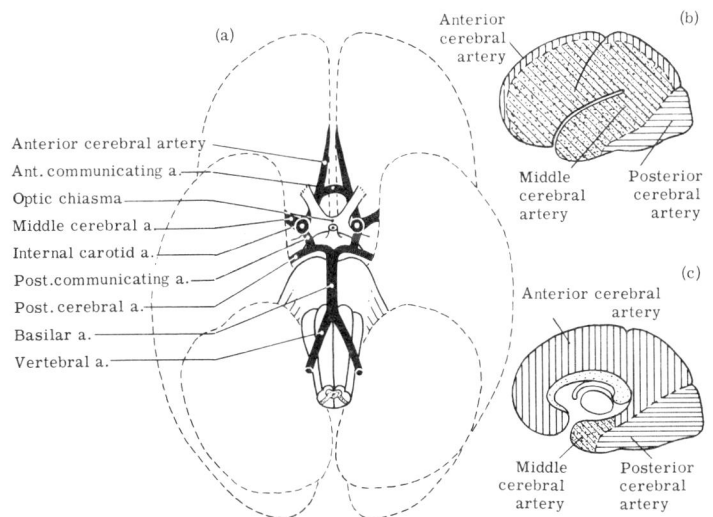

Anterior cerebral artery
Ant. communicating a.
Optic chiasma
Middle cerebral a.
Internal carotid a.
Post. communicating a.
Post. cerebral a.
Basilar a.
Vertebral a.

(a)

Anterior cerebral artery (b)

Middle cerebral artery
Posterior cerebral artery

Anterior cerebral artery (c)

Middle cerebral artery
Posterior cerebral artery

Figure 17.31 (a) The arrangement of the cerebral arteries. (b) The distribution of the cerebral arteries to the lateral surface of the cerebral hemisphere. (c) The distribution of cerebral arteries to the medial surface of the cerebral hemisphere.

hemisphere. This area of the hemisphere includes the primary motor and sensory area for the face, hand and arm; in the dominant hemisphere of the brain it also includes the speech centres. The penetrating branches of the middle cerebral artery supply much of the internal capsule and basal ganglia.

The anterior cerebral artery travels anteriorly from the Circle of Willis, enters the longitudinal fissure, then curves around the corpus callosum — that band of fibres connecting the right and left hemispheres. Each anterior cerebral artery supplies most of the medial surface of its respective hemisphere, the anterior aspect of the internal capsule and part of the basal ganglia. The area supplied by this artery thus includes the motor and sensory cortex for the leg and the foot, and the supplementary pre-motor cortex.

The two posterior cerebral arteries arise as terminal branches of the basilar artery. They first run at almost right angles from the basilar artery and then approach the medial surface of the temporal and occipital lobes, where they divide into their smaller terminal branches. Branches from these arteries supply the substantia nigra, the red nucleus, portions of the thalamus and the midbrain. The basilar artery and its major branches, the superior cerebellar arteries and the anterior and posterior inferior cerebellar arteries, supply much of the brainstem, the pons and the cerebellum.

The venous circulation was described in the Chapter on the circulatory system.

B. Regulation of the cerebral circulation

Blood flow through the brain is remarkably constant, averaging 750 ml/min. About 500 ml reaches the brain via the carotids, the other 250 ml via the vertebral and basilar arteries and their branches. One reason for this constancy is the fact that the vasomotor centre in the medulla of the brain regulates cardiac output and its distribution and is constantly informed on the brain's blood flow.

The vasomotor centre makes almost second-to-second adjustments, so brain blood flow is adequately maintained. Key factors in the vasomotor centre's ability to perform this function are the baroreceptors in the carotid sinus and aortic arch. Briefly, as blood flows through the sinus, the baroceptors will be stretched in rough proportion to the amount of blood flowing through the baroreceptors. The more they are stretched the greater will be the number of impulses generated by the receptors. Reduced flow through the sinus means reduced stretch and fewer impulses. Impulses travel to the vasomotor centre via a branch of cranial nerve IX. The vasomotor centre makes decisions appropriate to the information it receives from these receptors. Thus, if there is little flow through the baroreceptors, fewer impulses will be sent to the vasomotor centre. The centre is then less inhibited and can increase cerebral flow by increasing cardiac output and increasing peripheral resistance in blood vessels outside the brain. Thus, cardiac output could be increased and blood diverted from the viscera, so the flow to the brain is increased.

In atherosclerosis, the baroreceptors can become damaged and less sensitive to changes in flow. Patients with severe atherosclerosis often show postural hypotension; when they stand up, the cardiovascular system fails to compensate quickly for the volume of blood which pools in the legs. As a result of the fall in cardiac output, which can't be detected by the baroreceptors, brain perfusion is reduced. The patient may feel dizzy or nauseous and may even faint.

In healthy individuals, the baroreceptors are not the only story behind the constant flow to the brain. There are cerebral autoregulation mechanisms. This means that although there are changes in perfusion pressure, the brain and its blood vessels can react appropriately to keep flow constant. If blood pressure falls, the arterioles can dilate, so flow is increased, while flow may be decreased by arteriolar narrowing if pressure is increased. Even in mild or moderate heart failure, blood flow through the brain is constant.

Biochemical factors also work with the autoregulatory mechanism and influence the cerebral arterioles and resistance to flow. So it is that hypoxia and increases in carbon dioxide, lactic acid and hydrogen ion concentration (decreased pH) can all cause vasodilation. Decreased carbon dioxide can, to a limited extent, cause cerebral vasoconstriction. Adrenaline and noradrenaline have little direct effect on cerebral circulation, as there are only a few α receptors in the cerebral arterioles.

There is recent work suggesting that blood may be redistributed in the brain during talking and problem solving. The mechanism for this is not known.

C. Stroke

From the above material you should have an understanding of the mechanisms that nature employs to insure adequate blood flow to the brain. This is fortunate, for the brain does not tolerate ischaemia (a deficiency of blood). A stroke is a sudden interruption of the brain's circulation. The circulation may be interrupted by an occlusion of an artery due to a thrombus or an embolus or by haemorrhage or by any combination of them. Without an adequate blood supply, neurones will die and a cerebral infarct results. If the infarction is restricted to one hemisphere, weakness and paralysis will occur in the extremities on the one side opposite to the lesion; the affected extremities may feel numb or heavy or show some sensory disturbance. If the infarct is in the dominant hemisphere, speech may be affected. Often, if you know that and the anatomy and distribution of the cerebral circulation, you can determine where the stroke occured by observing the neurological deficit, i.e. with paralysis and sensory loss in the left leg, the lesion might be in that part of the cortex supplied with blood by the right anterior cerebral artery. (It is this artery which supplies blood to those portions of the motor and sensory hemisphere dealing with the motor and sensory aspects of the legs.)

Most strokes are the result of either a thrombus or an embolus in people with some degree of atherosclerosis. It is not uncommon for fragments of atherosclerotic plaque located in the bifurcation of the common carotid artery to break loose and lodge in one of the arteries of the brain. Hypertension predisposes to stroke.

The amount of paralysis which persists after a stroke is variable. With a willing patient and able therapists, considerable recovery is often possible.

WHAT IS A REFLEX?

A reflex is an involuntary response to a stimulus mediated by the nervous system; the relationship between the stimulus and the response is established by the anatomical connections between the receptor and the effector. Another way to look upon a reflex is to think of it as a mechanism by which sensory information quickly triggers an appropriate response. Clinically, reflexes are important because they can be used to test the integrity of neural pathways and localize lesions within the nervous system.

Although the examples presented in detail here involve the spinal cord, it should not be thought that the spinal cord is an essential component of all reflexes. For example, when you come home from a hard day at work and smell meat roasting in your kitchen, this sensory information from the nose will be relayed indirectly to neurones of the vagus nerves which in turn will stimulate gastric secretion. This may be termed a conditioned (learned) reflex, for you have learned to associate the smell with your subsequent pleasure as you eat the meat.

A. The withdrawal reflex

This reflex is perhaps the best known reflex and goes by a variety of names including the "hot stove reflex". The initial step in this reflex involves the stimulation of pain receptors, perhaps those on the hand as a result of touching a hot stove. Impulses are generated at the receptor and travel towards the spinal cord (afferent fibres) and enter it via the posterior (dorsal) roots. They synapse in the grey matter with interneurones, some of which cross the spinal cord and ascend to the thalamus while others synapse with motor neurones. Fibres from these motor neurones leave the spinal cord via the anterior root and travel to the flexor muscles of the limb. When the receptors are stimulated, the hand is quickly withdrawn from the injurious stimulus, so the reflex is essentially protective in nature.

The reflex does not involve conscious centres. An individual whose spinal cord has been completely separated from the brain will show the reflex — providing sufficient time has been allowed for recovery and the initial shock of the injury has worn off.

The fact that higher centres do not participate does not mean that they are not informed, or cannot influence its outcome. Pain receptors synapse in the cord, a second neurone crosses the cord and ascends to the thalamus and synapses with a third neurone which relays the information to the sensory cortex, at which point the individual becomes fully conscious of the pain and can localize it. Because of the number of synapses and the length of the pathway to the cortex, the reflex withdrawal begins before the individual becomes fully conscious of what is happening.

Reflex activity can be overcome however. When you place your hand upon the stove, pain receptors will generate impulses which will stimulate the motor neurones, but the higher centres in the brain will also send impulses whose effect will be to inhibit the motor neurone. As long as you choose to keep your hand there, the conscious inhibition will keep the motor neurones from reaching their threshold and prevent the movement.

Defaecation and micturition are reflexes which may be consciously inhibited. If the spinal cord has been damaged or the individual has not learned to inhibit them, the reflexes will be elicited whenever the colon or bladder are full; this involuntary action is called incontinence of the urine and faeces.

Much of an amoeba's behaviour may be predicted on the basis of reflexes — avoidance of temperature and pH extremes and attraction towards food. A person's behaviour may be predicted with less certainty, for occasionally he or she will choose to bear pain or discomfort for some higher end.

B. Stretch reflex — the knee jerk reflex

In the clinic, this reflex is commonly tested on a sitting individual by tapping the ligament between the patella and the tibia, the effect of which is to give the quadriceps muscle a short but sudden stretch. The pull on the quadriceps simultaneously stimulates the stretch receptors of the intrafusal fibres located within it. A volley of impulses is generated in the stretch receptors and travels to the spinal cord via the spinal nerves and posterior roots. Within the cord some fibres synapse with a second neurone whose fibres ascend and report the stretch to the cerebellum. Others synapse directly with motor neurones in the anterior horn which innervate the quadriceps. These neurones are stimulated so the muscle contracts and the leg kicks forward.

If either the anterior or posterior roots are injured, the reflex will be abolished. Of course, if the anterior roots are injured the muscle will be paralyzed, while if the posterior roots are injured, extending the leg will be possible, but a tapping on the tendon will not elicit the response. Often the dorsal roots and the area of the spinal cord where they synapse is injured in advanced forms of neurosyphilis. The reflex is also influenced by the facilitation of the lower motor neurones by impulses from the extrapyramidal system, and the reflex may be exaggerated if this facilitation is excessive or with certain lesions in the descending corticospinal tract.

The quadriceps muscle is not the only muscle in which it is possible to test stretch reflexes. These reflexes can be tested in muscles that are innervated by fibres from different levels of the brain and spinal cord. The Table below lists some of the other important stretch reflexes, and the cranial or spinal nerves responsible are also listed:

Reflex	Nerve responsible
Jaw jerk (masseter and pterygoid muscles)	cranial nerve V
Biceps reflex	cervical nerves 5 and 6
Triceps reflex	cervical nerves 7 and 8
Knee jerk (quadriceps muscle)	lumbar spinal nerves 2, 3 and 4
Ankle jerk (gastrocnemius and soleus muscle)	lumbar 5 and sacral spinal nerves 1 and 2

C. Superficial reflexes — the plantar reflex and Babinski's sign

Superficial reflexes do not involve muscle stretch receptors but require stimulation of receptors in the skin. The plantar reflex occurs after stimulating the sole of the foot by firmly drawing a key over the sole of the foot, in an arc, from heel to large toe. This area of skin is supplied by fibres of the lumbar nerve 5 and sacral spinal nerve 1. Although this is usually not a painful stimulus, it is usually uncomfortable. The normal reflex response is flexion of the foot and toes. The response should be the same for both feet if they are similarly stimulated.

Babinski's sign refers to an abnormal reflex in which, after adequate stimulation of the sole of the foot, there is dorsiflexion or upward movement of the big toe, fanning of the other toes and often withdrawal of the foot. Babinski's sign almost always indicates some lesion of the upper motor neurones or corticospinal tract. The actual mechanism for Babinski's sign has not clearly been worked out.

WHAT CAUSES PARALYSIS?

If you switch on a lamp but it fails to light, you are faced with the problem of determining where the fault is. It may be the bulb, the lamp, the cord, the plug or a power failure. When a muscle fails to contract, the fault may lie in the upper motor neurones in the cerebral cortex, in the muscle or at some point between (see Figure 17.32):

(1) The upper motor neurones may be injured directly because of trauma, but more commonly they are affected by stroke.

(2) The fibres may be severed or compressed by trauma or a tumour, or unable to conduct impulses because of a myelin defect.

(3) The lower motor neurones may be injured or infected. In poliomyelitis, the lower motor neurones are infected with polio virus and functionally destroyed.

(4) The fibres from lower motor neurones may be injured, particularly where they pass superficially. In contrast to

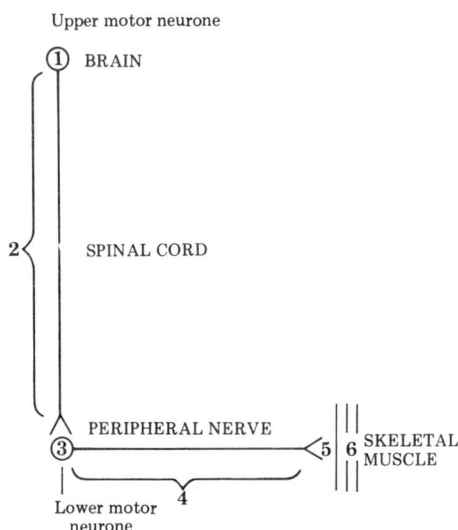

fibres within the CNS, peripheral fibres may regenerate, so some motor and sensory recovery is often possible.

(5) The myoneural junction may be affected so that acetylcholine is not sufficiently released or is ineffective. This happens with food poisoning by the botulinum toxin, or in myasthenia gravis.

(6) Finally, the muscle may be diseased so that it fails to contract in spite of adequate stimulation. Changes in the ionic environment or one of the muscular dystrophies may be involved.

WHAT IS AN ELECTRO-ENCEPHALOGRAM (EEG)?

An electro-encephalogram (EEG) is a recording of the electrical activity in the brain. Electrodes are placed on the skull and the electrical activity within different parts of the brain is recorded. Different patterns (rhythms) are recorded during sleep, dreaming, relaxing and the alert state, and the patterns are useful in the detection of some neural disorders such as epilepsy, and help in locating tumours and areas affected by stroke. In a sense, an EEG is somewhat like recording the sounds outside a giant stadium. One hears the tumult and the shouting of the thousands inside the stadium, but cannot be sure what is occurring inside. In some situations, however, an EEG may be clinically useful.

HOW DO WE REMEMBER?

Perhaps it might be better to ask: "How do we forget?" Evidence from hypnosis and electro-physiological studies indicates that we retain or store much more information than we can recall or bring to consciousness. It appears that there are two memory mechanisms; one for short term and one for long term memory. The latter appears to be dependent on molecular synthesis, for certain drugs which disrupt neuronal RNA synthesis prevent animals from remembering. Amnesia is the pathological inability to remember. There are some rare individuals who literally remember everything. This is not as advantageous as you might think. Often, when they are asked a question they recall so many facts that they fail to identify and emphasize the essential requirement of the answer. Memory is all the more amazing when you consider how quickly you locate the fact you need from among all the facts that you know. The mind's indexing system is truly phenomenal.

WHAT DOES THE BRAIN METABOLIZE?

The brain differs from other organs in that it normally derives most of its energy from glucose. Should blood glucose levels fall too low, brain metabolism is disturbed and confusion, loss of consciousness, convulsions and coma may result. Glucagon, growth hormone, adrenaline and the glucocorticoids all function to maintain adequate blood glucose. Brain cells are also unique in their great susceptibility to lack of oxygen. They will begin to die within minutes of being deprived of oxygen, so a steady flow of oxygenated blood is essential. Brain capillaries are in some ways less permeable than other capillaries of the body. When certain compounds are injected into the blood they will distribute themselves in

Upper motor neurone

① BRAIN

2 { SPINAL CORD

③ PERIPHERAL NERVE   5 | 6 SKELETAL MUSCLE

Lower motor neurone   4

Figure 17.32 Diagram indicating points of occurrence of lesions which may lead to paralysis.

all the tissues of the body save the brain; this phenomenon has given rise to the term "blood–brain barrier". The term is somewhat misleading, for the brain capillaries are permeable to many different molecules and there is also a great deal of variability of the capillaries within the brain; this fact is important for understanding the actions of some drugs which will be able to reach and affect only specific areas of the brain.

HOW DO DRUGS AFFECT THE BRAIN?

This is an exceedingly complex question without any clear answer. Not only does the brain have anatomically distinct areas, but different areas have unique chemical and pharmacological properties. Many of these differences result from the fact that different groups of neurones release different transmitters at their synapses. These transmitters include acetylcholine, adrenaline, noradrenaline, serotinin, γ-aminobutyric acid (GABA) and dopamine. One neurone releases only one type of transmitter.

Most drugs which have an effect on the brain work at the synapse. They may interfere with the synthesis, storage, release or re-uptake of the various transmitters by the presynaptic nerve endings, or imitate or block the action of the transmitter on the postsynaptic neurone. Attempts to discover and map the chemical and pharmacological anatomy of the brain are in their infancy.

In spite of our ignorance, some drugs are used with great efficacy. For example, some patients with the disease schizophrenia, a disorder in which the process of thinking is disturbed, have been helped by drugs known as phenothiazines. They are thought to influence synapses in the brain which release adrenaline, noradrenaline and dopamine, although the biochemical evidence is incomplete.

The problem of drugs and the brain cannot be restricted to a discussion of synapses. You are dealing with a person, not just a collection of synapses. Different people can react to the same drug in a variety of ways and, in fact, the same person can react to the same drug in very different ways over a period of time. In spite of the problems and uncertainties, the effect of drugs on the brain is one of the most important areas in all science. One is occasionally tempted to think that industries, subcultures and styles of life orbit around the pharmaceutical axis of the brain and spinal cord. There are drugs to keep you awake, to put you to sleep, energize or tranquilize the mind, increase or decrease the appetite, facilitate or inhibit aggression or reduce pain.

There are many legitimate uses for these drugs but the potential for abuse is quite high. In many societies, the problem of drug abuse has become a major social and medical problem. Drug abuse is a controversial area and difficult to deal with, for all too often in the past, well-meaning people have stretched or twisted facts to fit what they considered to be good ends. Until recent years, there has been little solid research, particularly in the area of neuro-pharmacology.

Finally, the problem of drug abuse is not restricted to certain socio-economic groups; in fact, the rate of drug abusers among workers in the health professions is higher than the rate in the general population. The following list of drugs is not comprehensive but it briefly covers the most commonly abused drugs.

a. Amphetamines

These drugs are classified as CNS stimulants. They can be used to increase alertness, elevate mood and can, for a short period of time, reduce appetite. Their mechanism of action is not known but they are thought to potentiate or imitate the action of adrenaline and/or noradrenaline in the brain. When abused, the drugs are usually taken intravenously or in many times the amount of the prescribed dose, and the user often experiences a brief pleasurable sensation and a feeling of euphoria. Amphetamine abusers show the property of tolerance. Tolerance means that increasing amounts are required to produce the same effect.

Methamphetamine, a member of the amphetamine family, is nicknamed "splash" or "speed", and the slogan "speed-kills" may be literally and figuratively true. In large doses, amphetamines may be fatal. In less-than-fatal doses euphoria, dizziness and confusion are produced and, occasionally, serious thought disorders may persist. Depression follows as the effects of the drug wear off.

b. Analgesic narcotics: heroin, morphine, meperidine (pethidine or demerol)

Generally, these drugs are used for brief periods under careful medical supervision for the relief of pain and, occasionally, to reduce cough and diarrhoea. These drugs have multiple effects within the brain.

With continued usage of the drugs, tolerance and physical dependence develop. Physical dependence refers to drug-induced changes in metabolic and physiological conditions which require repeated administration of the drug to prevent a withdrawal syndrome appearing when administration of the drug stops. In the case of the opiates and their derivatives (heroin, morphine and meperidine), the withdrawal syndrome is often characterized by depression, panic, painful muscle spasms, cramps, sweating and diarrhoea.

In addition to physiological changes, there are behavioural changes, so that the drug abuser cannot function unless he or she is taking the drug.

A drug addict is best defined as one whose life is centred on, or dominated by, the obtaining and using of a drug. It should be emphasized that not all people who abuse opiates become addicts, though the likelihood is great. One reason an addict continues to use drugs is to prevent the withdrawal syndrome. The reasons why the individual began using the drug in the first place are less clear. Initially, the opiates may induce a feeling of euphoria and well-being, but in many people they have unpleasant effects and cause feelings of nausea.

The opiates depress the respiratory centre in the medulla and, in large enough quantities, can cause death by respiratory depression. The non-sterile injection technique used by most addicts leads to frequent infections, and the many contaminants present in street-bought drugs add to the list of medical problems that the addict encounters.

Most of the narcotic analgesics are able to cross the placenta and enter the foetus. A pregnant addict may thus produce physical dependence in the unborn life within her. This tragedy highlights the problem of drug usage during pregnancy, and the particular tragedy of the use of addictive drugs during pregnancy.

c. Hallucinogenic drugs: lysergic acid diethylamide (LSD), mescaline, psilocybin, psilosin and marihuana

The characteristics which these drugs share is their ability to produce hallucinations, change perception and alter mood. These drugs do not create a state of physical dependence nor are they normally addictive.

Lysergic acid diethylamide (LSD) is not lethal but fatalities have resulted from traffic accidents and from successful suicide attempts while the individual was under the drug's influence. The drug may cause serious distortions of sense perception, visual hallucinations and a sense of depersonalization. Thought processes may become fragmented and irrational. Mood changes may range from euphoria to desperate panic; personality changes and personality disorders result. A person on a "bad trip" as a result of LSD ingestion needs medical attention and calm, helpful reassurance. That person should never be ridiculed or ignored. The mechanism of LSD action is not known but the molecule does share some structural similarities with a brain transmitter, serotonin. It is known that LSD is an extremely potent drug and that doses of only a few micrograms can produce significant effects.

Mescaline, psilocybin and psilosin may have effects similar to LSD; however, they are many times less potent.

Marihuana refers to parts, products or extracts of plants of the cannabis family and has a variety of popular names: Mary Jane, pot, reefer, grass, hashish, ganja, bhang and charas. Commonly, the users smoke the dried leaves of the cannabis plant, and the amounts inhaled are not sufficient to produce hallucinations. The drug is usually a mild euphoriant, with some slight sensory distortion and a feeling of enhanced sensitivity. An increase in heart rate and appetite are frequent occurrences. Individuals vary considerably in their response to the drug. There appear to be significant differences resulting from infrequent use and frequent high usage. The frequent user may suffer from intellectual impairment, show reduced productivity and have overall poorer health. There is evidence that the active agent in marihuana, L-Δ^9-*trans*-tetrahydrocannabinol, is fat soluble and is slowly removed from the lipids of the brain. With frequent usage, the concentration in the brain will build up.

The use, possession and sale of the above drug is strictly regulated by law. While the mechanism of action and some of the dangers of these drugs may be obscure and controversial, the law is usually clear and specific. Health workers should familiarize themselves with the law and its penalties. Frequently, conviction on a drug offence will seriously jeopardize the career of the health professional.

d. Sedatives

These drugs have a depressant action on the nervous system in that they reduce the responsiveness of the individual to a given level of environmental stimuli. They thus have a calming effect on the individual and are used clinically to promote sleep and reduce anxiety.

Barbiturates are a special class of sedatives and are sometimes called sedative-hypnotics. This is because in appropriate doses they may not only promote sleep but may also actually induce it. The mechanism of action is not fully understood but depression of the reticular system is thought to be involved. In high doses, the barbiturates produce an intoxication syndrome characterized by reduced mental alertness, relaxation and euphoria. In still higher doses, the barbiturates may so depress the respiratory centre that death follows. This property of barbiturates has given them the unfortunate title of "drug of choice" in suicide attempts.

Frequent use of high doses induces tolerance and physical dependence. The barbiturate-withdrawal syndrome is characterized by restlessness, anxiety, nausea and vomiting, possible circulatory collapse and convulsions.

In recent years, drugs in the benzodiazepine family have seen increasing use as sedatives. This family, which includes Librium and Valium, is apparently more effective than barbiturates in combating anxiety and is less likely to cause drowsiness. They may also be used to treat seizures and the alcohol-withdrawal syndrome.

Some idea of the widespread usage of benzodiazepines can be gained from the fact that in a 3-month period about 1 in 10 Americans will take these drugs. Overdosage usually causes a period of deep sleep. Deaths have rarely, if ever, occurred with an oral benzodiazepine taken alone. Physical dependence can take place with high dosage over a long period of time. The withdrawal syndrome is less severe than that encountered with barbiturates. Alcohol and the benzodiazepines may be a hazardous combination.

e. Alcohol

Ethyl alcohol (ethanol) is the most commonly abused drug in the world. The drug has both social uses and physiological effects. It can, in moderate doses, promote a feeling of relaxation and well-being. Actually, alcohol has a depressant action on the nervous system; this property becomes more pronounced as the dose is increased. Certain behavioural controls may be depressed and the individual may become uninhibited. In addition, speech and thought processes are slowed, and balance, co-ordination and perceptual judgement impaired.

Very large doses of alcohol may so depress the nervous system that death will follow from respiratory depression. The depressant effects of alcohol are addictive with the sedatives and opiates, so that severe depression of the nervous system may result. Mixing alcohol with either sedatives or opiates can produce a dangerous if not fatal combination.

Because beer, wine, whisky and other alcoholic beverages have such widespread social visibility, one can often forget that the alcohol they contain is a drug which, if used frequently in high doses, induces tolerance and physical dependence.

The alcohol-withdrawal syndrome is known as delirium tremens (the DTs) and is characterized by delusions, hallucinations, anxiety and excitement, trembling, fever and vomiting. Although the DTs are often the subject of humour, they constitute a medical emergency and should be taken very seriously. It is not uncommon for people to go into the DTs after they have been admitted to the hospital, as they are then suddenly cut off from their usual supplies of alcohol.

The ill effects of alcohol abuse are not limited to the withdrawal syndrome. Alcohol abuse and the associated nutritional deficiencies may cause gastritis, cirrhosis of the liver, increased susceptibility to infection or Wernicke–Korsakow syndrome with its severe impairment of memory. The alcoholic not only damages his or her own body but also frequently injures others in automobile accidents or violent acts. In addition, there is a tremendous social price paid in jobs lost, relationships destroyed and lives broken.

CONCLUDING THOUGHTS

No doubt, if you have come this far you are tired and perhaps confused. Topics like the pyramidal and extrapyramidal systems, the sensory mechanisms and pathways are neither easily learned nor easily understood. Some of the student's confusion is an appropriate response to a confusing situation. However, science has achieved a good understanding of many of the neural processes like reflexes and chemical transmission at autonomic ganglia; and yet many, more basic, processes are barely comprehended. Because of the often unsophisticated research techniques, great expense and ethical limits to human experimentation, modern research sometimes leads to a fragmented and contradictory picture of the nervous system. So far, our understanding of many neural processes approaches only their circumference; their secrets are hidden in the centre of nature's circle and freely given to no one.

18. The Eye and the Ear

INTRODUCTION

We can sometimes see the stars. Such a simple statement, yet such an incredible fact. The brightest star, after the sun, is Sirius, more than eight and a half light years away. A light year is the distance that light travels in a year. As light travels approximately 300 000 km per second (186 000 miles per second), it will travel about 9.46×10^{15} km in 1 year. If you were to see Sirius tonight, the light that would strike your eyes would have left the star more than eight and a half years ago. You will have to wait more than eight and a half years to see the light leaving the star this very instant. The wait would be longer if you wait for light from the Andromeda galaxy. This is the farthest group of stars that the human eye can see without a telescope and is more than two million light years away.

These facts tell us something about time, light and distance as well as about our eyes and ourselves. To the health professional, the eyes are important as they give him or her an opportunity to observe the blood vessels of the eye's retina by looking into the eye with an ophthalmoscope. The ability of the eye to move and its pupils to constrict or dilate provides information on the functioning of the nervous system.

We do not hear the stars. This is not because they are silent; in reality the stars are noisy and are continuously rocked with explosions, some of which last for centuries. That we cannot hear the stars without a radio telescope does reflect the distances of space and its emptiness, for sound cannot travel in a vacuum. Actually, the ear is useful in seeing the stars. The vestibular portion of the ear is concerned with balance, and it enables us to stand and look up to see the stars, maintaining our balance.

WHAT IS THE ANATOMY OF THE EYE?

In the eye, just as in the other organs of the body, structure and function are intimately united. A brief overview of the eye's functions might help make more sense of its anatomy (see Fig. 18.1). To function properly, the eye must be able to receive light and to focus it so that a sharp image is formed. The cornea and lens are important in focusing the light upon the retina, where the image is formed. Visual information must be sent to the brain; here "seeing" takes place. The retina can convert the visual image to neural impulses which are sent to the brain via the optic nerve and optic tract (see Figure 17.23). In the eye, there are also essential structures that move, moisten and protect the eye.

The eye or eyeball is spherical in shape; the diameter of a typical healthy eye being about 24 mm. The eyeball is

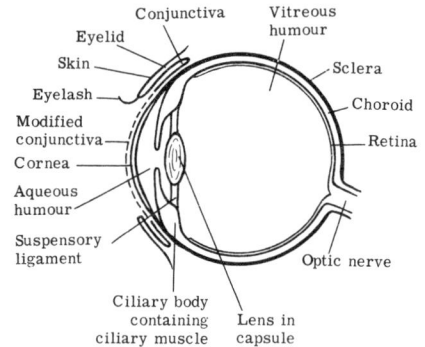

Figure 18.1 The eyeball and optic nerve — vertical section.

contained within a pear-shaped orbit. The space between the bony wall of the orbit and the eye is filled with fat and connective tissue which provide protection. In this space there are also glands which cleanse and moisten, as well as ligaments and muscles that support and move the eye.

The eyeball itself is composed of three layers and their enclosed contents. The layers are:
(1) The sclera and cornea.
(2) The choroid and ciliary body.
(3) The retina.
All three layers are not present in all parts of the eye. For light to reach the retina it must cross through:
(1) The cornea.
(2) The anterior chamber filled with a fluid called the aqueous humour.
(3) The lens.
(4) The vitreous humour, a clear jelly-like material filling the space between the lens and the retina known as the vitreous body.

A. The eyelids and lacrimal glands

The eyelids are two musculo-fibrous folds protecting each eye and giving it rest from light. The upper eyelid has attachments to the levator palpebrae superioris, a muscle that arises in the orbit from the sphenoid bone. Contraction of this muscle raises the eyelid and exposes the cornea and part of the sclera. This muscle is innervated by the oculomotor nerve (III); if this nerve is damaged, the upper lid will droop; a condition known as ptosis. The space between the upper and lower eyelid is known as the palpebral fissure. When the eye is closed the palpebral fissure becomes a slit. Muscular portions of both the upper and lower eyelids have muscle fibres which receive sympathetic nerve fibres; when the muscle fibres contract they widen the palpebral fissure. These sympathetic fibres come from the first thoracic segments of the sympathetic chain and, if they are injured, the loss of the normal sympathetic tone can cause ptosis. The eyelid also has specialized hairs — the eyelashes. A sty results when the glands of hair follicles become infected. The corners of the eye where the upper and lower eyelids join are known as the medial canthus and the lateral canthus. The small, fleshy mass of tissue which occupies part of the medial canthus is known as the caruncle.

The innermost lining of the eyelid is the conjunctiva, a thin mucous membrane which can be seen if the eyelid is everted (see Figure 18.1). The conjunctiva also covers the "white" of the eye which is formed by the sclera. Trachoma is a disease in which the conjunctiva becomes infected. This infection can lead to blindness. The disease is associated with poverty and personal hygiene; 400 million people in the world may be so infected. If a person has jaundice, the yellow colour of the sclera can be seen through the conjunctiva. The conjunctival sac is the capillary interval lying between the eyelids and the eyeball. Oedema, pallor and vascular injection can be noted by observing the conjunctiva.

The lacrimal gland lies in the upper outer corner of the orbit and is the main source of tears (see Figure 18.2). Tear formation is an almost continuous process. We are not

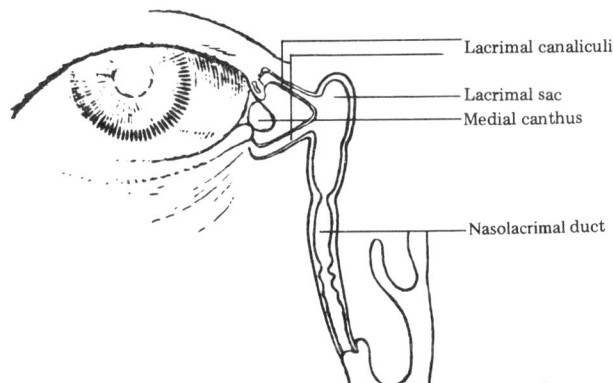

Figure 18.2   The lacrimal glands.

conscious of this because most of the tear fluid evaporates. The rest of the tear fluid washes over the eye, is absorbed into the lacrimal canaliculi at the medial border of the eyelids, then travels into the lacrimal sac and drains into the naso-lacrimal duct.

Tears function to:
(1) Provide lubrication for lid movements.
(2) Provide a moist optical surface for the cornea.
(3) Help wash away injurious agents and destroy certain bacteria (tear fluid contains lysozyme, an enzyme which attacks some of the bacterial cell walls).

When we cry, the rate of tear formation exceeds the rate at which the tears can be absorbed. The gland is innervated by both sympathetic and parasympathetic fibres. Various agents that are irritating to the eye can cause increased secretion of tears, as can emotion. In cases where tear formation is reduced, infection, irritation and injury to the cornea are common.

B. The sclera and cornea

The sclera forms the outermost posterior coat of the eye and is continuous with the transparent cornea anteriorly. The sclera is formed from dense connective tissue, is white in colour and, where visible, forms the white of the eye. The tendons of the eye muscles are attached to the sclera and, posteriorly, it is pierced by the optic nerve and blood vessels.

Anteriorly, the sclera gives rise to the transparent cornea (see Figure 18.1), which is about 5 mm thick at its centre and its shape is described as being convex anteriorly. The cornea is generally avascular and receives oxygen and nutrients by diffusion from surrounding structures. The dense connective tissue forming the cornea is made of specialized fibres which have an ordered arrangement so that the cornea is transparent because of this specialization and because of the lack of blood vessels; its transparency is also dependent on the maintenance of a normal pressure within the eye. The outer surface of cornea is lined with an epithelium of free nerve endings from the ophthalmic branch of the trigeminal nerve (V). If a person blinks when the cornea is lightly touched, you know that the sensory ophthalmic branch of trigeminal nerve (V) is intact.

The middle coat of the eyeball is the choroid, which comes between the sclera and the retina (see Figure 18.1). This is a complex, multi-layered structure, dark brown in colour and rich in blood vessels. These vessels are helpful in providing nourishment to the retina.

The anterior surface of the choroid gives rise to the ciliary body. The iris and the lens are attached to the ciliary body, which is a thickening of the choroid. The ciliary body contains the ciliary muscle, attached to the lens by means of the suspensory ligament. The 70 or so ciliary processes which arise from the ciliary body are attached in a circle behind the iris. The processes are very vascular and believed to produce the aqueous humour, a fluid similar but not identical to protein-free plasma.

The lens is a transparent bi-convex body containing neither blood vessels or nerves. When the lens loses its transparency and becomes opaque, the condition is known as cataract. The lens is formed by many layers of concentrically arranged fibrous cells, is more than 60% water and contains large amounts of protein. The lens is elastic and can change its shape when the ciliary muscle contracts. Contraction of the ciliary muscle pulls the suspensory ligament inward and anteriorly and thus permits the lens to assume a more rounded shape. Relaxation of the muscle lets the suspensory ligament draw the lens taut which reduces the thickness of the lens. These changes in the lens's thickness are important in focusing light and are part of the process of accommodation which will be discussed later. The ciliary muscle is innervated by parasympathetic fibres of the ciliary nerves.

When you say that someone has blue or brown eyes, you are stating that the individual's irises are either blue or brown. The iris is a pigmented, circular diaphragm lying in front of the lens and behind the cornea. In the centre of the iris is a circular aperture called the pupil. The iris is made of pigment-containing cells as well as circular and radiating smooth muscle fibres which surround and radiate from the pupil. These fibres have both a sympathetic and parasympathetic innervation via the ciliary nerves. Some of these muscles contract reflexly when light reaches the retina and when focusing on a near object as part of the process of accommodation. Other, more complex influences are also involved. When viewed under identical circumstances, photographs with a happy and pleasant pictorial content increase pupil size, whereas pictures of an unpleasant nature e.g. an automobile accident, lead to reduced pupil size. Contraction of the iris musculature is achieved by parasympathetic stimulation, while sympathetic fibres stimulate those muscles which cause the pupil to enlarge.

Normally, there is a balance between the sympathetic tone and parasympathetic tone. If a drug or lesion interrupts one system, the other system will act unopposed. If the effects of the parasympathetic stimulation are blocked by atropine or an atropine-like drug, the pupil will be enlarged and the retina will be easier to examine. Sympathetic stimulation or sympathomimetic drugs will also cause dilation. Dilation of the pupils is known as mydriasis; constriction of the pupils is miosis. Parasympathomimetic drugs and certain narcotics such as morphine and heroin can cause miosis. If the sympathetic nerve supply to the pupil is interrupted, ptosis and miosis will result.

The area between the iris and ciliary body and its attachments is known as the posterior chamber of the eye. The area between the cornea and the iris is known as the anterior chamber.

Finally, near the junction of the cornea and the sclera where the iris forms an angle with the cornea, there is a network of fine channels which drain into a larger channel called the canal of Schlemm, which in turn empties into the venous system of the eye. The aqueous humour is continuously produced at the ciliary processes and travels in the posterior chamber between the lens and the iris to enter the anterior chamber, where it circulates within the anterior chamber and is absorbed into the venous system via the canal of Schlemm. As is true with most other physiological processes, a balance must exist between the amount of fluid produced and the amount absorbed. Should any of the reabsorbtive or drainage channels be blocked so that more aqueous humour is produced than can be reabsorbed, pressure within the eye will increase. Any increase in intra-ocular pressure which endangers the eye is called glaucoma, which if untreated may lead to blindness.

C. The vitreous body and the retina

The vitreous body fills the large cavity between the retina and the lens and its associated structures. The vitreous body, which is mostly water, contains some collagen fibrils and mucopolysaccharide which give it the consistency of gelatin. The vitreous body transmits light rays, assists in holding the lens in place and keeps some of the layers of the retina together.

The retina is the innermost coat of the eye and is a complex structure. It contains the cones and the rods, light-sensitive cells that absorb and react to light. The cones function in bright light and are colour-sensitive while the rods function in dim light but cannot discriminate between different colours. Histologists describe a total of ten layers in the retina and a minimum of three different cell types through which information must pass to reach the optic nerve. Surprisingly enough, the cones and the rods are located in the posterior portion of the retina. This means that light leaves

the vitreous body and passes through most of the retina before reaching the light-sensitive cells.

The one area of the retina in which this is not true is known as the fovea centralis and is found within a yellow spot in the retina called the macula lutea. The fovea centralis contains a dense concentration of cones and no rods; many of the cells and blood vessels anterior to the cones appear to have been pushed aside so that light has an almost unimpeded access to the cones. Acuity refers to clearness or sharpness of vision; visual acuity is greatest in the fovea centralis, and many of the smaller eye movements are directed so that the visual image falls upon the fovea centralis.

If the cones are sufficiently stimulated, a bio-electric response will be generated which can stimulate the bipolar cells that synapse with the cones. The bipolar cells can then stimulate the ganglion cells. Axons of the ganglion cells leave the retina; for example, certain cells exchange information the lateral geniculate body of the thalamus. This pattern of cells and synapses is in general the same throughout the retina with one exception — in the non-foveal areas of the retina there is a convergence of rods and cones upon bipolar cells, and a convergence of bipolar cells upon ganglion cells. Thus, many rods and cones may synapse with a single bipolar cell, and many bipolar cells synapse upon a single ganglion cell. There are many other cells and synapses within the retina; for example, certain cells exchange information between ganglion cells. This is pointed out to illustrate the fact that the retina is not simply a passive receiver of the visual image, but an active processor of visual information.

Ganglion cells leave the retina by a single exit. They converge and leave the retina at the same point where the retinal arteries and veins leave the retina. This area of convergence, entry and exit is known as the optic disc. Since there are no receptors in the optic disc, this area of the retina is insensitive to light and is the cause of the blind spot, which is situated nasal to the macula lutea. The blind spot can be demonstrated by holding the page (see Figure 18.3) about 30 cm (12 inches) from the right eye while keeping the left eye closed. Look at the cross. You can still see the circle even though you are not staring at it. Now slowly bring it forward, then backward. At some distance, the circle will disappear because its image falls upon the blind spot.

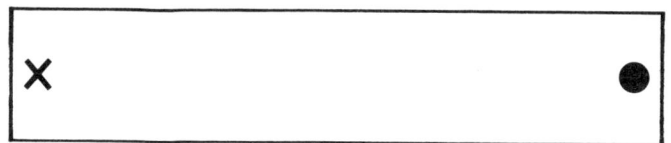

Figure 18.3 Diagram to demonstrate the optic disc.

Examination of the optic disc using an ophthalmoscope can provide clinical information. Papilloedema is a blurred or elevated optic disc caused by oedema fluid in the nerve fibres as they enter the optic nerve. This may be a very important clinical finding, for papilloedema usually results from increased intracranial pressure causing the ophthalmic vein, which enters the retinal end of the optic nerve, to be compressed and obstruct blood flow out of the retina. The retinal veins and capillaries enlarge and leak fluid into the optic nerve fibres as they leave the disc and enter the optic nerve. This causes the optic disc (papilla) to swell, hence papil-

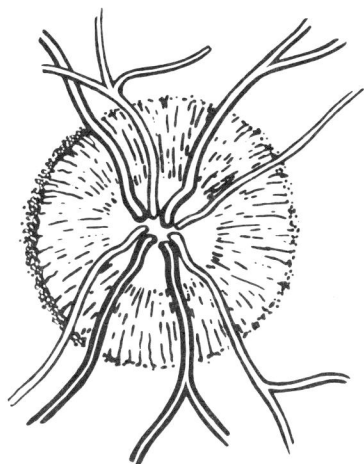

Figure 18.4 Blood vessels entering and leaving the retina at the optic disc as seen through an ophthalmoscope.

loedema. Tumours and sub-dural haematomas can cause papilloedema.

The arteries and the veins supplying the retina both enter and leave with the optic nerve. As the fundus (back portion of the interior of the eyeball) is not heavily pigmented, the blood vessels can be clearly seen with an ophthalmoscope (see Figure 18.4). The examination of the fundus and its arteries and veins with an ophthalmoscope provides a unique window through which to observe the circulatory system. The effects and severity of diabetes and hypertension can be ascertained by observing the fundus, as can information on many other diseases.

Before going on with the study of visual processes it is necessary to go over the physics of light and lenses.

REVIEW OF THE PHYSICS OF LIGHT AND LENSES

Light consists of electromagnetic energy. Visible light forms only a very small part of the electromagnetic spectrum, which includes X-rays, microwaves, radar and radio. The components of this spectrum can be described and differentiated in terms of wavelengths and frequencies. The wavelength is the distance between two successive wave peaks; the frequency is the number of wave peaks or cycles that pass a specific point in a given period of time. Frequency is generally expressed in cycles per second (cps). X-rays can have wavelengths that are 1 Ångstrom long, whereas radio waves can be more than 100 metres long. Those wavelengths capable of stimulating retinal receptors have wavelengths that range from 400 to 700 nm. (1 nm $= 10^{-9}$ metre.) Different colours of light have different wavelengths, blue being at the short end of the visible spectrum, red at the long end. Light waves are represented by a straight line drawn in the direction that the light is travelling.

The product of the frequency and the wavelength = the velocity.

The velocity of light in a vacuum is constant, but when light passes from one medium to another its velocity changes. When light travels from air to glass or water, its velocity decreases. This has important consequences and helps to explain refraction. When light passes at an angle from one medium to another there is a change in its direction; this bending of light rays as they pass from one medium to another is called refraction. The amount of refraction depends upon the angle at which the light enters the second medium and upon the physical nature of that medium. When light passes from air to glass at an angle other than 90°, it is refracted. When light enters the glass, the rays on one side of the light beam will be travelling more slowly in the glass, while rays on the other side of the beam will still be travelling at a more rapid rate in the air. This causes the rays to bend. If the light rays strike perpendicularly to the surface, they are not bent, the reason being that the rays will intersect the second medium at the same angle and will travel equal distances at reduced speed through that medium.

Lenses bend light rays towards the thickest part of the lens; the greater the curvature of the lens surface, the greater will be the bending. Convex lenses are thicker in the middle than at their edges and will therefore bend light towards the middle. The lenses cause light to converge and are also called "plus lenses". Concave lenses are thicker at their edges and thinnest in their centre. They cause light rays to diverge and bend towards the thickest parts of the lens.

The refractive power of a lens is described by a unit known as the diopter. When parallel rays of light pass through a converging lens, they are bent so that they all pass through a common point known as the principal focus. The distance between the lens and the principal focus is called the focal distance. A lens with a focal distance of 1 metre has a power of 1 diopter. The reciprocal of the focal distance of a lens expressed in metres is the power of the lens measured in diopters. A lens with a focal distance of 50 cm (0.5 metres) has a power of 2 diopters because

$$1/0.5 = 2 \text{ diopters}$$

The more powerful a lens is, the closer will be its principal focus to the lens and the higher will be its power in diopters. Thus, if the focal distance is 20 cm (0.2 metres), the power of the lens will be:

$$1/0.2 = 5 \text{ diopters}$$

The power of lenses used in most eye glasses ranges from 0.2 to 4 diopters.

Since a bi-concave lens causes light rays to diverge, it can have no principal focus. The lens's power is expressed in terms of its ability to counteract the converging ability of a bi-convex lens. The power of a bi-concave lens is expressed in minus diopters, that of a bi-convex lens in plus diopters.

The eye can be considered to be a compound lens system. The eye has one huge advantage over manufactured lenses, however, and that is the ability of the healthy lens to change its shape and thereby change its optic power. As stated earlier, the visual image must be focused upon the retina to be seen clearly. Light rays must be bent to focus on the retina, and the nearer the object, the greater the bending that is necessary. The ciliary muscle contracts when objects nearby are viewed and the lens becomes more spherical, simultaneously making the lens thicker and more convex and increasing its refractive power. When distant objects are viewed, the lens is drawn taut, its convexity and power are reduced.

If the image is focused in front of or behind the retina, vision is blurred.

WHAT ARE SOME OF THE FOCUSING DEFECTS OF THE EYE?

These defects are relatively common: the people who have been treated for them are usually wearing spectacles or contact lenses.

A. Hyperopia (hypermetropia)

This is probably the most frequently found error of refraction. In hyperopia, the image is focused behind the retina (see Figure 18.5). This occurs because either the eyeball is too short or the refractive power of the lens (its ability to bend light rays) is too weak. Individuals with this

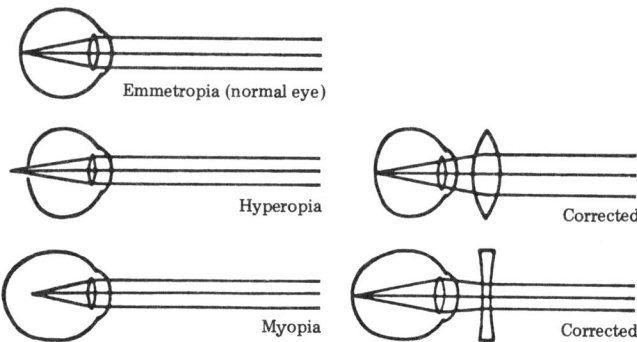

Figure 18.5   Common defects of the optical system of the eye and their correction.

disorder can focus distant objects on the retina and can see them clearly — these individuals are "far-sighted". As the objects come nearer to the eye, the light rays must be bent more, and blurring of the vision begins. This defect can be corrected by placing a converging lens in front of the eye; the lens would be convex.

As an individual ages, the lens loses some of its elasticity, and the nearest distance at which an object may be clearly seen gets farther and farther from the eye — so that reading-glasses are worn by many people over 45 years of age.

B. Myopia

Myopia is a result of the eyeball being too long or the refractive power of the lens being too great, so that even distant objects tend to be focused in front of the retina. When the ciliary muscle is relaxed and the lens is drawn taut, there is no way to reduce the thickness or convexity of the lens. Myopic persons are "near-sighted". They can focus nearby objects on the retina but distant objects are blurred. The defect is corrected by a concave (diverging) lens.

C. Astigmatism

This defect is usually caused by a fault in the cornea rather than in the lens, the result being that light rays are bent in

one plane more than they are bent in another. As an example, light rays falling in the vertical plane might be focused on the retina, while those in the horizontal plane could be focused behind or in front of the retina. Astigmatism tends to distort objects so that part of the image appears blurred; it may be corrected by cylindrical lenses placed in such a way that they equalize refraction in all planes.

HOW DOES LIGHT AFFECT THE RETINA?

This is a basic question and can be answered only partially.

A. Dim light and the rods

We do not actually see in the dark. If there is no light, there can be no physiological stimulation of the retina and therefore no vision. Most of the time we use the word dark, but we really mean dim light, as absolute or true darkness is rarely experienced.

In dim light, visual function depends mainly on the rods. Each of these long, thin cells contains millions of molecules of a light-sensitive pigment known as rhodopsin (visual purple). This molecule is formed by two other molecules — a large, protein molecule known as scotopsin, and a smaller molecule known as retinene, derived from vitamin A. (One of the first defects in vitamin A deficiency is night blindness.) There is some evidence that scotopsin and retinene have a rather close relationship. If sufficient light reaches the rods, the retinene absorbs some of its energy, undergoes a chemical transformation and changes its shape. This transformation causes the retinene to move apart from the scotopsin and generate the electric events leading to excitation of the rods and their bipolar cells. The transformed retinene proceeds through a series of reactions and is ultimately recycled back to retinene.

In the presence of continuous bright light, the close fit between retinene and scotopsin cannot develop and be maintained, and the rhodopsin is said to have been bleached. If you leave a brightly lit street and suddenly step into a darkened theatre, you are aware how difficult it is to see. The process whereby you become accustomed to the dim light and are able to see more clearly after leaving bright light is known as dark adaptation. Approximately 20 minutes are necessary for maximal dark adaptation, and part of this delay is due to the time required to synthesize and reform sufficient rhodopsin. As stated before, the rods are not concerned with colour vision. You can prove this by trying in dim light to differentiate between two objects which are identical in size and shape but have different colours. The cones do play a role in dim light vision and also in dark adaptation, but we are still in the dark as to their precise function in this situation.

B. The cones and colour vision

When sunlight passes through rain or mist, the light breaks into a band of varicoloured light known to us as a rainbow. An artist can make an infinite number of colours by mixing a few colours in different proportions. When coloured lights from different parts of the visual spectrum are put together, new colours can be produced; in fact, any three widely-spaced colours from the visual spectrum can be added together to produce all the other colours. One example: a mixture of red and green will give yellow. These physical principles are important, for colour vision depends upon the ability of receptors to respond to certain wavelengths of light and upon the visual system to process these responses so that most colours are perceived.

The cones are less numerous than the rods but they are concentrated in the fovea centralis and are responsible for your vision right now as you read this text. The difference between rods and cones is not one of shape, for the shape of the cones is quite variable, and some cones may even appear to be rod-shaped. Cones contain different light-sensitive pigments from those in rods. These pigments have a higher threshold than rhodopsin, that is, more light must be absorbed by the pigment before a change can occur and a response generated. There are believed to be three different photopigments, each residing in a different class of cone. These photopigments are like rhodopsin in that they contain an opsin, a protein which interacts with vitamin A derived from a retinene molecule. There are three different opsins and each opsin–retinene complex is especially sensitive to a particular wavelength of light.

The pigment in certain cones responds to light in the blue area of the spectrum, whereas others respond to light in the red–yellow area of the spectrum. This ability to respond to specific frequencies of light gives rise to the names — blue cones, green cones, red cones. There is a certain amount of overlap in the wavelengths to which the blue, green and red cones respond (see Figure 18.6). It is thought that the molecular response of the pigments to light is similar to that

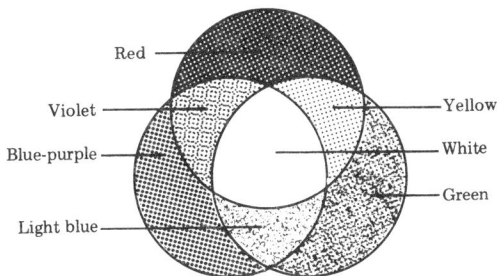

Figure 18.6 The primary wavelengths of light which give rise to the colour sensations of red, blue and green.

of rhodopsin. Of course, we do not see only three colours. The perception of a multicoloured universe depends upon the stimulation of a combination of receptors by many different wavelengths of light. A wavelength of 560 nm, for example, would stimulate both red and green cones and give rise to the sensation of yellow. The same sensation would occur if red and green lights were simultaneously shone into the retina. If all three types of cones are stimulated equally, the sensation of white results. Finally, some cones are thought to respond to light regardless of its wavelength.

These facts do not explain colour vision but are useful in understanding a part of the total process. Nerve fibres from the retina synapse in the lateral geniculate body of the thalamus. If red cones in the retina are stimulated, specific cells in the lateral geniculate body will be stimulated simultaneously. Other cells in the lateral geniculate body will be inhibited. There seems to be a complex pattern of response involving

both excitation and inhibition of cells in the lateral geniculate body.

Defects in colour vision can be partially understood on the basis of defects in one or more of the light-sensitive pigments in the cones of the retina. Colour blindness is an inability to distinguish between different colours. The defect can be classified as red blindness, blue blindness or green blindness because of an inability to distinguish among colours in the red, blue or green area of the spectrum. A classic illustration of a red blindness defect was demonstrated by a man who attended a funeral wearing a bright red tie he thought was black. Inability to discriminate red from green is the most common defect, and for genetic reasons males are affected more frequently than females. Individuals may also have more than one defect.

WHAT ARE THE OPTIC PATHWAYS?

A. The visual pathway

Light stimulates the rods and cones, which then stimulate the bipolar cells of the retina. The bipolar cells stimulate the ganglion cells. Axons from the ganglion cells form the optic nerve and leave the retina to synapse in the lateral geniculate body of the thalamus. Some fibres stay on the same side of the brain, while others cross over to synapse in the lateral geniculate body on the opposite side of the brain. Thus, fibres from the right eye will synapse in both the right and left lateral geniculate bodies (see Figure 17.23). The area where fibres cross over to go to the opposite side of the brain is known as the optic chiasma. Fibres from the lateral geniculate body sweep back to the occipital lobe and synapse in an area referred to as the visual cortex. The sensation of sight takes place in the visual cortex.

Figure 18.7 outlines the visual pathway. Knowledge of this pathway is important because a lesion or injury to the nervous system can be located from a description of a defect in the visual field. The entire area of vision in each eye is

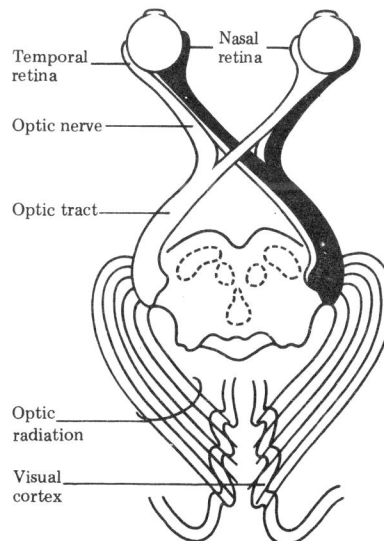

Figure 18.7 The visual pathway.

called the visual field. The visual field of each eye is slightly different. You can confirm this by looking at an object and blinking one eye, then the other. (The difference in visual fields is believed to be important in the ability to perceive depth.) To understand the relationship between the optic pathway and a possible defect in the visual field, certain facts must be clear:

(1) The visual field of each eye has a right half and a left half; it can also be said to have a nasal (closer to the nose) field, and a temporal (lateral) field. The words right, left, nasal and temporal must be used carefully to avoid confusion.

(2) Light rays cross over in the eye so that the image of objects in the right visual field of each eye falls on the left side of each retina. The image of objects in the left visual field of each eye falls on the right side of each retina.

(3) Information in the left half of both visual fields is projected to the visual cortex in the right occipital lobe. Conversely, information about objects in the right half of both visual fields is projected to the visual cortex in the left occipital lobe.

This happens because fibres from the temporal part of each retina proceed to the optic cortex on the same side of the brain. Fibres from the nasal portion of the retina cross at the optic chiasma to synapse in the lateral geniculate body on the opposite side of the brain.

Knowing these facts you should be able to predict the effect of several lesions:

(1) If the optic nerve is severed before the optic chiasma, the individual will lose the sight in one and keep the sight in the other eye.

(2) If the fibres which cross at the optic chiasma are destroyed, the individual will not be able to see objects in the temporal field of each eye. This is called a bitemporal hemianopsia and may be caused by tumours of the pituitary gland which can exert pressure on the optic chiasma.

(3) If the cut or injury is behind the chiasma on the right side, the left visual field of each eye will be lost. If the cut or injury is on the left side, the right visual field of each eye will be lost. This defect is called either a right or left homonymous hemianopsia.

The visual process is much more than a series of impulses following an anatomical path. Many unknown factors are important.

B. The reflex pathways

If an individual is seriously injured, ill or not responsive, one of the first things a health professional will do is observe and note the size of the pupils, whether the pupils are dilated or constricted and whether they are both the same size. The examiner will shine a bright light into the patient's pupils and test the visual reflexes. These reflexes can provide vital information on the nature of a possible brain injury.

When light is shone on the retina of one eye, both pupils will constrict. The response of the eye which receives the light is called the direct pupillary response; the response in the eye which is not stimulated by the light is known as the consensual pupillary light reflex. Fibres involved in this reflex leave the retina via the optic nerve, and synapse near the superior colliculus in the pretectal area. Axons from the pretectal area synapse with cells in the nucleus of the oculo-motor nerve (III) complex. Some fibres from the pretectal area cross to the oculomotor nerve complex on the opposite side of the brain and are responsible for the consensual pupillary light reflex.

The accommodation–convergence reaction occurs when you shift your focus from a distant object to one nearby. This reflex is not a true one, for components of this reaction are a willed movement. There are three components to this reaction:

(1) Both medial recti contract to draw the eyeball nasally.

(2) The contraction of the ciliary muscle is reduced, so the lens becomes more convex and better able to focus nearby objects upon the retina.

(3) The pupils constrict, reducing the light which must be focused on the retina.

Part of the pathway involves fibres going from the retina to the lateral geniculate body to the visual cortex. Fibres leave from the visual cortex to synapse in the pretectal area and the oculomotor nerve (III) complex. The pupil can fail to respond to light but responds during accommodation. This is termed an Argyll Robertson pupil and is often found in neurosyphilis.

WHAT ARE THE MUSCLES OF THE EYE AND HOW DO THEY FUNCTION IN VISION?

Although we tend to think of the eye as a sense receptor, we should not forget that it is a dynamic, active organ. As you read this book, your head is relatively motionless while your eyes are rapidly jumping back and forth across the page. Even if you stare at the stop at the end of this sentence, your eyes will make many small movements. (During deep sleep the eyes make big, rapid movements — REM.) If your eyes stop looking at this book and focus on an object across the room, your eyes move, and the reduction in contraction of the ciliary muscles changes the shape of the lens.

The eyes must not only move but also their movements must be co-ordinated precisely so that the visual image falls on corresponding parts of each retina. When the image does not fall on corresponding points, double vision (diplopia) results. You can demonstrate diplopia by extending your right arm and staring at your right finger tip. Press gently on either eyeball with your finger and vary the pressure until you "see double". Pathological diplopia may be caused by many conditions ranging from lesions in the nerves of the eye or its muscles to hypertension or tumours in the orbit.

If the centre of the cornea moves laterally (away from the nose), the movement is described as abduction; movement of the centre of the cornea toward the nose is adduction; upward movement of the cornea is elevation, and downward motion is depression. If the cornea rotates about an anterior–posterior axis so that the top part (12 o'clock) moves medially, the motion is called intorsion, while if the top part rotates laterally, the motion is called extorsion.

The annular tendon is a ring of dense connective tissue lying in the rear of the orbit. Two pairs of voluntary muscles arise from this ring and insert in the sclera (see Figure 18.8). The lateral rectus inserts on the lateral surface of the sclera and abducts the eye, while the medial rectus adducts the eye and inserts on the medial surface of the sclera. The superior rectus inserts on the upper surface of the sclera and elevates

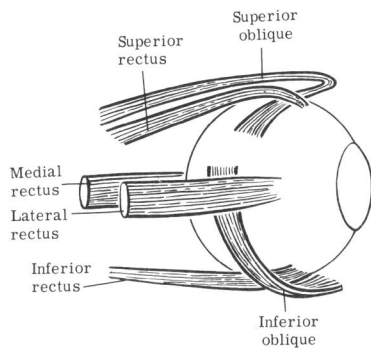

Figure 18.8 Muscles moving the right eyeball.

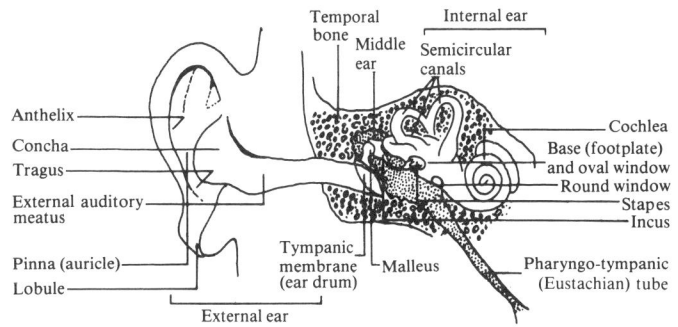

Figure 18.9 The three divisions of the ear.

the eye, while the inferior rectus depresses the eye and inserts on the lower surface of the eye.

The superior oblique arises above the annular ring and passes anteriorly near the superior rectus. Before inserting on the sclera, the muscle's tendon passes through a small loop of connective tissue which functions as a pulley and is called the trochlea. The tendon then reverses its direction to insert on the upper surface of the sclera below the superior rectus. The effect of this arrangement is such that when the superior rectus contracts, the eyeball can be depressed, abducted and intorted.

The inferior oblique arises from the floor of the orbit, passes obliquely below the lateral rectus and inserts below the inferior rectus. This muscle aids in elevation, adduction and extorsion of the eye.

Most movements of the eye require more than one muscle to contract and these muscular contractions must be carefully co-ordinated. When you look to your left, your left eye is abducted by its lateral rectus muscle. The right eye is adducted by its medial rectus. The strength of these contractions must be balanced so the image falls on corresponding points of each retina. The eye muscles are tested by having the patient keep his eye still and focus on the examiner's finger which is about 50 cm in front of the eye. The examiner forms an "H" with his finger and the patient follows with his eyes so that the eyes are adducted, then elevated and then depressed. The patient is asked if at any time he experiences double vision.

The trochlear nerve (IV) innervates the superior oblique and the abducent nerve (VI) innervates the lateral rectus. The oculomotor nerve (III) innervates the rest.

WHAT IS THE ANATOMY OF THE EAR?

The ear, like other sensory structures, must be able to receive a specific form of energy and convert this energy to neural impulses which can be interpreted by the brain. The ear is uniquely sensitive to the energy of sound waves. It translates this energy into neural impulses which give rise to the sensation of sound when these impulses reach the auditory cortex of the brain. The ear plays an important part in the maintaining of balance. The ear provides information about how the head is orientated in space with respect to gravity and provides information on movement of the head. The part of the ear which functions in balance and movement is referred to as the vestibular apparatus.

Impulses generated by the vestibular apparatus ultimately reach the cortex, the cerebellum, the motor nuclei controlling the movements of the eye, and also reach neurones in the spinal cord.

Each ear has three major parts and each of these parts is itself called an ear; thus there is the external ear, the middle ear and the inner ear (see Figure 18.9):

A. The external ear

This part of the ear has two components, an outer pinna (auricle) and a tube leading away from the pinna called the external auditory meatus.

The external ear functions to help protect the inner parts of the ear and aids in directing sound waves towards the ear drum. In man, the auricle can be moved but slightly, in contrast to many other animals who can actually point the auricle towards the source of a sound. The auricle is made of yellow elastic fibrocartilage covered with skin on both of its sides. It is a deeply grooved and ridged structure. The outermost groove is called the helix, and the depression in front of the helix is called the anthelix. The lowest part of the ear is the lobule. This lacks cartilage, is formed from fibrous tissue and fat and may be used to obtain blood samples because it is vascular and easily accessible. The deepest part of the auricle is the concha, while the tragus is a small cartilaginous projection immediately anterior to the entrance to the external auditory meatus.

The external auditory meatus is a canal extending from the auricle to the ear drum, a distance of about 25 mm. The outer (lateral) third of the canal is continuous with the cartilage of the auricle, while the inner part of the canal is formed by the temporal bone. The cartilaginous portion of the meatus is slightly curved so the auricle must be pulled backward and upward when the meatus and ear drum of an adult are being examined. This pulling helps to straighten out the canal and makes observation easier. The skin lining the meatus contains hair follicles and glands which secrete cerumen (ear wax).

The external ear is separated from the middle ear cavity by the ear drum (tympanic membrane). This is cone-shaped and is formed from three layers of tissue. The outermost layer is stratified squamous epithelium and is continuous with the lining of the external auditory meatus. The tough, middle layer is made of collagen fibres. The innermost layer is continuous with the lining of the middle ear and is formed from cuboidal epithelium. The ear drum is about 1 cm in diameter and is attached to the temporal bone by means of a layer of collagen. It provides a large surface for sound-transmitting airwaves to pound against, and these waves cause it to vibrate. The membrane is normally shiny and pearly-grey in colour, though this may change with infection and inflammation or other disease processes. The membrane and the external auditory meatus both contain a rich sensory nerve supply, so care must be taken when examining them.

B. The middle ear

The middle ear is an irregularly shaped, air-filled cavity within the petrous portion of the temporal bone (see Figure 18.9). The "U"-shaped floor and the roof of the cavity are formed by the petrous portion of temporal bone, the lateral wall is formed by the tympanic membrane, and the medial wall is formed by a thin strip of bone separating the middle ear cavity from the inner ear. There is also a small opening from this cavity into the hollowed-out mastoid portion of the temporal bone. The cavity of the middle ear is lined with a cuboidal epithelium.

The pharyngo-tympanic (Eustachian) tube opens into the middle ear. This tube is about 4 cm long and extends from the floor of the cavity into the posterior wall of the nasopharynx. From a functional viewpoint it serves an important purpose in that it is the means by which pressure in the middle ear cavity can equalize (equilibrate) with atmospheric pressure. Every time you yawn or swallow, air moves in or out of the middle ear cavity via the pharyngeal slits of the Eustachian tube. This is necessary because the tissues of the middle ear will absorb gases and a partial vacuum will develop which can hinder sound transmission.

You may have experienced a temporary, partial loss of hearing if you have ever had a "head cold" or other infection in which the Eustachian tube becomes blocked and air cannot move into the middle ear through the tube. Throat infections can spread via the Eustachian tube to the middle ear and even infect and form abscesses within the mastoid air cells which are in communication with the middle ear cavity. Treatment with modern antibiotics has reduced the probability of this happening.

In infants and young children the Eustachian tube is short, its entrance is wide open and its horizontal position hinders drainage, particularly when the infant or child spends much of the time lying on his or her back. These factors tend to promote bacteria from the mouth which enter the Eustachian tube and can cause infection within the middle ear (otitis media). The blockage of the Eustachian tube because of oedema or hypertrophy of the lymphoid tissues can cause effusions within the ear; these effusions can cause the tympanic membrane to bulge, have a dull colour and have dilated blood vessels. If the fluid persists, it can cause permanent damage to the middle ear and result in deafness. In pus-forming infections within the middle ear, it may be necessary to drain the pus by means of an incision in the tympanic membrane.

The smallest bones in the body are the three auditory ossicles, the malleus, the incus and the stapes (see Figure 18.9). These structures form a chain which transmits and amplifies the vibrations of the tympanic membrane to the oval window. The synovial joints uniting these three bones are movable. Movement of the malleus causes movement of the incus which causes movement of the stapes.

The malleus resembles a hammer with a head, a neck and a handle. The handle of the malleus is imbedded in the tympanic membrane, while the head articulates with the incus. The incus is the middle bone in the ossicular chain and is thought to resemble an anvil. It has a body and two processes and articulates with the stapes by means of its long process (crus). The stapes is the most medial of the ossicles and resembles a stirrup. The base (footplate) of the stapes fits into and fills the oval window, a small opening in the bony medial wall of the middle ear cavity.

The tensor tympani is a muscle that arises from the Eustachian tube and attaches to the handle of the malleus. The stapedius arises from the wall of the middle ear cavity and attaches to the neck of the stapes. When these muscles contract they put tension on the tympanic membrane and the ossicles, restricting their movement, which has the effect of reducing sound transmission through the middle ear (the significance of this will be discussed later).

The thin, bony medial wall of the middle ear has two openings. The upper opening is called the oval window and it is covered by the base of the stapes. Beneath the oval window is the round window. This window is covered with an elastic membrane said to "fill in" the round window like a flexible window pane. This elastic membrane is sometimes referred to as the second tympanic membrane. The oval window opens into the vestibule leading to the scala vestibuli, a fluid channel within the inner ear. When the tympanic membrane vibrates and the stapes moves inward, the fluid within the scala vestibuli must also move because fluid, unlike gas, cannot be compressed. The scala vestibuli is continuous with the scala tympani and is filled with the same fluid, which is called perilymph, a fluid similar to cerebrospinal fluid. The base of the scala tympani is the round window covered with the second tympanic membrane. When the stapes moves medially or inward, the perilymph in the scala vestibuli moves, causing the perilymph in the scala tympani to move, and this in turn causes the second tympanic membrane to move outward. The anatomical and physiological relationships between these structures will become more clear after studying the anatomy of the inner ear, and the physiology of hearing.

C. The inner ear

This complex structure is located within the petrous portion of the temporal bone (see Figure 18.10). The bone is

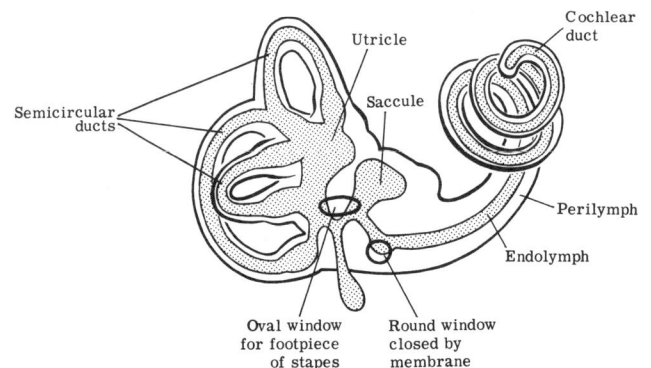

Figure 18.10 The inner ear.

hollowed out so that a complicated network of connecting channels is formed within the bone. Because of the twisting and turning nature of these channels, they are called the bony (osseous) labyrinth; the word labyrinth is derived from a Greek word meaning "maze" or "a building with intricate passages". The bony labyrinth contains perilymph, a fluid similar to cerebrospinal fluid, and also contains the membranous labyrinth.

The membranous labyrinth has an epithelial lining attached to a tough membrane of connective tissue and is a system of tubes and pouches conforming more or less to the shape of the bony labyrinth. It produces and contains a specialized fluid, the endolymph, and is attached to the bony labyrinth by fibrous bands.

The bony labyrinth can be considered to have three main parts: the cochlea, the semicircular canals and the vestibule. The cochlea is the most anterior, the semicircular canals the most posterior, and the vestibule is between the two.

The vestibule is immediately medial to the middle ear. (A micro-sized visitor could enter the vestibule by going through either the round or oval window.) The membranous labyrinth of the vestibule contains two pouches or sacs: the saccule and the utricle.

Three separate round tubes leave each utricle, take a looping semicircular path and return to the utricle. These curved tubular portions of the membranous labyrinth are the semicircular ducts, and the channels they travel in are the semicircular canals.

One end of each semicircular duct is enlarged and forms the ampulla. The ampullae contain cells which respond to movements of the head; they will be discussed in the Section on balance. The anterior and posterior ducts are both arranged in vertical planes and are at right angles to each other. The lateral duct is horizontal when the head is flexed about 30°. The utricle and saccule are connected by a small duct, and the saccule is connected to the cochlear duct by the ductus reuniens.

The cochlea is that part of the bony labyrinth which contains the structures essential for hearing. The cochlea is shaped like the shell of a snail; it is a helical channel that coils into a spiral of about two and a half turns. The cochlea is broadest at its base, near the vestibule, and narrowest at the completion of its turns, this part being termed the apex.

The modiolus is the centrally located bony core of the cochlea. The cochlea spirals around the modiolus, which contains fibres of the acoustic branch of cranial nerve VIII. Projecting from the modiolus into the cochlear cavity is a small winding shelf of bone, the bony spiral lamina. The cochlear duct is part of the membranous labyrinth and lies within the cochlea; it extends from the spiral lamina and is attached to the wall of the cochlea by the spiral ligament. There is some evidence that a part of the spiral ligament known as the stria vascularis produces the potassium-rich endolymph which fills the membranous labyrinth. The cochlear duct is surrounded by perilymph and goes up the winding turns of the cochlea in such a way that there is perilymph above and below the duct. The compartment above the cochlear duct is the scala vestibuli; the beginning of the scala vestibuli is in the vestibule near the oval window. The lower compartment is the scala tympani, whose origin is near the round window. The cochlear duct ends very near the

apex of the bony cochlea so there is no partition to separate the two scalae. This area of communication, the perilymph of which can flow between the scala vestibuli and the scala tympani, is the helicotrema. Because the cochlear duct is between the scala vestibuli and the scala tympani it is sometimes termed the scala media. It is filled with endolymph as are the other parts of the membranous labyrinth.

The floor of the cochlear duct is the basilar membrane extending from the spiral lamina to the spiral ligament and is made of a dense mat of collagen and elastic fibres. The stiffness of the basilar membrane presumably varies with the content of collagen and elastic fibres. The membrane increases in width and decreases in stiffness from the base to the apex of the cochlea. The significance of this will become more apparent later on in the Chapter. The roof of the cochlear duct is dissimilar to the basilar membrane because it contains only two layers of squamous epithelial cells. Known as either the vestibular membrane or Reissner's membrane, the roof separates the scala vestibuli from the cochlear duct.

The organ of Corti (see Figure 18.11) is the specialized receptor organ which is essential for hearing. It is a complex

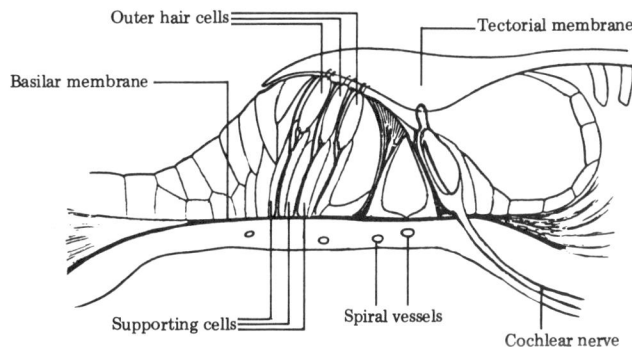

Figure 18.11 The organ of Corti.

network of cells resting upon the basilar membrane and follows the membrane up its spiralling course. The actual receptors are hair cells. The base of the hair cells is anchored to the basilar membrane, while the free surface of each cell has hair-like processes extending from it. The hair-like processes are embedded in a delicate gelatinous mass termed the tectorial membrane. Nerve endings also extend into each hair cell. These nerve endings are from bipolar neurones whose cell bodies are located in the spiral or cochlear ganglion within the modiolus. These cells are the first link in the chain of neurones connecting the organ of Corti with the auditory cortex in the temporal lobe of the brain.

Before progressing to the physiology of hearing it is necessary to review the physics of sound.

REVIEW OF THE PHYSICS OF SOUND

You remember that the sound of your voice is produced when air leaving the lungs forces the vocal cords to vibrate. Sound has its source in vibrating bodies. A simple illustration of sound production and transmission is provided by the tuning fork. At rest, the tuning fork produces no sound. When it is struck so that its arms vibrate, it produces sound. As the arms move together they produce a region in which the air molecules are pushed together into what is known as an area of compression. When the arms swing back, a region of reduced pressure called a rarefaction is produced. As the arms swing together again, another area of compression is produced. A sound wave therefore consists of a series of alternate compressions and rarefactions.

The sound waves "travel" because the molecules in an area of compression bump into the molecules ahead of them, pushing them together to form a new area of compression. Although the individual molecules travel only very short distances, the sound waves can travel for many kilometres, as the molecular disturbance is transmitted from one molecule to another. The sound waves die out only after their energy has been dissipated or reduced so that they can no longer significantly disturb the air molecules around them.

The frequency with which the tuning fork vibrates is what determines the pitch (the note that we hear). The faster the frequency of vibration of the sound source, the higher the pitch. The ear of a typical young adult can detect vibration with a frequency of from 20 cycles per second (cps) to 20 000 cps, but it is most sensitive to those frequencies in the 1000–4000 cps range. In a quiet conversation, the pitch of the typical male voice is about 120 cps, and that of the typical female voice is about 250 cps.

You can tell the difference between a piano and a trumpet even though they are playing the same note having the same frequency at the same loudness, because neither sound source, in contrast to the turning fork, produces a single frequency, a pure tone. The lowest frequency produced by the musical instrument is called the fundamental, and it is this frequency which primarily determines the pitch. In addition to the fundamental, many higher frequencies are present — they are the overtones. When two notes differ in quality they differ in the frequency and relative intensities of the various overtones. Most of the sounds we hear are not simple, regularly spaced waves of compression and rarefactions but are complex waves with many different fundamentals and overtones. The frequency with which the tuning fork vibrates will be the same if you strike it either gently or forcefully; however, the loudness of the sound will vary.

If the arm of the tuning fork moves forcefully, the molecules in the zone of compression will be more densely compressed because of the greater energy imparted to them. The sound wave will have more energy and therefore have a greater amplitude. The loudness of a sound is related to the amplitude of the sound wave. The units which are commonly used to express loudness are decibels. These units have a logarithmic derivation, with zero decibels being near the threshold of hearing. A value greater than 140 decibels can cause pain in the ear and is potentially damaging to the organ of Corti. People who are exposed to excessively loud noise can be said to live in a polluted environment just as bad as an environment filled with noxious fumes that they are forced to breathe.

Finally, sound waves, unlike light, cannot travel in a vacuum. They need a medium to travel in. The velocity of sound in air at 0 °C at sea level is 331.4 metres/s (1087 ft/s); in water it is 1500 metres/s.

HOW DOES THE EAR RESPOND TO SOUND?

Sound waves reaching the ear are transmitted through the external auditory meatus to the tympanic membrane. The sound wave has areas of compression as well as rarefaction. When an area of compression reaches the tympanic membrane, it pushes against the membrane and causes it to move inward. Some authorities claim that the membrane is so sensitive that at certain frequencies it can respond to a vibration which is less than the diameter of a hydrogen molecule. The tympanic membrane returns to its original position when an area of rarefaction arrives. The greater the frequency of the sound wave, the greater the frequency of the membrane's movement. The greater the amplitude of the sound wave, i.e. the louder the sound, the greater will be the movement of the membrane. In this manner, the tympanic membrane reproduces the sound wave. The malleus, incus and stapes transmit the vibrations of tympanic membrane to the oval window. The surface area of the tympanic membrane is many times that of the oval window. The significance of this fact is often illustrated by the pin analogy.

If you take a hat-pin or a drawing-pin and push its head against a cork board, the pin will probably not penetrate into the board; however, if you reverse the pin so that the sharp point is against the cork, and then press the pin with exactly the same force you pressed its other end, the sharp end of the pin will pierce the cork, because the force is now concentrated on a much smaller area. The large surface area of the tympanic membrane, the smaller surface area of the oval window and the lever arrangement of the ossicles all have the effect of significantly increasing the pressure (force per unit area) which is exerted against the oval window. This is fortunate, as it compensates for the increased resistance offered by the perilymph in the scala vestibuli.

When the stapes moves into the oval window, the pressure in the scala vestibuli is increased. This increased pressure is transmitted by the perilymph to the endolymph in the cochlear duct, causing a downward movement of the basilar membrane. The increased pressure is then transmitted to the scala tympani which causes the round window to bulge outward. When the oval window moves outward, these processes are reversed, the final effect being an inward bulging of the round window.

The response of the basilar membrane to rapid cyclic pressure changes caused by sound waves is complex. You will recall that the part of the membrane nearest the oval window is quite stiff, but the part near the helicotrema is wide and more flexible. Therefore, when the pressure changes in the inner ear, energy is absorbed by the basilar membrane and a wave of vibrations travels down the basilar membrane. The part of the basilar membrane that will vibrate the most is dependent upon the frequency with which the oval window vibrates, which in turn depends upon the frequency of the original sound. Movement of the basilar membrane in response to different frequencies of sound has been observed. The most distant, flexible part of the membrane near the apex of the cochlea vibrates chiefly in response to low frequency tones, while the stiff, proximal parts of the membrane respond to low frequencies but vibrate maximally in response to high frequencies. When the basilar membrane vibrates, the relationship between the hair cells and the tectorial membrane is changed so that the hairs are bent. This bending leads to the generation of neural impulses in the nerve fibres which innervate the hair cells.

This mechanism provides a means whereby the nervous system can discriminate different frequencies of sound. High frequencies will stimulate nerve fibres in that part of the membrane close to the oval window, while low frequencies will stimulate fibres in the basilar membrane near the helicotrema. These neurones will relay impulses to different parts of the auditory cortex. How the cortex interprets these impulses as different frequencies is not known. Other factors are involved. It is known that some nerve fibres respond with the same frequency as the frequency of the sound. If the sound is 100 cps, certain fibres will respond by generating 100 impulses/s. It is also thought that the numbers of impulses generated by a specific fibre increase with the loudness of a sound. Presumably, this is correlated with a greater movement of the basilar membrane and greater bending of the hairs against the tectorial membrane.

B. The auditory pathway

Impulses generated in the inner ear must eventually reach the auditory cortex. The nerve fibres which innervate the hair cells of the organ of Corti form the cochlear nerve. The cell bodies of this nerve are located within the modiolus in a ganglion known as either the spiral ganglion or the cochlear ganglion (see Figure 17.25a). Cochlear nerve fibres leave the cochlear nucleus to enter the brain at the level of the medulla. In the medulla they synapse in either the dorsal or ventral cochlear nucleus. There is much crossing over of fibres between the cochlear nuclei on the right and on the left. Cells from the cochlear nuclei send their axons across the medulla and then ascend to synapse in the inferior colliculus via a tract named the lateral lemniscus. Again, in the inferior colliculus there is a crossing over of fibres from right to left and left to right. Fibres leave the inferior colliculus and synapse in the medial geniculate body of the thalamus. Fibres also cross over and connect the right and left medial geniculate bodies. Neurones in the medial geniculate body relay impulses to the auditory cortex on the superior surface of the temporal lobe. The function of these synaptic stops in the various nuclei of the auditory pathway is not fully known, but they are believed to process auditory information — emphasize certain sounds, reduce certain others. For example, you can "hear" an orchestra but only "listen" to the violins and other instruments.

Because of the extensive crossing over of fibres in the auditory pathway, the effects of a lesion in the brain are quite different from those within the optic pathway. If there were, for instance, a large lesion in the temporal lobe on one side, the person would not be completely deaf in either ear; in fact, deafness in one ear is more often due to a lesion in the peripheral apparatus of hearing on the affected side, that is, a lesion on the cochlear nerve, the ossicles, the ear drum or even a blockage of the auditory meatus.

C. Auditory reflexes

The ear, like the eye, is more than a simple sensory receiver. It even has its own protective reflexes. The acoustic reflex helps to protect the inner ear against the consequences of very loud sound. When the tensor tympani muscle contracts, it pulls the handle of the malleus medially and tightens the tympanic membrane so it is less responsive to sound waves. Contraction of the stapedius muscle pulls the stapes laterally out of the oval window.

These two muscles work together to reduce the transmission of sound energy through the oval window to the basilar membrane. The tensor tympani is innervated by fibres from cranial nerve V, while the stapedius is innervated by fibres from cranial nerve VII. The reflex pathway has not been definitively worked out, but it has been determined that reflex contraction of these muscles is initiated by irritation of the auditory meatus, by swallowing and by loud sounds. The response time of the reflex is from 10 to 20 ms; therefore, although the reflex cannot protect against the noise of sudden explosions, it can protect when there is prolonged loud sound. Certain diseases abolish the reflex capability and the patient is bothered by the intensity of certain sounds.

A crude estimate of hearing may be obtained through use of the auditory-palpebral reflex. When people hear loud sounds, they involuntarily blink. If a person being tested hears a loud sound without expecting it and he or she then blinks, you know that some auditory function is present; however, if the person does not respond, you cannot always assume a hearing defect.

HOW IS HEARING TESTED?

Earlier in the Chapter it was stated that the organ of Corti is the essential structure for hearing. It is possible to bypass the outer and middle ears and still hear. This can be demonstrated by placing a vibrating tuning fork on the mastoid process of the temporal bone. The bone will transmit the vibrations to the inner ear, the basilar membrane will vibrate, neural impulses will be generated in the cochlear nerve, and the person will hear the tone. This can occur even though the auditory meatus is blocked and the ossicles are nonfunctional. The organ of Corti and the cochlear nerve must, however, be intact.

In testing hearing, it is first necessary to find out if the patient can hear. A patient's hearing can be tested crudely by rubbing your fingers a few centimeters from the patient's ear. Each ear is tested and the patient is asked to say at once when the sound is heard and what it is like. Should there be a hearing deficit, it must be established whether the loss is caused by a failure of sound to be conducted through the external and middle ears, or whether the loss is due to a defect in the neurosensory apparatus, namely, the organ of Corti and cochlear nerve.

Normally, air-borne conduction of sound through the external and middle ears is more efficient than bone conduction through the mastoid process. The Rinne test is used to measure the relative efficiency of two pathways. A tuning fork is gently set vibrating, and its base is placed against the mastoid process. When the person being tested says he or she can no longer hear the tuning fork, it is immediately removed from the mastoid process, and the vibrating ends are held about 2 cm from the external auditory meatus. Since air conduction is superior to bone conduction, the person should now still be able to hear the tuning fork and hear it for the same length of time that he or she heard it when the tuning fork was held against the mastoid process. When air conduction is better than bone conduction, the Rinne test is said to be positive. A person with a conduction defect will not be able to hear the sound from the external auditory meatus when he or she can hear it from the mastoid process; this is called a negative Rinne test. It should be noted that in disease of the cochlea or auditory nerve, both air and bone conduction will be diminished and the Rinne test may remain positive. Conduction defects frequently result from chronic otitis media (infection of the middle ear) in which the ossicles are damaged.

If a vibrating tuning fork is placed in the middle of the forehead, a person with normal hearing will hear the sound equally loud in both ears. If a person has a *neurosensory* defect — a lesion in the organ of Corti or cochlear nerve — the sound will seem to be louder on the side where the nerve is intact. If the person has a *conduction* defect, the sound will seem louder on the impaired side. It can be assumed that this occurs because of the masking effect — environmental noise is reduced or absent on the impaired side, and more attention can be focused on the sound caused by the vibrating tuning fork, making the sound seem louder on the affected side. This test, the Weber test, is performed by placing a vibrating tuning fork on the middle of the forehead or on the vertex of the skull and then asking the patient where the sound seems to come from.

There are many other, more sophisticated, hearing tests. It is a standard practice to test the threshold of hearing over a wide range of frequencies.

HOW DOES THE VESTIBULAR SYSTEM FUNCTION?

In more ways than one, life is a balancing act. Balance is important to the ice skater, the pirouetting ballerina and even for such mundane but complex acts as arising from bed and standing up. Balance is a sense just as seeing and touching are. We really become conscious of it only when we "lose our balance" and fall or can't get up. Balance is a complex sense, as information from many different receptors is involved — the eye, touch and pressure receptors as well as the proprioceptors all contribute to it. Receptors in the semicircular ducts provide information which is uniquely important in maintaining a sense of balance. Information from all receptors must ultimately be relayed to the muscles.

Factors other than the large muscles of the limbs and trunk are important in balance. The muscles of the neck and those which move the eyes are likewise essential. These movements ensure that there is some stability to the visual world we see and that our vision, which depends on the movements of the head and eyes, is "balanced" and also appropriate to our posture and our actions.

A. The semicircular ducts and angular acceleration

Acceleration refers to a change in velocity. If you are running at a constant rate of speed you are moving but you are not accelerating. Positive acceleration occurs from the time you start to run till the time you run at a constant rate; negative

acceleration occurs from the time you decrease your rate of speed till the time you stop running.

Angular motion is motion that is not in a straight line. An example of angular motion with which you are familiar is the spinning of a record on a record player; this is angular motion in a horizontal plane. You will note that the velocity of angular motion is not expressed in miles or kilometres per unit of time but in revolutions per unit of time. Thus, the speed of a record may be $33\frac{1}{3}$ revolutions per minute (rpm) or the speed may be 45 rpm. The record undergoes angular acceleration when you turn the record player on or off but not when the record is turning at a constant speed.

If you turn cartwheels you undergo angular acceleration in a transverse plane, while you experience angular rotation in a medial plane when you turn somersaults head over heels; turning around can constitute angular acceleration in a horizontal plane.

The gross anatomy of the semicircular canals and the semicircular ducts contained within them was discussed earlier in the Section on the inner ear. You will recall that each ear has three semicircular ducts filled with endolymph and that each duct is perpendicular to the other two ducts. This arrangement enables the ear to respond to rotation in all planes.

The actual receptor for rotation is in the ampulla, the enlargement of the semicircular duct before it returns to the utricle. On the wall of each ampulla is a transverse ridge of neuro-epithelial cells, the crista. These cells have hairs projecting into a gelatinous structure, the cupula. On both sides of the crista and the cupula is the endolymph. The hair cells of the crista are innervated by fibres forming the vestibular portion of cranial nerve VIII (see Figure 18.12). Bending of the hairs of the cells in the crista in one direction

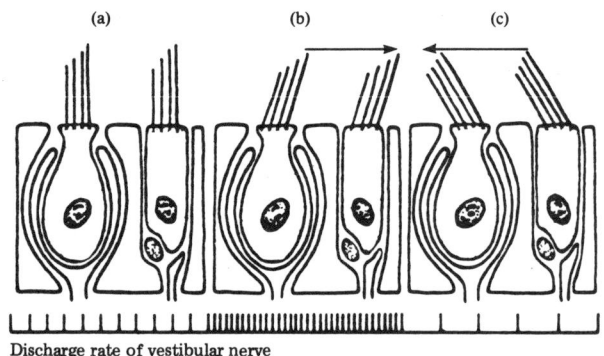

Discharge rate of vestibular nerve

Figure 18.12 The relation between the position of hairs and activity in the different nerve. (a) Resting state, (b) Movement in one direction, (c) Movement in the opposite direction.

stimulates the cells and leads to an increased number of impulses in fibres of the vestibular nerve. Bending of the hairs of the same cells in the opposite direction leads to a reduction in the number of impulses generated by the hair cells, and to fewer impulses travelling down the vestibular branch of cranial nerve VIII.

B. Physiology of the canals

Because of the complexity of the anatomy, it might be best to concentrate on one pair of semicircular ducts — the horizontal ducts in the right and left inner ear. Although these two ducts are orientated in the same plane, their response to rotation in a horizontal plane is not identical.

To understand why the hair cells of the crista are bent during angular acceleration, you have to recall the property of inertia. In physics, inertia is the tendency of a body at rest to remain at rest or, if moving, to keep moving in the same direction unless acted upon by some external force. When you are riding in a car that is brought to a sudden stop, you continue moving because of your inertia, until you are stopped. When you rotate or turn your head to the right, your head and the cristae of the ampullae also move to the right. The crista and the cupula are surrounded by the liquid endolymph.

When the head rotates, the endolymph does not immediately move, because of its inertia, and is displaced in the direction opposite to the direction of rotation. If you rotate to the right, the endolymph is displaced to the left. This movement causes the endolymph to press against the hair cells and to bend the cells to the left. The hair cells of the crista in the right horizontal ampulla will be bent toward the midline, while those in the left horizontal ampulla will be bent away from the midline. The hair cells in the right crista will generate more impulses, while those in the left crista will generate fewer. The brain will interpret the increased response from the right ear and the decreased response from the left as rotation to the right.

As the acceleration is reduced, the crista and cupula will return to their original position, and the rate of discharge from their hair cells will return to its original resting level of discharge. When the rotation stops, the inertia of the endolymph will carry it in the direction of the rotation. This will cause the hair cells and cupula in the left ampulla to be bent toward the midline, and those in the right ampulla away from the midline. The left ampulla will generate more impulses, the right fewer. The brain interprets this differential discharge as rotation to the left.

Evidence for this comes from observing the optic nystagmus. The optic nystagmus has two components: a rapid motion in one direction and a slow motion in the opposite direction. When an individual rotates to the right, the eyes will rapidly jerk to the right, fix on a point and slowly move to the left, then rapidly jerk to the right again. This occurs during the acceleration phase of the rotation. These eye movements are not caused by visual cues because they occur in blind persons. They also take place when the person has suddenly stopped rotating — post-rotatory nystagmus. These eye movements are caused, in part, by the movement of the endolymph and by subsequent bending of the hair cells in the ampulla. You can demonstrate this by having someone spin slowly in a swivel-chair for less than a minute, then suddenly stopping the chair and observing the movement of the person's eye. The fast component of the nystagmus will be in the direction opposite to that of the rotation. Thus, after rotation to the right, the rapid component of the nystagmus will be to the left, while the displacement of the endolymph will be to the right.

Immediately after rotation has stopped, the individual may still experience the sensation of rotation. Vertigo is the sensation of rotation in the absence of actual rotation and may be accompanied by nausea and vomiting. Stimulation of the semicircular ducts can cause vertigo. To avoid vertigo,

the individual should not try to stand up immediately after rotating in a chair, because the labyrinth is signalling the muscles that rotation is taking place. The person's postural adjustments will be inappropriate to his position and actions. The cause of this is the inertia of the endolymph which bends the hair cells in the crista.

The semicircular ducts can be stimulated without rotation by simply irrigating the external auditory meatus with either hot or cold water. The temperature differential between the water and the endolymph in the inner ear will cause currents in the endolymph which will bend the hair cells of the crista.

The previous examples have shown rotation in a horizontal plane which leads to maximal stimulation of the ducts located in a horizontal plane. Rotation causes maximal stimulation of the ducts which are most nearly in the plane of rotation.

C. The anatomy and physiology of the utricles

These structures are not as complicated as the ducts, and their function is more straightforward. The macula which lines part of the utricle contains the sensory apparatus of that structure. It is similar to the organ of Corti, as it contains many neuro-epithelial cells with hair-like projections. There is no tectorial membrane, however, for the hair cells are embedded in a gelatinous membrane containing dense particles of calcium carbonate called otoliths. The orientation of the hair cells is not in a single plane but in virtually every axis. The relationship between the otoliths and the macula has been compared to that between stones resting upon a plate. If the plate is tilted with respect to gravity, the stones will slide downhill. Similarly, if the plate is suddenly pulled forward, the inertia of the stones will displace them in a direction opposite to the plate's acceleration. Because gravity is a constantly acting force, some otoliths will always be pressing down on the hairs of the neuro-epithelial cells of the macula. This bending of the hairs causes impulses to be generated by the cells and be conducted down the vestibular branch of cranial nerve VIII. When the head is tilted, there is movement of the otoliths and different receptors or cells in the macula are stimulated.

The same happens when the head is accelerated in a straight line — the otoliths are displaced in a direction opposite to the acceleration, and different receptors are stimulated. Information from these receptors ultimately reaches skeletal muscle, so the appropriate postural adjustments are made. Because of the responses of the macula to changes in gravitational forces (linear acceleration), the head is always able to know its position.

The saccule has a macula-like structure but the function of the saccule is not known.

D. The vestibular pathway

The fibres which innervate the crista of the semicircular ducts and the macula of the utricle have their cell bodies in the vestibular ganglion located at the inner end of the inner auditory meatus. Fibres of the vestibular nerve leave the temporal bone by passing through the meatus to enter the brainstem with acoustic fibres of cranial nerve VIII (see Figure 17.25b). Within the brain, most of these fibres ascend or descend a short distance before synapsing in one of four nuclei: the superior, lateral, medial or inferior (spinal) vestibular nucleus. The connections of all these nuclei are beyond the scope of this book; however, some of them should be mentioned:

(1) Many fibres from the vestibular nuclei project to the nuclei in the cerebellum which are involved with such muscular co-ordination as help to maintain equilibrium.

(2) Fibres from the lateral vestibular nucleus descend in the brain stem and spinal cord as the lateral vestibulo-spinal tract. This tract is believed to exert a facilitory influence chiefly on the motor neurones innervating the extensor muscles. In this way the vestibular apparatus, which detects whether or not the body is balanced, can exert influence on those muscles which can maintain or restore upright posture.

(3) Fibres from the vestibular nuclei join the medial longitudinal fasiculus (MLF). This tract co-ordinates and connects the motor nuclei of the oculomotor (III), trochlear (IV) and abducent (VI) nerves, and many of the neck and some of the trunk muscles. In this way, balance information is sent to those structures which move the head and the eyes. The optic nystagmus is also controlled through this pathway.

(4) Some fibres from the vestibular nuclei synapse in the reticular formation and others in the thalamus.

19. The Skin

INTRODUCTION

It may seem strange to find a medical text-book that ends with a Chapter on the skin. Logic could have it that, since the skin is the outermost organ, it is the logical place to begin, not end. One might think that, inasmuch as the skin is an outer covering, it is itself almost superfluous, something like the wrapper on a bar of soap. Many advertisements convey the impression that the skin is only of cosmetic importance — to be lightened or darkened, powdered and scented — and that failure to do so leads to a lifetime of pimples, wrinkles and unhappiness. Wherever there is an anatomical structure there is a function and many substantial reasons why. The skin is presented at the end of this book because it cannot be properly understood without some understanding of the body systems heretofore discussed.

The skin, like the eye and the ear, can be considered a sense organ, as it is crowded with sense receptors providing information on touch, pressure, pain and temperature. The colour and texture of the skin are influenced by hormones and the skin also produces hormones. The skin plays a role in homeostasis, particularly in the regulation of temperature and in the maintenance of a constant internal environment.

Finally, there are diseases unique to the skin and changes in the skin that are responses to systemic diseases.

WHAT IS THE ANATOMY OF THE SKIN?

In a typical 70 kg adult there are almost 2 m^2 of skin. The total weight of the skin even exceeds that of the liver. The skin is formed from two layers; the epidermis and the dermis (see Figure 19.1). Skin is classified as either thick skin or thin skin. Thick skin is found on the palms of the hands and the soles of the feet; thin skin covers the rest of the body.

A. The epidermis

This is the outer, thinner part of the skin. In thin skin, there are four layers:

(1) The stratum germinativum (basal cell layer).
(2) The stratum spinosum (malphigian cell layer).
(3) The stratum granulosum (granular cell layer).
(4) The stratum corneum (horny layer).

Thick skin also contains the stratum lucidum, a thin homogeneous layer between the stratum corneum and the stratum granulosum (see Figure 19.2).

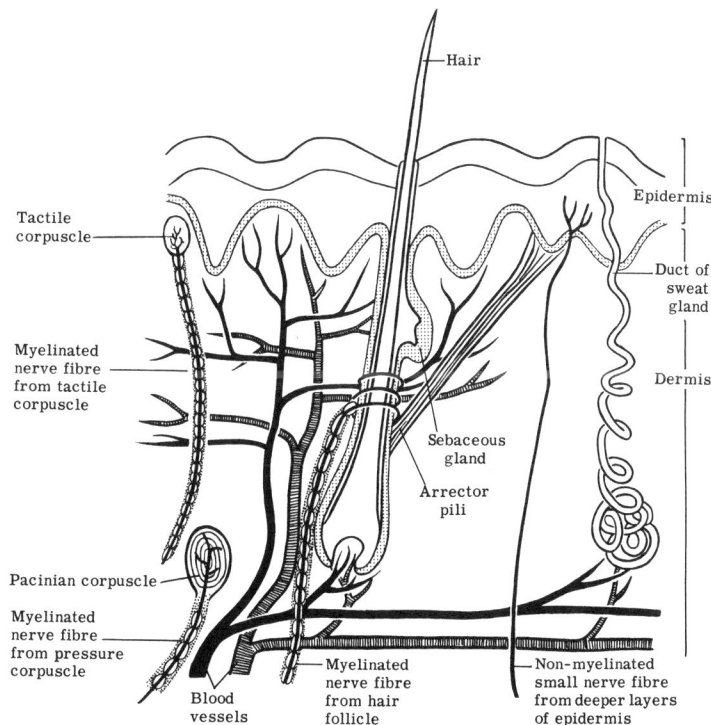

Figure 19.1 Cross-section through the skin.

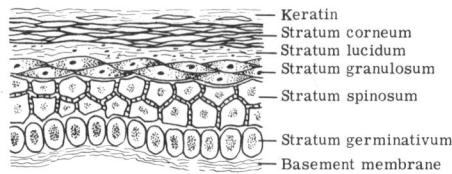

Figure 19.2 Compound (stratified) epithelia.

To understand the histology of the skin, it is necessary to understand the process of keratinization. Keratin is a tough, fibrous protein found in the epidermis, predominantly in its outer layer, the stratum corneum. Because keratin is relatively waterproof, it prevents the body fluids from leaking out of the body and helps keep water from entering the body through the skin. It protects the underlying epithelial tissues and offers a relatively impermeable barrier against bacterial invasion. Keratinization is a form of cell differentiation in which metabolically active epithelial cells pass through a series of chemical, structural and physiological changes to become inert and filled with keratin. The cells which form keratin are the keratinocytes, and the process of keratinization begins in the stratum germinativum.

The stratum germinativum is the deepest layer of the epidermis, rests upon the dermis and contains two important types of cells, the keratinocyte and the melanocyte. The keratinocytes in the stratum germinativum have a high degree of mitotic activity. Keratinocytes formed from this mitotic activity are pushed upward into the stratum spinosum. The cells in the stratum spinosum contain tonofibrils, which are condensations of protein fibrils that have been synthesized by the keratinocyte and are believed to be the first stage in the development of keratin. As cells are pushed from the stratum spinosum into the stratum granulosum, they accumulate granules of keratohyalin, a complex material that includes material from the tonofibrils. When cells are pushed from the stratum granulosum upwards into the stratum corneum, all cellular structures seem to disintegrate, leaving only cellular debris and keratin, which is somehow derived from keratohyalin. The dead cells and keratin are constantly flaking off, only to be replaced by cells from the layers beneath. It is estimated that every day approximately 1 gram of protein is lost in the shed skin of an adult.

Twenty-eight days are usually required for a keratinocyte to progress from the stratum germinativum to the stratum corneum. This rate is accelerated in the disease of psoriasis when the migration takes place in only 4 days. This disease is characterized by inflamed, elevated patches of skin with thick silvery scales. Other parts of the body besides the skin can be affected in psoriasis.

The stratum germinativum of the epidermis also contains melanocytes. These cells synthesize melanin and are distributed in all parts of the body. Melanin is a complex, brown or black pigment produced by oxidation of the amino acid, tyrosine, and then bound to a protein. There is no racial difference in the number of melanocytes but dark-skinned people do synthesize more melanin. The only persons who do not synthesize any melanin at all are albinos. The melanocytes synthesize melanin in a cellular body known as a melanosome, which contains the enzyme, tyrosinase. Processes from the melanocytes transfer the melanosome to the keratinocytes, where the melanosome loses all enzymatic

activity and becomes an inactive granular inclusion. Melanin has a protective function in the skin and is particularly useful in protection against high levels of ultra-violet (UV) light or sunlight.

Melanin synthesis can be stimulated by UV light and this is the physiological basis of the "sun tan". There is also a melanin-stimulating hormone (MSH) produced by the pituitary gland which causes increased synthesis and dispersion of the melanin. This protein hormone has a certain structural similarity to part of the ACTH molecule, and the secretion of MSH is increased by low levels of cortisol. MSH is believed to be responsible for the increased pigmentation of the skin seen in adrenal insufficiency.

The darker the skin of an individual, the greater the rate of melanin synthesis and dispersion. Some of the creams used to lighten the skin work by inhibiting the enzyme, tyrosinase, which is responsible for synthesizing melanin from tyrosine. Those skin-lightening creams containing mercury are dangerous, as the toxic effects of mercury are not limited to the skin.

B. The dermis (corium)

The dermis functions to support the epidermis and give the skin strength and elasticity. There are two layers to the dermis: the papillary layer and the reticular layer. The papillary layer projects into the dermis and consists of a loose network of collagen and elastic fibres with a scattering of fibroblasts, macrophages and mast cells. Beneath the papillary layer is the thicker reticular layer, which is made up of numerous dense rows of collagen fibres, many of which run parallel to the surface of the skin. Some of these collagen fibres enter the subcutaneous tissues where they form bundles between the lobules of fat. The dermis also contains blood vessels and lymphatics, sensory nerve endings, sebaceous and sweat glands and their ducts, and hair follicles and their associated structures.

In thin skin, the dermis projects irregularly into the epidermis. The dermis of thick skin projects into the epidermis more regularly in a series of peaks and valleys called dermal ridges. The thick epidermis of the thick skin closely adheres to these dermal ridges. Epidermal grooves and ridges can be observed on the soles of the feet and the palmar surface of the hand and are responsible for fingerprint patterns.

C. Specialized structures of the skin

a. Hair follicles. Although most of the body is covered with hair, humans as a species are not particularly hairy. Hair formation begins in the foetus with a downgrowth of epidermal cells into the underlying dermis to form pockets of epithelial cells which then form the germinal matrix of the hair follicle. The germinal matrix becomes fitted over a papilla, a projection of connective tissue containing capillaries and nerve endings. The external root sheath connects the germinal matrix with the outer surface. The bottom of the external root sheath surrounds and becomes continuous with the germinal matrix.

Since the germinal matrix was derived from the epidermis, it is not surprising that the matrix contains cells similar to the keratinocytes and the melanocytes, and that the formation of a hair occurs by a modified process of keratinization. The cells at the base of the germinal matrix are mitotically active. Growing cells are pushed upward into the external root sheath. As the cells are forced away from the papilla, they lose contact with their nutrient source and become keratinized. The hair shaft is that part of the follicle extending beyond the epidermis. The shaft has a scaly outer cuticle and a cortex containing pigment and a special, tough form of keratin, and a small medulla, which has keratin similar to that found in the skin. The colour of the hair depends upon the kind and amount of melanin produced. Grey hair results when little or no melanin is deposited in the hair shaft.

Alopoecia is the medical term for the absence of hair from where it is usually present. There is some evidence that the combination of a genetic predisposition and male sex hormone cause the common forms of baldness. Hirsutism is the term used for hair growth on a woman, a growth that would be normal on a man but is abnormal on a woman. A hirsute woman does not have more hair follicles than normal, but her hair follicles may be uniquely sensitive to hormones or there may be excessive amounts of androgens which stimulate the hair follicles. Tumours or excessive activity of the adrenal gland or ovary may produce androgens which stimulate the follicles. Thus, on occasion, hirsutism may be a sign of a tumour or endocrine disorder.

Many people are curious to know if frequent shaving or cutting of the hair accelerates its growth. It doesn't.

Extending from the deep part of the hair follicle to the dermis is a poorly developed bundle of muscle fibres known as the arrector pili muscle (see Figure 19.1). These muscles have a sympathetic innervation. When the muscles contract it makes the follicle more perpendicular to the surface so it appears to "stand up", and it pulls upon the dermis causing "goose pimples".

b. Sebaceous glands. These glands develop from, and empty their secretions into, the hair follicle (see Figure 19.1). Their chief secretion is sebum, a lipid that serves to lubricate the skin. These glands are most plentiful on the face and scalp. At puberty, the sebaceous glands hypertrophy as a result of hormonal stimulation, mainly the androgens. The blackhead (comedone) results when sebum, keratin and certain bacteria fill and plug up the hair follicle. The inflammatory lesions of acne result when sebum escapes from the follicle into the dermis. Sebum irritates the dermis and facilitates infection.

c. Sweat glands. These glands are found over most of the body and are particularly numerous in thick skin. Each gland has a secretory part which may be located in the dermis or subcutaneous tissues, and a coiled excretory duct that opens by a pore on the surface of the skin (see Figure 19.1). Their secretion is 99% water and some salts, especially sodium chloride, with a trace of urea. Sweat is originally isotonic to plasma but becomes hypotonic because of the reabsorption of sodium chloride by the cells of the ducts of the sweat glands.

Large sweat glands are found in the axilla (armpit), in the anal region, and scrotum and labia majora. These can be called apocrine sweat glands because the secretion is produced by partial disintegration of glandular cells. The secretion of these glands contains water, salt and portions of glandular cells which have disintegrated. It is this organic material which is acted upon by bacteria and thus contributes to the characteristic odour associated with these regions.

Sweat glands are innervated by sympathetic nerve fibres. The postganglionic sympathetic fibres, which innervate these glands, release acetylcholine rather than noradrenaline. The sympathetic fibres stimulating sweat glands increase their discharge in response to heat or stress. Often, people who are stressed break into a "cold sweat". Sympathetic stimulation causes the sweat glands to secrete and also constricts the arterioles in the skin, so that less blood flows through the skin and this leads to a reduction in the skin's temperature. A cool, moist skin is often seen in cardiovascular shock and its associated sympathetic stimulation. In fact, some intensive care and cardiac care wards have devices for monitoring the temperature of the big toe. This relatively simple device can provide useful information on the cardiovascular status of the patient.

d. Nails. On the dorsal aspect of the distal phalanges the stratum corneum of the skin is hardened into a plate of keratin which forms the nail. The lunula is the crescent-shaped white area near the root of the nail and is most often seen in the thumb and first finger but seldom seen in the little finger. With the exception of the lunula, the body or visible part of the nail appears pink because the keratin forming the nail is transparent, and the vascular plexus in the dermis beneath the nail shows through. If you press on the nail it becomes white due to blood being forced out of the dermal blood vessels beneath the nail. The proximal, hidden portion of the nail is the nail root which is covered by the cuticle (eponychium).

D. Descriptive terms applied to findings in the skin

As stated at the beginning of this Chapter, there are specific diseases of the skin, and other systemic diseases can have manifestations in the skin. Everyone cannot be a dermatologist (skin specialist), yet most health professionals need to be able to describe findings in the skin. Occasionally, dermatologists are accused of speaking their own language. Certain terms used in describing findings in the skin are presented here to ensure accurate communication and to let more people speak this language.

a. Primary skin lesions

A primary skin lesion is a pathological discontinuity in the skin which develops without any preceding manifest skin changes.

(1) Macule. This is a discolouration (change in colour) of the skin. There is no elevation or palpable change in a macule. A freckle is a macule.

(2) Papule. A papule is a small, less than 1 mm in diameter, circumscribed, solid, elevation of the skin. Many warts are papules.

(3) Vesicle and Bulla. A vesicle is a fluid-filled, elevated lesion less than 1 cm in diameter, while a bulla is a fluid-filled elevated lesion greater than 1 cm in diameter. In varicella (chicken-pox), a crop of small, red papules appears and quickly develops into oval-shaped vesicles on an erythematous (red) base. These lesions have been described as tear-drops on rose petals.

(4) Wheal (hive). A wheal is a temporary, localized, raised area of oedema in the skin; the elevated area of skin is pale

and is usually surrounded by a macular erythematous flare. Wheals are evidence of an allergic response with histamine release taking place in the skin.

b. Secondary skin lesions

A primary skin lesion may change in character and appearance as a result of natural evolution, or of scratching, infection or treatment, and become a secondary skin lesion.

(1) *Crusts.* These are formed by ruptured or unruptured vesicles as they dry up. Crust is made of dried body fluid such as serum, blood or purulent exudate.

(2) *Pustule.* This is an elevated lesion in the skin and contains white blood cells, cellular debris and/or micro-organisms.

c. Special dermatological terms

(1) *Alopoecia.* This refers to baldness (hair loss).

(2) *Ecchymosis.* An ecchymosis is a bleeding in a large area of tissue beneath the skin. Lay people often refer to an ecchymosis as a bruise.

(3) *Excoriations.* These are scratch marks or other linear lesions caused by trauma.

(4) *Petechiae.* Petechiae are round, pin-point, non-raised, purplish-red spots that are caused by haemorrhages from superficial blood vessels in the skin. They can be caused by septic emboli released in subacute bacterial endocarditis and are also found in persons with bleeding disorders.

(5) *Telangiectasia.* This term refers to a condition in which the small blood vessels in the skin become permanently dilated and visible.

WHAT ARE THE FUNCTIONS OF THE SKIN?

A. Protection

It is often said that the skin serves a protective function and at the same time raises the question — protection against what? One answer is: protection against micro-organisms. You are certainly aware that your finger is more likely to become infected when the skin is cut or abraded than when the skin is intact. A less obvious but equally important function is protecting the internal environment. By retaining most of the body fluids within the body, the skin prevents the tissues from drying out.

More important, it protects the fluid volumes from falling below critical levels. This is illustrated in the case of severe or third-degree burns, which destroy the skin and injure the tissues beneath it. So much fluid can leak out of the injured capillaries that blood volume is depleted, and this may cause circulatory shock and even death. The immediate treatment of burn victims requires fluid replacement; subsequent problems involve bacterial infection of the burned area, and the spread of this infection throughout the body.

B. Vitamin D synthesis

Vitamin D is not a single molecule but is actually a series of molecules with similar chemical structures which differ in their potency. The synthesis of vitamin D begins in the skin when ultraviolet light causes a molecular rearrangement in a molecule called 7-dehydrocholesterol, which becomes cholecalciferol (vitamin D_3). This compound promotes calcium absorption in the intestine and it facilitates normal calcium and phosphorus metabolism. Vitamin D_3 undergoes further chemical additions in the liver and kidney which enhance its activity. Ergosterol, a molecule similar to 7-dehydrocholesterol, is converted to ergocalciferol (vitamin D_2) in the skin by the action of UV light. This is the reason why sunlight is said to prevent rickets. Since these compounds are synthesized in the skin, liver and kidneys, and work in the bones and intestine, they can be classified as either hormones or vitamins.

C. Temperature regulation

There is an old experiment in which a man would carry a beefsteak on a platter and walk into a room heated to a high temperature. The man would smile, sweat, watch the steak broil and walk out when the steak had been done to his taste. In emphasising the significance of this experiment, the body's ability to maintain its temperature, it should be pointed out, however, that the brain tissue cannot survive if the body temperature is sustained above 42 °C.

Before going into the skin's role in temperature regulation, pertinent facts should be reviewed.

As a result of its metabolism, the body is constantly producing heat. The rate of heat production can be increased by thyroid hormones, progesterone, adrenaline and muscular activity. Heat can be exchanged with the external environment by means of radiation, conduction, convection and water evaporation. When you walk into the sunshine and feel its warmth, you are receiving its warmth by radiation — the transfer of heat energy by electromagnetic waves. Heat can be lost from the body via radiation if the temperature of the skin is greater than the average temperature of the other surfaces in the surrounding environment. The amount of heat that is lost depends on the temperature difference between the skin and the other surfaces.

Conduction is the process whereby heat is transferred from molecules to different molecules as a result of molecular collisions or contact. If you jump into an ice-cold lake, your body loses heat because heat is conducted away from your skin by the water molecules. Conduction contributes to the process of convection, but other than that, it usually is unimportant in temperature regulation unless you happen to be a skin diver.

Convection is the process of heat transfer by the actual movement of the heated material. The air surrounding the skin is warmed by the body's heat because of conduction. This warm air will rise and move away from the skin because the air is warmer and therefore less dense than the other cooler air. The process of convection continues as cooler air moves in close to the skin, is warmed, rises and moves away.

Since heat is gained or lost from the skin, it is logical to ask what controls the temperature of the skin. To answer this, it may be helpful to think of the skin as a heat-exchanging unit and the internal viscera as a central heat-producing core. The temperature of this vital central core is kept relatively constant by regulating the amount of blood which flows through the skin. These changes are controlled by the hypothalamus.

You know that if you leave a warm room and walk outside

when it is cold, your hands become cold. This does not occur because the body is producing any less heat, for in fact, heat production remains the same or even increases. Rather, less blood flows through the skin and less heat is lost from the skin. The hypothalamus receives information from temperature receptors in the skin but also contains cells responsive to the temperature of the blood which perfuses it. Since more blood flows through the internal viscera than through the skin, the arterial blood which reaches the hypothalamus will reflect the temperature of the central core more than the temperature of the skin. If the temperature of the blood reaching the hypothalamus is lowered, certain cells become more active. This increased activity leads to an increased activity in the sympathetic nerve fibres innervating the arterioles of the skin. This causes the arterioles to constrict and reduces the flow of blood through the skin especially in the skin of the hands and the feet. If the blood does not flow through the outer parts of the skin, the amount of heat that can be lost to the colder external environment is reduced and the critical temperature of the internal core is protected.

If the blood reaching the hypothalamus is warmed, different cells are activated. As a result of their activation, the arterioles of the skin dilate, more blood flows through the skin and heat can be exchanged with the external environment. The amount of blood which can flow through the skin is quite variable, ranging from 2% to more than 25% of the cardiac output. Hypothalamic cells are also activated which leads to the stimulation of the sweat glands via their sympathetic nerve innervation. It is not the formation of sweat which cools the body, but the use of body heat to convert the sweat to vapour. This change from the liquid to gaseous state requires considerable heat. In fact, it takes more than five times as much energy to convert 1 gram of water at 100 °C to steam, than it does to heat 1 gram of water from 0 to 100 °C, and still more heat if the water temperature is below 100 °C. The efficiency of sweating as a mechanism for heat loss depends on the amount of water vapour in the air. If it is humid, that is, if the air is highly saturated with water vapour, much of the sweat will not evaporate but will simply drip off

the body or be absorbed by its clothing. This helps to explain why many people are more comfortable in dry, desert-like climates than in humid, tropical climates. Desert air has little water vapour in it and sweating is an efficient mechanism for heat loss.

A certain amount of water is vaporized at all times; this is known as insensible perspiration. Normally, the insensible loss of water from the skin and lungs varies from 300 to 800 ml/day.

Finally, the colour of the skin depends upon the amount of melanin it contains, as well as upon the rate and oxygen saturation of the blood flowing through it. The skin becomes paler as blood flow is reduced; in Caucasian people the skin tends to redden as flow increases.

D. Sense receptors of the skin

The story of how structures within the skin provide information is a familiar one, only the names of specific anatomical structures are new. There are specific receptors for each type of sensation with the exception of pain receptors which can respond to mechanical, chemical or temperature stimuli, provided they are intense enough. The actual receptors are fine, unmyelinated nerve endings which branch freely and end between and beneath the deep layers of the epidermis.

Before going on with the specifics of the sense receptors, it might be good to comment on the overall organization of sense receptors in the skin, and their relation to the spinal nerves (see Figures 19.3 and 19.4). This gives you one last chance to revise some neuro-anatomy.

You recall that there are 31 pairs of spinal nerves:
  8 Cervical nerves
 12 Thoracic nerves
  5 Lumbar nerves
  5 Sacral nerves
  1 Coccygeal nerve.

Each spinal nerve is formed by the dorsal (posterior) root filaments which carry sensory information, and by the ventral (anterior) root filaments which carry motor impulses. The

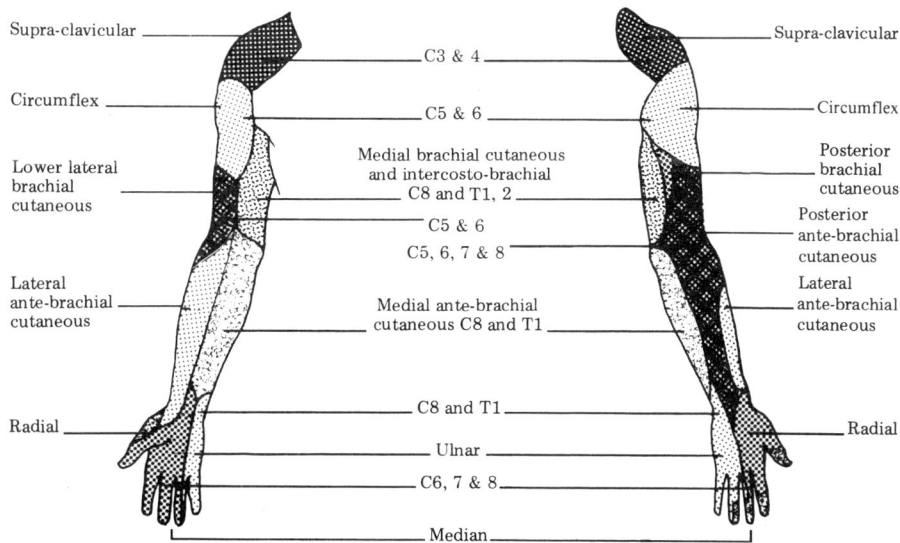

Figure 19.3 Cutaneous nerves with dermatomes and spinal nerve contribution.

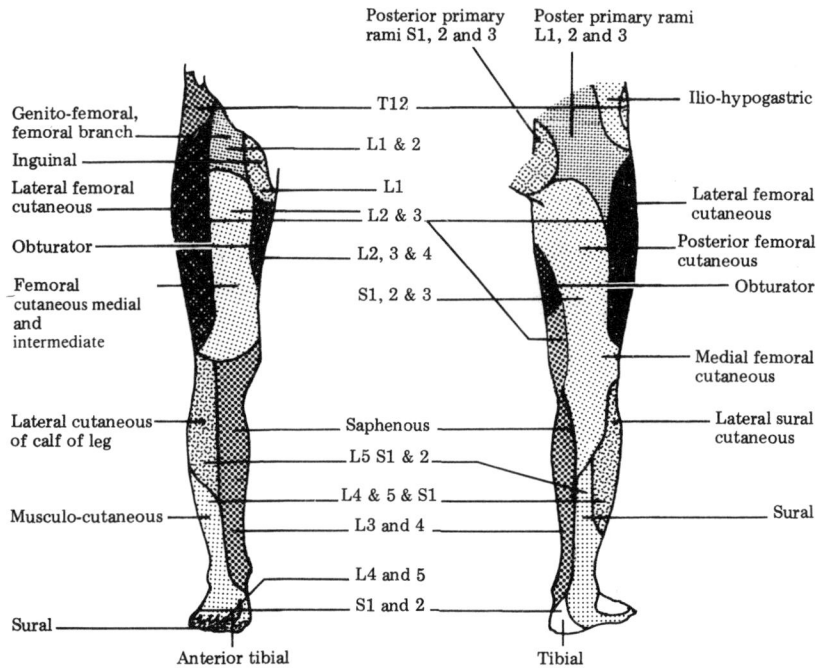

Figure 19.4   Peripheral nerves with dermatomes and spinal nerve contribution.

dorsal and ventral root filaments from a segment of the spinal cord come together to form one of the 31 spinal nerves. After leaving the vertebral column, some spinal nerves group together, then separate to form distinct peripheral nerves which have both efferent nerve fibres which relay information to skeletal muscle, and afferent sensory nerve fibres which relay information from the skin. And so it is possible to trace the path that sensory information takes as it leaves the skin and ultimately enters the spinal cord via one or more of the 31 spinal nerves.

A dermatome is the area of skin supplied by the afferent sensory nerve fibres from a single spinal nerve. Figure 19.5 shows the innervation of dermatomal areas of the skin. C stands for cervical; T for thoracic; L for lumbar; and S for sacral. You can see that in the thoracic and abdominal areas, there is a small serial relationship between the thoracic nerves and the area of the thorax they supply. In the limbs, this simple relationship does not apply, for reasons having to do with embryology and the early development of the brachial and lumbo-sacral plexus. (In reality, the dermatomes shown in Figure 19.5 are somewhat idealized, and there is a certain amount of overlap.) If the dorsal sensory roots of a single spinal nerve are cut, there may be a decrease of sensation but not an elimination of it in the affected dermatome. Figure 19.5 shows the relationship between the dermatomes and the peripheral nerves which supply the limbs. A knowledge of dermatomes can be useful in trying to locate a lesion at a particular level of the spinal cord. For instance, if a person has a loss of sensation all around the abdomen at the level of the umbilicus, you can postulate a lesion at or about the dorsal roots of thoracic spinal nerve 10. The peripheral nerves supplying the skin have specialized receptors for translating environmental information into neural impulses that can be interpreted within the brain.

The end bulb of Krause has been termed the cold receptor,

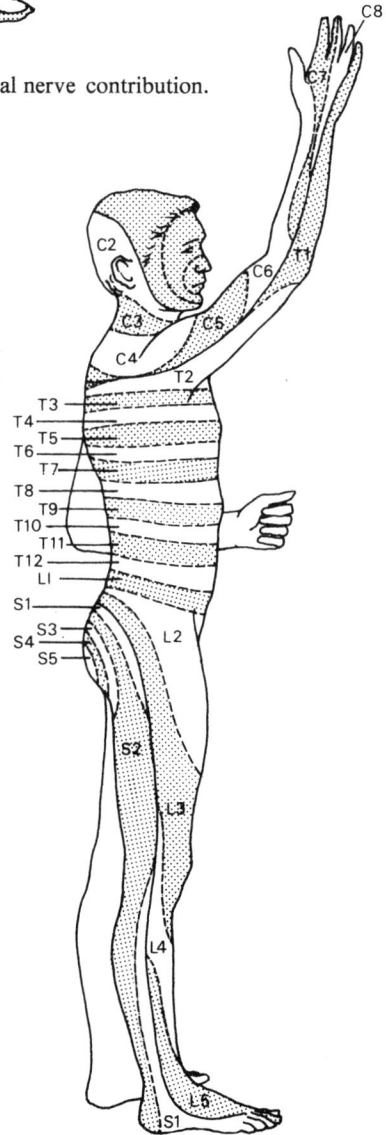

Figure 19.5   Dermatomes.

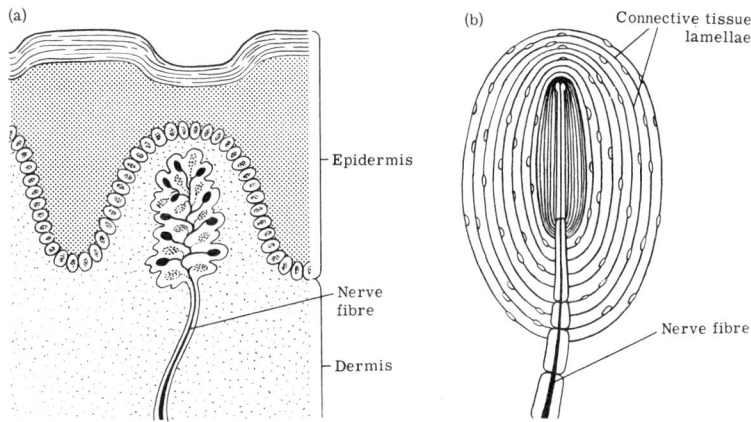

Figure 19.6 (a) Meissner's corpuscle. (b) Pacinian corpuscle.

and the Ruffini end organ, the warm receptor. These receptors are located in the dermis (subcutaneous tissues) and are essentially nerve endings which are surrounded and supported by a connective tissue covering of varying thickness. Warm receptors increase their rate of discharge as the temperature rises, while the cold receptors increase their rate of discharge when the temperature falls. The structural reasons for their different responsiveness are not known.

There is a variety of receptors sensitive to mechanical stimulation, and these are separated into those which are responsive to light touch, and those that require more forceful stimulators in order to respond to deep pressure. The deep pressure receptors are called Pacinian corpuscles and have a wide distribution, particularly in the subcutaneous tissue. They consist of a nerve ending wrapped in layers of connective tissue, which appears, when sectioned, to resemble a sliced onion (see Figure 19.6b). Many elegant studies have been performed using the Pacinian corpuscle, and much is known about it. As pressure is put upon the Pacinian

corpuscle, the membrane potential changes, and if the receptor is sufficiently bent, action potentials will be generated and will travel down the nerve fibre which synapses in the spinal cord.

The sensation of light touch can be tested by gently touching the skin with a wisp of cotton. Some free nerve endings and Meissner's corpuscles can respond to this stimulation. Meissner's corpuscles are especially numerous in the lips and in the palmar surface of the fingers. These corpuscles are located in the papillae of the dermis and consist of swollen nerve endings surrounded by a delicate, connective tissue capsule (see Figure 19.6a). Many hair follicles are surrounded by a basket-like arrangement of nerve endings which respond to light touch or movement of the hair shaft.

Information from all these receptors is relayed to the spinal cord, to the thalamus and lastly to the cortex, where the neural pathways end and the mystery of consciousness begins.

Index

Main references shown in **bold** type